ISSUES IN KIDNEY DISEASE

DIALYSIS

Issues In Kidney Disease Series

Stephen Z. Fadem – Series Editor

Selzman Institute for Kidney Health, Section of Nephrology,
and Michael E. DeBakey Veterans Affairs Medical Center,
Baylor College of Medicine, Houston, TX, USA;
Kidney Associates, Houston, TX, USA

Issues in Kidney Disease – Transplantation
Bhamidipati V. R. Murthy and Stephen Z. Fadem (Editors)
2021. ISBN: 978-1-53619-960-4 (Hardcover)

Issues in Kidney Disease – Dialysis
Stephen Z. Fadem and José A. Moura-Neto (Editors)
2021. ISBN: 978-1-68507-000-7 (Hardcover)

Issues in Kidney Disease – Acute Kidney Injury
Stephen Z. Fadem and Ahmed Arslan Yousuf Awan (Editors)
2021. ISBN: 978-1-68507-002-1 (Hardcover)

Issues in Kidney Disease – Chronic Kidney Disease
Stephen Z. Fadem and Samaya Javed Anumudu (Editors)
2021. ISBN: 978-1-68507-001-4 (Hardcover)

ISSUES IN KIDNEY DISEASE SERIES

ISSUES IN KIDNEY DISEASE

DIALYSIS

STEPHEN Z. FADEM
AND
JOSÉ A. MOURA-NETO
EDITORS

nova
Medicine & Health
New York

https://doi.org/10.52305/WMRB2438

Additional color graphics may be available in the e-book version of this book.

Library of Congress Cataloging-in-Publication Data

ISBN: 978-1-68507-000-7

Published by Nova Science Publishers, Inc. † New York

To my lovely wife, Joyce

Stephen Z. Fadem

To Thor, Leto and Maya, and my dear wife, Ana Flavia

José A. Moura-Neto

CONTENTS

FOREWORD

Jeffrey Giullian, MD

DaVita Kidney Care, Denver, CO, USA

The earliest written record of renal failure may date back to biblical times. The Book of Numbers in the Old Testament recounts the massive death of Israelites associated with the consumption of quail. Quail in Northern Africa are known to subsist on hemlock seeds. Theodore Ouzounellis postulated in a 1970 Journal of the American Medical Association (JAMA) editorial that the biblical story's cause of death of Moses's people would have been consistent with acute myoglobinuric syndrome from ingesting hemlock-laced meat [1].

Fortunately, kidney failure—acute or chronic–is no longer a death sentence due to centuries of painstaking research, often following a course of trial and error and subsequent success, edging our great medical specialty ever closer to the Holy Grail of finding a cure to this menacing disease. As outlined in the first chapter of this book, we stand on the shoulders of giants, from Richard Bright to Belding Scribner to George Schreiner, including the lineage of great nephrologists with whom we each could train and learn. Although we owe much to their achievements, the genuine heroes are the brave and unfortunate patients they served. They are the ones to whom we owe so much. In the chapters of this book, we readers get to explore major advancements in dialysis, from the basics to the nuanced and from the well-established to the novel. The authors of each chapter are, in their own right, the next standard-bearers of nephrology.

In a subsequent JAMA two weeks after the quail article was published, appeared an editorial on the merits of home dialysis. "Home dialysis allows a more normal life and more complete vocational rehabilitation, as well as making the patient more responsible for his own well-being [2]." Perhaps this sentence, more than any other in the care of persons with End-Stage Kidney Disease (ESKD), is proof that the more things change, the more they stay the same.

To be sure, much has changed in the care of patients requiring dialysis in the subsequent 51 years. Access to care has increased in the US and around the world; mortality has declined, and peritoneal dialysis has become the dominant form of self-care. Even since the last publication of this book in 2012, rates of hospitalizations for patients in the US have declined over 15% [3]; renal transplant rates have increased by almost 40% [4]. Nephrology has done more to improve the lives of patients on dialysis than many other specialties for their dominant morbidity. While survival from heart failure increased just over 6% in the first 10-16 years of this millennium [5, 6], mortality in the first year of dialysis decreased 28% in a shorter period of time [7]. Importantly, this survival improvement included "both men and women, and in all five races."

Yet, much more must be done to reduce health disparities and engage patients in their own care. For the population of patients that we serve, that means greater shared decision making in modality choice and palliative care. It means better access to kidney transplants, both from living and deceased donors; and it means fair representation in clinical trials.

Together, we stand on the cusp of the next great advancement in kidney care. With changing reimbursement paradigms, there is no longer a role for dialysis care or even kidney care in a silo. Rather, we are each tasked with providing holistic care to our patients with kidney failure. Care for the whole person includes incorporating social determinants of health into our treatment plans, improving patient experience, overcoming the limitations of Kt/V, and providing individualized care.

As a nephrology fellow, I recall a phenomenal Grand Rounds given by Dr. Paul Teschan. Far removed from direct patient care at that point, Dr. Teschan regaled us with stories from his time treating soldiers during the Korean War. Using the Kolff-Brigham dialyzer, mortality from advanced acute kidney injury dropped from ~90% to ~50%. But the numbers themselves were not what Dr. Teschan seemed most proud. What struck me was the way he talked about *his* soldiers, *his* men - the heroes he was honored to serve.

The horizon for kidney care is bright and offers us innovative ways to improve the lives of patients living with kidney failure. Nephrology is a specialty where we have the opportunity to serve the most vulnerable and the most heroic among us. In this book, Drs. Fadem and Moura-Neto have brought together esteemed collaborators from around the globe, and their output will help us serve patients better, more holistically, and with an even greater emphasis on evidence-based practices.

References

[1] Ouzounellis T. Some notes on quail poisoning. *JAMA*. 1970;211(7):1186-7.

[2] Hemodialysis: who and where. *JAMA*. 1970;211(9):1535.

[3] System USRD. *2020 USRDS Annual Data Report: Epidemiology of kidney disease in the United States*. National Institutes of Health, National Institute of Diabetes and Digestive and Kidney Diseases, Bethesda, MD, 2020.

[4] *USA: US Department of Health and Human Services Organ Procurement and Transplantation Network*; 2021 [April 25, 2021]. Available from: https://optn.transplant.hrsa.gov.

[5] Taylor CJ, Ordóñez-Mena JM, Roalfe AK, Lay-Flurrie S, Jones NR, Marshall T, et al. Trends in survival after a diagnosis of heart failure in the United Kingdom 2000-2017: population based cohort study. *BMJ*. 2019;364:l223.

[6] Conrad N, Judge A, Canoy D, Tran J, Pinho-Gomes AC, Millett ERC, et al. Temporal Trends and Patterns in Mortality After Incident Heart Failure: A Longitudinal Analysis of 86 000 Individuals. *JAMA Cardiol.* 2019;4(11):1102-11.

[7] Shah S, Leonard AC, Meganathan K, Christianson AL, Thakar CV. Temporal Trends in Incident Mortality in Dialysis Patients: Focus on Sex and Racial Disparities. *Am J Nephrol.* 2019;49(3):241-53.

PREFACE

Stephen Z. Fadem*[1,*]*, MD, FACP, FASN
and José A. Moura-Neto*[2]*, MD
[1]Selzman Institute for Kidney Health, Section of Nephrology,
and Michael E. DeBakey Veterans Affairs Medical Center,
Baylor College of Medicine, Houston, TX, USA;
Kidney Associates, Houston, TX, USA
[2]Department of Internal Medicine, Bahiana School of Medicine and Public Health,
Salvador, Bahia, Brazil

For over 100 years after its discovery by Richard Bright, the diagnosis of kidney failure was a death sentence. Even with the flourishing and advancements of renal replacement therapy, it did not become widely available to patients for 13 years. Because of economic and regulatory barriers, patients died with no access to therapy in the initial years of dialysis development and history, which sadly is still a reality in some countries. Currently, less than one century after the technical development of dialysis, over three million people are on maintenance renal replacement therapy worldwide. While considered commonplace, dialysis therapy is still fraught with complications and has a high mortality rate.

Issues in Kidney Disease–Dialysis is a collection of nineteen updated chapters written by renowned authors, covering a wide range of topics, from the history to the future, in different renal replacement therapy modalities, such as hemodialysis, online hemodiafiltration, and peritoneal dialysis. It brings timely and updated reviews and addresses trends, challenges, and controversies of dialysis therapies. It will appeal to renal fellows, nephrologists, and healthcare professionals involved with chronic kidney disease patients on maintenance dialysis, including all those interested in the advances and challenges still facing medicine.

[*] Corresponding Author's E-mail: fadem@bcm.edu.

ACKNOWLEDGMENTS

Editing and revising this book was a gratifying experience, in which we have been able to interact with an expert team of colleagues and learn from them. Indeed, this book was a collective international effort. We would like to thank all authors who kindly took part in this book. We put together authors from Africa, North America, Latin America, Asia, Europe, and Oceania. In particular, we would like to thank Michelle (Misha) L. Nguyen for her masterful work and help in proofreading and copy editing all chapters—her attentive eye and expertise was a strength for this project.

We also would like to acknowledge kidney disease patients on dialysis - the main and ultimate reason for this academic and editorial effort. Our aim is that the knowledge and fulfillment that readers gain will translate into more informed care and better outcomes for those who must receive renal replacement therapy.

We fondly appreciate the unwavering support of our families—in the United States and Brazil—and would like to thank them for unselfishly lending us to this project for almost two years.

Editors' Contact Information

Stephen Z. Fadem, MD, FACP, FASN
Selzman Institute for Kidney Health, Section of Nephrology,
and Michael E. DeBakey Veterans Affairs Medical Center,
Baylor College of Medicine, Houston, TX, USA;
Kidney Associates, Houston, TX, USA
fadem@bcm.edu

José A. Moura-Neto, MD, MS, MBA, FASN
Department of Internal Medicine, Bahiana School of Medicine and Public Health,
Salvador, Bahia, Brazil
moura@nephrologyworldwide.com

List of Contributors

John W. M. Agar, MBBS, FRACP, FRCP (Lond)
Renal Services, University Hospital Geelong, Geelong, Australia

Abdullah Khalaf Al-Hwiesh, MD
King Fahd University Hospital, Imam Abdulrahman Bin Faisal University, Dammam, Saudi Arabia

Fahad Aziz, MD
Department of Medicine, Division of Nephrology, University of Wisconsin School of Medicine and Public Health, Madison, WI, USA

André Luís Balbi, MD, PhD
Department of Internal Medicine, University of São Paulo State - UNESP, Botucatu, Sao Paulo, Brazil

Silvio Barberato, MD, PhD
School of Medicine, Pontifical Catholic University of Parana, Curitiba, Brazil

Kleyton Bastos, MD, PhD
Department of Medicine, Federal University of Sergipe, Aracaju, Brazil
Latin American Chapter (LAC-DD)-International Society for Peritoneal Dialysis

Harini Bejjanki, MD
The University of Texas MD Anderson Cancer Center, Houston, TX, USA

Brendan Bowman, MD
University of Virginia School of Medicine, Charlottesville, VA, USA

Viviane Calice-Silva, MD, PhD
Research Department, Pro-Rim Foundation, Joinville, Brazil
and Department of Medicine, UNIVILLE, Joinville, Brazil

Bernard Canaud, MD, PhD
Senior Medical Scientist, Global Medical Office FMC, Bad Homburg, Germany
and Emeritus Professor of Nephrology, University of Montpellier, School of Medicine, Montpellier, France

Rosana Chaud, MD
Latin American Chapter (LAC-DD)-International Society for Peritoneal Dialysis
FISSAL Comprehensive Health Insurance, Ministerio de Salud, Peru

Joseph Chilcot, PhD
Institute of Psychiatry, Psychology, and Neuroscience, King's College, London, UK

Andrew Davenport, MD
UCL Department of Renal Medicine, Royal Free Hospital,
University College London, London, UK

Bianca Davidson, MD
Division of Nephrology, Medicine, University of Cape Town, Cape Town, South Africa

Anas Diab, MD
Department of Medicine, Section of Nephrology,
West Virginia University School of Medicine, Morgantown, West Virginia, USA

Marcela Ávila Diaz, PhD
Unidad de Investigación Médica en Enfermedades Nefrológicas.
UMAE Hospital de Especialidades Bernardo Sepúlveda Gutiérrez, Centro Médico Nacional Siglo XXI, Instituto Mexicano del Seguro Social, Mexico City, Mexico

José Carolino Divino-Filho, MD, PhD
Division of Renal Medicine, Department of Clinical Science, Intervention and Technology, CLINTEC, Karolinska Institutet, Campus Flemingsberg, Stockholm, Sweden
Latin American Chapter (LAC-DD)-International Society for Peritoneal Dialysis

Natália Maria da Silva Fernandes, MD, PhD
Departments of Internal Medicine and Nephrology, Juiz de Fora Federal University, Juiz de Fora, Minas Gerais, Brazil

Jeffrey Giullian, MD, MBA, FASN
Chief Medical Officer, DaVita Kidney Care, Denver, CO, USA

Thomas Golper, MD
Vanderbilt University Medical Center, Nashville, TN, USA

Talerngsak Kanjanabuch, MD
Division of Nephrology, Department of Medicine and Center of Excellence in Kidney Metabolic Disorders, Faculty of Medicine, Chulalongkorn University, Bangkok, Thailand
Peritoneal Dialysis Excellence Center, King Chulalongkorn Memorial Hospital, Bangkok, Thailand

Omar Mamlouk, MD
The University of Texas MD Anderson Cancer Center, Houston, TX, USA

Susana Marcos, RN
Latin American Chapter (LAC-DD)-International Society for Peritoneal Dialysis
Argentina Society of Nephrological Nursing, Argentina

Ikuto Masakane, MD, PhD
Yabuki Hospital, Yamagata City, Japan

Devin McKelvey, DO
Perelman School of Medicine at the University of Pennsylvania, Philadelphia, PA, USA

Carmen Arias Minaya, RN
Latin American Chapter (LAC-DD)-International Society for Peritoneal Dialysis
National Coordinator of PD Hersil, Peru

Madhukar Misra, MD, FRCP (UK), FASN, FACP
Department of Medicine, Division of Nephrology, University of Missouri-Columbia, Columbia, MO, USA

Anju Mohan, MD
Department of Internal Medicine, Division of Nephrology, North Shore University Health System, University of Chicago, Pritzker School of Medicine, Evanston, IL, USA

Joan Araujo Oliveira Moitinho, MD
Department of Nephrology, Rio de Janeiro State University – UERJ, Rio de Janeiro, Brazil

Andrew Mooney, MD
Leeds Teaching Hospitals, Leeds, UK

Celso Souza de Moraes Junior, PhD
Departments of Financial and Accounting and FADEPE (Foundation for Development, Teaching, Research and Extension), Juiz de Fora Federal University, Juiz de Fora, Minas Gerais, Brazil

Gustavo Moretta, MD, PhD
Latin American Chapter (LAC-DD)-International Society for Peritoneal Dialysis
Escuela de Educación, San Andrés University, Buenos Aires, Argentina

Ana Flávia Moura, MD, MBA, MSc
Department of Internal Medicine, Bahiana School of Medicine and Public Health, Salvador, Bahia, Brazil

Vo Nguyen, MD
Memorial Nephrology Associates, Olympia, WA, USA

Ramón Paniagua, MD
Unidad de Investigación Médica en Enfermedades Nefrológicas. UMAE Hospital de Especialidades Bernardo Sepúlveda Gutiérrez, Centro Médico Nacional Siglo XXI, Instituto Mexicano del Seguro Social, Mexico City, Mexico

Roberto Pecoits-Filho, MD, PhD
School of Medicine, Pontifical Catholic University of Parana, Curitiba, Brazil
and DOPPS Program, Arbor Research Collaborative for Health, Ann Arbor, MI, USA

Federica Picariello, PhD
Institute of Psychiatry, Psychology, and Neuroscience, King's College, London, London, UK

Andreas Pierratos, MD
Humber River Hospital, University of Toronto, Toronto, Canada

Daniela Ponce, MD, PhD
Department of Internal Medicine, University of São Paulo State - UNESP, Botucatu, Sao Paulo, Brazil

Hugh Rayner, MD
University Hospitals Birmingham NHS Foundation Trust, Birmingham, UK

Johan Rosman, MD, PhD, FRACP
Professor of Medicine, Curtin University Medical School, Nephrologist Royal Perth Hospital, Perth, Western Australia, Australia

Athanasios Roumeliotis, MD, PhD
Division of Nephrology and Hypertension, 1st Department of Internal Medicine, AHEPA Hospital, Aristotle University of Thessaloniki, Thessaloniki, Greece

Stefanos Roumeliotis, MD, PhD
Division of Nephrology and Hypertension, 1st Department of Internal Medicine, AHEPA Hospital, Aristotle University of Thessaloniki, Thessaloniki, Greece

Megha Salani, MD
Vanderbilt University Medical Center, Nashville, TN, USA

Rebecca Schmidt, DO, FACP, FASN
Department of Medicine, Section of Nephrology,
West Virginia University School of Medicine, Morgantown, WV, USA

Rebecca Kurnik Seshasai, MD, MSHP
Perelman School of Medicine at the University of Pennsylvania, Philadelphia, PA, USA

Ankur Shah, MD
Warren Alpert Medical School of Brown University, Providence, RI, USA

Cassiano Augusto Braga Silva, MD
Hospital Dom Pedro de Alcântara, Santa Casa de Misericórdia de Feira de Santana,
Feira de Santana, Bahia, Brazil

Stuart M. Sprague, DO, FACP, FASN, FNKF
Department of Internal Medicine, Division of Nephrology, North Shore University
Health System, University of Chicago, Pritzker School of Medicine, Evanston, IL, USA

José Hermógenes Rocco Suassuna, MD, PhD
Department of Nephrology, Rio de Janeiro State University – UERJ, Rio de Janeiro, Brazil

James Tattersall, MD
Leeds Teaching Hospitals, Leeds, UK

Nicola Wearne, MD
Division of Nephrology, Medicine, University of Cape Town, Cape Town, South Africa

Biruh T. Workeneh, MD
The University of Texas MD Anderson Cancer Center, Houston, TX, USA

Welder Zamoner, MD
Department of Internal Medicine, University of São Paulo State - UNESP, Botucatu,
Sao Paulo, Brazil

In: Issues in Kidney Disease – Dialysis
Editors: Stephen Z. Fadem and José A. Moura-Neto ISBN: 978-1-68507-000-7

Chapter 1

MILESTONES IN DIALYSIS

Stephen Z. Fadem**, MD, FACP, FASN
Selzman Institute for Kidney Health, Section of Nephrology,
and Michael E. DeBakey Veterans Affairs Medical Center,
Baylor College of Medicine, Houston, TX, USA;
Kidney Associates, Houston, TX, USA

ABSTRACT

In 1861, kidney failure was a terminal disease, but keen observations by Thomas Graham identified not only a mechanism for disease but also a means of treatment. For the next 100 years, investigators waited for the technology to come through and enable therapy to commence. The development of cellophane and the discovery of heparin made it possible to advance care. Willem Kolff's ingenious device and follow-up contributions led to physicians in the United States refining his invention. Using technology designed for water purification, small portable dialyzers could then be built. Teflon and silastic made the first chronic dialysis possible, but it was the surgical development of the Brescia Cimino fistula and the Tenckhoff Catheter that made hemodialysis and peritoneal dialysis practical. Once dialysis was developed, financial coverage was required to meet the needs of patients. The passage of the Social Security Amendment extending Medicare coverage for thousands of patients was a major milestone. The development of an equilibrium equation had a major impact on care, as did the development of recombinant erythropoietin. The understanding that bone disease associated with CKD also causes vascular calcification and cardiac disease is likewise a milestone.

Keywords: history of dialysis, Willem Kolff, dialysis, heparin, hollow fiber, John Merrill, Medicare, Thomas Graham, Belding Scribner, AV fistula, Tenckhoff catheter, peritoneal dialysis, Kiil Board, Nils Alwall, Leonard Skeggs, A. Peter Lundin, Richard Bright

* Corresponding Author's E-mail: fadem@bcm.edu.

Introduction

To watch the advancements in the management of kidney disease is to witness a miracle. To appreciate this journey, one must reflect that, not just during the time of Richard Bright (1789-1858), but in the late 1950s, the diagnosis of chronic renal failure was a death sentence. Each achievement and milestone in care is set upon the one preceding it (See Table 1). Reviewing these milestones should inspire the next generation that enters our profession, as our journey is far from over. Chronic dialysis therapy has been a compilation of science and technology, industry advancements, and commerce. But it has always centered on the needs of the patients on whom the burden of kidney disease has fallen.

Milestone 1: Dialysis Projected as a Treatment for Bright's Disease (1861)

In the 1820s and 1830s, the English physician Richard Bright did pioneering work on the etiology and clinical signs and symptoms of kidney failure. Ultimately, this terminal disease became known as Bright's disease. By 1839, it was clearly established that it was caused by the retention of urea, a nitrogenous substance known to be present in urine. Around the same period, Thomas Graham of Glasgow discovered that colloids could be separated from crystalloids using a "semipermeable membrane" or "dialyzer." The term dialysis was coined in 1861. Graham demonstrated that urea and sodium chloride could pass through a membrane, were both elements of urine, and could be separated from blood. Together, Bright and Graham projected that dialysis would someday be a form of therapy for uremia, yet success was still 100 years away. Graham's membrane experiments were performed with tissues from animal internal organs, and decay and putrefaction precluded the peritoneal membranes that worked quite well *in vitro* from effectively separating blood from electrolytes and urea *in vivo*. The application of the early principles of dialysis would have to await the emergence of suitable synthetic or chemically altered substances.

Medical science turned to nutrition as an alternative means of treating patients with Bright's disease after recognizing that it was impossible to remove "azote" or the nitrogen causing azotemia or uremia using a device or machine. The focus was on identifying ways to restrict the dietary intake of protein. The prescient low-protein diet to reduce albuminuria was introduced in the late 1800s by Mariano Semmola (1831-1895), the first Italian professor of pharmacology [1]. This culminated in a popular therapy, the Giovannetti diet, introduced in 1964 [2]. This diet, designed for patients with renal failure, consisted of 2000-3000 calorie consumption per day of fruits and vegetables having the lowest nitrogen content, ("pears, apples, peaches, oranges, plums, tomatoes, peppers, pumpkins, lettuce, carrots, etc."), spaghetti, essential amino acids, butter, coffee and liquor for flavoring, bread substitutes, and small amounts of beer and wine. While a successful adjunct to the formative hemodialysis therapy of the time [2], it was not effective as a standalone diet for patients with end-stage disease, but it did set the stage for the low-protein diet as a worthwhile therapeutic option to slow kidney disease progression.

MILESTONE 2: HEPARIN (1916)

The greatest advancement in kidney was the realization of Graham and Bright's prescient notion that dialysis would someday be a practical therapy, sparking a search for a suitable form of dialysis. In 1913, John Jacob Abel (1859-1938) of Johns Hopkins University attempted to direct blood outside the body through collodion membranes. It attracted the press, as it was the first time the term "artificial kidney" was mentioned. The story was reproduced in the New York Times [3]. Collodion was a flammable solution of nitrocellulose in ether. It was used in photography to coat glass photographic plates, reducing exposure time. It was also used as a surgical dressing. The anticoagulant Abel used, hirudin, was prepared from leeches, but it was found to be too toxic for practical human use. In 1924, George Haas (1886-1971) also tried to perform dialysis in humans using collodion membranes; in 1925, he was the first to use heparin [4].

Table 1. Milestones in dialysis

1. Dialysis Projected as a Treatment for Bright's Disease (1861)
2. Heparin (1916)
3. Cellophane for Dialysis (1937)
4. The First Dialysis Machine (1943)
5. Kidney Transplantation (1954)
6. Developing the Arteriovenous Access (1960)
7. Home Dialysis
8. Hollow Fibers and Membrane Technology (1960s)
9. Infrastructure for Dialysis Development – National Medical Care
10. Social Security Amendment of 1973 (1973)
11. Kt/V (1985)
12. Erythropoiesis Stimulating Agents (1989)
13. Chronic Kidney Disease Mineral Bone Disorders (CKD-MBD)

The original edition of this book listed 20 milestones. This has been revised downward for continuity

The sulfated glycosaminoglycan, heparin, was first isolated from the canine liver in 1916, hence its name – hepar, and its odyssey in revolutionizing health care as we know it today can be the subject of another treatise. It is actually a misnomer that it should be called heparin in that the yield is much higher from lung and intestines. It has a strong negative charge and occurs naturally in vertebrates and some invertebrates. Its isolation was first accomplished by a medical student, Jay McLean (1890-1957) in the laboratories of William Henry Howell (1860-1945) at Johns Hopkins University. Howell was searching for thromboplastins at the time and sent his student to look for natural anticoagulants. Howell was initially surprised and disappointed that the liver "phoshatid" was not a procoagulant as he had anticipated. Heparin was not a phosphorus containing lipid but actually a highly sulfated glucosaminoglycan. That it was not primarily from the liver but the intestines was not determined until 1928, and until then thwarted efforts at purification. Its therapeutic value was being explored during the period when better techniques for its production were being developed. Leonard Rowntree (1883-1959) moved from Johns Hopkins to the Mayo Clinic, and maintained his interest using anticoagulants to manage pulmonary emboli. He had previously worked with Abel while at Johns Hopkins, and even collaborated with him to devise the "artificial kidney." Despite its experimental success, heparin was not commercially practical for clinical use until 1937, with its introduction paralleling the practical use of cellophane as a dialyzer membrane that same year. Charles Best (1889-1978), who was renowned for discovering insulin, played a role in developing methods for standardization and purification of heparin, and confirmed that it should be isolated from the intestines and lung, not the liver [5].

MILESTONE 3: CELLOPHANE FOR DIALYSIS (1937)

Collodion is made by the reaction of nitric acid with cellulose in cotton or wood, creating the highly explosive component of dynamite, gun-cotton, or nitrocellulose. When dissolved in ether and ethyl alcohol, the product dries as a thin film. This film, though flammable, was used in early photography and the early film industry. Cellophane was just being developed at the time of Abel's work and, in fact, the manufacturing techniques for manufacturing cellulose film were patented in 1913 and 1918 by Jacques E. Brandenberger (1872-1954) (US Patents 1,049,658 and 1,266,766). It was used primarily at that time to wrap Whitman candy in the well-known and still popular Whitman Sampler. Abel probably chose collodion because Adolph Fick (1829-1901) had previously used it for *in vitro* dialysis in 1855. Collodion was used to impregnate filter paper in 1907. Abel's experiments with collodion were in animals, but his intent was to develop a device that could be used in humans. His efforts, as well as those of his team, Benjamin Turner and Leonard Roundtree, were noteworthy in demonstrating that endogenous substances could be removed from the body by dialysis, and that the dialyzer they developed became an early prototype for future devices. Collodion stability is poor, as it is fragile. It could only be prepared immediately prior to use and was not practical for commercial application. In 1923, DuPont purchased the patents and rights to produce cellophane from Brandenberger. In 1924, DuPont opened a US plant to manufacture cellophane, but their process was not perfected until 1927. Having a US rather than a European manufacturer accelerated its use in commercial packaging. By 1930, cellophane accounted for 10% of DuPont's sales. Around this time, it was also identified to be suitable for sausage casing by Erwin O. Freund, founder of the Visking Company of Chicago. As its price dropped and its popularity rose, cellophane became the logical choice as a potential dialysis membrane substitute for collodion. Perhaps this should seem less a coincidence in that heparin forms a suitable anticoagulant on the surface of medical materials such as glass and plastics. In 1937, William Thalhimer demonstrated that dialysis worked well with the cellophane sausage casing he acquired from the Visking Company. His major interest was in blood transfusion and exchange transfusion. In fact, he pioneered exchange transfusion with heparinized blood as a potential treatment for uremia in dogs. His construction of an artificial kidney of cellophane that would work for 3 to 5 hours in dogs to remove urea was a vital contribution to the field of dialysis [5].

MILESTONE 4: THE FIRST DIALYSIS MACHINE (1943)

The first dialysis machine was developed by Willem "Pim" Kolff (See Figure 1) of the Netherlands between 1939 and 1943. It consisted of a rotating drum wrapped with 20 meters of cellophane sausage casing. The dimensions of this membrane were calculated by Kolff to be sufficient to remove an adequate amount of urea. During the time of its development, the Nazis invaded the Netherlands. Kolff is credited with setting up the first blood bank in Europe, and claimed his experiences of handling blood outside the body gave him added confidence when working with the artificial kidney. In 1943, the first person, a 29-year-old housewife with malignant hypertension, was treated with 12 courses for kidney failure with this prototype, but ultimately died. Kolff did not achieve success until 1945 [6]. This machine used glucose to increase the osmotic gradient across the membrane, creating the risk that serum glucose level could rise and that the patient could go into pulmonary edema. Later research would lead to more ideal dialysates. Kolff's dialysis machine became popular in the USA. In 1948, Isadore Snapper, a legendary physician in his own right, invited Willem Kolff to visit Mt. Sinai Hospital in New York and to set up a dialysis program. George Thorn (1906-2004), the Hersey Professor of Medicine at the Peter Bent Brigham Hospital, visited Mt. Sinai Hospital to witness the Kolff machine and then invited him to "The Brigham" to help develop a second-generation machine. Many of the duties related to dialysis management were assigned to his resident, John Merrill (1917-1984) (See Figure 2). The result was the Kolff-Brigham Kidney. This redesigned machine was built of stainless steel by Edmund Olson and Carl Walter (1905-1992) (See Figure 3). John Peters and Louis Welt were two highly prominent academicians in the early days of nephrology. They were skeptical about the early dialysis machine of Merrill's and considered this a "deluxe toy," questioning its utility. Despite this skepticism, the device was ultimately shipped to several worldwide centers. During the Korean War, many soldiers developed acute kidney injury. Early hemodialysis proved itself successful in treating them. John Merrill went on to help shape and develop the new specialty of nephrology, not only serving as a pioneer in dialysis and transplantation, but also in training future physicians who would not only apply this new, innovative technology, but also assure its widespread adoption [7]. Initially, in addition to acute care, Merrill's dream was that dialysis would be useful as a stopgap measure for a revolutionary procedure, known as transplantation, developed at his hospital.

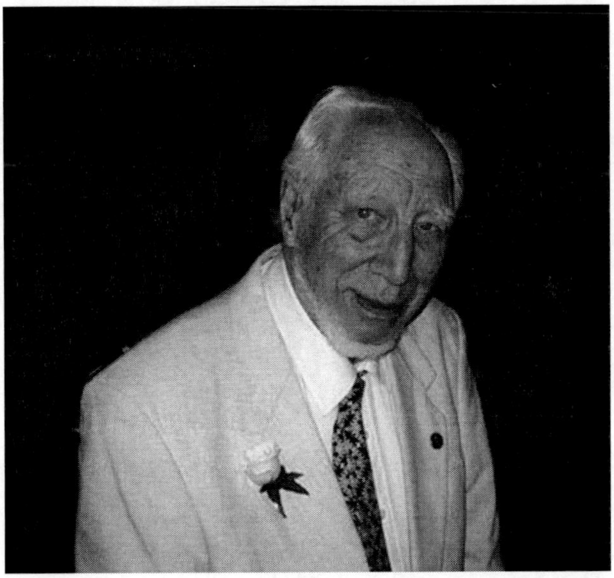

Figure 1. Willem Kolff – taken at the 2003 AAKP Medal of Excellence Award Dinner (Photo by Stephen Z. Fadem, MD)

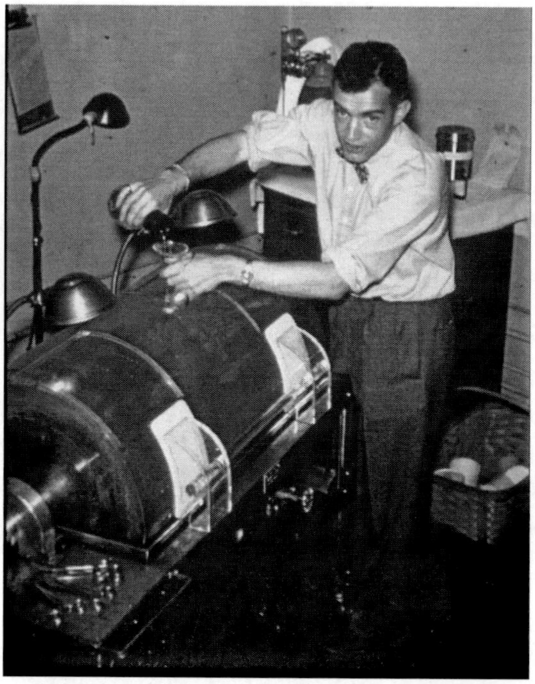

Figure 2. John P. Merrill preparing the dialysate bath for the Kolff-Brigham Kidney. (Photo used with permission from Eli A. Friedman, MD)

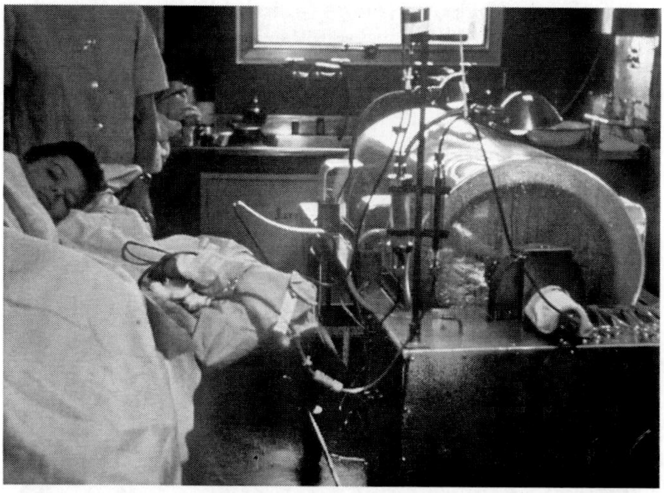

Figure 3. The Brigham Kolff Kidney in use. (Photo used with permission from Eli A. Friedman, MD)

MILESTONE 5: KIDNEY TRANSPLANTATION (1954)

The next advancement was the development of kidney transplantation, and the discovery of the role the immune system would play in its success or failure.

This milestone took place in 1954, with the successful transplant of a kidney in an identical twin by Joseph Murray (1919-2012) and his team at The Peter Bent Brigham Hospital in Boston

[8], substantiating that it was immune system rejection that was causing previous kidneys to fail. To tackle these immune system challenges, the team performed a series of transplants using various combinations of irradiation and corticosteroids. It was the development of tissue typing, and by 1962, the introduction of immunosuppressive medications that made kidney transplantation a more reliable option [9]. The next milestone of the Brigham team was to successfully perform a cadaveric kidney transplant, which was accomplished in 1963. Transplantation opened the door to an entirely new field of medicine. Joseph E. Murray was awarded the Nobel Prize in Physiology or Medicine in 1990.

MILESTONE 6: DEVELOPING THE ARTERIOVENOUS ACCESS (1960)

Although viable for acute therapy, dialysis in the 1950s was not conducive for chronic therapy. Initial dialysis treatments would last for 24 hours. The major challenge to the care of the end-stage renal disease patient was access to the circulation. After World War II, the plastics industry catapulted. In the years prior, cellophane and Bakelite were top choices in plastics. Bakelite, formed from a chemical combination of phenol and formaldehyde, could be molded and machined. It was used for radios, combs, jewelry, hairbrushes, and ashtrays. Bakelite revealed uses of plastic never previously imagined and ushered in a new era of manufacturing into America. The disadvantage of Bakelite was that once it hardened, it could not be remelted and used again. Other plastics polymerized before being injected into a mold. These thermoplastics eclipsed Bakelite, which is no longer produced [10]. There were many products developed before the war such as cellulose acetate, polystyrene, nylon, polyethylene, and polytetrafluoroethylene. Were it not for the emergence of "plastic" polymers, starting with cellophane, dialysis as we know it today would not exist.

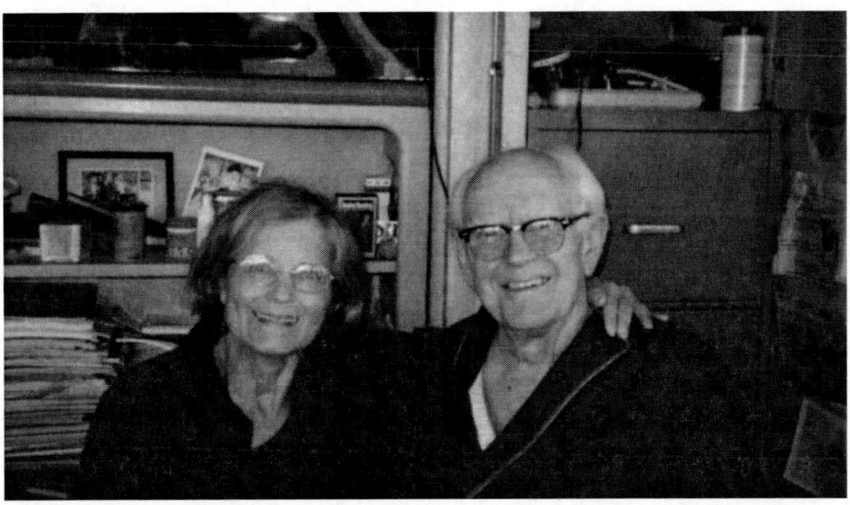

Figure 4. Nancy, Hewlitt Spaeth, RN along with Belding Scribner. Spaeth started dialysis in 1966 and used the Kiil Dialyzer. "Scrib" was beloved by his patients as well as his colleagues. (Photo courtesy of Nancy Hewlitt Spaeth. Used with permission).

For dialysis to be repeated several times a week, one needed a conduit between the dialysis pumps and the patient's circulation. This would have to resist clotting, connect with ease to existing equipment, and would have a low incidence of infection. In 1950, Belding Scribner (1921-2003) (See Figure 4), then at the Mayo Clinic, was planning to golf with colleagues, but instead attended a lecture by John Merrill. Although convinced that dialysis would be a valuable tool in the future, the Mayo Clinic did not share his enthusiasm, and he moved to Seattle. In 1960, "Scrib", then a professor at the University of Washington in Seattle, in collaboration with Wayne Quinton (1921-2015), an instrument maker, developed a U-shaped shunt devised of a slippery fluorinated ethylene plastic that was becoming widely used in industry, as well as the kitchen, as a non-stick coating. This DuPont plastic was polytetrafluoroethylene (PTFE), now well known as Teflon®, and had been used to coat valves and seals during the Manhattan Project. In the 1950s, its use expanded from being an insulator to being used in fishing tackle. It was soon used as a coating to form nonstick cooking utensils. Scribner felt it would be ideal because it would not react with body tissues, but its nonstick properties made it invaluable. On March 9, 1960, a Boeing machinist, Clyde Shields became the first patient ever initiated on dialysis with this prototype access. His first treatment was 76 hours, and the 300 liters of dialysate were stored in a Sears Roebuck freezer. His survival heralded a new era in managing kidney failure. This shunt only lasted two months before it had to be replaced, but Shields lived for 11 more years. Teflon was too stiff, irritating the intima of the artery and vein whenever the patient moved the forearm [11]. It was replaced as Quinton discovered a more flexible plastic – a silicone elastomer trademarked Silastic,® when combined with Teflon tips greatly extended the life of the "Scribner Shunt" [12]. The shunt achieved wide use well into the late 1970s.

In 1961, Stanley Shaldon, who started his career as a hepatologist at the Royal Free Infirmary in London, was placed in charge of the hospital's dialysis machine by his professor, Sheila Sherlock. His initial patients were connected via the "Scribner Shunt," but he pioneered the use of a silicone-Teflon femoral catheter to facilitate treatment. Economic necessity combined with advancing technology as the demand for dialysis grew. Shaldon's hospital would only budget three twin-coil dialyzers per month, forcing him to develop a protocol to reuse dialyzers [13].

An arterio-venous communication that develops during the healing of military wounds inspired James Cimino. These would create traumatic arteriovenous fistula. James Cimino, who had worked as a phlebotomist, observed that soldiers returning from the Korean War with traumatic fistulae were easily cannulated. Working with Kenneth Appel and Michael Brescia, the Brescia-Cimino fistula was developed at the Bronx Veterans Administration Hospital in 1962 and refined by 1966 [14, 15]. It is still the preferred access for dialysis today, replacing the need for the temporary access catheters that had been developed by Quinton. The AV fistula has a low injection rate and decreased propensity to clot or stenose. Its disadvantage is that is sometimes requires a second step of surgery and takes several weeks to be ready for use.

In 1969, Wilbert H. Gore, patented his work on tetrafluoroethylene polymers as a sealant. Later, along with Rowena Taylor and his son Robert Gore, discovered the process for making these polymers porous and "breathable" yet water resistant. As the story goes, they attempted to stretch the polymer as far as possible, but instead of fracturing, it returned to its former shape more porous and with highly unique properties. Gore patented their product, GORE-TEX. (USPTO 3,953,966), and initially promoted it as ideal for electrical insulation, and as a pipe-sealant. GORE-TEX is widely used in sportswear and raingear but is also suitable for implantable devices. In 1981, Gore developed a cardiovascular patch using GORE-TEX and later developed the arterio-venous graft for hemodialysis patients. Although it does not last as long as a well-placed AV fistula, it is still a mainstay of dialysis care when the fistula is not suitable [16]. In 2006, the FDA approved Flixene, a third-generation porous polytetrafluoroethylene laminate. Its advantage is that it can be cannulated within 24 to 72 hours [17].

MILESTONE 7: HOME DIALYSIS

The university-based machines were devised to mix concentrates centrally and proportion them to each machine. This proportioning technology was developed by Albert 'Les' Babb, a nuclear engineer. The in-center machine and proportioning system was known as "The Monster." The capacity to provide in-center dialysis was greatly exceeded by the demands of emerging patients with kidney failure. From this necessity, home dialysis machines were born and became the prototype for all dialysis machines used today.

Carolyn Helms (See Figure 5) was a 15-year-old girl who had developed renal failure as the result of lupus nephritis. The selection committee in Seattle rejected her, claiming she was too young to qualify for dialysis. This young girl was the daughter of a family friend of Babb, hence asked for his help. To enable her to receive dialysis at home, he developed a single patient proportioning system with monitors and safety devices. This became the "Mini-1", and was built by the Milton Roy Company in 1964. It used a Kiil Dialyzer (Figure 6) and was designed exclusively for home dialysis. The "Mini-1" had a wood veneer front so that it would match furniture in the house. Milton-Roy ultimately joint-ventured with Extracorporeal and was acquired by Johnson & Johnson, but then sold to Delmed in 1984. This negative pressure machine evolved into Baxter-Travenol SPS machines that culminated in the Baxter Arena dialysis machine [18-20].

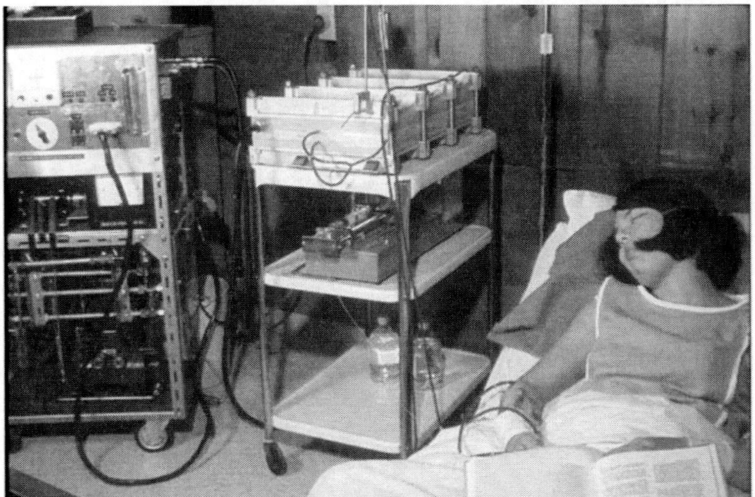

Figure 5. Carolyn Helms dialyzing at home, 1965. (Photo courtesy of the University of Washington).

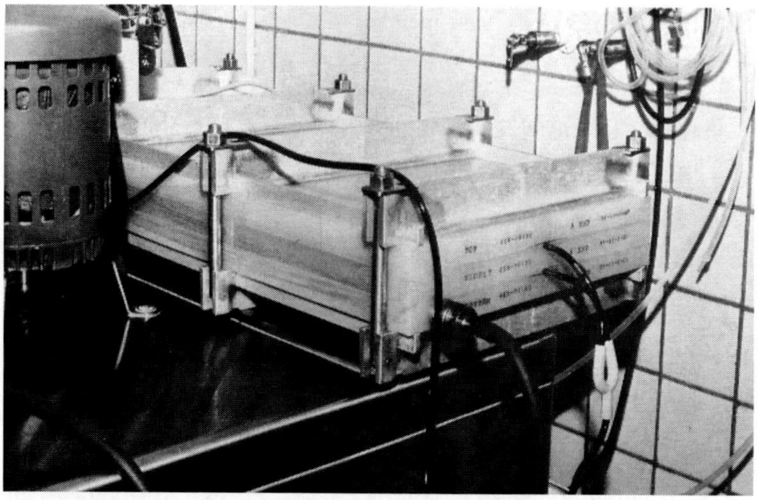

Figure 6. Alternate photo - Kiil Dialyzer – as modified by Belding Scribner. (Photo courtesy Chris Blagg, MD, University of Washington, Seattle).

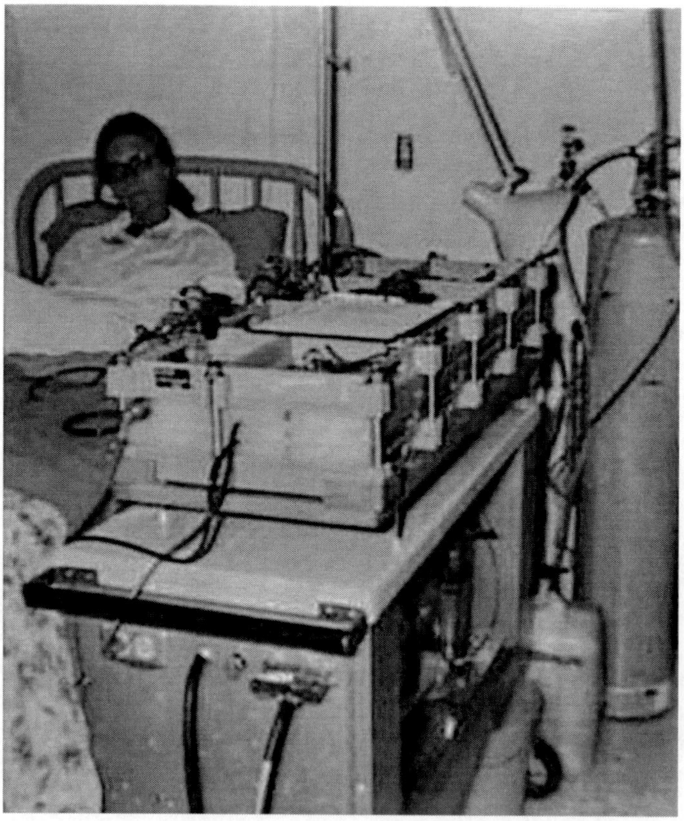

Figure 7. Nancy Hewlitt Spaeth, a young nurse, dialyzing with a modified Kiil dialyzer at home. (Photo courtesy of Nancy Hewlitt Spaeth. Used with permission).

The design and concept behind the dialysis machines used today in dialysis centers were based upon original machines intended for home use. Recently, interest in home dialysis has been reborn, not only out of economic necessity, but because of patient preference. Home dialysis requires not only the appropriate equipment, but also the education and training of the patient and, in the case of hemodialysis, a significant other or friend. This was first reported in 1963. A 30-year-old draftsman, after becoming uremic, was referred to the Royal Free Hospital in London and was treated with a low-sodium diet and daily dialysis. He improved and was discharged on twice weekly 12-hour dialysis, dialyzing by himself using reusable coil dialyzers. He was maintained on a 22 mEq sodium diet, and returned to work [21]. In 1965, Shaldon also reported that he underwent unattended overnight self-care dialysis using the pump-free Kiil dialyzer and the Scribner Shunt [12]. His patient remained healthy and functional. In the second year of care, the patient fathered another child. His success underscored the value of dialysis, the feasibility of self-care, and the value of the low sodium diet in kidney patients.

Chronic peritoneal dialysis did not become successful as home therapy until 1976. This procedure was first attempted on guinea pigs and rabbits in 1923 by Georg Ganter [22], who was able remove non-protein nitrogen, resulting improvement in the animals' uremic symptoms. His attempts to apply this procedure in humans was not successful, but by the1940s [23] and throughout the 1950s, it became a preferred technique for the treatment of acute renal failure [24]. Catheters in use during this period were stiff and not practical. A flexible catheter was first developed by Arthur Grollman in 1952. In 1959, Paul Doolan developed a polyethylene catheter for chronic use, but it was not until 1968 that Henry Tenckhoff developed the implantable peritoneal catheter that bears his name. The tubing was made of silicone and the cuff of polyester [25-27]. In Austin, Texas, RP Popovich and Jack Moncrief developed chronic ambulatory peritoneal dialysis (CAPD) based upon calculations of the contact time of dialysate with the peritoneal membrane (the dwell time). The concept called for fluid to constantly remain in the peritoneal space, and a major barrier to its usefulness was peritonitis. This was addressed by Dimitrios Oreopoulos (1936-2012) in 1978, with the development of dialysis containers made of plastic bags instead of glass bottles. As peritoneal dialysis became more popular, it was championed Zbylut Twardowski and Karl Nolph (1937-2014), major contributors to its development [28]. Renown inventor, Dean Kamen, developed the Home ChoiceTM peritoneal dialysis system for Baxter International. By automating the dialysis procedure, this device made it easier for patients to undergo convenient, nightly peritoneal dialysis. Peritoneal dialysis is more economical to provide than hemodialysis, shares similar outcomes with respect to mortality, and enables patients to have a more flexible schedule. It is ideal for patients who continue to work and is very popular in cities such as Hong Kong. In recent years, it has become very popular as a modality in the USA.

MILESTONE 8: HOLLOW FIBERS (1960S) AND MEMBRANE TECHNOLOGY

Advancements in plastics technology enabled both reverse osmosis, widely used to generate pure water, and the dialyzer. The history of dialyzers as recounted by Zbylut Twardowski, one of the premier pioneers in dialysis technology, is fascinating [29].

Nils Alwall (1904-1986) had been working on a dialysis technique in Lund, Sweden since the 1940s. His efforts were independent and parallel to those of Kolff insofar as he also developed an artificial kidney and an early prototype dialyzer. With this dialyzer, cellophane was wrapped around a coil over which was placed a support. The Alwall method introduced a means to treat fluid overload, known as ultrafiltration [30]. This was not present in the Kolff rotating drum dialyzer.

Leonard Skeggs and Jack Leonard of Case Western Reserve University in Cleveland, Ohio collaborated to develop a more portable, compact dialyzer. By 1948, they were able to modify the earlier prototypes by wrapping cellulose between parallel plates. The parallel plate dialyzer was the first to use negative pressure, also an advancement that enabled volume control. This was the dialyzer used in 1960 by Scribner to dialyze Clyde Shields; however, it was difficult to use in practice.

Skeggs worked in a hospital laboratory. He is also remembered as the inventor of the SMA-12 autoanalyzer, which he sold to Technicon. This revolutionary device automated the analysis of blood chemistries. Ironically, advancements in nephrology would not have been possible were it not for this concomitant contribution to laboratory science. Flame photometry had been applied by John Peters of Yale in the 1940s, but was adapted to the autoanalyzer by Skeggs, enabling the measurement of sodium and potassium. This practical measurement of electrolytes was essential for the new specialty of nephrology [31].

Kolff was brought to the Cleveland Clinic by Irvine Page (1901-1991). In 1954, Kolff developed a prototype kidney by coiling cellophane around orange juice cans and using wood slats and a cellophane membrane. He was able to prevent the pressure drop across dialyzers by using two lengths of cellophane, and named his device the "twin coil kidney." It was used to describe the first disposable dialyzer. The dialyzer was produced by Travenol and became commercially available in 1955. Travenol later became Baxter. Kolff wanted to use Maytag washing machines as the tank for his new artificial kidney, and even sent patients home with the retrofitted devices. Maytag feared litigation, and forbade its use, refusing further sales of washing machines to Kolff. Kolff then found a supply of abandoned rocket nose cones and, although this product worked, it never became commercially available [32].

Cellulose is the structural component of green plants and algae, and the most abundant organic compound on earth. It is more familiarly known as cotton and paper. Cellophane and rayon are regenerated cellulose, made by shredding wood pulp, treating it with sodium hydroxide or lye. It is then processed into sheets or filaments. Cellulosics were developed in 1862, and the original products were cellulose acetate, celluloid, and rayon. Cellophane was developed in the early 1900s, and the more porous cupraphan in 1937. Although they became popular polymers in the early days of dialysis, their poor ability to clear beta microglobulins contributed to long-term patients developing amyloidosis. They have since been replaced by more biocompatible membranes.

Frederic Kiil (1921-2015), a Norwegian urologist, modified the Skeggs-Leonard flat plate dialyzer using cupraphan instead of cellophone and replaced rubber pads with plastic. In 1961, Scribner learned of it and started using it in Seattle for home dialysis patients. No blood pump was needed [33] and it was ideal for overnight treatment. He modified the design, had local machinists at Western Gear Corporation mill the boards, and used this dialyzer for over 10 years. Cupraphan was later used in coil dialyzers.

In the early 1960s, Twardowski concluded that the ideal dialyzer would require high efficiency and would not rupture easily when obtaining a high transmembrane pressure, and thus should be made of capillary tubing as opposed to plates or coils. In 1965, he patented his device in Poland. Although hollow fiber extrusion had actually been developed in the 1940s, it was not commercialized until the 1960s when Dow Chemical Company started manufacturing fibers for desalination plants using reverse osmosis. Richard Stewart, at the University of Michigan, recognized its potential in dialysis. In collaboration with Joseph Cerny and Henry Mahon, he pursued the idea for a hollow fiber dialyzer. The hollow fiber effort was developed as a joint effort with Ben Lipps and John Sargent of Dow Chemical Company, along with the Western Division Research Laboratories, Marquette University School of Medicine, and the Wood Veteran's Administration Hospital. Dow and the Cordis Company formed a joint venture to manufacture hollow fiber dialyzers [34]. As concerns with biocompatibility grew, other plastics were tried. By 1981, it was estimated that there were 23 companies manufacturing 100 different dialyzers, mainly cupraphan and cellulose acetate [29]. Polysulfones are high performance thermoplastic polymers. They were introduced by Union Carbide in 1965, have a high permeability, as well as a better clearance of beta macroglobulin. Thus, they have a higher biocompatibility profile. Fresenius collaborated and supported the development of this polymer. Polysulfones are in use today by Fresenius and polyarylethersulfones are used by Baxter. Polyflux, another popular membrane, is a blend of polyamide and polyarylethersulfone. Baxter acquired Gambro AB in 2013. New membranes are engineered to provide highly efficient, stable, and biocompatible dialysis treatments.

Reverse Osmosis

The concept of osmosis was first observed by Abbe Nottet, a French cleric, in 1748. A difference in solute concentrations across a semipermeable membrane creates a pressure, the osmotic pressure, that drives solutions to the compartment with the highest concentration. Although the quantitative relationships of osmotic pressure were studied in 1887 by van't Hoff, it was not until the twentieth century that pressure was recognized as the driving force in the movement of fluids across a membrane. While conventional osmotic pressures will move fluids from the compartment with a lower to that with the higher concentration, this osmotic pressure can be overcome by increasing the pressure on the other side of the membrane. This drives fluids backward from the higher to the side of the lower concentration. By applying several passes, one can achieve a very pure sample of a fluid.

In the late 1940s and 1950s, reverse osmosis was attempted, but its evolution to a commercially practical method of purifying water depended upon the advancement in thin-film membrane technology. Spiral wound polyamide membranes have been available and in use since 1977 and are available through many manufacturers. These membranes generally do not tolerate chlorine, and while this presents a vexing dilemma for community water purification systems, is quite convenient for dialysis facilities that routinely remove chlorine prior to processing with reverse osmosis. Currently RO is the major source of pure water for dialysis facilities [35, 36].

Milestone 9: Infrastructure for Dialysis Development – National Medical Care

Initially, hemodialysis was adopted and developed by academic centers of excellence. In 1962, Merrill started his own dialysis program at the Brigham, recruiting fellows to purchase and boil the cellophane, wrap the dialyzers and mix the chemicals. Three of the fellows, Edward "Ted" Hager, Eugene "Gene" Schupak (1931-2008) and Constantine "Gus" Hampers became famous as founders of what would become the largest dialysis company in the world. Their story is well recounted in Tim McFeely's *The Price of Access* [37].

By 1965, the Peter Bent Brigham Hospital's 6 stations were the only source of dialysis for the growing numbers of patients. Those without insurance were not turned away, but it was not long before dialysis services consumed a disproportionate share of the hospital's resources, becoming a burden to the hospital. As a major academic institution adjacent to Harvard Medical School, the provision of routine chronic services was not aligned with being a major innovative research center. By 1966, the hospital's dialysis center was at capacity, and the Brigham, along with the Massachusetts Department of Public Health, offered support to Hager and Hampers to establish a program in Boston's Normandy House, an extended care facility. Their outpatient center was able to provide dialysis services at a fraction of the cost of the hospital. They next set up a center on Babcock Street. The new company, National Medical Care began to grow as the three founders planned to replicate their dialysis center model across the country. By 1971, the enterprise, also included Biomedical Applications in Queens, New York, managed by Schupak; it was successfully capitalized. Centers were opened in Bethesda, Maryland, Philadelphia, Pennsylvania and Dallas, Texas, as well as Miami, Torrance, Pittsburgh, Beverly Hills, San Francisco, Portland, Tampa and other cities. During this period, dialysis was largely funded through insurance and for some, Medicaid, as this preceded the passage of legislation creating a Medicare coverage benefit.

However, in 1971, their success was marred as their association with the Brigham brought unfavorable press in a series of stories published by the Boston Globe. The attack on this venerable institution created a backlash against the key NMC executives, and the hospital and university disassociated from them.

As the company grew, it was purchased by W.R. Grace, and later sold to Fresenius. In its wake, NMC developed an infrastructure for cost effective, accessible and efficient dialysis care [37].

Milestone 10: Social Security Amendment of 1973 (1973)

The God Committee

As word of Scribner's success grew, it became apparent in Seattle that the hospital per se would be short lived as an ongoing site for dialysis. The original dialysis program in Seattle was funded by the National Institute of Health, but it was soon discovered that other funding would be necessary. The dialysis center would have to be moved out of the hospital. In January 1962, Scribner established a three-station non-profit outpatient center. Initially known as the Seattle Artificial Kidney Center, it was the first dialysis center in the country. Ultimately, it became the world-renown Northwest Kidney Center.

When the center reached capacity, a serious ethics conundrum was born. It was estimated that 10,000 persons were in need of dialysis in the USA, and strict criteria were established to determine who would be deemed eligible. Some were unfit for therapy and never considered because they were too young - under 15, or too old - greater than 55, had comorbid conditions, or no rehabilitation potential. An admissions and policy committee was established to decide which patients could undergo dialysis. Comprised of 6 community leaders and a non-nephrologist physician, the committee only considered patients who met stringent criteria for review. Thirty candidates were considered in Seattle, but only 17 were judged suitable. They were reviewed by a panel to determine whether or not they would be able to undergo therapy or would be consigned to die. Only 10 could be selected for the 3 station program; the other 7 would die. Criteria among those medically fit included net worth, marital status, nature of occupation, extent of education, number of children, and church attendance.

In November 1962, Life Magazine ran a feature story by Shana Alexander, "They Decide Who Lives, Who Dies," which achieved national attention [38]. As dialysis spread as a viable treatment option, controversy over the balance of scarcity vs. rationing continued. In some areas, IQ tests and personality tests were administered to determine who would qualify for treatment. In Los Angeles, candidates were selected by lottery. It was circumstances such as this that sparked the controversies that ultimately led to the passage of legislation to cover dialysis [39].

Legislation Passes

Despite the pressure placed on Congress in 1963, they would not decide to cover dialysis costs and make therapy available for another decade. In 1963 and 1964, the Veterans Hospital and the Public Health Service both announced plans to build dialysis centers. In 1965, the Budget Bureau established a committee headed by Carl Gottschalk (1922-1997) to study its feasibility and cost, as well as to make recommendations. Although dialysis legislation was delayed, an act was passed to provide coverage to Americans over 65 years old.

During the 1960s, dialysis was becoming widely accepted. National Medical Care was incorporated in 1968 to provide dialysis care using outside funding. As in Seattle, the Peter Bent Brigham Hospital in Boston was also unable to bear the financial hardships of providing dialysis. The small program that the NMC founders established – the Babcock Unit - in a neighboring hospital was replicated throughout the nation. Young physicians trained at major academic centers became dialysis pioneers.

National Association of Patients on Hemodialysis NAPH (1969)

The Brooklyn Kings County Hospital Dialysis Unit was started by Eli Friedman with an old Kolff machine rusting in the basement. He received a three-year federal grant and built a 14-station unit. Samuel Orenstein, a CPA, had been dialyzing 18 hours a day in the Brooklyn Unit since its start. Together with William Blackton, a psychology major on dialysis since 1965, they had a vision to "get all kidney patients together." In September 1969, they sent a flier to 200 dialysis units, and by October the first issue of NAPHNews was published. Their dream was to appeal to Congress to enact legislation to cover dialysis benefits; many had gone through selection committees. The newsletter is now a magazine, AAKP Renalife, and exists today.

A Peter Lundin III and NAPH

In 1966, a junior college student, Andrew Peter Lundin III (1944-2001), developed kidney failure and enrolled in the home training program at the University of Washington in Seattle where he was trained by Joseph Eschbach (1933-2007). He dialyzed 10 hours a day thrice weekly overnight on the Milton Roy Mini II, the second generation of a machine developed for Carolyn Helms. After completing his pre-med education at Stanford University, he was accepted into medical school, despite having only one kidney. In 1963, Eli Friedman began a program in Brooklyn that would serve as a nidus for the development of patient-centered health care and took a chance on the young applicant. Lundin became the first dialysis patient to graduate from medical school and had a distinguished career as a nephrologist.

NAPH and Capitol Hill

The National Association of Patients on Hemodialysis would later become The American Association of Kidney Patients, but in the interim served to convince Congress to enact legislation covering dialysis costs. The prediction to Congress was that there would never be more than 35,000 persons on dialysis, and that the program would never cost more than 250 million dollars became the nidus legislation to make all ESRD patients eligible for health coverage. Congress also advised that most people who underwent a kidney transplantation would return to work and thus be able to afford immunosuppressive therapy [40].

The Bill Passes

The combined efforts of scientists, patients, physicians such as George Schreiner, and the public brought increasing pressure on Congress. It was a fortuitous coincidence that the powerful Ways and Means Committee wanted to expand Medicare to cover disability. In 1970, the House sent the Senate a proposed draft of the amended Medicare bill. Although the Senate passed and returned an amended bill to the House, it occurred during the week between Christmas and New Years, making it impossible to review. It was well known that the Ways and Means Committee Chairman, Wilbur Mills (1909-1992) would hear any citizen who wanted to speak. On November 4, 1971 Bill Litchfield (1940-2014), an engineer from Houston; June Crowley, a mother of four; Abraham Holtz, a CPA; and Lundin joined Shep Glazer, a salesman with two young children, in the Ways and Means Committee Room. Samuel Orenstein, the founder of NAPH, had passed away before the meeting. Schupak, the nephrologist from Queens provided a machine and Glazer briefly dialyzed before Mills and his committee while Schreiner nervously stood by (personal communication). James Carey, the renal fellow who was nearby, noted that he had ventricular tachycardia and immediately clamped the lines. Although he only dialyzed 5 minutes, Mills commented "I don't know of any testimony that I have heard in such a short period of time that has made a more dramatic impact on me."

It was George Schreiner, NKF president who, working with Charles Plante, his neighbor, devised the idea to put dialysis care in the Medicare Trust Fund. Plante and Schreiner toiled together untiringly at their homes to craft legislation, (usually fueled by scotch – personal communication), and worked tirelessly on Capitol Hill to "proselytize" for this bill.

In 1972, the Senate Finance Committee chaired by Russell Long considered the legislation, but when released in September it did not have a provision for kidney disease. Plante was able to intercede and get the provision introduced, but the bill also had a drug provision which Long wanted. Mills did not think his Ways & Means Committee would accept Long's drug provision but compromised that if the drug provision were removed the kidney provision would be allowed. The bill passed. One of the reasons it passed was the human face of the issue that presented itself to Russell Long and Wilbur Mills – Richard Rettig wrote: "Ultimately, the ESRD entitlement was added to Medicare because the moral cost of failing to provide lifesaving care was deemed to be greater than the financial cost of doing so" [40].

In a unique experiment, Medicare amended its coverage policy to include a single disease, rather than basing eligibility upon age. In this same act, it also extended coverage for disability. Tragically for some, it fell short of continuing long-term eligibility for the expensive and necessary immunosuppressive agents required maintaining a kidney transplant. This would not become law until December 2020. In October 1972, when Congress enacted legislation that amended The Social Security Act, there were 10,000 persons on dialysis, of whom 40% were on home therapy [41].

OBRA 1981

During the first ten years of therapy, dialysis availability greatly expanded. No longer were patients restricted by age or comorbidities. In 1974, the Health Care Financing Administration (HCFA) reported the prevalence of dialysis at 15,993; but by 1983, it increased to 86,354. That year the incidence of new patients rose to 25,155. Total Medicare expenditures for all dialysis patients in 1974 was $229 million USD, but by 1983 it had jumped to $1.898 billion USD. When corrected for inflation, this was a 331% change. During this time Medicare reimbursement payment policy for outpatient dialysis services was based upon reasonable charges, set at $138.00 per treatment.

Congressional hearings were held in 1976, 1977, and 1978 in an effort to reduce reimbursement. In 1978, PL 95-292 passed a law to implement a prospective payment rate (PPR) for dialysis providers. A Notice of Proposed Rulemaking was not issued until 1980 and rejected by the Reagan administration. The passage of the Omnibus Budget Reconciliation Act (OBRA) of 1981 mandated the PPR, and after a Notice of Rulemaking the following year, the composite rate was established in a Final Rule effective August 1, 1983. The consolidated dialysis rates averaged between $127 and $131 per treatment based on geographic wage adjustment. In 1986, HCFA proposed a $6.00 decrease by calculating dialysis rates on the basis of the median treatment cost per treatment for all dialysis facilities in the entire sampled patient population, arguing this would be a more accurate reflection than by median per facility. This was a response to pressure from the Office of Management and Budget to reduce the ESRD program by $100 million dollars. Although only cut by 2 dollars in 1986, between 1986 and 1991, the composite rate fell regularly. In 1991, it was $124 per treatment. HCFA used the argument that dialysis rates were initially set too high, as was evidenced by the growth and profitability of companies like NMC. However, it did not consider that as primary payer,

Medicare only paid 80% of the rate. Primary insurance payments were higher resulting in a shift of costs from Medicare to private health insurers.

In 1990, the Institute of Medicine (IOM) issued a report highlighting several issues – that while dialysis reimbursement rates were lowered, facilities remained financially solvent by obtaining lower supply costs, reducing treatment times, reusing dialyzers, and decreasing patient to staff ratios. Concerns were raised that the quality of core medical services was threatened. HCFA countered the IOM argument by showing that in cost reports from 1985 and 1987, payment for treatment exceeded unaudited costs by 8 dollars. HCFA was criticized for not adjusting dialysis prices for inflation but argued back that price drops in dialyzers offset raises in salaries. HCFA claimed that as long as dialysis facilities were expanding capacity, they must have been making a profit. They also maintained that vertical integration of large chains allowed the offset of negative costs from profits in other aspects of their business, such as manufacturing. Likewise, they debated that physician-owned facilities could be offset by professional fees. Concerns by regulators were that facility profits were at the expense of quality because quality was not systematically monitored.

The price change of 1983 had a sobering effect upon dialysis care. NMC was already looking for a buyer prior to the establishment of a composite rate. By 1984, W.R. Grace had agreed, closing the deal on December 20 [37]. The strain between providing services for those in need conflicted with the availability of discretionary resources, challenging the quality of care provided. Providers contended the reimbursement rate declines forced compromised care, adversely affecting patient outcomes. The 1990 IOM Report expressed concerns that as real payments decreased, units would survive by reducing services and quality to the point of reducing standards. They recommended that the composite rate not be reduced, but that the rate be updated yearly, rebased only when an ESRD quality assessment program was in place, and that payment policy be reviewed on a regular basis [42].

For the first four years after the ESRD program was established, it was administered by the Bureau of Health Insurance and the Public Health Service Bureau of Quality Assurance, resulting in a lack of coordinated data management. In 1977, the Health Care Financing Administration (HCFA) was established. Public Law 95-292 of 1978 created a specific program for ESRD information management – the ESRD Program Management and Medical Information System, which was fully implemented by 1980. It established several source documents, including the uniform billing bill (UB-82), the Medical Evidence Report (Form 2728) and the ESRD death notification (2746). It also established forms for report health cost information (2552) and to record the facility survey (2744).

USRDS

After much discussion with stakeholders, Congress passed OBRA 1986, establishing an ESRD registry. In 1988, the United States Renal Data System (USRDS) was established, in which the contract was awarded to the University of Michigan. The USRDS contract was shifted to University of Minnesota and is now back in Ann Arbor. Its goals (http://www.usrds.org) are to characterize the ESRD population, as well as to describe the prevalence and incidence of ESRD along with trends in mortality and rates of disease; investigate demographic, treatment, and morbidity relationships; identify areas for special studies and support research; and provide data sets and samples of national data to support research by special studies centers.

The KDOQI Guidelines

In 1950, the National Nephrosis Foundation (NNF) was started by Ada and Harry DeBold in an attempt to save their child, stricken with kidney disease. In 1958, the name was changed to the National Kidney Disease Foundation, then to the National Kidney Foundation (NKF) in 1964. NKF was instrumental in providing resources to the kidney community. In March 1995, under the leadership of Garabed Eknoyan, the NKF launched the Dialysis Outcome Quality Initiative (DOQI), an effort to create evidence-based clinical practice guidelines to aid providers in caring for patients. Multidisciplinary workgroups were established to methodologically review published literature on hemodialysis, peritoneal dialysis, anemia and vascular access [60, 61]. After expert and public review, the DOQI Guidelines were published in time for the 1997 American Society of Nephrology/NKF meeting in San Antonio, Texas. An internet version was also established under the direction of this author. This meeting was to have historical significance in that the MDRD Study equation for Glomerular Filtration Rate was also presented by Andrew Levey at the same meeting. The web version was originally created by this author along with Brian Rosenthal, and now exists at http://mdrd.com.

The guidelines were widely disseminated and accepted by the renal community. Further guidelines were later published, first in nutrition, but later in bone disease, hypertension [43] and lipid management [44]. By 2002, the guidelines had been extended to chronic kidney disease. By consolidated terminology they eliminating vagueness, establishing a lexicon and classification system for kidney disease [45]. These classifications were based upon the calculated GFR presented in 1997. The GFR was initially only available as a web tool on kidney.org and mdrd.com. Ultimately, it was integrated into standard laboratory testing. As the guidelines expanded, DOQI became KDOQI – the Kidney Disease Outcomes Quality Initiative. The CKD guidelines helped to integrate better care between primary physicians and specialists, and increased the understanding of CKD by referral groups [46]. The guidelines have been updated regularly (http://kidney.org). An international iteration of clinical guidelines, Kidney Disease: Improving Global Outcomes (KDIGO) (http://www.kdigo.org) has developed 12 sets of guidelines (acute kidney injury, anemia of CKD, blood pressure in CKD, CKD evaluation and management, CKD-MBD, Diabetes in CKD, glomerulonephritis, hepatitis C in CKD, lipids in CKD, living kidney donor, transplant candidate, and transplant recipient).

Conditions for Coverage

In 1997, Conditions for Coverage for dialysis facilities (41 Fed. Reg. 22503-22522, June 3, 1976) were created to specify the fulfillment of services, furnishing of data and information, compliance with laws and regulations, governance, a care plan, patient rights, medical records, the physical environment, medical director responsibilities, staff responsibilities, and minimal service requirements. It also established that a social worker and dietitian should be available, and that state surveys be performed under contract of HCFA. The statute paved the way for the formation of ESRD Networks in 1977, and required each network have a medical review board. These conditions for coverage remained in effect for over 30 years.

By 2005, a new set of regulations for Medicare coverage of dialysis services were completed and went to final review after extensive public comment. After revision and approval by the necessary components of HHS, they were released in active form on April 8, 2008, becoming effective October 14, 2008 [47].

These conditions, along with attendant interpretive guidelines and tools, created a uniform survey environment with the expressed desire to eliminate variations in quality between dialysis facilities. They dealt mainly with general compliance and patient safety, with special attention to infection control, water and dialysate systems, reuse and the physical environment, providing for updated infection and water quality control guidelines. They required cardiac defibrillators in dialysis facilities, better fire safety and disaster management standards, and created a requirement for dialysis technician certification.

They also dealt with specifics of patient care, including improved patient rights, responsibility, grievance and involuntary discharge provisions. They provided structure for improved patient assessments at chairside and during interdisciplinary team conferences. The program provided for a patient assessment at least once yearly for stable, but monthly for patients who were unstable. The patient plan of care was to be completed and dated by interdisciplinary team members with 30 days of initiating treatment and adjusted as frequently as monthly if achieved outcomes were not being met. Additionally, the new conditions specified medical director responsibilities, giving more authority to the medical director, providing for a tight structure in which to assess, trend, and improve a series of quality measures.

The Conditions established a Quality Assessment and performance Improvement (QAPI) program requiring dialysis centers to achieve measurable improvement in health outcomes and reduce medical errors by measuring, analyzing, and tracking quality indicators. This became an essential tool to assure quality after the enactment and implementation of legislation to achieve payment reform by bundling separately billable ancillary services with the composite rate.

MIPPA 2008

OBRA 1981, Public Law 97-35 established the prospective payment system and required payments to be based on a composite weighted formula. However, substantial expenditures were excluded from this rate, particularly erythropoiesis stimulating agents and vitamin D analogues. As dialysis organizations billed separately for these products, expenses grew around 40% of total dialysis expenditure by 2008. The Medicare Payment Advisory Commission (MedPac) and the Government Accountability Office (GAO) reviewed the Medicare payment system and suggested a bundled prospective payment methodology that would combine the composite rate with separately billable services under a single payment [47]. The passage of MIPPA (Medicare Improvement for Patients and Provider Act) in 2008 offered compromising legislation to dialysis stakeholders. First, it tied an adjustment to the composite rate to inflation, enabling costs to maintain pace with salary changes. This was necessary in a service-based operation. It also legislated that payment reform based upon MedPac and GAO recommendations be implemented January 1, 2011. The Final Rule was published after much debate with respect to the possibility of including calcium binders and calcimimetics. The expanded bundle of services also included dialysis related laboratory studies as well as the oral equivalents to injectable medications (vitamin D analogs) phosphate binder therapy and calcimimetics.

The demand for services is constrained by available funding. Like the composite rate in 1983, the prospective payment reform created an environment where cost reduction strategies competed with quality service. Protocols that stressed comparative effectiveness became based on least costly alternatives. The IOM report of 1990 and the NIH Consensus report of 1993 demonstrated the quality of US dialysis care worsened in response to the institution of the composite rate in 1983. This was sure to happen again.

MIPPA 2008 directed Medicare to establish payment methodology for education sessions to be provided by office-based nephrology teams to patients who had Stage 4 CKD. This offered opportunities for cost savings coupled with quality improvement through proactive care and patient preparedness. The costs for transitioning patients into a hemodialysis program were highest in populations where patient care was not previously managed by a nephrologist. These patients generally had a poor understanding of their condition, presented in an emergency center with ESRD, and required a central venous catheter plus emergency dialysis. Furthermore, this population of patients was most often discharged to chronic in-center dialysis without the educational opportunity to select an alternate modality that might have been more suitable to their lifestyle. Data confirmed that 83% of incident dialysis patients presented for their first dialysis treatment with a central venous catheter.

Kidney X

In February 2017, the VA Center for Innovation (VACI) and the American Society of Nephrology (ASN) convened to meet the challenges faced by kidney disease patients. The summit was divided into three divisions, renal replacement therapy, transplantation, and chronic kidney disease. The program focused on CKD detection, prevention and treatment, better education for persons at risk, data science developments to improve care, and rehabilitation. In addition, the ASN and VACI collaboration targeted early CKD patients [48]. In November 2017, Kidney X was launched as private-public partnership between the ASN and the Department of Health and Human Services (DHHS). With John Sedor appointed chair of the steering committee, the program set up competitions and offered prizes for the most innovative kidney projects. The categories were artificial kidney, COVID-10, Redesign Dialysis Phases 1 and 2, and the Patient Innovator Challenge. The Phase 2 Redesign Dialysis contestants were required to have a prototype to demonstrate. Winning innovations were a bioresorbable shape memory polymer wrap to improve dialysis access site maturation and patency, a novel device to reduce PD touch contamination, a pro-regenerative vascular access graft, an intracorporeal hemodialysis system, vascular hemodialysis grafts with self-renewable endothelia, and a nitric oxide hemodialysis cap to prevent infection and thrombosis.

The integration of health care to have multidisciplinary services address preventive modalities has the best odds for preparing the patient for renal replacement care. In July 2019, Donald Trump established policies that would increase home dialysis; establish awareness initiates for education; prevent kidney failure through better diagnosis, treatment and incentives; increase patient choice through affordable alternative treatments; encourage the development of artificial kidneys; and increase kidney transplantation. The policy also aimed at achieving outcomes by creating incentives to provide care for patients not yet on dialysis, and advanced payments to support management, coordination, and care.

Milestone 11: Kt/V (1985)

The optimal time for a dialysis treatment was initially determined by the Seattle team, [49, 50] but a true mathematical relationship between urea equilibrium was not established until 1985. Its development, the single pool (Kt/V, spKt/V) to define the equilibrium kinetics of solute clearance in dialysis procedures was a major advance in kidney health care. The spKt/V formula states that the logarithmic expression of urea reduction equals the urea clearance of the dialyzer multiplied by the contact time of dialysis divided by the volume of distribution of urea [51]. Measuring the Kt/V immediately post dialysis is not accurate because different compartments or pools in the body each have urea transfer characteristics. Thus, the urea measured in the immediate period is artificially low, and it takes around 30 to 60 minutes to calibrate back. It is not practical for patients and staff to wait for this to occur. Calibration for the time that it takes urea to rebound back into equilibrium between the vascular, intercellular, and the intracellular space immediately after dialysis back to the extracellular space was taken into consideration by later modifications of the formula, hence the more accurate eKt/V used in the HEMO Study [52-56]. The therapeutic goal was initially designed to maintain the spKt/V in balance with protein catabolic rate, i.e., maintain sufficient dialysis to remove wastes products generated through the combination of food breakdown and muscle turnover. The National Cooperative Dialysis Study (NCDS) first reported that increased urea clearance during dialysis was associated with better patient outcomes [57, 58]. Using these data, Gotch and Sargent predicted that a single pool spKt/V lower than 0.8 was associated with worse clinical outcomes [51].

Dialysis services were molded by the confluences of commerce, technology, and necessity. Necessity was determined by the economic challenge of providing for a growing population of ESRD patients in an environment where available resources were in stiff competition for other medical disciplines. The message that a spKt/V < 0.8 amidst the budgetary and economic constraints of 1983 translated to shorter and efficient dialysis. The institution of reuse was also gaining in popularity as a cost-saving measure.

However, as the cottage industry of dialysis care burgeoned, a reality check was needed. By the end of the 1980s, inadequate dialysis dosing in the United States was accounting for inferior patient outcomes compared to other nations [59]. This was noted in a key stakeholder meeting in Dallas in 1989 and resulted in a multicenter study initiated by Dallas Nephrology Associates (DNA) to capture key observational data. As the DNA nephrologists increased the Kt/V from 1.18 to 1.46 between 1989 and 1992, their mortality fell from 21.8 to 19.5%, which was superior to that of the rest of the USA. Similar observations were noted at NMC, which between 1990 and 1992 increased its urea reduction ratio from 57.1 to 62.5% and achieved a standard mortality rate of .77 when referenced to the rest of the USA [60].

As these were not a randomized trial, the debate continued as to what was optimal dialysis, and whether or not increasing the Kt/V could extend patient life. A large, multi-center, randomized, controlled trial, the HEMO study was undertaken, but failed to demonstrate an improvement in mortality in the group with the higher eKt/V. In fact, it was not shown that an eKt/V greater than the original DOQI recommendation improved mortality [61]. The HEMO study showed a survival advantage of Kt/V for women over men, but this was based upon an ad hoc analysis, hence not strictly evidence based. Thus, measures by CMS merely call for an acceptable spKt/v of 1.2. It is unknown, though strongly suggested, that men and women have different body characteristics that might determine a more selective determination of their dose, [55, 62, 63] in which further studies are needed to demonstrate this.

Other analyses revealed that shortening the dialysis times to under 240 minutes were associated with an increase in all-cause mortality (HR 1.26) [64]. The HEMO study demonstrated that increased volume derived from modeled urea kinetics was associated with mortality, recent hospitalizations, and decreased serum albumin [65]. Data from the HEMO study demonstrated that the ultrafiltration rate during dialysis was associated with mortality. Patients who had rates > 13 ml/h/kg had an increased all-cause mortality of 1.59. The HR for cardiovascular-related death was 1.71 [66].

MILESTONE 12: ERYTHROPOIESIS STIMULATING AGENTS (ESAS) (1989)

Erythropoietin is produced in the kidney in healthy patients and maintains the bone marrow production of red blood cells in a steady state. In kidney disease, renal mass decreases, as does the production of erythropoietin. Anemia is almost universal in ESRD patients. A major technological advance has been to clone the gene that transcribes erythropoietin and genetically engineer the immortal cells from the Chinese Hamster ovary to commercially produce it. Previous efforts at managing anemia included stimulating red blood cell production with anabolic steroids such as nandrolone. These were met with limited success. Blood transfusions were often the only option to manage anemia.

Since 1974, it was known that dialysis was associated with accelerated cardiac disease. 74% of patients presented with abnormal cardiac dysfunction and anemia, along with hypertension; accelerated atherosclerosis was considered a causative factor. When Palfrey studied 434 dialysis patients for 41 months during a period between 1982 and 1991, he and his group demonstrated that 31% had congestive heart failure at the onset of disease and another 25% developed it. Those with heart failure had a survival time of 36 months as compared with 62 months for the rest. Anemia was identified as one of the risk factors [67]. During this period, the mean hb was 8.5 g/dL ± 1.5. After adjusting for age, diabetes, blood pressure, serum albumin and ischemic heart disease, each 1 gm decrease in hemoglobin was associated with worsening left ventricular hypertrophy and worsening mortality [68].

A recombinant erythropoietin was thus welcomed by nephrology in the late 1980s. The phase III clinical trials for this product targeted the hematocrit between 33 to 38%. In the multicenter trial, 33% hemodialysis patients with a hematocrit of at least 30% at initiation showed that with a rise in hematocrit, there was the elimination of blood transfusions, improvement in quality of life and control of iron overload [69]. These results were submitted to the FDA, which approved epoetin alfa in June 1989 at a target of 30 to 33%. In 1994, they widened their target to 30 to 36%.

In 1993, the mean hematocrit recorded in the USRDS data registry was 30.2%, still with 43% of patients having hematocrits below this value. The National Anemia Cooperative Project was established in 1994 and set the target for hematocrit at 30%. When the National Kidney Foundation Dialysis Outcome Quality Initiative (DOQI) was released in the autumn of 1997, the average hematocrit was already up to 32.4% (USRDS). The DOQI Guidelines raised the targets to between 33 and 36%. Clinical Performance Measurements established by HCFA were based upon these guidelines.

In 1998, the Normal Hematocrit Study was published. It is the only hard evidence against normalizing the hematocrit using ESA. In this study of dialysis patients with cardiac disease, 618 were assigned to receive ESA to maintain a target of 42% and the remaining 615 to maintain a target of 30%. Although the study never reached statistical significance, it was terminated when the higher hematocrit target group had a higher mortality. This group also required more intravenous iron and had poorer adequacy outcomes. Nevertheless, it was recommended that dialysis patients not be targeted to a normal hematocrit [70].

Despite this study, the next eight years saw a steady rise in the average hematocrit of dialysis patients; by 2007, the mean hb was 12 g/dL. The CPM project also demonstrated that the ratio of ESA/hb levels also rose during the years of 1998-2004, indicating an increase in EPO hyporesponsiveness [71].

By 2000, the updated KDOQI guideline target was 11-12 gm/dL. The Normal Hematocrit Study was challenged by observational data such as a study in 2002 by Collins, whose team reported that the risk of death was not different in groups who had higher (36 to 39%) vs. lower (33 to <36%) hematocrits. The higher hematocrit arm also had a lower hospitalization rate, hence lower costs [72]. Randomized clinical trials to determine the benefits of ESAs were thus initiated.

Two such trials, CREATE Study in Europe and the CHOIR Study in the USA were reported in November 2006, and failed to demonstrate an advantage to targeting high hemoglobin levels. In both trials, study subjects were targeted to higher or baseline hemoglobin levels. In 2006, the NKF KDOQI anemia guideline specified a target > 11 gm/dL and urged caution when maintaining a hb > 13gm/dL.

Those patients with a higher hemoglobin target actually did worse in the CHOIR Trial resulting in an FDA advisory and a Congressional Hearing the following month. An FDA Black Box warning was revised to allow a target hb of 10 to 12 gm/dL. Early in 2007, the NKF revised the KDOQI guideline to specify a hb target between 11 and 12 gm/dL and advised that hb levels should not exceed 13 gm/dL. In 2009, the TREAT trial was published. This was a randomized controlled trial comparing a placebo arm with an arm targeted to achieve a hb of 13 gm/dL. Although outcomes were similar, the higher target group had slightly worse outcomes. In 2011, Medicare conducted a MEDCAC hearing to determine whether ESA reimbursement needed to change. In June 2011, the FDA modified its labeling recommendation to remove the target hb levels of 10 to 12 gm/dL, and substituted language that non-dialysis patients should commence treatment with the hb level falls < 10 gm/dL. For dialysis patients, it was suggested for the dose to be interrupted if the hb rises above 11 gm/dL. The following month, CMS stated that the new guidelines would require the lowest dose to prevent blood transfusions, and that dialysis facilities would be penalized should the hemoglobin exceed 12 gm/dL.

Milestone 13: Chronic Kidney Disease – Mineral Bone Disorders (CKD-MBD) (2005)

As part of the Kidney Disease – Improving Global Outcomes (KDIGO) initiative, a consensus conference was held to redefine and classify the renal osteodystrophy associated with advanced disease. The serum phosphorus has emerged as an independent risk factor for mortality in kidney disease, and its association with vascular calcification and mortality has also been established. The relationships between calcium and phosphorus elevations, mortality rates, and extraskeletal vascular calcification established the need for a classification to encompass all the diverse manifestations of this disease process. The disorder was defined as a triad of laboratory abnormalities, bone abnormalities, and vascular calcification. The morbidities were identified as cardiovascular disease, fractures, and mortality. This has opened a field of discovery that enabled us to visualize the relationship between skeletal and vascular mineralization [73-75].

Conclusion

In the past 160 years, we have journeyed through the history of dialysis from its discovery to what is now a routine procedure that keeps thousands of people alive each day. That journey was fraught with obstacles and barriers, but for each one there was a milestone. We have seen how the invention of cellophane and heparin made dialysis possible, and how the advent of technological development in thermoplastic made it practical. Technology is just one part of the tale that also includes the bright scientists who make amazing observations and discoveries, the legislators who witness the human side of the dialysis procedure and create sound policies, and the entrepreneurs who once expanded the therapy from a small room in a Boston hospital to a worldwide procedure that continually saves lives. Key players are patients like Sam Orenstein, Shep Glazer, Bill Litchfield, and Peter Lundin. These are the people who did not let dialysis stop them from moving forward with their lives. They inspired each other, their doctors, and the nation. The milestone list is not complete. With technology blazing, the distribution of prizes and incentives for novel inventions, and a therapy that is far from perfect, we should see an acceleration in innovation, and we should anticipate more milestones on the horizon.

References

[1] De Santo NG, Bisaccia C, De Santo RM, Perna AF, Manzo M, Di Stazio E, et al. Mariano Semmola (1831-1895): the effect of low protein diet in primary albuminuria. *J Nephrol.* 2006;19 Suppl 10:S48-57.

[2] Giovannetti S, Maggiore Q. A low-nitrogen diet with proteins of high biological value for severe chronic uraemia. *Lancet.* 1964;1(7341):1000-3.

[3] Eknoyan G. The wonderful apparatus of John Jacob Abel called the "artificial kidney". *Semin Dial.* 2009;22(3):287-96.

[4] Benedum J. [The early history of the artificial kidney]. *Anasthesiol Intensivmed Notfallmed Schmerzther.* 2003;38(11):681-8.

[5] Cameron JS. Practical haemodialysis began with cellophane and heparin: the crucial role of William Thalhimer (1884-1961). *Nephrol Dial Transplant*. 2000;15(7):1086-91.
[6] Kolff WJ. 50th anniversary ASAIO speech. *Asaio j*. 2004;50(6):xxii-xxiii.
[7] Epstein M. John P. Merrill: The Father of Nephrology as a Specialty. *Clin J Am Soc Nephrol*. 2009;4(1):2-8.
[8] Guild WR, Harrison JH, Merrill JP, Murray J. Successful homotransplantation of the kidney in an identical twin. *Trans Am Clin Climatol Assoc*. 1955;67:167-73.
[9] Murray JE, Tilney NL, Wilson RE. Renal transplantation: a twenty-five year experience. *Ann Surg*. 1976;184(5):565-73.
[10] Fadem L, Fadem SZ. Bakelite: A Revolutionary Early Plastic. *Deco Echoes*. 1996.
[11] Scribner BH. A Personalized History of Chronic Hemodialysis. *American Journal of Kidney Diseases*. 1990;16(6):511-9.
[12] Shaldon S. 40 Years of Dialysis. *Nephron Information Center*. 2001.
[13] Shaldon S, Silva H, Pomeroy J, Rae AI, Rosen SM. Percutaneous femoral venous catheterization and reusable dialysers in the treatment of acute renal failure. *Trans Am Soc Artif Intern Organs*. 1964;10:133-5.
[14] Cimino JE, Brescia MJ. Simple venipuncture for hemodialysis. *N Engl J Med*. 1962;267:608-9.
[15] Brescia MJ, Cimino JE, Appel K, Hurwich BJ. Chronic hemodialysis using venipuncture and a surgically created arteriovenous fistula. *N Engl J Med*. 1966;275(20):1089-92.
[16] Giacchino JL, Geis WP, Buckingham JM, Vertuno LL, Bansal VK. Vascular access: long-term results, new techniques. *Arch Surg*. 1979;114(4):403-9.
[17] Sutaria R, Gilbert JA. Single-centre experience of an early cannulation graft for haemodialysis access. *J Vasc Access*. 2020;21(6):883-91.
[18] Blagg CR. The first dialysis for chronic renal failure 50 years ago. Preface. *Hemodial Int*. 2010;14(1):1-2.
[19] Blagg CR. Belding Hibbard Scribner--better known as Scrib. *Clin J Am Soc Nephrol*. 2010;5(12):2146-9.
[20] Blagg CR. The early history of dialysis for chronic renal failure in the United States: a view from Seattle. *Am J Kidney Dis*. 2007;49(3):482-96.
[21] Rae AI, Rosen SM, Silva H, Pomeroy J, Bienenstock J, Shaldon S. Rehabilitation of terminal uraemic patients by periodic haemodialysis. *Proc R Soc Med*. 1963;56(8):760-1.
[22] Teschner M, Heidland A, Klassen A, Sebekova K, Bahner U. Georg Ganter--a pioneer of peritoneal dialysis and his tragic academic demise at the hand of the Nazi regime. *J Nephrol*. 2004;17(3):457-60.
[23] Odel HM, Ferris DO, Power MH. Peritoneal lavage as an effective means of extrarenal excretion; a clinical appraisal. *Am J Med*. 1950;9(1):63-77.
[24] Maxwell MH, Rockney RE, Kleeman CR, Twiss MR. Peritoneal dialysis. 1. Technique and applications. *JAMA*. 1959;170(8):917-24.
[25] Tenckhoff H, Schechter H. A bacteriologically safe peritoneal access device. *Trans Am Soc Artif Intern Organs*. 1968;14:181-7.
[26] Tenckhoff H, Shilipetar G, Van Paasschen WH, Swanson E. A home peritoneal dialysate delivery system. *Trans Am Soc Artif Intern Organs*. 1969;15:103-7.
[27] Tenckhoff H, Curtis FK. Experience with maintenance peritoneal dialysis in the home. *Trans Am Soc Artif Intern Organs*. 1970;16:90-5.

[28] Twardowski ZJ. History of peritoneal access development. *The International journal of artificial organs*. 2006;29(1):2-40.
[29] Twardowski ZJ. History of hemodialyzers' designs. *Hemodial Int*. 2008;12(2):173-210.
[30] Shaldon S. *40 Years of Dialysis*. Nephron Information Center; 2001.
[31] Peitzman SJ. The flame photometer as engine of nephrology: a biography. *Am J Kidney Dis*. 2010;56(2):379-86.
[32] Broers H. *Inventor of Life, The Story of W.J. Kolff, Father of Artificial Organs*: B & V Media Publishers, Montreal; 2007.
[33] Kiil F. Development of a parallel-flow artificial kidney in plastics. *Acta chirurgica Scandinavica Supplementum*. 1960;Suppl 253:142-50.
[34] Mclain EA, inventor; Dow Chemical Co, assignee. *Wound Hollow Fiber Permeability Apparatus and Process of Making the Same*. USPTO. 1969.
[35] Glater J. The early history of reverse osmosis membrane development. *Desalination*. 1998;117(1):297-309.
[36] Yang Z, Zhou Y, Feng Z, Rui X, Zhang T, Zhang Z. A Review on Reverse Osmosis and Nanofiltration Membranes for Water Purification. *Polymers (Basel)*. 2019;11(8).
[37] M'cFeeley T, L. The Price of Access. Nashua, New Jersey: MDL Press; 2001.
[38] Alexander S. They Decide Who Lives, Who Dies. *Life Magazine*. 1962 November 9, 1962:102-25.
[39] Satel S. *The God Committee*. American Enterprise Institute for Public Policy Research [Internet]. 2008 June 17, 2008. Available from: http://www.aei.org/article/28156.
[40] Rettig RA. Special Treatment , The Story of Medicare's ESRD Entitlement. *N Eng J Med*. 2011;364(7):596-8.
[41] Foley RN, Parfrey PS, Morgan J, Barre PE, Campbell P, Cartier P, et al. Effect of hemoglobin levels in hemodialysis patients with asymptomatic cardiomyopathy. *Kidney Int*. 2000;58(3):1325-35.
[42] Medicine Io. *Kidney Failure and the Federal Government*. Rettig RA, Levinsky NG, editors. Washington, DC: The National Academies Press; 1991. 440 p.
[43] K/DOQI clinical practice guidelines on hypertension and antihypertensive agents in chronic kidney disease. *Am J Kidney Dis*. 2004;43(5 Suppl 1):1-290.
[44] Eknoyan G, Levin NW. Impact of the new K/DOQI guidelines. *Blood Purif*. 2002;20(1):103-8.
[45] K/DOQI clinical practice guidelines for chronic kidney disease: evaluation, classification, and stratification. *Am J Kidney Dis*. 2002;39(2 Suppl 1):S1-266.
[46] Eknoyan G. Meeting the challenges of the new K/DOQI guidelines. *Am J Kidney Dis*. 2003;41(5 Suppl):3-10.
[47] *2009 PFS Final Rule with Comment Period* [19.90 MB] US Government Printing Office; 2009. Available from: http://edocket.access.gpo.gov/2008/pdf/E8-26213.pdf.
[48] Crowley ST, Meyer L. Sparking Innovation To Improve the Lives of People with Kidney Disease. *Clin J Am Soc Nephrol*. 2017;12(9):1548-50.
[49] Parsons FM, Hobson SM, Blagg CR, Mc CB. Optimum time for dialysis in acute reversible renal failure. Description and value of an improved dialyser with large surface area. *Lancet*. 1961;1(7169):129-34.
[50] Scribner BH, Cole JJ, Ahmad S, Blagg CR. Why thrice weekly dialysis? *Hemodial Int*. 2004;8(2):188-92.

[51] Gotch FA, Sargent JA. A mechanistic analysis of the National Cooperative Dialysis Study (NCDS). *Kidney Int*. 1985;28(3):526-34.

[52] Pflederer BR, Torrey C, Priester-Coary A, Lau AH, Daugirdas JT. Estimating equilibrated Kt/V from an intradialytic sample: effects of access and cardiopulmonary recirculations. *Kidney Int*. 1995;48(3):832-7.

[53] Daugirdas JT. Simplified equations for monitoring Kt/V, PCRn, eKt/V, and ePCRn. *Adv Ren Replace Ther*. 1995;2(4):295-304.

[54] Priester-Coary A, Daugirdas JT. A Recommended Technique for Obtaining the Post-Dialysis BUN. *Semin Dial*. 1997;10(1):23-5.

[55] Depner T, Daugirdas J, Greene T, Allon M, Beck G, Chumlea C, et al. Dialysis dose and the effect of gender and body size on outcome in the HEMO Study. *Kidney Int*. 2004;65(4):1386-94.

[56] Depner T, Beck G, Daugirdas J, Kusek J, Eknoyan G. Lessons from the Hemodialysis (HEMO) Study: an improved measure of the actual hemodialysis dose. *Am J Kidney Dis*. 1999;33(1):142-9.

[57] Lowrie EG, Laird NM, Parker TF, Sargent JA. Effect of the hemodialysis prescription of patient morbidity: report from the National Cooperative Dialysis Study. *N Engl J Med*. 1981;305(20):1176-81.

[58] The National Cooperative Dialysis Study. *Kidney Int Suppl*. 1983(13):S1-122.

[59] *Morbidity and mortality of dialysis*. NIH Consensus Statement Online 1993 1993. p. 1-33.

[60] Parker TF, 3rd, Husni L, Huang W, Lew N, Lowrie EG. Survival of hemodialysis patients in the United States is improved with a greater quantity of dialysis. *Am J Kidney Dis*. 1994;23(5):670-80.

[61] Eknoyan G, Beck GJ, Cheung AK, Daugirdas JT, Greene T, Kusek JW, et al. Effect of dialysis dose and membrane flux in maintenance hemodialysis. *N Engl J Med*. 2002;347(25):2010-9.

[62] Daugirdas JT, Greene T, Chertow GM, Depner TA. Can rescaling dose of dialysis to body surface area in the HEMO study explain the different responses to dose in women versus men? *Clin J Am Soc Nephrol*. 2010;5(9):1628-36.

[63] Daugirdas JT, Finn WF, Emmett M, Chertow GM. The phosphate binder equivalent dose. *Semin Dial*. 2011;24(1):41-9.

[64] Flythe JE, Curhan GC, Brunelli SM. Shorter length dialysis sessions are associated with increased mortality, independent of body weight. *Kidney Int*. 2012.

[65] Daugirdas JT, Greene T, Depner TA, Levin NW, Chertow GM. Modeled urea distribution volume and mortality in the HEMO Study. *Clin J Am Soc Nephrol*. 2011;6(5):1129-38.

[66] Flythe JE, Kimmel SE, Brunelli SM. Rapid fluid removal during dialysis is associated with cardiovascular morbidity and mortality. *Kidney Int*. 2011;79(2):250-7.

[67] Harnett JD, Foley RN, Kent GM, Barre PE, Murray D, Parfrey PS. Congestive heart failure in dialysis patients: prevalence, incidence, prognosis and risk factors. *Kidney Int*. 1995;47(3):884-90.

[68] Foley RN. The impact of anemia on cardiomyopathy, morbidity, and mortality in end-stage renal disease. *Am J Kidney Dis*. 1996;28:53-61.

[69] Adamson JW, Eschbach JW. Management of the anaemia of chronic renal failure with recombinant erythropoietin. *Q J Med*. 1989;73(272):1093-101.

[70] Besarab A, Bolton WK, Browne JK, Egrie JC, Nissenson AR, Okamoto DM, et al. The effects of normal as compared with low hematocrit values in patients with cardiac disease who are receiving hemodialysis and epoetin. *N Engl J Med.* 1998;339(9):584-90.

[71] Wish JB. Past, present, and future of chronic kidney disease anemia management in the United States. *Adv Chronic Kidney Dis.* 2009;16(2):101-8.

[72] Collins AJ. Influence of target hemoglobin in dialysis patients on morbidity and mortality. *Kidney Int Suppl.* 2002(80):44-8.

[73] Moe SM. Vitamin D, cardiovascular disease, and survival in dialysis patients. *J Bone Miner Res.* 2007;22 Suppl 2:V95-9.

[74] Fadem SZ, Moe SM. Management of chronic kidney disease mineral-bone disorder. *Adv Chronic Kidney Dis.* 2007;14(1):44-53.

[75] Fadem SZ, Moe SM. Management of chronic kidney disease-mineral bone disorder. *Adv Chronic Kidney Dis.* 2007;14(1):2.

In: Issues in Kidney Disease – Dialysis
Editors: Stephen Z. Fadem and José A. Moura-Neto
ISBN: 978-1-68507-000-7

Chapter 2

Transitional Care Units and Incident End-Stage Kidney Disease

Brendan Bowman**, MD
University of Virginia School of Medicine, Charlottesville, VA, USA

Abstract

Over 120,000 Americans initiate dialysis each year. The vast majority of these patients will receive either modest or no pre-dialysis care. Their transition from advanced Chronic Kidney Disease (CKD) to End-Stage Kidney Disease (ESKD) is often sudden and difficult to predict. The result is a majority of patients initiating dialysis with a high-risk central venous catheter and within an outpatient dialysis center or inpatient setting. Incident dialysis patients also suffer from high rates of anxiety, depression and poor health literacy. The cumulative effect of this situation is a particularly vulnerable subset of dialysis patients with markedly higher mortality and hospitalization rates in the first months of dialysis versus prevalent patients. Dialysis providers and professionals have responded to this scenario by providing dedicated transitional care programs to ease the first few weeks and months of ESKD. A Transitional Care Unit (TCU) provides multiple educational and clinical interventions delivered by a dedicated interdisciplinary team. The goal of a TCU is the medical stabilization of the patient in parallel with education and empowerment that allows patients to make truly informed decisions about weighty matters such as modalities, access, transplant, and conservative care options. Such interventions can significantly increase patient satisfaction and comfort with ESKD, while improving abysmal home therapy adoption rates.

Keywords: transitional care units, incident dialysis, end-stage kidney disease, home dialysis

* Corresponding Author's E-mail: btb5k@hscmail.mcc.virginia.edu.

Introduction and Background

The advent of widely available renal replacement therapy in the 1960s and 1970s brought life-saving treatment to thousands of patients previously beyond the reach of medical care. The technical components of dialysis from that period remain familiar to the modern practitioner; however, our current paradigm of care for new dialysis patients might seem foreign to yesteryear's professional. The historical goal of dialysis therapy was the gentle "rehabilitation" of the patient from a holistic perspective; essentially, a return to a near normal life including gainful employment. In fact, policies justifying government financing of dialysis treatment estimated 60% of patients would return to employment [1].

During the early days of dialysis therapy, large outpatient dialysis units, dominant in many countries today, were not the norm. A patient was treated in a hospital-based program and a transition to outpatient dialysis meant, effectively, home dialysis. The machine itself was complex and safety features left much to be desired. These facts necessitated extensive training to allow patients to competently manage an outpatient treatment. Dedicated renal nurses, technicians, and nephrologists provided individualized care and training to patients. A strong therapeutic bond was formed. Over time, this dynamic would necessarily change as provisioning dialysis at scale required consolidation of services around dedicated outpatient dialysis clinics. By the 1970s, outpatient in-center hemodialysis was the dominant modality in the United States [2]. Care then was still provided by a highly-skilled staff under the overall direction of a nephrologist. However, highly protocolized in-center care did not require the same degree of in-depth patient education. As such, the intensive patient training that characterized early dialysis programs of the 1960s faded. Patients were able to initiate rapid and effective dialysis therapy, but incident patients were subsumed into the general prevalent population with fairly homogenous educational offerings.

Recognizing that rates of home dialysis therapy adoption were dropping during the 1970s and 1980s, physicians and nurses at the Northwest Kidney Centers established a "Hemodialysis Orientation Unit" to promote home therapy through supportive education during the first several weeks of dialysis initiation. The program was characterized by strong nursing-led education by a small team, a multi-week duration and emphasis on home or in-center self-care. The unit was successful in placing the vast majority of patients into home therapy training and an early version of in-center self-care. Typical in-center outpatient dialysis was the exception, chosen by only 10 of 93 first year participants [3].

In the modern era, many of the same justifications support creation of dedicated ESKD transition programs. The most recent US data shows continuation of decades old patterns: few patients initiate dialysis on a home therapy, nearly a third of patients initiate without preceding nephrology care and those that do obtain pre-dialysis care often receive less than 12 months [4]. In addition, significant disparities persist between socioeconomic and ethnic groups with minorities significantly less likely to have had nephrology care in advance of dialysis initiation [5]. Long term pre-ESKD nephrology care is important as it is generally associated with superior clinical outcomes such as higher rates of dialysis initiation out of hospital with an arteriovenous fistula (optimal start) and improved first year mortality [6]. Even in a highly effective integrated care environment, patients in the first month of dialysis experience the highest cost, hospitalization and a mortality rate 2-3 times that of prevalent patients at initiation

[4]. This incredibly high-risk period argues strongly that incident dialysis patients are an even more vulnerable subset of the overall dialysis cohort and require specialized care.

Despite a growing number of patients receiving some degree of pre-dialysis care, most will not obtain an "optimal start," defined as initiating dialysis as an outpatient in a home dialysis program or an in-center program with an arteriovenous fistula (AVF) or graft (AVG) as the primary access. Much of this missed opportunity is driven by high initial central venous catheter (CVC) rate. Rates of CVCs in incident dialysis patients have remained, essentially, unchanged for over a decade at around 80% [4]. The reasons for this are complex, but one driving factor may be the difficulty in predicting the actual transition time to ESKD. Several studies have looked at pre-dialysis rates of estimated glomerular filtration rate (eGFR) loss and found that those with rapid/accelerated eGFR loss in the months prior to dialysis start are at an increased risk of catheter use and suffer higher rates of first-year hospitalization and mortality [7, 8]. This rapid decline in a previously stable patient is familiar to the nephrologist as acute kidney injury (AKI) on chronic kidney disease (CKD). Once in the dialysis program, the majority of patients will transition to an AVF or AVG within the first year [4]. However, if initiating dialysis with a CVC is a proxy for the value of pre-dialysis care, the health system has strides to make. The development of more accurate ESKD prediction equations such as the Kidney Failure Risk Equation is an exciting development, but the effect of incorporating such equations into pre-dialysis preparation remains under study [9, 10].

To address the complex needs of incident patients with varying levels of pre-dialysis care, Transitional Care Units (TCUs) have been established in various forms in the United States and Canada [11]. The overarching goal of a TCU program is support and education of the dialysis patient during the vulnerable first few weeks and months of therapy. The output of a TCU program should be a patient with a well-defined plan for renal replacement or supportive therapy based on a shared decision-making framework, a personalized access plan (if appropriate), and a basic understanding of how to care for oneself in the setting of ESKD. Figure 1 provides a conceptual example of a TCU program curriculum and output. A TCU program is not necessarily an intervention in and of itself, but rather a consolidation of multiple proven educational and support interventions. In this way – whether a "virtual TCU" or an actual physical location, the TCU provides a kind of organizing framework of interventions. While the tools of an incident dialysis education program may have evolved from the original "Hemodialysis Orientation Unit," there are similarities to the modern TCU: a dedicated team, high staff to patient ratio, and individualized care delivered in an empathetic and compassionate environment. The end result should be a patient empowered to make decisions on modality, access, transplant, and supportive care.

Elements of a Transitional Care Program

Patients: Inclusion and Exclusion Criteria

The most important component of any transitional dialysis program is the patient. Patients initiating dialysis suffer high rates of anxiety and depression while those with advanced CKD also suffer from low levels of health literacy [12, 13]. Given the vulnerable picture of the incident patient, broad inclusion criteria for a TCU seem appropriate; however, in order to target educational benefits while preserving clinical resources, it is important to develop general admission criteria. For example, an incident patient with severe cognitive deficits that precludes capacity for decision-making will derive little benefit from a TCU. On the opposite spectrum, a highly motivated patient with extensive pre-dialysis care in a supportive home therapy training program will also see little benefit from a TCU. Other relative contra-indications include: unstable living situation/transient status, mental health conditions severe enough to impair education, active substance abuse, inclusion in a hospice program, permanent residency in a skilled nursing facility or dialysis dependent acute kidney injury. Aside from the above scenarios, the vast majority of incident patients should be eligible for inclusion in a TCU. Essentially, all incident patients not already enrolled in a home therapy training program at dialysis start should be considered for the TCU.

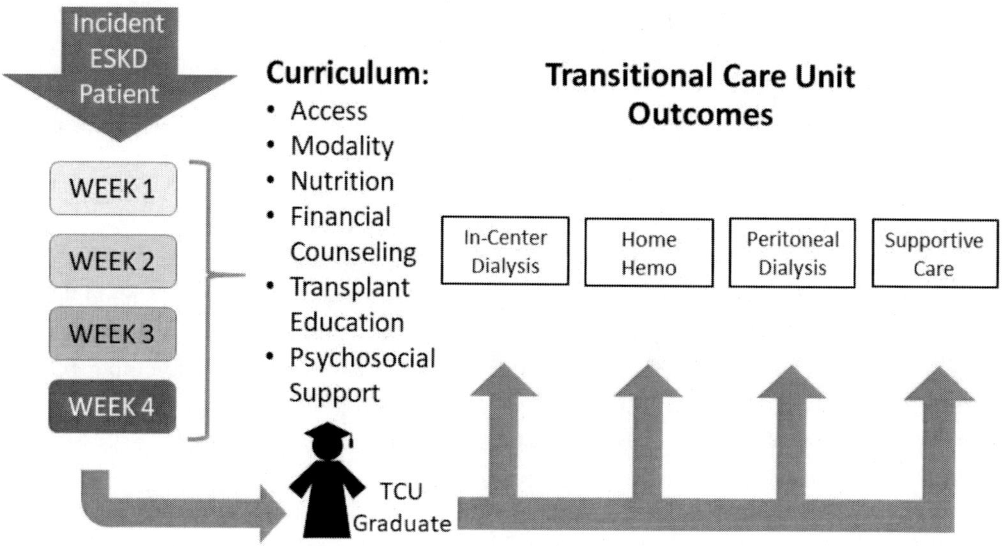

Figure 1. Conceptual Flow Diagram of for a Transitional Care Unit Participant.

Educational Curriculum

Dialysis clinics and nephrology professionals are required to provide education and counseling to new dialysis patients regarding kidney disease and associated topics. However, education efforts often become ineffectual when abridged in favor of direct clinical care. Simply providing access to education or handouts does not yield effective knowledge transfer, and so the manner in which education is delivered is as important as the content itself. Even among those that have received pre-dialysis education and counseling, survey data have shown high levels of dissatisfaction with earlier education when surveyed after their transition to ESKD [14]. This suggests a broad curriculum (an "educational reset") is best suited for a TCU. The efficacy of the delivered education intervention should be assessed via intermittent assessment tools – typically patient content quizzes combined with a review of TCU patient clinical outcomes.

Patient engagement assessments, both before and after the educational intervention, should be performed. Few tools to measure patient engagement have been validated specifically in ESKD, but there are many with extensive validation in other chronic disease states and good correlation with improved clinical outcomes. For example, the Patient Activation Measures (PAM) tool – a nine question instrument has been selected as the main patient engagement evaluation tool for CKD and ESKD in the Advancing American Kidney Health Initiative [15]. In general, the following minimum topics should be covered in a TCU program:

- Insurance and finances of ESKD
- Overview of dialysis therapies and side effects / complications
- Nutrition in ESKD
- Dialysis access options and care
- Modality options: pros and cons
- Conservative/supportive care
- Transplant

Optional topics may include: common medications used in dialysis, hands-on experience with peritoneal dialysis equipment and/or home hemodialysis machines and time with patient peer mentors.

Dialysis providers have already proven that dedicated incident ESKD educational interventions can yield improved home therapy uptake [16, 17]. Unfortunately, many educational curricula are often proprietary. Vetted and freely available resources are available from a number of reputable sources including the National Kidney Foundation and the Medical Education Institute [18, 19]. The latter has produced a series of recently updated educational modules with associated patient assessments. An educational curriculum that is available in multiple languages and in audio format for those with low literacy rates or visual impairment is ideal.

Staffing

Like many elements of the TCU, staffing may be quite variable depending on availability of personnel and the physical location where a TCU is housed. For example, a TCU that consists of 1-2 chairs in an existing dialysis center may draw from existing unit staff; whereas, a separate free-standing high volume TCU may have a dedicated staff. Regardless, it is crucial that staff members are provided adequate time for clinical support and educational tasks. A typical TCU includes:

- Social Worker
- Dialysis nurse/RN
- Dietician
- Nephrologist

Optional team members include:

- Dialysis technician
- Advance practice nurse / Physician's Assistant
- Dialysis peer mentor
- Palliative Care Professional
- Transplant educator
- Dialysis Pharmacist

While individuals with the knowledge base to teach in a TCU can be found within the pool of dialysis professionals listed above, it is also possible to provide adequate teaching with a limited pool of educators. For example, a Canadian program successfully drove increased adoption of home therapy by urgent start dialysis patients utilizing a nurse practitioner delivering all sessions [20]. In addition to knowledge base, it is important that consistent staff members are dedicated to the TCU. This allows for standardization of teaching, continuous improvement, and consistency. Ideally, staff members should also possess the emotional intelligence to assess the best time and methods to approach educating the individual patient on a session-by-session basis. The ability to build rapport and trust in the clinical task set carries over into a trusting educational/mentoring relationship.

Operational Aspects of a Transitional Care Program

Dialysis and Education Schedule

The main decisions regarding a TCU schedule include the number of days per week a patient will be in the educational program, as well as the overall length of the program. These decisions will be highly local and specific to the TCU sponsoring organization. Organizational factors that should be considered include: availability of staff, the type of dialysis machine used for treatment, and increase in costs if considering more than a typical thrice-weekly dialysis schedule. Clinical considerations include the acuity of patients transitioning into the TCU, anticipated degree of fluid overload and uremia on program entry, and potential risks of a long interdialytic break.

The simplest TCU schedule is a typical thrice-weekly dialysis plan where a dialysis chair or chairs is set aside for incident patients. In this model, there is usually no need to utilize home training staff, as the machine is a typical in-center dialysis machine. Weaknesses of this schedule include exposure of the patient to the long interdialytic break – a period of high risk for mortality and clinically significant arrhythmias [21]. Other programs have utilized a four or five day per week schedule [22]. The advantages of these programs include greater flexibility in educational delivery, ability for gentler more frequent ultrafiltration, flexibility to use home hemodialysis machines, and potential to eliminate the typical long break. Disadvantages include increased staffing needs, increased costs due to extra treatments, and inconvenience to the patient in the form of extra dialysis sessions. A typical first week schedule for a four day per week TCU is shown in Table 1.

Table 1. Sample first week schedule – four sessions/week TCU model

Session Number	Clinical Tasks	Assigned Team Member(s)	Educational Tasks	Assigned Team Member(s)
1	Medication Reconciliation	Dialysis RN / Dialysis Pharmacist	Pre-dialysis education Assessment	Dialysis RN
	Target Weight Assessment / Establishment	Dialysis RN / Nephrologist	Health Literacy Assessment	Social Worker
	Finalize Initial Prescription	Dialysis RN / Nephrologist	Basics of Dialysis Access Care	Dialysis RN / Access Specialist
2	Target Weight Assessment	Dialysis RN / Nephrologist	Finances / Insurance in Dialysis	Social Worker or Financial Counselor
	Develop Initial Anemia and Nutrition Plans	Dialysis RN / Nephrologist / Dietician		
3	Target Weight Assessment	Dialysis RN / Nephrologist	Treatment Expectations – Side Effects and Complications	Dialysis RN
	Access & Transplant Referral Status Assessment	Dialysis RN / Nephrologist		
4	Target Weight Assessment	Dialysis RN / Nephrologist	Additional Topic if patient wishes or catch up Day for Topics 1-3 if missed	Nephrologist / Access Specialist
	Expedite Access / Transplant referrals if necessary	Dialysis RN / Nephrologist		

RN – Registered Nurse;

Another key decision for planners is the duration of a TCU program. In many ways, this is driven by the number of topics necessary for patients to master prior to discharge from the TCU. The original Hemodialysis Orientation Unit covered not only basics of dialysis but blended with home hemodialysis training. This produced a prolonged training program lasting 2-4 months [3]. A more measured goal – determining the patient's favored modality while medically stabilizing the patient, may allow a shorter three to four week stay. Logistical factors such as the number of stations and staff available versus the anticipated annual number of incident patients eligible for the TCU should also play a part in determining the duration of the program.

Dialysis Machine Selection

TCU dialysis machine selection is dependent upon factors such as schedule, expertise of available staff, and an individual organization's available machines.

A TCU would ideally utilize a dialysis machine that seamlessly moves from inpatient/outpatient and in-home dialysis. As such, a machine is not available. Currently, providers choose between typical in-center machines or a home dialysis machine. A thrice-weekly schedule necessitates using an in-center approved machine as the need to maintain adequacy is paramount. For those providers that opt for a four-or-five treatment per week schedule, home dialysis machines can be used as an alternative. The benefits of using home dialysis machines are mostly theoretical. For example, by providing dialysis treatments on a home hemodialysis machine, it is possible patients will be less intimidated and more likely to opt for a home hemodialysis option. This could even reduce home hemodialysis training times after patients exit the TCU. These concepts have yet to be studied rigorously. However, a case series of a four-day per week TCU with a typical weekend long break suggests that this schedule significantly reduces interdialytic weight gain over the long break versus the same patients when crossed over to in-center hemodialysis [23].

Educational Delivery

Staff members working in a TCU are necessarily operating both in a clinical role and an educational role. The key educator is typically the dialysis RN, but many others will provide specialized knowledge throughout a patient's course. To avoid duplication of topics and effectively assign educators to topics, a simple checklist can suffice to keep staff members on task. By referencing a patient's checklist, an educator meeting the patient mid-course can quickly review which topics have been covered in prior sessions and stay on track. During the TCU intake procedure, the initial task is to assess the patient's interest and engagement with the program, determine his/her priorities, and assess general health literacy levels. As noted earlier, dialysis patients frequently possess low health literacy and simple screening tools with as few as one to two questions can discriminate between those at risk [24, 25]. Following the intake assessment, a tailored education program can be devised that meets the patient's priorities and learning style.

In order to avoid overwhelming already anxious patients, a goal of two to three topics per week in the TCU seems a realistic goal. Educational sessions can utilize multiple types of media for reference including texts, pamphlets, or web-based education provided on tablets. Ideally, education is active when the educator engages with the patient and uses validated techniques such as the "teach back" method. Formal teaching sessions should be relatively brief; i.e., thirty minutes as a reasonable guideline, to avoid exceeding the attention span of a potentially uremic adult learner. In addition to the patient, care partners such as family members should be invited to participate in chairside teaching sessions if infection control protocols allow. As patients progress through the curriculum, an assessment tool to ensure knowledge is acquired, such as simple topic quizzes or the like, may suffice to evaluate the efficacy of teaching. The overall proof of efficacy will be in hard clinical outcomes like home therapy adoption rates out of the TCU. In addition, a patient engagement assessment such as the PAM-9 survey may be useful before and after the TCU experience to assess improvements in patient comfort with self-care.

Clinical Tasks

The majority of incident patients begin dialysis on in-center hemodialysis [4]. While most dialysis centers provide protocols for new patients, a TCU can provide enhanced care navigation and expedited medical stabilization in place of standard unit startup protocols. The goals of the clinical care in a TCU are overall medical stabilization of the patient. These may include:

- Establishing target weight
- Medication reconciliation
- Reduction of blood pressure medications
- Expediting referrals for access and transplant if clinically appropriate
- Develop and implement anemia and nutritional care plans

Clinical care occurs in parallel and is complementary to educational tasks. For example, most patients will arrive with a central venous catheter (CVC) and require a permanent access plan after determining their modality of choice. Modality selection may follow quickly after that portion of the education curriculum is completed. The TCU staff then assists in expediting permanent access placement. In this setting, there is no need to provide handoff of care to a separate access coordinator as the educational staff and clinical team are one in the same. While these tasks are common to all new dialysis patients, the TCU educational program compresses the time frame in which these occur. By utilizing a small program-specific care team, standardization is achieved and best practices, such as continuation of diuretics and strict adherence to gentle ultrafiltration, can be ensured.

One area where TCU treatment plans may require modification is in the application of incremental dialysis for new starts. The incremental dialysis concept suggests a subset of patients maintain a significant degree of residual renal function and may safely dialyze with decreased frequency versus the typical thrice-weekly schedule. This type of dialysis initiation is suggested to provide advantage by reducing the decrement in quality of life and therapy associated side effects [26]. A TCU plan can incorporate this concept in a couple of ways. First, a patient may initiate a transitional program for a set number of weeks and then shift to a long-term incremental approach. The short duration of a TCU schedule (4-8 weeks) coupled with high diuretic utilization and gentle ultrafiltration may help prevent worrisome loss of residual renal function [27]. Another method involves the patient coming to the TCU for planned incremental sessions (typically twice weekly) but also attending for "education only" dates where the patient may engage with the designated educator for that day but does not receive dialysis therapy. In either scenario, it is important the TCU remains flexible to accommodate a variety of patient-centric dialysis initiation concepts.

Conclusion

Transitional Care Units are one aspect of a comprehensive ESKD transitions program. A TCU provides a soft landing approach to patients that have either ineffective or little pre-dialysis care. As unexpected conversions from normal renal function or CKD to ESKD will continue to occur, there will always be a need for such post-dialysis initiation programs. A TCU, however, should be part of a comprehensive transitions program. It is best paired with a dedicated high-risk CKD clinic and a supportive / palliative care program for those that opt out of dialysis therapy. In this scenario, educational materials and staff can be shared and result in improved economies of scale and smooth patient handoffs.

Providers considering establishing a transitional care unit should evaluate the limitations and costs of such programs carefully. While post-dialysis initiation education programs have clearly demonstrated improvements in home therapy uptake, data supporting fully integrated TCUs comes mostly from small retrospective case series. This is partially to due to the fact that these programs are typically initiated within a quality improvement framework where data is kept internal to organizations. However, limited data (mostly from abstracts) suggests TCU graduates may adopt home therapies at 30-50% [12, 13]. Costs are not insignificant and are best addressed in planning stages. It is important to consider the expected patient volume and allocate staff appropriately. Effective staff-to-patient/learner ratios are higher than in a usual in-center dialysis scenario. In addition, dedicating precious square footage of a dialysis center to a low volume TCU may not be an effective use of resources. However, on balance, the potential upsides of a TCU, are significant. Improved home dialysis uptake and educated, empowered patients capable of self-care are proximal outcomes. Longer-term improvements may be seen in the form of reduced hospitalizations and, hopefully, reduced mortality. As medicine moves towards outcomes-based payments, it is hoped that investment in a TCU program will be accounted for by cost savings in other areas. This remains to be evaluated as a high quality trial of the short and long term outcomes of the TCU concept is desperately needed.

In the future, the TCU may serve as a flexible "hub" for additional programs. For example, urgent start peritoneal dialysis can be integrated into a transitional care unit. A TCU may also serve as a soft landing for those with failing transplants or an opportunity for respite care when patients on home hemodialysis suffer caregiver fatigue or burnout. Patients with acute kidney injury have improved rates of renal recovery with dedicated protocols similar to TCU volume management concepts, and they may be able to share the infrastructure of a TCU [28].

References

[1] Institute of Medicine (US) Committee to Study Decision Making; Hanna KE, editor. Biomedical Politics. Washington (DC): National Academies Press (US); 1991. Origins of the Medicare Kidney Disease Entitlement: *The Social Security Amendments of 1972*. Available from: https://www.ncbi.nlm.nih.gov/books/NBK234191/.

[2] United States Renal Data System. 2010 USRDS *Annual Data Report: Atlas of chronic kidney disease and end-stage renal disease in the United States*. National Institutes of Health, National Institute of Diabetes and Digestive and Kidney Diseases, Bethesda, MD, 2010.

[3] Eschbach JW, Seymour M, Potts A, Clark M, Blagg CR. A hemodialysis orientation unit. *Nephron.* 1983;33(2):106-110. doi:10.1159/000182922.

[4] United States Renal Data System. *2019 USRDS Annual Data Report: Epidemiology of kidney disease in the United States.* National Institutes of Health, National Institute of Diabetes and Digestive and Kidney Diseases, Bethesda, MD, 2019.

[5] Purnell TS, Bae S, Luo X, et al. National Trends in the Association of Race and Ethnicity With Predialysis Nephrology Care in the United States From 2005 to 2015. *JAMA* Netw Open. 2020;3(8):e2015003.

[6] Gillespie BW, Morgenstern H, Hedgeman E, et al. Nephrology care prior to end-stage renal disease and outcomes among new ESRD patients in the USA. *Clin Kidney J.* 2015; 8(6): 772-780.

[7] Chin AI, Nguyen TA, Dinesh KP, Morfin JA. Late acceleration of glomerular filtration rate decline is a risk for hemodialysis catheter use in patients with established nephrology chronic kidney disease care. *Hemodial Int.* 2015;19(3):379-385. doi:10.1111/hdi.12253.

[8] Soohoo M, Streja E, Obi Y, et al. Predialysis Kidney Function and Its Rate of Decline Predict Mortality and Hospitalizations After Starting Dialysis. *Mayo Clin Proc.* 2018;93(8):1074-1085.

[9] Harasemiw O, Drummond N, Singer A, et al. Integrating Risk-Based Care for Patients With Chronic Kidney Disease in the Community: Study Protocol for a Cluster Randomized Trial. *Can J Kidney Health Dis.* 2019;6:2054358119841611.

[10] Green JA, Ephraim PL, Hill-Briggs FF, et al. Putting patients at the center of kidney care transitions: PREPARE NOW, a cluster randomized controlled trial. *Contemp Clin Trials.* 2018;73:98-110.

[11] Lockridge Jr R, et al. A Systematic Approach to Promoting Home Hemodialysis During End Stage Kidney Disease. *Kidney* 360. 2020; 1(9):993-1001 10.34067/KID. 0003132020.

[12] Ng HJ, Tan WJ, Mooppil N, Newman S, Griva K. Prevalence and patterns of depression and anxiety in hemodialysis patients: a 12-month prospective study on incident and prevalent populations. *Br J Health Psychol.* 2015; 20 (2): 374-395.

[13] Taylor DM, Fraser SDS, Bradley JA, et al. A Systematic Review of the Prevalence and Associations of Limited Health Literacy in CKD. *Clin J Am Soc Nephrol.* 2017;12(7):1070-1084. doi:10.2215/CJN.12921216.

[14] Fadem S Z. Satisfaction with renal replacement therapy and education: the American Association of Kidney Patients survey. *Clin. J. Am. Soc. Nephrol.* 2011; 6(3):605-612.

[15] *Centers for Medicare & Medicaid Services (CMS)* Center for Medicare and Medicaid Innovation (CMMI) Kidney Care Choices (KCC) *Model Request for Applications.* Accessed at: https://innovation.cms.gov/files/x/kcc-rfa.pdf.

[16] Wingard RL, Chan KE, Lazarus JM, Hakim RM. The "right" of passage: surviving the first year of dialysis. *Clin J Am Soc Nephrol.* 2009; 4(1): S114-S120.

[17] Wilson SM, Robertson JA, Chen G, Goel P, Benner DA, Krishnan M, Mayne TJ, Nissenson AR. The IMPACT (Incident Management of Patients, Actions Centered on Treatment) program: a quality improvement approach for caring for patients initiating long-term hemodialysis. *Am J Kidney Dis.* 2012; 60 (3): 435-443.

[18] *National Kidney Foundation Treatment and Support.* Accessed at: https://www.kidney.org/treatment-support.

[19] Kidney School Learning Modules. Accessed at: https://kidneyschool.org/mods/.

[20] Rioux JP, Cheema H, Bargman JM, Watson D, Chan CT. Effect of an in-hospital chronic kidney disease education program among patients with unplanned urgent-start dialysis. *Clin J Am Soc Nephrol.* 2011; 6(4):799-804.

[21] Wong MC, Kalman JM, Pedagogos E, Toussaint N, Vohra JK, Sparks PB, Sanders P, Kistler PM, Halloran K, Lee G, Joseph SA, Morton JB. Temporal distribution of

arrhythmic events in chronic kidney disease: highest incidence in the long interdialytic period. *Heart Rhythm.* 2015; 12: 2047-2055.

[22] Morfín JA, Yang A, Wang E, Schiller B. Transitional dialysis care units: A new approach to increase home dialysis modality uptake and patient outcomes. *Semin Dial.* 2018;31(1):82-87. doi:10.1111/sdi.12651.

[23] Bose S, Bowman BT, McPhatter L, Wentworth D, Daniel CL, Abdel-Rahman EM. A Transitional Start Unit (TSU) Improves Home Dialysis Adoption by Incident ESKD Patients. *American Society of Nephrology Kidney Week.* Washington, DC, 2019.

[24] Brice JH, Foster MB, Principe S, et al. Single-item or two-item literacy screener to predict the S-TOFHLA among adult hemodialysis patients. *Patient Educ Couns.* 2014;94(1):71-75. doi:10.1016/j.pec.2013.09.020.

[25] Taylor DM, Bradley JA, Bradley C, et al. Limited health literacy in advanced kidney disease. *Kidney Int.* 2016;90(3):685-695. doi:10.1016/j.kint.2016.05.033.

[26] Kalantar-Zadeh K, Crowley ST, Beddhu S, et al. Renal Replacement Therapy and Incremental Hemodialysis for Veterans with Advanced Chronic Kidney Disease. *Semin Dial.* 2017;30(3):251-261. doi:10.1111/sdi.12601.

[27] Li T, Wilcox CS, Lipkowitz MS, Gordon-Cappitelli J, Dragoi S. Rationale and Strategies for Preserving Residual Kidney Function in Dialysis Patients. *Am J Nephrol.* 2019;50(6):411-421. doi:10.1159/000503805.

[28] Gautam SC, Brooks CH, Balogun RA, Xin W, Ma JZ, Abdel-Rahman EM. Predictors and Outcomes of Post-Hospitalization Dialysis Dependent Acute Kidney Injury. *Nephron.* 2015;131(3):185-190. doi:10.1159/000441607.

In: Issues in Kidney Disease – Dialysis
Editors: Stephen Z. Fadem and José A. Moura-Neto ISBN: 978-1-68507-000-7

Chapter 3

ANEMIA MANAGEMENT IN DIALYSIS PATIENTS

Ana Flávia Moura[1], MD, Joan A. Oliveira Moitinho[2], MD and José H. R. Suassuna[2,*], MD, PhD

[1]Department of Internal Medicine, Bahiana School of Medicine and Public Heath, Salvador, Bahia, Brazil

[2]Department of Nephrology, Rio de Janeiro State University, UERJ, Rio de Janeiro, Brazil

ABSTRACT

Anemia is one of the cardinal manifestations of chronic kidney disease. It has a high incidence in dialysis patients and is associated with significant morbidity. The pathophysiology of the anemia of kidney disease is complex as it involves several mechanisms, erythropoietin deficiency being the main one. For patients with chronic kidney disease, recombinant human erythropoietin therapy and IV iron supplementation brought about a striking improvement in their quality of life and a significant reduction in blood transfusion needs. Nevertheless, current strategies for anemia management are not exempt from side effects. Hyporesponsiveness to erythropoietin therapy and the eventual need for blood transfusions are still part of the routine of dialysis patients. Several studies sought to define the optimal target of hemoglobin, pursuing the balance between optimal oxygen carriage capacity and the risks of side effects by overtreatment. Research aimed at the development of drugs that not only stimulate erythropoietin production but also interfere with iron metabolism has renewed the prospects of more effective approaches to control the anemia of chronic kidney disease.

Keywords: anemia, iron, erythropoiesis-stimulating agents, chronic kidney disease, dialysis

* Corresponding Author's E-mail: suassuna@mac.com.

INTRODUCTION

Richard Bright is usually credited for describing the anemia of chronic kidney disease, although he just remarked on the fading of healthy skin color of his patients [1]. The seminal clinical and laboratory description of anemia of kidney disease was by Dr. Robert Christison, of Edinburgh, in 1839 [2]. Anemia is one of the cardinal manifestations of chronic kidney disease (CKD), being associated with increased mortality, hospitalization, heart failure, and reduced quality of life [3-5]. It affects roughly 75% of patients in stage 5, and up to 90% of those on dialysis [6].

The pathogenesis of anemia in CKD is largely multifactorial (Table 1) [2, 7], although the predominant causes are reduced renal erythropoietin production and impairment in the absorption and utilization of iron [7, 8]. The hormone hepcidin also plays a key role in the pathogenesis of CKD. It is produced in the liver and mainly eliminated by the kidney. Hepcidin production increases with inflammation, in patients with CKD, and after iron loading, such as following IV iron therapy [9, 10]. At high levels, hepcidin decreases the availability of iron by binding to the iron export channel ferroportin and inducing its endocytosis and subsequent proteolysis. Since ferroportin is the sole conduit for the transfer of iron from cells to the plasma, iron becomes trapped into stores of enterocytes (decreasing intestinal iron absorption), of macrophages (compromising iron recycling from senescent red blood cells), and of hepatocytes (preventing the release of iron stores) [10]. Other factors, such as malnutrition, uremic toxicity, and the shortened half-life of erythrocytes are also operative [3, 11, 12].

Table 1. Main causes of anemia in CKD patients

Erythropoietin deficiency
Iron deficiency
Bleeding
Vitamin B12/folate deficiency
Hemoglobinopathies
Hypothyroidism
Hyperparathyroidism
Underdialysis
Infection or inflammation
Malignancy
Malnutrition
Bone marrow disorders
Hemolysis
ACEi/ARB
Poor adherence to therapy

ACEi: angiotensin-converting enzyme inhibitor; ARB: angiotensin-receptor blocker.

Until the 1990s, treatment of CKD-associated anemia was based on iron replacement supplemented with androgen therapy, with most patients needing blood transfusions [6]. The availability of recombinant human erythropoietin (rHuEPO) forever changed the management of anemia in CKD [13, 14]. The regular administration of erythropoiesis-stimulating agents (ESAs) increases hemoglobin (Hb) levels, reduces transfusion requirements, and improves quality of life [15].

Over the past decade, several studies attempted to define the optimal hemoglobin target levels in patients with CKD; pursuing the balance between optimal oxygen carriage capacity and the risks of side effects by overtreatment [16-18]. In 2017, 65% of patients on hemodialysis and 56% of those on peritoneal dialysis (PD) had hemoglobin levels within stipulated targets [19].

In spite of undeniable progress, anemia management in CKD is still a challenge [20]. There is hope in new approaches in the clinical pipeline. Drugs that explore the regulatory interplay between iron metabolism and hypoxia-inducible factor (HIF) stabilizers, also known as HIF-prolyl hydroxylase inhibitors (PHIs), are emerging as a new therapy option for the treatment of anemia associated with CKD [21-23].

Diagnosis and Evaluation of Anemia

Anemia is defined by hemoglobin (Hb) concentration levels below 13 g/dL for adult males and postmenopausal women, and under 12 g/dL for premenopausal women [24]. Anemia in CKD is generally normochromic, normocytic and hypoproliferative [3]. Iron deficiency is common and may occur in over 50% of the patients on dialysis [25].

Anemia should be evaluated independently of CKD stage, so as to identify potential reversible processes that might be causing or contributing to its generation. The initial assessment includes: complete blood and reticulocyte count, serum ferritin, transferrin saturation (TSAT), serum vitamin B12, and folate levels (25). A more comprehensive workup may occasionally be needed, including serum albumin and aluminum levels, thyroid and parathyroid assessment, hemolysis assays, and occasionally bone marrow biopsy, particularly in patients with a poor response to ESAs [11, 25].

Treatment of Anemia with Iron Agents

As with any disease condition, the first step in the treatment of anemia is to try and determine its etiology. In patients with kidney failure, iron deficiency should always be investigated before treatment is started, as it is a very common cause of hyporesponsiveness to ESAs.

Besides the impairment of iron absorption due to hepcidin production mediated by chronic inflammation, several other factors may contribute to iron depletion in patients with kidney failure: blood sampling for frequent laboratory testing, gastrointestinal bleeding, medication interference with iron absorption (*e.g.,* gastric acid inhibitors and phosphate binders), bleeding associated with surgical and catheter implantation procedures, and blood loss in the dialysis circuit [26-28].

Iron replacement is widely used in the treatment of anemia in patients with ESKD, being considered an essential adjuvant to ESAs therapy [29]. Studies have consistently demonstrated the superiority of the hemoglobin response with intravenous (IV) iron in comparison with oral replacement, especially in patients on hemodialysis [30]. In addition, IV iron therapy allows a reduction in the dose and frequency of use of ESAs, with an attendant favorable impact in the cost of treatment [31].

In addition to serum hemoglobin levels, iron replacement decisions rely on two parameters: TSAT and serum ferritin [25]. Guidelines agree on the cut-off for initiation of therapy, but the recommended limit for withholding therapy is quite varied, especially in regard to the level of ferritin.

The Kidney Disease Improving Global Outcomes (KDIGO) guidelines suggest the same conditions for starting iron supplementation in patients on peritoneal dialysis or hemodialysis, whether or not using ESAs: TSAT ≤ 30% and ferritin ≤ 500ng/mL [25]. Once iron replacement has started, TSAT and ferritin should be evaluated at least every 3 months to determine dose adjustments or interruption of replacement. In cases of initiation of use or adjustment of the dose of an ESA, a new evaluation of ferritin and TSAT is recommended after 30 days. Also, according to the guidelines, hemoglobin should be measured monthly in all patients undergoing dialysis, and iron supplementation should be withheld in patients with TSAT > 30% and ferritin > 500ng/mL [25].

The 2013 position paper from the European Renal Best Practice group recommended that patients on hemodialysis, and not on ESAs, should receive iron supplementation if TSAT ≤ 25% and ferritin ≤ 300ng/mL. For patients on peritoneal dialysis (PD), and not on ESAs, iron could be administered orally for 1 to 3 months, but converted to IV therapy, in case of poor response [32]. For those already on ESAs, IV iron supplementation was recommended for patients with TSAT < 30% and ferritin <300ng/mL, but could be maintained at higher levels of ferritin, on an individual assessment basis [32]. Iron replacement was to be withheld at TSAT > 30% and ferritin levels > 500ng/mL [32].

Additionally, in 2013, the Kidney Disease Outcomes Quality Initiative (KDOQI) review of the KDIGO recommendations agreed with the KDIGO proposed cut-off for initiation of IV iron supplementation (TSAT ≤ 30% and ferritin ≤ 500ng/mL, on either HD or PD). The upper limit for IV iron discontinuation was not clearly defined, as there was insufficient evidence to establish a ferritin cut-off rule for IV iron discontinuation. Their recommendation was to maintain IV iron supplementation whenever TSAT ≤ 30%, even when ferritin levels were already above 500ng/mL [33].

In 2015, the updated guidelines from the National Institute for Health and Care Excellence (NICE) for the management of anemia in patients with CKD, stated that IV iron should be initiated in patients with TSAT < 20% and ferritin < 100ng/mL. In hemodialysis patients, markers of iron status were to be measured every 1 to 3 months. For PD patients, this assessment could be made on a quarterly basis [34]. The suggestion was that IV iron should be discontinued whenever ferritin > 800ng/mL. The need for IV iron is questionable whenever serum ferritin levels become greater than 500ng/mL [34].

Iron can be potentially toxic when in its free form. Aggressive intravenous iron administration strategies have largely been associated with higher odds of mortality and with infection-related morbidity and mortality [35]. For this reason, it is important to avoid excessive supplementation that may cause tissue accumulation of iron. Most guidelines recommend stopping IV iron administration at ferritin levels between 500ng/mL to 1200ng/mL [35]. It is considered prudent to withhold IV iron therapy whenever ferritin levels rise above 800ng/mL.

Iron Agents

The main agents available for IV iron supplementation are depicted on Table 2.

Iron sucrose has a low rate of adverse reactions and does not require a testing dose. It can be administered undiluted as an IV bolus at an infusion rate of 1mL/min or diluted in saline. In this case, it is recommended to dilute the vial in 100mL saline with an infusion time of 15 minutes [36].

Table 2. Intravenous Iron

	Trade Name	Formulation	Maximum dosage	Minimal administration time
Iron Sucrose	Venofer, Sucrofer, Hemacit, Noripurum, Ferropurum	20mg/mL in 2.5mL or 5mL ampoules	200mg	10-30min
Iron Dextran	Cosmofer	50mg/mL in 2mL, 5mL or 10mL ampoules	20mg/Kg	4-6h
Sodium Ferric Gluconate	Ferrlecit	12.5mg/mL in 5mL ampoule	125mg	10-60min
Ferric Pyrophosphate	Triferic	5,44mg/mL in 5mL or 50mL ampoules	110mcg/L	For the duration of HD procedure
Ferric Carboxymaltose	Ferinject or Injectafer	50mg/mL in 2mL, 10mL or 20mL ampoules	1000mg (up to 200mg if CKD-HD patient)	15min
Ferumoxytol	Feraheme	30mg/mL in 17mL ampoule	10mg	15min

HD: hemodialysis; CKD: chronic kidney disease.

Adapted from "Roger SD. Practical considerations for iron therapy in the management of anemia in patients with chronic kidney disease. *Clin Kidney J.* 2017(1): i9-i15."

Iron dextran is less frequently used due to a higher risk of severe hypersensitivity reactions. For this reason, it needs a testing dose of 25mg, infused over 5 minutes. The patient must remain under observation for 60 minutes, the first 15 minutes post-infusion being the most critical period. It can be administered diluted in 500 to 1000mL saline or undiluted, with the maximum infusion rate of 50mg/min [37].

Sodium ferric gluconate is less associated with adverse reactions than the previously mentioned agents, requiring no testing dose. Its infusion should not exceed 1mL/min. If opted for non-dilution, up to 125mg can be administered during 10 minutes [38].

Even lesser used than the above stated, ferric pyrophosphate has aroused interest in dialysis patients due to its ability to reduce serum phosphorus. Another advantage is that it can be added to the dialysate, in addition to having a low rate of adverse reactions [39, 40]. The recommended dosage is 5mL ampoule of ferric pyrophosphate solution to each 2.5 gallons of bicarbonate concentrate. It should be administered during each dialysis procedure for as long as patients are receiving maintenance hemodialysis therapy. Hemodialysis solutions should be used within 24 hours of the preparation of the bicarbonate concentrate mixture [39].

Ferric Carboximaltose is a ferric hydroxide core stabilized by a carboxymaltose. A test dose is not required because of its low risk of hypersensitivity reactions. A single high dose of ferric carboxymaltose can be infused in a short time frame [41].

Sucroferric oxyhydroxide (SOH), an iron-based phosphate binder whose use has been expanded since 2014, has been recently approved by the U.S. Federal Drug Administration (FDA) for the treatment of patients on hemodialysis. Some studies point to a favorable effect on ferritin and transferrin saturation levels following SOH administration [42, 43]. However, the follow-up period was short. A recent long-term study failed to show significant differences in hemoglobin, ferritin and transferrin saturation levels in comparison with other phosphate binders [44]. It is unclear whether long-term administration of SOH may cause iron overload.

Complications and Long-Term Safety of IV Iron

The risks associated with long-term use of IV iron still need to be investigated further. The PIVOTAL (Proactive IV iron therapy in hemodialysis patients) trial was set up to evaluate the safety of high doses of IV iron. It was a large multicenter RCT that enrolled 2141 patients. PIVOTAL compared a high-dose regimen (iron proactively administered at a dose of 400mg monthly up to a TSAT of 40% or a serum ferritin of 700ng/mL) with a low-dose supplementation schedule (routine iron replacement from 0 to 400 mg monthly with a TSAT target of 20% and a serum ferritin of 200ng/mL). After 5 years of follow-up (2013-2018), there was a significantly lower incidence of major adverse cardiovascular events (MACE) in the proactive regimen group. Importantly, the incidence of infections was similar in the two groups [45].

Findings of the PIVOTAL trial contrast with several other studies in which a minor increase or a lack of association between cardiovascular risk and a proactive regimen was shown (46-50). It is worth mentioning that none of these studies have reported MACE as a clinical end point. Furthermore, the possible association between high-dose IV iron and a higher incidence of infections was often reported [46, 50, 51]. Other complications associated with IV iron supplementation include: acute hypersensitivity reactions, iron overload, exacerbation of chronic inflammatory states and worsening established infection.

Acute hypersensitivity reactions associated with iron infusions are rare but can be life-threatening. Although its mechanisms are not entirely known, it is believed that iron may activate the complement system through the alternative route, in a process that may be triggered by genetic predisposition or by other non-specific factors [52, 53]. All iron agents in current use are associated with hypersensitivity reactions, the occurrence of which are generally unpredictable. For this reason, IV iron should be administered slowly, respecting the recommended infusion rate for each agent [53].

The prescription of IV iron should always be individualized, with the aim of providing the lowest dose to provide adequate stores to maintain erythropoiesis while preventing oversaturation that may potentiate inflammation and lead to organ toxicity [54-56].

Several studies suggest withholding IV iron supplementation in case of bacterial infections. This is because most human pathogens use iron as a substrate for their growth. Thus, the increased availability of serum iron may cause an exacerbation of the infectious episode and may impair the response to treatment [25, 51, 57, 58].

Personalizing the recommendations of the guidelines is essential for the success of the proposed therapy. The choice of IV iron replacement and the prescribed dose depends on the evaluation of the set of comorbidities and risks presented by each patient and of the type of renal replacement therapy.

Role of ESAs in Anemia in ESKD Patients

ESAs are key elements in the treatment of anemia in ESKD patients. Since their 1989 approval by the FDA, these agents have completely changed the care of dialysis patients, improving their quality of life and preventing the need for regular blood transfusions [59]. However, the hemoglobin target levels for starting and stopping ESAs have evolved over the years [60-63].

Target Hemoglobin Levels

Before the availability of rHuEPO, the treatment of anemia in dialysis patients relied on androgen therapy and blood transfusions, usually indicated when the hematocrit fell below 30% [64]. The 1989 phase III trial that evaluated the effect of rHuEPO on CKD-associated anemia, was the harbinger of a new era when it recorded a striking drop in blood transfusion requirements, from 0.52 units per patient per month to less than 0.03 units after just 2 months of ESA therapy [65].

In its original approval the FDA recommended a target hematocrit between 30 to 33%, with the advice to withhold treatment whenever it surpassed 36% [66]. Over the years, the ideal hematocrit/hemoglobin target for patients on hemodialysis has been a matter of debate, addressed by several studies and guidelines [60-63]. Arguments in favor of higher targets close to those of the general population included an improvement in the quality of life, better exercise tolerance, increased survival, reduced progression of CKD, and regression of left ventricular hypertrophy [60, 62, 67-72]. There were, however, concerns with the potential risks brought about by higher hemoglobin levels and increased blood viscosity, including the risk of thrombotic cardiac and cerebral events, and reduced solutes clearance [73, 74].

The Normal Hematocrit Study (NHS) was key to the establishment of current hemoglobin target levels in hemodialysis patients. Dialysis-dependent patients with congestive heart failure or ischemic heart disease were allocated to either a high or a low hemoglobin target level (14.0 vs. 10.0 g/dL). The trial was held before completion due to a higher rate of adverse events in the high hemoglobin group, including vascular access thrombosis, acute myocardial infarction, and cardiovascular death [8].

After NHS, cardiac disease became an exclusion criterion in studies evaluating events associated with higher hemoglobin targets. Nevertheless, several other clinical trials and meta-analyses have confirmed the higher odds for overall mortality and thrombotic events in hemodialysis patients treated to reach normal hemoglobin levels, as well as the lack of significant quality of life benefits [16, 18, 73, 75, 76]. On the basis of these findings and with only small variations in their exact values, the main guidelines revised their targets, with the advice to keep hemoglobin levels above 9.0 g/dL, with a target range between 10 and 12 g/dL [25, 32-34]. The guidelines were also unanimous in cautioning about the increased risk of thrombotic events when Hb is maintained above 12 g/dL.

ESAs Therapy Recommendations

The decision of whether or not to initiate ESA therapy should be based on individual patient assessment. Risks associated with ESAs, such as worsening hypertension, hyperviscosity-associated thrombotic events, and the potential for tumor progression must be considered in light of its known benefits on blood transfusion requirements, quality of life, and anemia-related myocardial ischemia [59, 68-70, 73, 74-78].

All current guidelines recommend that alternative causes for anemia should be ruled out before initiating ESAs (Table 1). For instance, in CKD patients with anemia and iron deficiency, ESAs should not be initiated without the provision of adequate iron substrate. Serum hemoglobin levels should be monitored monthly in order to achieve the minimum ESA dose to reach the target hemoglobin and to prevent overshooting.

After individual assessment of risks and benefits, the KDIGO guidelines advise starting ESAs for patients with a hemoglobin < 10.0 g/dL, without allowing levels to fall below 9.0 g/dL. Conversely, continuation of ESA therapy in patients with hemoglobin greater than 11.5g /L is not considered appropriate, being strongly discouraged in patients with hemoglobin > 13.0 g/dL. The target maintenance range is 10.0-11.5 g/dL, with dose adjustment according to the response to treatment [25, 66].

The KDOQI group and the FDA diverge minimally from KDIGO. There is agreement in the threshold for the initiation of therapy (Hb < 10.0 g/dL). However, on the basis of the NHS study, the KDOQI group and the FDA recommend a lower maintenance target hemoglobin, in the range between 10.0 and 11.0 g/dL [8].

Both the European Renal Best Practice and the NICE initiatives consider the same parameters for initiation of ESAs therapy: hemoglobin < 10.0 g/dL, provided that the risks and benefits are properly assessed. However, target hemoglobin has a slightly higher tolerance, ranging between 10.0 to 12.0 g/dL. As with the other guidelines, the use of ESAs in patients with hemoglobin greater than 13.0 g/dL is not endorsed [32, 34].

Hyporesponsiveness and failure of ESAs therapy

Even with the provision of ESAs, there are patients with a low response or even failure to achieve the recommended targets. Some may need very high doses of ESAs or even require blood transfusions. The definition of hyporesponsiveness to ESAs varies between the guidelines. According to KDIGO, hyporesponsiveness to ESAs is diagnosed when there is a lack of response after one month of treatment with an optimized dose [25]. The KDOQI guidance recommends waiting at least two months before labeling the patient as hyporesponsive [33].

The diagnosis of hyporesponsiveness to ESAs therapy should always be preceded by a thorough investigation for alternative causes of the anemia. These render the diagnosis of ESAs resistance temporary, requiring a reassessment after the associated comorbidity has been addressed. Table 1 presents a summary of alternative diagnoses associated with an unsatisfactory response to ESAs therapy.

Both in cases of primary as well as in acquired hyporesponsiveness (need for two subsequent 50% escalations of the dose of an ESA after a period of previous Hb stability), it is not advisable to further increase the dose of ESAs beyond twice the usual dose (25). Higher doses are costly, have no associated advantages, and may increase the risks associated with ESA therapy [25].

RED BLOOD CELL TRANSFUSIONS

Red blood cell transfusion (RBC) is associated with potential adverse effects and is preferably avoided in patients with ESKD [25]. RBC transfusion has the risk of viral infections, as well as of bacterial or parasite contamination [79, 80]. It is also associated with a variety of reactions that include febrile non-hemolytic transfusion reactions, transfusion-related acute lung injury (TRALI), transfusion-associated circulatory overload (TACO), acute hemolytic transfusion reactions, delayed hemolytic transfusion reactions (DHTR), and anaphylactic transfusion reactions [80-85]. In patients with ESKD, special attention should be paid to additional adverse effects such as iron overload, hyperkalemia, and alloimmunization [79, 80].

Although the availability of ESAs has drastically reduced the need for repeated RBC transfusion in patients with ESKD, transfusions were not entirely eliminated [80]. During 2016 in the United States of America, at least 16.6% of patients on hemodialysis and 15.1% of patients on peritoneal dialysis received at least one RBC transfusion, for a variety of indications [19]. RBC transfusions are still required in particular clinical situations such as acute severe hemorrhage and unstable coronary artery disease, when preoperative hemoglobin correction is urgently needed, and when ESA therapy is not effective (hemoglobinopathies, bone marrow failure, rHuEPO resistance, etc.). In this latter circumstance, the recommendation is to adhere to a restrictive transfusion strategy that targets symptomatic patients, instead of an arbitrary hemoglobin threshold [25, 32, 86].

Alloimmunization against red blood cells and/or HLA antigens is a major concern in ESKD patients. Alloantibodies to RBC may make it difficult to find compatible, antigen-negative RBC units, particularly if multiple alloantibodies are present, and may also increase the risk of DHTR [80].

In candidates for kidney transplantation, transfusions increase the risk of sensitization to HLA antigens, leading to increased transplantation waiting time and reduced graft survival [79]. Commonly used strategies such as leukoreduction of RBC transfusions do not seem to protect potential kidney transplant candidates against allosensitization [82]. Whenever possible, RBC transfusions are better avoided in patients eligible for kidney transplantation.

NOVEL THERAPIES

Hypoxia-Inducible Factor Prolyl Hydroxylase Inhibitors

Hypoxia-inducible factor prolyl hydroxylase inhibitors (HIF-PHIs), also known as hypoxia-inducible factor stabilizers (HIF stabilizers), are promising drugs for the treatment of CKD-related anemia. Drug candidates for this new class include roxadustat, molidustat, daprodustat and vadadustat [23, 87-90]. HIF-PHIs act by mimicking the cellular response to reduced oxygen levels, with attendant increase in HIF activity, which in turn activates endogenous EPO production and, ultimately, stimulates erythropoiesis [87, 91]. In addition, levels of hepcidin are indirectly decreased [92, 93], which results in increased absorption of intestinal iron and release of iron from macrophages and hepatocytes. This results in increased transferrin levels and better supply of iron to the bone marrow [87, 88].

Several phase II placebo-controlled or rHuEPO comparative studies have shown that HIF-PHIs are effective in maintaining adequate levels of hemoglobin and decreased levels of hepcidin [21, 87, 90, 94-96]. Phase III trials in hemodialysis patients have also shown that these drugs were not inferior when compared to epoetin alfa and darbopoetin [97, 98]. In a study in PD patients, roxadustat was effective in maintaining hemoglobin levels within the stipulated range, with a favorable safety profile [99]. These agents may also eliminate the risk of developing cross-reactive antibodies against EPO [100].

HIF-PHIs are oral agents, with lower production costs, used with once-daily or thrice-weekly dosing schedules, and with a likely positive impact in treatment adherence [100]. They stimulate the intermittent production of erythropoietin close to the physiological level and, therefore, have the potential to avert adverse side-effects observed with higher doses of ESAs [87, 91, 98, 101]. In addition, increased iron availability may decrease or eliminate the need for IV iron replacement and its associated side effects [87]. Daprodustat and roxadustat also significantly reduce low-density lipoprotein cholesterol levels [102, 103].

Potential adverse effects of HIF-PHIs include: pulmonary artery pressure increase, vascular calcification, tumor progression, higher risk of thrombosis, and hyperkalaemia [104, 105].

Activin Receptor Ligand Traps

Activins are dimers of β-type chains that belong to the transforming growth factor beta (TGF-β) superfamily [106]. Sotatercept and luspatercept are recombinant human fusion proteins containing the extracellular domain of the human activin receptor IIA. They are able to bind and inhibit activin and other members of the TGF-β superfamily that are also involved in erythropoiesis [107, 108]. The mechanism of action that underlies an increased production and liberation of mature erythrocytes is poorly understood. Apparently, it is related to the inactivation of soluble proteins of the TGF-β family. In addition, at least sotatercept can inhibit hepcidin production [108]. In phase II placebo-controlled studies of sotatercept in hemodialysis-dependent ESKD patients, the hemoglobin response was discrete. However, there was a positive trend in the slowing of vascular calcification [109].

Erythropoietin Gene Therapy

Attempts have been made to boost erythrocyte production by the induction of extra-renal EPO by DNA transmission in a variety of genetic platforms. The only one that reached the clinical trial phase employed the TARGT technology (transduced autologous restorative gene therapy), an autologous protein-delivery platform set up as small autologous dermal implants. In phase I and II studies, this approach achieved EPO levels that matched the physiological range, with a sustained effect [110, 111]. As current guidelines recommend lower and narrower hemoglobin targets, the unprecise nature of the EPO response has made this approach less appealing, and clinical studies are currently halted.

Other Approaches

A variety of approaches with different mechanisms of action may in the future increase the therapeutic arsenal for patients with kidney disease-related anemia. GATA-2 inhibitors that act by depressing EPO synthesis, anti-hepicidin drugs and ferroportin agonists/stabilizers may in the future contribute to better management of CKD-associated anemia [112-114].

CONCLUSION

The treatment of anemia in dialysis patients with rHuEPO is one of the milestones in the history of nephrology. EPO clinical application in association with adequate iron replacement, has improved the quality of life and decreased the exposure to repeated blood transfusions in millions of patients. In spite of the remarkable success, adverse effects and resistance to ESAs may still be a limitation for a fraction of patients. Hypoxia-inducible factor prolyl hydroxylase inhibitors appear to be promising agents by regulating, in a more physiological way, the production of erythropoietin, and also allowing better management of the iron metabolism.

REFERENCES

[1] Bright R. Cases and observations, illustrative of renal disease accompanied with the secretion of albuminous urine. *Guys Hosp Rep.* 1836;2(1):1-64.

[2] Cameron JS. Towards the millennium: a history of renal anaemia and the optimal use of epoetin. *Nephrol Dial Transplant.* 1999;14 Suppl 2:10-21.

[3] Babitt JL, Lin HY. Mechanisms of anemia in CKD. *J Am Soc Nephrol.* 2012;23(10):1631-4.

[4] Li S, Foley RN, Collins AJ. Anemia and cardiovascular disease, hospitalization, end stage renal disease, and death in older patients with chronic kidney disease. *Int Urol Nephrol.* 2005;37(2):395-402.

[5] Soni RK, Weisbord SD, Unruh ML. Health-related quality of life outcomes in chronic kidney disease. *Curr Opin Nephrol Hypertens.* 2010;19(2):153-9.

[6] Nair S, Trivedi M. Anemia management in dialysis patients: a PIVOT and a new path? *Curr Opin Nephrol Hypertens.* 2020;29(3):351-5.

[7] Nurko S. Anemia in chronic kidney disease: causes, diagnosis, treatment. *Cleve Clin J Med.* 2006;73(3):289-97.

[8] BESAsrab A, Bolton WK, Browne JK, Egrie JC, Nissenson AR, Okamoto DM, et al. The effects of normal as compared with low hematocrit values in patients with cardiac disease who are receiving hemodialysis and epoetin. *N Engl J Med.* 1998;339(9):584-90.

[9] Coyne DW. Hepcidin: clinical utility as a diagnostic tool and therapeutic target. *Kidney Int.* 2011;80(3):240-4.

[10] Panwar B, Gutierrez OM. Disorders of Iron Metabolism and Anemia in Chronic Kidney Disease. *Semin Nephrol.* 2016;36(4):252-61.

[11] Elliott J, Mishler D, Agarwal R. Hyporesponsiveness to erythropoietin: causes and management. *Adv Chronic Kidney Dis.* 2009;16(2):94-100.

[12] Nangaku M, Mimura I, Yamaguchi J, Higashijima Y, Wada T, Tanaka T. Role of uremic toxins in erythropoiesis-stimulating agent resistance in chronic kidney disease and dialysis patients. *J Ren Nutr.* 2015;25(2):160-3.

[13] Semenza GL, Wang GL. A nuclear factor induced by hypoxia via de novo protein synthesis binds to the human erythropoietin gene enhancer at a site required for transcriptional activation. *Mol Cell Biol.* 1992;12(12):5447-54.

[14] Takeuchi M, Kobata A. Structures and functional roles of the sugar chains of human erythropoietins. *Glycobiology.* 1991;1(4):337-46.

[15] Stone WJ, Graber SE, Krantz SB, Dessypris EN, O'Neil VL, Olsen NJ, et al. Treatment of the anemia of predialysis patients with recombinant human erythropoietin: a randomized, placebo-controlled trial. *Am J Med Sci.* 1988; 296(3):171-9.

[16] Drueke TB, Locatelli F, Clyne N, Eckardt KU, Macdougall IC, Tsakiris D, et al. Normalization of hemoglobin level in patients with chronic kidney disease and anemia. *N Engl J Med.* 2006;355(20):2071-84.

[17] Pfeffer MA, Burdmann EA, Chen CY, Cooper ME, de Zeeuw D, Eckardt KU, et al. A trial of darbepoetin alfa in type 2 diabetes and chronic kidney disease. *N Engl J Med.* 2009;361(21):2019-32.

[18] Singh AK, Szczech L, Tang KL, Barnhart H, Sapp S, Wolfson M, et al. Correction of anemia with epoetin alfa in chronic kidney disease. *N Engl J Med.* 2006; 355(20):2085-98.

[19] United States Renal Data System. Chapter 2: Clinical Indicators and Preventive Care. USRDS *Annual Data Report: Epidemiology of kidney disease in the United States.* Bethesda, MD,: National Institutes of Health, National Institute of Diabetes and Digestive and Kidney Diseases; 2018.

[20] Barbieri C, Molina M, Ponce P, Tothova M, Cattinelli I, Ion Titapiccolo J, et al. An international observational study suggests that artificial intelligence for clinical decision support optimizes anemia management in hemodialysis patients. *Kidney Int.* 2016;90(2):422-9.

[21] Akizawa T, Tsubakihara Y, Nangaku M, Endo Y, Nakajima H, Kohno T, et al. Effects of Daprodustat, a Novel Hypoxia-Inducible Factor Prolyl Hydroxylase Inhibitor on Anemia Management in Japanese Hemodialysis Subjects. *Am J Nephrol.* 2017;45(2):127-35.

[22] Bernhardt WM, Wiesener MS, Scigalla P, Chou J, Schmieder RE, Gunzler V, et al. Inhibition of prolyl hydroxylases increases erythropoietin production in ESRD. *J Am Soc Nephrol.* 2010;21(12):2151-6.

[23] Haase VH. Regulation of erythropoiesis by hypoxia-inducible factors. *Blood Rev.* 2013;27(1):41-53.

[24] Nutritional anaemias. Report of a WHO scientific group. *World Health Organ Tech Rep Ser.* 1968;405:5-37.

[25] KDIGO Anemia Work Group. KDIGO Clinical Practice Guideline for Anemia in Chronic Kidney Disease. *Kidney Int Suppl.* 2012;2(4):279-335.

[26] Ganz T. Hepcidin and iron regulation, 10 years later. *Blood.* 2011;117(17):4425-33.

[27] Rosenblatt SG, Drake S, Fadem S, Welch R, Lifschitz MD. Gastrointestinal blood loss in patients with chronic renal failure. *Am J Kidney Dis.* 1982;1(4):232-6.

[28] Sargent JA, Acchiardo SR. Iron requirements in hemodialysis. *Blood Purif.* 2004;22(1):112-23.

[29] DOPPS. *IV iron use.* The DOPPS Practice Monitor Available at: https://www.dopps.org/DPM/ Accessed September 08, 2020: DOPPS; 2020

[30] Shepshelovich D, Rozen-Zvi B, Avni T, Gafter U, Gafter-Gvili A. Intravenous Versus Oral Iron Supplementation for the Treatment of Anemia in CKD: An Updated Systematic Review and Meta-analysis. *Am J Kidney Dis.* 2016;68(5):677-90.

[31] Thamer M, Zhang Y, Kaufman J, Kshirsagar O, Cotter D, Hernan MA. Major declines in epoetin dosing after prospective payment system based on dialysis facility organizational status. *Am J Nephrol.* 2014;40(6):554-60.

[32] Locatelli F, Barany P, Covic A, De Francisco A, Del Vecchio L, Goldsmith D, et al. Kidney Disease: Improving Global Outcomes guidelines on anaemia management in chronic kidney disease: a European Renal Best Practice position statement. *Nephrol Dial Transplant.* 2013;28(6):1346-59.

[33] Kliger AS, Foley RN, Goldfarb DS, Goldstein SL, Johansen K, Singh A, et al. KDOQI US commentary on the 2012 KDIGO Clinical Practice Guideline for Anemia in CKD. *Am J Kidney Dis.* 2013;62(5):849-59.

[34] Padhi S, Glen J, Pordes BA, Thomas ME, Guideline Development G. Management of anaemia in chronic kidney disease: summary of updated NICE guidance. *BMJ.* 2015;350:h2258.

[35] Li X, Cole SR, Kshirsagar AV, Fine JP, Sturmer T, Brookhart MA. Safety of Dynamic Intravenous Iron Administration Strategies in Hemodialysis Patients. *Clin J Am Soc Nephrol.* 2019;14(5):728-37.

[36] Hayat A. Safety issues with intravenous iron products in the management of anemia in chronic kidney disease. *Clin Med Res.* 2008;6(3-4):93-102.

[37] Sunder-Plassmann G, Horl WH. Safety aspects of parenteral iron in patients with end-stage renal disease. *Drug Saf.* 1997;17(4):241-50.

[38] Michael B, Coyne DW, Fishbane S, Folkert V, Lynn R, Nissenson AR, et al. Sodium ferric gluconate complex in hemodialysis patients: adverse reactions compared to placebo and iron dextran. *Kidney Int.* 2002;61(5):1830-9.

[39] Fishbane SN, Singh AK, Cournoyer SH, Jindal KK, Fanti P, Guss CD, et al. Ferric pyrophosphate citrate (Triferic) administration via the dialysate maintains hemoglobin and iron balance in chronic hemodialysis patients. *Nephrol Dial Transplant.* 2015;30(12):2019-26.

[40] Keating GM. Ferric carboxymaltose: a review of its use in iron deficiency. *Drugs.* 2015;75(1):101-127.

[41] Shah HH, Hazzan AD, Fishbane S. Ferric Pyrophosphate Citrate: A Novel Iron Replacement Agent in Patients Undergoing Hemodialysis. *Semin Nephrol.* 2016;36(2):124-9.

[42] Floege J, Covic AC, Ketteler M, Mann JF, Rastogi A, Spinowitz B, et al. Long-term effects of the iron-based phosphate binder, sucroferric oxyhydroxide, in dialysis patients. *Nephrol Dial Transplant.* 2015;30(6):1037-46.

[43] Covic AC, Floege J, Ketteler M, Sprague SM, Lisk L, Rakov V, et al. Iron-related parameters in dialysis patients treated with sucroferric oxyhydroxide. *Nephrol Dial Transplant.* 2017;32(8):1330-8.

[44] Lioulios G, Stangou M, Sarafidis PA, Tsouchnikas I, Minasidis I, Vainas A, et al. Chronic Therapy with Sucroferric Oxyhydroxide Does Not Affect Iron and Anemia Markers in Dialysis Patients. *Blood Purif.* 2020;49(4):440-7.

[45] Macdougall IC, White C, Anker SD, Bhandari S, Farrington K, Kalra PA, et al. Randomized Trial Comparing Proactive, High-Dose versus Reactive, Low-Dose Intravenous Iron Supplementation in Hemodialysis (PIVOTAL): Study Design and Baseline Data. *Am J Nephrol.* 2018;48(4):260-8.

[46] Bailie GR, Larkina M, Goodkin DA, Li Y, Pisoni RL, Bieber B, et al. Data from the Dialysis Outcomes and Practice Patterns Study validate an association between high intravenous iron doses and mortality. *Kidney Int.* 2015;87(1):162-8.

[47] Hougen I, Collister D, Bourrier M, Ferguson T, Hochheim L, Komenda P, et al. Safety of Intravenous Iron in Dialysis: A Systematic Review and Meta-Analysis. *Clin J Am Soc Nephrol.* 2018;13(3):457-67.

[48] Kshirsagar AV, Freburger JK, Ellis AR, Wang L, Winkelmayer WC, Brookhart MA. Intravenous iron supplementation practices and short-term risk of cardiovascular events in hemodialysis patients. *PLoS One.* 2013;8(11):e78930.

[49] Kuo KL, Hung SC, Lin YP, Tang CF, Lee TS, Lin CP, et al. Intravenous ferric chloride hexahydrate supplementation induced endothelial dysfunction and increased cardiovascular risk among hemodialysis patients. *PLoS One.* 2012;7(12):e50295.

[50] Miskulin DC, Tangri N, Bandeen-Roche K, Zhou J, McDermott A, Meyer KB, et al. Intravenous iron exposure and mortality in patients on hemodialysis. *Clin J Am Soc Nephrol.* 2014;9(11):1930-9.

[51] Brookhart MA, Freburger JK, Ellis AR, Wang L, Winkelmayer WC, Kshirsagar AV. Infection risk with bolus versus maintenance iron supplementation in hemodialysis patients. *J Am Soc Nephrol.* 2013;24(7):1151-8.

[52] Fadem SZ. Comprehensive review of iron therapy in chronic kidney disease. In: Moura-Neto JA, editor. *Renal Replacement Therapy: Controversies and Future Trends.* New York: Nova; 2018. p. 33-41.

[53] Szebeni J, Fishbane S, Hedenus M, Howaldt S, Locatelli F, Patni S, et al. Hypersensitivity to intravenous iron: classification, terminology, mechanisms and management. *Br J Pharmacol.* 2015;172(21):5025-36.

[54] Gabrielsen JS, Gao Y, Simcox JA, Huang J, Thorup D, Jones D, et al. Adipocyte iron regulates adiponectin and insulin sensitivity. *J Clin Invest.* 2012;122(10):3529-40.

[55] Wish JB, Aronoff GR, Bacon BR, Brugnara C, Eckardt KU, Ganz T, et al. Positive Iron Balance in Chronic Kidney Disease: How Much is Too Much and How to Tell? *Am J Nephrol.* 2018;47(2):72-83.

[56] Wlazlo N, van Greevenbroek MM, Ferreira I, Jansen EH, Feskens EJ, van der Kallen CJ, et al. Iron metabolism is associated with adipocyte insulin resistance and plasma adiponectin: the Cohort on Diabetes and Atherosclerosis Maastricht (CODAM) study. *Diabetes Care.* 2013;36(2):309-15.

[57] Cassat JE, Skaar EP. Iron in infection and immunity. *Cell Host Microbe.* 2013;13(5):509-19.

[58] Zitt E, Sturm G, Kronenberg F, Neyer U, Knoll F, Lhotta K, et al. Iron supplementation and mortality in incident dialysis patients: an observational study. *PLoS One.* 2014;9(12):e114144.

[59] Bazeley J, Wish JB. The Evolution of Target Hemoglobin Levels in Anemia of Chronic Kidney Disease. *Adv Chronic Kidney Dis.* 2019;26(4):229-36.

[60] Kuriyama S, Tomonari H, Yoshida H, Hashimoto T, Kawaguchi Y, Sakai O. Reversal of anemia by erythropoietin therapy retards the progression of chronic renal failure, especially in nondiabetic patients. *Nephron.* 1997;77(2):176-85.

[61] Roth D, Smith RD, Schulman G, Steinman TI, Hatch FE, Rudnick MR, et al. Effects of recombinant human erythropoietin on renal function in chronic renal failure predialysis patients. *Am J Kidney Dis.* 1994;24(5):777-84.

[62] Silberberg JS, Rahal DP, Patton DR, Sniderman AD. Role of anemia in the pathogenesis of left ventricular hypertrophy in end-stage renal disease. *Am J Cardiol.* 1989;64(3):222-4.

[63] Walls J. Haemoglobin--is more better? *Nephrol Dial Transplant.* 1995;10 Suppl 2:56-61.

[64] Eschbach JW, Egrie JC, Downing MR, Browne JK, Adamson JW. Correction of the anemia of end-stage renal disease with recombinant human erythropoietin. Results of a combined phase I and II clinical trial. *N Engl J Med.* 1987;316(2):73-8.

[65] Eschbach JW, Abdulhadi MH, Browne JK, Delano BG, Downing MR, Egrie JC, et al. Recombinant human erythropoietin in anemic patients with end-stage renal disease. Results of a phase III multicenter clinical trial. *Ann Intern Med.* 1989;111(12):992-1000.

[66] Procrit [package insert]. *Thousand Oaks,* CA: Amgen Inc.; 1993.

[67] NKF-DOQI clinical practice guidelines for the treatment of anemia of chronic renal failure. National Kidney Foundation-Dialysis Outcomes Quality Initiative. *Am J Kidney Dis.* 1997;30(4 Suppl 3):S192-240.

[68] Auer J, Simon G, Stevens J, Griffiths P, Howarth D, Anastassiades E, et al. Quality of life improvements in CAPD patients treated with subcutaneously administered erythropoietin for anemia. *Perit Dial Int.* 1992;12(1):40-2.

[69] Paganini EP. In search of an optimal hematocrit level in dialysis patients: rehabilitation and quality-of-life implications. *Am J Kidney Dis.* 1994;24(1 Suppl 1):S10-6; discussion S31-2.

[70] Revicki DA, Brown RE, Feeny DH, Henry D, Teehan BP, Rudnick MR, et al. Health-related quality of life associated with recombinant human erythropoietin therapy for predialysis chronic renal disease patients. *Am J Kidney Dis.* 1995;25(4):548-54.

[71] Ritz E, Zeier M, Schneider P, Jones E. Cardiovascular mortality of patients with polycystic kidney disease on dialysis: is there a lesson to learn? *Nephron.* 1994;66(2):125-8.

[72] Silberberg J, Racine N, Barre P, Sniderman AD. Regression of left ventricular hypertrophy in dialysis patients following correction of anemia with recombinant human erythropoietin. *Can J Cardiol.* 1990;6(1):1-4.

[73] Foley RN, Curtis BM, Parfrey PS. Hemoglobin targets and blood transfusions in hemodialysis patients without symptomatic cardiac disease receiving erythropoietin therapy. *Clin J Am Soc Nephrol.* 2008;3(6):1669-75.

[74] Junor BJ. Hematocrit above 30% in continuous ambulatory peritoneal dialysis patients treated with erythropoietin is harmful. *Perit Dial Int.* 1993;13 Suppl 2:S535-7.

[75] Coyne DW. The health-related quality of life was not improved by targeting higher hemoglobin in the Normal Hematocrit Trial. *Kidney Int.* 2012;82(2):235-41.

[76] Phrommintikul A, Haas SJ, Elsik M, Krum H. Mortality and target haemoglobin concentrations in anaemic patients with chronic kidney disease treated with erythropoietin: a meta-analysis. *Lancet.* 2007;369(9559):381-8.

[77] Krapf R, Hulter HN. Arterial hypertension induced by erythropoietin and erythropoiesis-stimulating agents (ESAs). *Clin J Am Soc Nephrol.* 2009;4(2):470-80.

[78] Tonia T, Mettler A, Robert N, Schwarzer G, Seidenfeld J, Weingart O, et al. Erythropoietin or darbepoetin for patients with cancer. *Cochrane Database Syst Rev.* 2012;12:Cd003407.

[79] Brenner N, Kommalapati A, Ahsan M, Ganguli A. Red cell transfusion in chronic kidney disease in the United States in the current era of erythropoiesis stimulating agents. *J Nephrol.* 2020;33(2):267-75.

[80] Tanhehco YC, Berns JS. Red blood cell transfusion risks in patients with end-stage renal disease. *Semin Dial.* 2012;25(5):539-44.

[81] Alam A, Lin Y, Lima A, Hansen M, Callum JL. The prevention of transfusion-associated circulatory overload. *Transfus Med Rev.* 2013;27(2):105-12.

[82] Carson JL, Guyatt G, Heddle NM, Grossman BJ, Cohn CS, Fung MK, et al. Clinical Practice Guidelines From the AABB: Red Blood Cell Transfusion Thresholds and Storage. *JAMA.* 2016;316(19):2025-35.

[83] Kleinman S, Caulfield T, Chan P, Davenport R, McFarland J, McPhedran S, et al. Toward an understanding of transfusion-related acute lung injury: statement of a consensus panel. *Transfusion.* 2004;44(12):1774-89.

[84] Oakley FD, Woods M, Arnold S, Young PP. Transfusion reactions in pediatric compared with adult patients: a look at rate, reaction type, and associated products. *Transfusion.* 2015;55(3):563-70.

[85] Tobian AA, King KE, Ness PM. Transfusion premedications: a growing practice not based on evidence. *Transfusion.* 2007;47(6):1089-96.

[86] Obrador GT, Macdougall IC. Effect of red cell transfusions on future kidney transplantation. *Clin J Am Soc Nephrol.* 2013;8(5):852-60.

[87] BESAsrab A, Chernyavskaya E, Motylev I, Shutov E, Kumbar LM, Gurevich K, et al. Roxadustat (FG-4592): Correction of Anemia in Incident Dialysis Patients. *J Am Soc Nephrol.* 2016;27(4):1225-33.

[88] BESAsrab A, Provenzano R, Hertel J, Zabaneh R, Klaus SJ, Lee T, et al. Randomized placebo-controlled dose-ranging and pharmacodynamics study of roxadustat (FG-4592) to treat anemia in nondialysis-dependent chronic kidney disease (NDD-CKD) patients. *Nephrol Dial Transplant.* 2015;30(10):1665-73.

[89] Flamme I, Oehme F, Ellinghaus P, Jeske M, Keldenich J, Thuss U. Mimicking hypoxia to treat anemia: HIF-stabilizer BAY 85-3934 (Molidustat) stimulates erythropoietin production without hypertensive effects. *PLoS One.* 2014; 9(11):e111838.

[90] Holdstock L, Meadowcroft AM, Maier R, Johnson BM, Jones D, Rastogi A, et al. Four-Week Studies of Oral Hypoxia-Inducible Factor-Prolyl Hydroxylase Inhibitor GSK1278863 for Treatment of Anemia. *J Am Soc Nephrol.* 2016;27(4):1234-44.

[91] Hasegawa S, Tanaka T, Saito T, Fukui K, Wakashima T, Susaki EA, et al. The oral hypoxia-inducible factor prolyl hydroxylase inhibitor enarodustat counteracts alterations in renal energy metabolism in the early stages of diabetic kidney disease. *Kidney Int.* 2020;97(5):934-50.

[92] Dhillon S. Roxadustat: First Global Approval. *Drugs.* 2019;79(5):563-72.

[93] Locatelli F, Fishbane S, Block GA, Macdougall IC. Targeting Hypoxia-Inducible Factors for the Treatment of Anemia in Chronic Kidney Disease Patients. *Am J Nephrol.* 2017;45(3):187-99.

[94] Haase VH, Chertow GM, Block GA, Pergola PE, deGoma EM, Khawaja Z, et al. Effects of vadadustat on hemoglobin concentrations in patients receiving hemodialysis previously treated with erythropoiesis-stimulating agents. *Nephrol Dial Transplant.* 2019;34(1):90-9.

[95] Macdougall IC, Akizawa T, Berns JS, Bernhardt T, Krueger T. Effects of Molidustat in the Treatment of Anemia in CKD. *Clin J Am Soc Nephrol.* 2019;14(1):28-39.

[96] Provenzano R, BESAsrab A, Wright S, Dua S, Zeig S, Nguyen P, et al. Roxadustat (FG-4592) Versus Epoetin Alfa for Anemia in Patients Receiving Maintenance Hemodialysis: A Phase 2, Randomized, 6- to 19-Week, Open-Label, Active-Comparator, Dose-Ranging, Safety and Exploratory Efficacy Study. *Am J Kidney Dis.* 2016;67(6):912-24.

[97] Akizawa T, Iwasaki M, Yamaguchi Y, Majikawa Y, Reusch M. Phase 3, Randomized, Double-Blind, Active-Comparator (Darbepoetin Alfa) Study of Oral Roxadustat in CKD Patients with Anemia on Hemodialysis in Japan. *J Am Soc Nephrol.* 2020;31(7):1628-39.

[98] Chen N, Hao C, Liu BC, Lin H, Wang C, Xing C, et al. Roxadustat Treatment for Anemia in Patients Undergoing Long-Term Dialysis. *N Engl J Med.* 2019;381(11):1011-22.

[99] Akizawa T, Otsuka T, Reusch M, Ueno M. Intermittent Oral Dosing of Roxadustat in Peritoneal Dialysis Chronic Kidney Disease Patients with Anemia: A Randomized, Phase 3, Multicenter, Open-Label Study. *Ther Apher Dial.* 2020;24(2):115-25.

[100] Sugahara M, Tanaka T, Nangaku M. Prolyl hydroxylase domain inhibitors as a novel therapeutic approach against anemia in chronic kidney disease. *Kidney Int.* 2017;92(2):306-12.

[101] Li ZL, Tu Y, Liu BC. Treatment of Renal Anemia with Roxadustat: Advantages and Achievement. *Kidney Dis (Basel).* 2020;6(2):65-73.

[102] Olson E, Demopoulos L, Haws TF, Hu E, Fang Z, Mahar KM, et al. Short-term treatment with a novel HIF-prolyl hydroxylase inhibitor (GSK1278863) failed to improve measures of performance in subjects with claudication-limited peripheral artery disease. *Vasc Med.* 2014;19(6):473-82.

[103] Provenzano R, BESAsrab A, Sun CH, Diamond SA, Durham JH, Cangiano JL, et al. Oral Hypoxia-Inducible Factor Prolyl Hydroxylase Inhibitor Roxadustat (FG-4592) for the Treatment of Anemia in Patients with CKD. *Clin J Am Soc Nephrol.* 2016;11(6):982-91.

[104] Mokas S, Lariviere R, Lamalice L, Gobeil S, Cornfield DN, Agharazii M, et al. Hypoxia-inducible factor-1 plays a role in phosphate-induced vascular smooth muscle cell calcification. *Kidney Int.* 2016;90(3):598-609.

[105] Sanghani NS, Haase VH. Hypoxia-Inducible Factor Activators in Renal Anemia: Current Clinical Experience. *Adv Chronic Kidney Dis.* 2019;26(4):253-66.

[106] Biggar P, Kim GH. Treatment of renal anemia: Erythropoiesis stimulating agents and beyond. *Kidney Res Clin Pract.* 2017;36(3):209-23.

[107] Carrancio S, Markovics J, Wong P, Leisten J, Castiglioni P, Groza MC, et al. An activin receptor IIA ligand trap promotes erythropoiesis resulting in a rapid induction of red blood cells and haemoglobin. *Br J Haematol.* 2014;165(6):870-82.

[108] Jelkmann W. Activin receptor ligand traps in chronic kidney disease. *Curr Opin Nephrol Hypertens.* 2018;27(5):351-7.

[109] Coyne DW, Singh HN, Smith WT, Giuseppi AC, Connarn JN, Sherman ML, et al. Sotatercept Safety and Effects on Hemoglobin, Bone, and Vascular Calcification. *Kidney Int Rep.* 2019;4(11):1585-97.

[110] Blum S, Shapir N, Miari R, Lerner B, Koren B, Doenyas-Barak K, et al. TARGT Gene Therapy Platform for Correction of Anemia in End-Stage Renal Disease. *N Engl J Med.* 2017;376(2):189-91.

[111] Shapir N, Miari R, Blum S, Schwartz D, Chernin G, Neil GA, et al. Preclinical and Preliminary Clinical Evaluation of Genetically Transduced Dermal Tissue Implants for the Sustained Secretion of Erythropoietin and Interferon alpha. *Hum Gene Ther Clin Dev.* 2015;26(4):216-27.

[112] Locatelli F, Del Vecchio L, Luise MC. Current and future chemical therapies for treating anaemia in chronic kidney disease. *Expert Opin Pharmacother.* 2017;18(8):781-8.

[113] López-Gómez JM, Abad S, Vega A. New expectations in the treatment of anemia in chronic kidney disease. *Nefrología* (English Edition). 2016;36(3):232-6.

[114] Schmid H, Jelkmann W. Investigational therapies for renal disease-induced anemia. *Expert Opin Investig Drugs.* 2016;25(8):901-16.

In: Issues in Kidney Disease – Dialysis
Editors: Stephen Z. Fadem and José A. Moura-Neto
ISBN: 978-1-68507-000-7

Chapter 4

CHRONIC KIDNEY DISEASE-MINERAL BONE DISORDER AND VASCULAR CALCIFICATION

Anju Mohan, MD and Stuart M. Sprague*, DO
Department of Internal Medicine, Division of Nephrology,
North Shore University Health System, University of Chicago,
Pritzker School of Medicine, Evanston, IL, USA

ABSTRACT

Chronic kidney disease-mineral bone disease (CKD-MBD) is frequently encountered during the management of patients with chronic kidney disease (CKD). The systemic phenomenon of CKD-MBD results in derangements in mineral metabolism, disturbances in bone mineralization, or renal osteodystrophy and extraskeletal calcification, resulting in significant morbidity and mortality, especially cardiovascular complications. Classically, metabolic derangements include the vitamin D-PTH axis with more recently FGF-23 and Klotho being identified as important regulators. This chapter explores the complex interplay between the mineral-associated hormones and proteins in CKD along with the pathophysiology and clinical aspects of CKD-MBD.

Keywords: parathyroid hormone, vitamin D, fibroblastic growth factor 23, renal osteodystrophy, osteoporosis, calciphylaxis

INTRODUCTION

The three hormones that play a key role, along with the kidneys, in maintaining normal serum concentrations of calcium and phosphorus are fibroblast growth factor 23 (FGF-23), parathyroid hormone (PTH), and 1,25-dihydroxyvitamin D, which is the active metabolite of vitamin D. The four primary targets for these hormones are bone, kidney, intestine, and parathyroid glands. Kidneys play a critical role in maintaining calcium and phosphorus

* Corresponding Author's E-mail: ssprague@northshore.org.

homeostasis, and hence derangements in mineral homeostasis is common in chronic kidney disease (CKD) patients. The imbalance occurs early in the development of CKD and, by the time patients approach end stage renal disease (ESRD), these abnormalities are universally observed. With the progression of CKD, the body attempts to maintain normal serum concentrations of calcium and phosphorus by altering the production of FGF-23, PTH, 1,25-dihydroxyvitamin D and klotho, an enzyme necessary for activation of FGF23 at its receptor. In due course, the compensatory responses fail to maintain normal mineral homeostasis. This results in (1) altered serum concentrations of calcium, phosphorus, PTH, 1,25-dihydroxyvitamin D, FGF-23, and klotho; (2) disturbances in bone remodeling and mineralization (often referred to as "renal osteodystrophy"); and (3) extraskeletal calcification in soft tissues and arteries. The term chronic kidney disease-mineral bone disease (CKD-MBD) was defined in 2006 by the National Kidney Foundation Kidney Disease Outcomes Quality Initiative (NKF-KDOQI) to describe this triad of abnormalities [1]. All three components of CKD-MBD are associated with increased risk of fractures, cardiovascular disease, and mortality in patients with advanced CKD. Treatment of CKD-MBD focuses on the prevention and correction of these hormonal abnormalities.

Abnormalities in Mineral Metabolism

Calcium, Phosphate and 1,25-Dihydroxyvitamin D

Calcium and phosphate homeostasis as CKD progresses is complex, and dysregulation of calcium is directly related to the dysregulation of serum phosphate and 1,25-dihydroxyvitamin D, which develops early as renal disease progresses. With the progression of renal disease, there is a tendency to develop hypocalcemia as well as phosphate retention. Early in the development of CKD, there is decreased renal production of 1,25-dihydroxyvitamin D, both as a result of loss of renal parenchyma and increasing concentrations of FGF-23 resulting in decreased 1α-hydroxylase (CYP27B1) activity, resulting in decreased vitamin D mediated gastrointestinal calcium absorption [2-4].

Phosphate retention and ultimately hyperphosphatemia is another accompanying biochemical abnormality seen as CKD progresses. When there is resultant nephron loss, there is reduction in filtered phosphate. Increased production of FGF23 and PTH promotes phosphaturia in the remaining nephrons during early CKD; however, hyperphosphatemia eventually develops [2-4]. Hyperphosphatemia itself can contribute to hypocalcemia by causing calcium-phosphate deposition in the vasculature or extra skeletal tissues and by further suppressing CYP27B1 activity [4]. Elevated phosphorus concentrations can also have a direct stimulatory effect on the parathyroid gland [5]. Regulation of serum concentrations of calcium, phosphate and 1,25-dihydroxyvitamin D is thus influenced by circulating hormones, which comprise the PTH-Vitamin D-FGF23 axis [2, 4].

Parathyroid Hormone

The major physiological role of parathyroid gland is to function as a "calciostat" [6]. Hence PTH secreted by the chief cells of the parathyroid gland, works in regulating serum concentrations of calcium and phosphate. PTH acts mainly via the PTH receptor (PTH1R) which is expressed in high concentrations in bones and kidneys. In mammals, PTH1R is located in cells of the osteoblast lineage, where it increases osteoclast formation and activity via the receptor activator of the NF-κB ligand (RANKL) and its receptor RANK pathways [7].

In order to maintain calcium homeostasis, PTH acts by increasing bone mineral dissolution, thus releasing calcium and phosphate, increasing renal absorption of calcium and excretion of phosphate, increasing the activity of the renal CYP27B1 enzyme to convert 25-hydroxyvitamin D to 1,25-dihydroxyvitamin D, and enhancing the gastrointestinal absorption of both calcium and phosphate indirectly through its effects on the synthesis of 1,25-dihydroxyvitamin D [8]. Hypocalcemia further stimulates PTH secretion while high calcium concentrations provide a negative feedback mechanism for PTH. Calcium action on parathyroid gland is mediated through a calcium sensing receptor (CaSR) expressed in chief cells [9]. When hypocalcemia stimulates PTH, in short term, there is exocytosis of PTH packaged in granules, and longer term stimulation can result in an increase in number of cells that secrete PTH [10]. CaSR expression has been shown to be reduced by 1,25-dihydroxyvitamin D deficiency and stimulated by vitamin D receptor activators (VDRA) administration [10].

Phosphate exerts a stimulatory effect on PTH through stabilization of PTH mRNA and thereby increases secretion when hyperphosphatemia occurs [11]. 1,25-dihydroxyvitamin D is known to exert negative feedback on PTH secretion through binding of the parathyroid vitamin D receptor (VDR) and direct suppression of the PTH gene transcription [12, 13]. FGF-23 also acts to negatively inhibit PTH secretion through down regulation of PTH gene expression, decreased PTH secretion, and decreased PTH cell proliferation through the parathyroid klotho-FGF receptor [14].

FGF-23 and Klotho

FGF-23 is 32-kDa protein located on chromosome 12p13.3 in humans [15]. The main sources of FGF-23 are osteocytes and osteoblasts in the skeleton, but low concentrations of unclear significance can be detected in the ventrolateral thalamic nucleus, the thymus, small intestine, and heart [6, 16]. It causes urinary phosphate excretion by suppressing the expression of sodium/phosphate co-transporter, Na-Pi 2a cotransporters, in the proximal tubules [17, 18]. It also inhibits CYP27B1 resulting in decreased concentrations of 1,25-dihydroxyvitamin D and stimulates 24-hydroxylase (CYP24) that converts both 1,25-dihydroxyvitamin D and 25-hydroxyvitamin D to inactive metabolites in the proximal tubule of the kidney [17, 18]. It has been found that in patients with hypophosphatemic rickets the circulating FGF-23 concentrations were increased by 10 to 20 fold when compared to normal healthy adults [19, 20]. Thus FGF-23 in excess results in renal phosphate wasting, low 1,25-dihydroxyvitamin D concentrations and osteomalacia [21-23]. While in contrast, the depletion of FGF-23 leads to hyperphosphatemia, high concentrations of 1,25-dihydroxyvitamin D, and soft tissue calcification [24-26].

FGF-23 exerts its biological actions by binding to fibroblastic growth factor receptor (mainly FGFR-1) in the presence of its coreceptor klotho. Klotho proteins produced by the kidney can be found as both membrane bound, which acts as co-receptor for FGF-23, or soluble proteins. Klotho determines the tissue specificity of FGF-23 [15]. The N-terminal region of FGF-23 binds to and activates FGFR whereas the C-terminal region of FGF-23 interacts with klotho [27, 28]. The soluble form of klotho, which is freely circulating, has also been shown to effect calcium homeostasis. It can increase calcium reabsorption in distal convoluted tubules and connecting tubules through enzymatically cleaving the extracellular domain of TRPV5 calcium channels, which keeps TRPV5 calcium channels in the cell membranes [29, 30]. This results in calcium entry into the cells down the electrochemical gradient. Serum elevations in 1,25-dihydroxyvitamin D also can upregulate klotho expression, which in turn works in conjunction with FGF-23 to suppress 1,25-dihydroxyvitamin D concentrations [31]. Both progressive CKD and decreases in 1,25-dihydroxyvitamin D result in decreased klotho production thus decreased FGF-23 activity at the parathyroid gland [31].

FGF 23 secretion is regulated by several factors including serum phosphate and 1,25-dihydroxyvitamin D concentrations. Gutierrez et al. in 2005 demonstrated that FGF-23 concentrations increase early in CKD before the development of serum mineral abnormalities and are independently associated with serum phosphate, fractional excretion of phosphate and calcitriol deficiency. They also demonstrated that increased FGF-23 may contribute to maintaining normal serum phosphate concentrations in the face of advancing CKD but may decrease 1,25-dihydroxyvitamin D concentrations and hence play a central role in early pathogenesis of secondary hyperparathyroidism (SHPT) [32]. Elevated PTH tends to increase FGF-23 concentration in the blood and serum FGF-23 decreases PTH secretion [33, 34]. However, the effect of FGF-23 on decreasing PTH secretion may be limited by decreased klotho. This interaction completes a bone parathyroid hormonal axis [33].

In posttransplant hypophosphatemia, FGF-23 may be contributing more than previously thought. FGF-23 is excessively increased in the pre-transplant period but fails to exert its effects due to lack of functioning kidney. However, posttransplant, this FGF-23 acts on the allograft to promote renal phosphate wasting and suppress 1,25-dihydroxyvitamin D production contributing to posttransplant hypophosphatemia [35, 36].

Summary of the Physiologic Response

The physiologic response to hyperphosphatemia is a very complex system of multiple integrated feedback loops. Below is deconstructed version of the loops that occur in order to maintain homeostasis of calcium, phosphate and 1,25-dihydroxyvitamin D.

PTH-FGF23-1,25-Dihydroxyvitamin D Loop

Both PTH and FGF-23 simulate phosphate excretion but have different effects on the vitamin D axis. PTH stimulates CYP27B1 activity, thereby increasing the production of 1,25-dihydroxyvitamin D, which in turn negatively feeds back on the parathyroid gland. In contrast, FGF-23 inhibits CYP27B1 and stimulates CYP24, thereby decreasing the production and increasing the degradation of 1,25-dihydroxyvitamin D, thus feeding back to limit further secretion of FGF-23. However, both PTH and 1,25-dihydroxyvitamin D stimulate the production of FGF23.

Phosphate-PTH-FGF 23 Loop

As phosphate concentrations increase both PTH and FGF-23 increase, causing urinary phosphate excretion through downregulation of NaPi transporters. PTH by increasing renal calcium reabsorption, minimizes the chances of high calcium and phosphate concentrations in urine during the period were there is desire to increase phosphate excretion. PTH stimulates the secretion of FGF-23 from osteocytes, and increased FGF-23 inhibits PTH by decreasing both PTH gene expression and PTH secretion [37, 38]. However, decreased klotho may limit the ability of FGF-23 to inhibit PTH production and secretion.

Calcium-PTH-FGF 23

As mentioned above, hypocalcemia is a potent stimulator of PTH, blunts FGF-23 release [39]. With down regulation of FGF-23, its inhibitory effect on PTH and 1,25-dihydroxyvitamin D is removed. Thus, PTH effects to maintain normal serum calcium would be maximized. In contrast, hypercalcemia stimulates FGF-23 and directly inhibits 1,25-dihydroxyvitamin D synthesis and PTH secretion [40]. The result is decreased intestinal calcium absorption, renal reabsorption of calcium, and bone resorption.

Secondary and Tertiary Hyperparathyroidism

Secondary hyperparathyroidism (SHPT) is initially an adaptive and in many cases ultimately becomes a maladaptive process which occurs in response to declining renal function. Due to the latter, there is impaired phosphate excretion, failure of formation of 1,25-dihydroxyvitamin D leading to dysregulation of calcium and phosphorus homeostasis. This leads to a cascade of changes which increases synthesis and secretion of PTH, parathyroid hyperplasia, contributing to a vicious cycle [41]. By definition, secondary hyperparathyroidism (SHPT) is characterized by increased concentrations of PTH secretion required for the maintenance of normal serum calcium concentrations in the setting of renal impairment. This elevation of PTH simulation is multifactorial caused by hypocalcemia, decreased 1,25-dihydroxyvitamin D, and hyperphosphatemia which occurs as renal disease progresses.

There is continuous stimulation of parathyroid gland by a combination of elevated serum phosphate, decreased ionized calcium and reduced calcitriol leading to increased PTH synthesis and release. Simultaneously, elevated FGF-23 leads to downregulations of residual renal CYP27B1 which worsens the deficiency of 1,25-dihydroxyvitamin D, thus acting as a driver to SHPT. Correlations between high FGF-23 concentrations in dialysis patients, refractory SHPT, and increased mortality have been observed [42, 43].

During the early stages of renal failure, several studies have documented the reduction in 1,25-dihydroxyvitamin and increasing PTH concentrations before there are any changes to the serum phosphate and calcium [44-46]. In majority of the patients, 1,25-dihydroxyvitamin D concentrations drops to the lower end of reference range in late CKD stage 2 and, by the time the disease has progressed to CKD stage 3, many patients have low 1,25-dihydroxyvitamin D and elevated PTH concentrations. This compensatory rise in PTH is primarily from low vitamin D and not to the substantial changes in serum calcium or phosphate [47]. Approximately 40% of patients with stage 3 CKD and 70% with stage 4 CKD have elevated PTH concentrations [47].

Although FGF-23 is known to decrease PTH secretion, cell proliferation and increase CaSR and VDR in normal parathyroid gland, it fails to exert these effects on hyperplastic parathyroid glands [14, 48, 49]. This could be due to the reduced expression of FGFR1 and Klotho protein were markedly reduced in hyperplastic parathyroid glands in humans compared to normal parathyroid glands [50]. Hence, this mechanism precludes control of hyperparathyroidism by FGF-23 in the presence of renal failure [49].

As mentioned above, SHPT is accompanied by parathyroid hyperplasia [51, 52]. Hyperphosphatemia enhances parathyroid hyperplasia. If there are no therapeutic interventions at this point, the parathyroid glands can develop areas of micronodular change which can then progress to macronodular adenomas. This development of nodularity is irreversible and as mentioned above is associated with decreased concentrations of VDRs and CaSRs with the development of autonomous function [53]. The nodular changes seen in parathyroid gland is often refractory to medical therapy and may warrant parathyroidectomy. Ultimately, prolonged hyperparathyroidism results in increased bone remodeling and loss of bone density and structural integrity. As a result of the parathyroid-induced changes, excess bone resorption leads to loss of bone mineral, furthering the release of calcium and phosphorus from bone, increasing risk of vascular and visceral calcification, and increased risk of cardiovascular complications and mortality in patients receiving dialysis [54, 55]. Hence, interventions to prevent and/or treat SHPT should be initiated early in patients with CKD.

Therapeutic interventions for SHPT consists of management of calcium, phosphate, 1,25-dihydroxyvitamin D dysregulation. However, lowering PTH while simultaneously controlling serum concentrations of calcium and phosphorus can become challenging. Current treatment modalities include management of calcium and phosphorus balance by dietary intake and dialysis, VDRAs like calcitriol, phosphate binders and calcimimetics [53, 56].

CKD patients have a deficiency of endogenous calcitriol which can be managed by treatment with calcitriol or one of its prodrugs, alfacalcidol, doxercalciferol, and extended release calcifediol, or other VDRAs, 22-oxacalcitriol and paricalcitol. Active vitamin D sterols suppress PTH by 2 mechanisms: preventing parathyroid gland enlargement and decreasing PTH synthesis [57-59]. The activation of VDRs can also decrease PTH indirectly by increasing the serum calcium and thereby activating CaSR and directly stimulating the expression of CaSR within the parathyroid gland [60]. However, higher pharmacologic doses could lead to hypercalcemia and hyperphosphatemia, which can lead to ectopic or vascular calcifications [61, 62]. Yet another challenge is concern for resistance to active vitamin D compounds in patients with nodular hyperplasia of parathyroid gland [63]. Size of the parathyroid glands may also play a role, with moderately increased glands being more responsive to vitamin D and enlarged glands less so [64-66].

Hyperphosphatemia is associated with cardiovascular mortality in SHPT [67]. Management of hyperphosphatemia is key through dietary control, oral phosphate binders in CKD patients, and via dialysis in ESRD patients. It is known that dialysis removal of phosphate is poor [68]. The use of calcium salts increases the risk for hypercalcemia, calciphylaxis, and vascular calcification [69]. While calcium free binders are effective in lowering phosphorus, they do not significantly affect the PTH concentrations [70]. Hence phosphate binders have limited utility in SHPT therapy, even though hyperphosphatemia is an important factor in the pathogenesis of early SHPT.

Calcimimetics such as cinacalcet and etecalcetide are positive allosteric modulators of CaSR that can reduce PTH concentrations by increasing sensitivity to extracellular calcium

[71]. Several studies have shown that calcimimetics can inhibit development and progression of parathyroid hyperplasia [72]. Hypocalcemia is a common side effect, which is commonly managed by dose adjustment or by concomitant use of VDRAs in patients with moderate to severe SHPT [73].

Tertiary hyperparathyroidism, commonly seen in long-standing CKD and post renal transplant, is characterized by the semi-autonomous hypersecretion of PTH leading to hypercalcemia. Etiology is postulated to be monoclonal expansion of a clone of parathyroid cells, which have acquired an altered set point of calcium-sensing receptor (CaSR) of that PTH continuously secreted despite high serum calcium concentrations [74]. The clinical presentation is similar to primary hyperparathyroidism and is dependent on the serum calcium and PTH concentrations. The features include decreased bone mineral density (BMD), bone pain, fractures, pruritis, nephrolithiasis, vascular calcifications, peptic ulcer disease, pancreatitis, muscle weakness and impaired allograft function [75].

The primary treatment modality is surgery; the strategies are divided as subtotal or total parathyroidectomy with or without auto transplantation [76]. The approach is determined on a case-by-case basis and there is limited evidence favoring one method to another. In one study, those undergoing total parathyroidectomy had lower serum calcium and higher serum phosphate concentrations compared to subtotal parathyroidectomy, hence the latter is preferred as it reduced risk of hypocalcemia [77]. In contrast, in another study total parathyroidectomy without auto transplantation appears to be protective against persistent and recurrent diseases [78].

Abnormalities in Bone Turnover, Mineralization, Volume, Linear Growth, and Strength

Renal Osteodystrophy

Renal osteodystrophy is an alteration of bone morphology in patients with CKD. It is one measure of the skeletal component of the systemic disorder of CKD-MBD that is quantifiable by histomorphometry of bone biopsy [1]. Traditionally five major histopathologic patterns were described: osteitis fibrosa, mild lesion, osteomalacia, mixed uremic osteodystrophy, and adynamic bone disease.

Bone remodeling is a very complex and dynamic process with distinct phases: osteoclast resorption, reversal, pre-osteoblast migration and differentiation, osteoblast matrix formation, mineralization and quiescent stage. The process of remodeling in a single bone unit can take up to 3-6 months. The receptor activator of nuclear-factor kB (RANK) is located on the osteoclasts and the osteoprotegerin-ligand (OPG-L) on the osteoblasts. These latter cells secrete the protein OPG which can bind to OPG-L and inhibit the subsequent binding of OPG-L to RANK on osteoclasts, thus inhibiting bone resorption. Alternatively, if OPG production is decreased, the OPG-L can bind with RANK and can induce bone resorption [79]. This pathway is regulated by numerous cytokines and hormones including PTH.

Deficiency of 1,25-dihydroxyvitamin D plays an important role in pathophysiology of renal osteodystrophy. As in ESRD, this leads to decreased intestinal calcium and phosphorus absorption and increased PTH secretion [80]. Persistent elevation in PTH concentrations can produce an abnormal phenotype of osteoblast function with less type 1 collagen and more RANK ligand production than anabolic osteoblasts leading to high-turnover osteodystrophy and excess bone resorption. Thus, secondary hyperparathyroidism plays a major role in the pathogenesis of the high-turnover bone disease osteitis fibrosa, which is characterized by marrow fibrosis caused by fibroblast-like cells secreting fibrous tissue occupying peri-trabecular space. Both osteoclast and osteoblast activity are increased resulting in increased bone resorption and bone formation, the latter reflected by the increased amounts of osteoid and non-lamellar bone which is weaker than its lamellar counterpart. This is predominantly found in the cortical osteons of long bones. In long bones, increases in cortical resorption tends to reduce bone mass. Hence osteitis fibrosa may be associated with osteopenia and risk of fractures [79, 80]. Although SHPT is common in early renal failure, osteitis fibrosa is rarely seen prior to development of ESRD [81]. The mild lesion is characterized by a slight increase in the bone remodeling but without significant peri-trabecular fibrosis. It is seen commonly prior to development of ESRD [82], as a result of mild or early secondary hyperparathyroidism or following therapy for hyperparathyroidism.

Osteomalacia is defined by low rates of bone turnover, defect in mineralization, and accumulation of unmineralized osteoid (bone matrix). It was predominantly associated with aluminum intoxication or with other heavy metals like iron. Sources of aluminum included dialysis water and aluminum containing phosphate binders [83]. Aluminum intoxication can cause defective mineralization and increased matrix synthesis by existing osteoblasts but with long-term inhibition of osteoblast differentiation, as well as inhibition of osteoclast function. The incidence of osteomalacia has decreased with elimination of aluminum exposure in patients with ERSD, but still occurs, which points towards other factors such as severe vitamin D deficiency, iron intoxication, other heavy metals, and metabolic acidosis [80, 81, 84].

Mixed uremic osteodystrophy has features of both osteitis fibrosa and osteomalacia, characterized by high bone turnover and mineralization defects. It is present in varying degrees in different individuals. Pathogenesis is related to SHPT, aluminum intoxication, and other unknown factors [79-81].

Another form of low turnover bone disease is adynamic bone disease (ABD), which is characterized by marked reduction in bone formation and cellular activity without an increase in osteoid thickness [81, 85]. It is associated with relatively low concentrations of PTH following parathyroidectomy, from exposure to high concentrations of calcium (phosphate binders and dialysate fluid), and active VDRAs like calcitriol. Peritoneal dialysis patients are at increased risk due to prolonged exposure to high peritoneal dialysate calcium concentration [81, 85, 86]. The clinical significant of ABD is controversial; however, low turnover diseases are associated with increased rates of fracture, brittle calcium control, increased vascular calcification and calciphylaxis [87-90]. A prospective observational study showed that in patients commencing dialysis, normal PTH was associated with twice the mortality risk when compared to patients with iPTH concentrations three times the upper limit of normal [91]. One explanation was poor nutritional status, but these patients could also be at high risk for ABD and vascular calcifications [85].

In order to appropriately diagnose renal osteodystrophy, a bone biopsy is required. With the updated NKF-KDOQI guidelines, the appropriate interpretation of bone biopsies should no longer be classified descriptively as described above, but should be based on three key histologic quantitative measurements: bone turnover, mineralization, and volume (TMV system) [1]. Turnover would be either low, normal or increased, mineralization either normal or abnormal, and volume as either low, normal, or increased [1, 92]. Treatment of renal osteodystrophy involves controlling serum calcium and phosphorus concentrations in order to prevent severe hyperparathyroidism and its complications. Dietary phosphorus control along with phosphate binders is integral. When using calcium-based binders, it's pertinent to balance the need for controlling serum phosphorus, calcium phosphate product, and SHPT against vascular calcifications and development of adynamic bone disease. Serum calcium should be maintained in the upper end of normal limits in order to suppress PTH [80]. However, if the patient is receiving calcium-based phosphate binders, then the dialysate calcium might need to be reduced in order to prevent developing hypercalcemia. The dialysate calcium concentration can be reduced to 1.25 mmol per liter and this should allow for sufficient oral intake of calcium-based binders [93]. The timing of intake of oral calcium is also important; if taken between meals it acts more like a calcium supplement than a binder. Calcitriol and other VDRAs are used to control PTH, but their use should be avoided in hyperphosphatemia due to concern for increased calcium phosphate product and in low turnover bone disease. Nutritional vitamin D or Vitamin D preparations like extended release calcifediol, which are associated with lower incidence of hypercalcemia and hyperphosphatemia in CKD prior to the initiation of dialysis, can assist in prevention of osteodystrophy [94-96]. The Kidney Disease: Improving Global Outcomes (KDIGO) guidelines in 2017 do not recommend the uniform use of active vitamin D analogues in CKD 3a to 5 and should only be considered in severe and progressive SHPT [97].

Osteopenia/Osteoporosis

Osteoporosis is defined as a condition of impairment in bone strength due to low bone mineral density and poor bone quality and predisposes individuals to an increased risk of fractures. Compared to the general population, in patients with CKD, there is a high incidence of both vertebral and hip fractures (4.4 fold more) [98, 99]. The mortality rate was also 2.4 fold higher in CKD populations following hip fractures when compared to general population [99]. There are several causes for bone loss in CKD patients including traditional risk factors that apply to general populations like age, gender, chronic illness, low body mass index and factors that are specific to uremia and its treatment. Factors specific to CKD, including but not limited to: longer time on dialysis, metabolic bone disease, PTH concentrations (lower concentrations associated with higher risk of fractures), β2 microglobulin-related amyloidosis, aluminum intoxication, hypogonadism, avascular necrosis, and chronic acidosis [100-102].

The Kidney Disease: Improving Global Outcomes (KDIGO) guidelines in 2017 recommends the use of dual energy x-ray absorptiometry to assess fracture risk in patients with CKD-MBD and/or risk factors for osteoporosis [97]. World health organization T score can also be used for fracture risk classification as several longitudinal studies demonstrated that T scores performed similarly in patients with or without CKD [103-106]. Bone biopsy is the gold standard for assessment of renal osteodystrophy, and is recommended in patients when there are questions about the type of bone disease amongst other indications. In contrast to the 2009 KDIGO guidelines, in 2017 the requirement for bone biopsy prior to the initiation of anti-resorptive therapy was removed [56]. This was likely due to limited centers experienced in performing bone biopsies, along with growing evidence that antiresorptive therapies are effective in patients with CKD G3a to G3b and G4. However, it is advised that the underlying renal osteodystrophy be addressed first [56].

The first step in treatment of CKD-associated osteoporosis is management of CKD-MBD through addressing vitamin D deficiency, hyperphosphatemia, and hyperparathyroidism. 25-hydroxyvitamin D concentration of >30 ng/ml has been shown to optimize mineralization in patients with ESRD [107]. In a study of dialysis patients, cinacalcet not only reduced PTH concentrations and bone formation rate but effectively normalized bone histology in a portion of the population by study completion [108]. Non-pharmacologic strategies which has proven benefit in osteoporosis should be adapted for all patients irrespective of their CKD status; these include appropriate calcium and vitamin D supplementation, smoking cessation, weight-bearing exercise, fall prevention, improved nutrition and moderating alcohol intake [109].

Pharmacological management aimed at treating osteoporosis includes anti-resorptive agents and anabolic agents. Anti-resorptive agents, which inhibit osteoclast-mediated bone resorption, may be helpful in preventing bone loss and fracture in patients with normal to high-turnover bone disease. They comprise of calcitonin, estrogens, selective estrogen receptor modulators, bisphosphonates and denosumab. Bisphosphonates, cleared mainly by the kidneys, are avoided in adynamic or low-turnover bone disease and in eGFR <30 ml/min due to excessive accumulation and resultant over suppression of bone remodeling. Intravenous bisphosphonates, especially zoledronic acid, can cause a tubular lesion mimicking acute tubular necrosis and is possibly related to the dose and rate of administration [110-112]. Some studies have suggested their safety in eGFR ranging from 15-59 ml/min per 1.73 m^2 when the kidney dysfunction is due to age-related factors and without CKD-MBD [109, 113]. The use of bisphosphonates in CKD stages 4, 5 would be an off-label use and if given should be administered very slowly (e.g., over 60 minutes) [112]. Denosumab is a monoclonal antibody against receptor activator of NF-kB ligand, and not cleared by kidneys hence can be used safely in CKD without concern for accumulation. The main adverse effect is hypocalcemia with a reactive increase in PTH, requiring post-treatment, close monitoring, and management with vitamin D and calcium supplementation, and high-calcium dialysate bath [114-116]. Osteoanabolic agents are forms of recombinant PTH or PTH-related peptide. These agents increased bone turnover and BMD in adynamic or low-bone turnover disease, and should be avoided in high bone-turnover disease from hyperparathyroidism [109]. Teriparatide is the first FDA approved osteoanabolic agent and has been found to be both safe across CKD populations and efficacious in terms of improving bone mineral densities [117-119]. Abaloparatide is a newer parathyroid hormone-related peptide analog and is believed to be more anabolic that teriparatide, but has not yet been studied in patients with CKD [109]. Finally, romosozumab, a monoclonal antibody to sclerostin, is a new anabolic agent that is an effective anabolic treatment, but also has not yet been evaluated in patients with CKD [109].

Extraskeletal Calcification

Vascular Calcification

It has been well established that cardiovascular mortality is the leading cause of death in CKD population [120]. Since the presence of traditional risk factors such as hypertension, aging, smoking, diabetes, and abnormal lipid metabolism does not fully explain the propensity of cardiovascular disease, the presence of other pathophysiology contributing to this has been postulated [121, 122]. Many studies have shown that a high percentage of patients with CKD had vascular calcifications stressing its impact on the high morbidity and mortality in this population [123, 124].

Vascular calcification is defined as the inappropriate and pathological deposition of mineral in the form of calcium phosphate salts into the vascular tissues [125]. There are 2 distinct types of vascular calcifications based on their location and association with atherosclerotic plaque formation. One affects intimal layer and occurs within atherosclerotic plaques. The other affects the medial layer. The consequences of the 2 types of the calcification differ [126]. The intimal lesions compromise the lumen of the arteries and block the blood supply during advanced stages. These atherosclerotic lesions are associated with disturbances in lipid metabolism, inflammation, and cellular necrosis [126, 127]. Atherosclerotic calcification is patchy and discontinuous, seen more prominently in larger, more mature lesions. The calcium content in the atherosclerotic lesions is greater in patients undergoing dialysis compared to people of same age with normal renal function [128]. As lesions progress, osteogenesis, which includes osteoblast induction and lamellar bone formation, occurs [129]. The second type of calcification, medial wall calcification or Mönkeberg's sclerosis, is commonly seen in patients with CKD and diabetes mellitus. Here mineral deposition occurs throughout tunica media, which is rich in elastic collagen and results in increased vascular stiffness, reduction in vessel compliance, rise in systolic blood pressure leading to left ventricular hypertrophy and reduced coronary artery blood flow during diastole [126, 130].

Traditionally, vascular calcification was thought to be a passive process with elevated serum phosphate and deposition of calcium-phosphate product resulting from over saturated plasma [55, 131, 132]. While dysregulation of calcium and phosphorus metabolism does play a critical role, recent studies have shown that calcification is more of an active and complex process resembling skeletal bone formation, with key regulators of bone formation and bone structural proteins expressed in both calcified medial arterial layers and atherosclerotic plaques [129].

Pathophysiology of Vascular Calcification

Phenotypic changes in the vascular smooth muscle cells- Ectopic vascular calcification formation closely resembles the physiologic bone formation. Vascular smooth muscle cells (VSMCs) are of mesenchymal origin and under stress can differentiate into different mesenchymal cells like osteoblasts, chondrocytes or adipocytes. At the sites of calcification, VSMCs undergo phenotypical change and become similar to bone formative cells. Then there is a downregulation of smooth muscle specific genes such as smooth muscle (SM) α-actin and SM22α [125]. Simultaneously, these cells upregulate expression of mineralization-regulating proteins that are normally confined to bone and cartilage [133, 134]. These proteins include RUNX Family Transcription Factor 2 (RUNX2), Osterix, MSX2, and SRY-BOX transcription Factor-9 (SOX9), that induce differentiation of VSMCs to an osteochondrocytic phenotype [135, 136]. VSMCs are able to produce matrix vesicles, which under normal circumstances, contain mineralization inhibitors such as matrix γ-carboxy glutamic acid protein (MGP) and Fetuin-A [137]. Coupled with high extracellular calcium and low concentration of mineralization inhibitors, matrix vesicles serve as nucleation sites for hydroxyapatite [138,

139]. The source of phosphorus to potentiate the crystal growth is supplied by alkaline phosphatase contained in the vesicles [140]. RUNX2 is a crucial component for transdifferentiation of VSMCs, in the absence of which the morphological change and mineralization does not occur [125].

Elastin Degradation

Elastin is abundant in the aortic wall. In animal studies, elastin breakdown in the setting of uremia and high calcium-phosphate milieu increases risk of calcification of VSMCs [141]. Matrix metalloproteinases (MMP), specifically MMP-2 and MMP-9, are upregulated in CKD and degrade elastin [142]. This degradation of elastin induces overexpression of TGF-β, which are involved in osteoblast differentiation and also accelerates calcification of VSMCs [142].

Abnormal Calcium and Phosphate Balance

The uremic environment contains numerous factors which allows for initiation and progression of vascular calcification. *In vitro* and animal models demonstrated that initiation of calcification requires increased uptake of calcium and phosphate by VSMCs. Phosphate entry occurs via sodium dependent phosphate co-transporters, PiT-1 and PiT-2 [144]. Calcium uptake by VSMCs is regulated by CaSR and voltage-gated calcium channels. *In vitro* exposure of VSMCs to high extracellular calcium can downregulate CaSR [145]. Loss of CaSR can lead to increase in VSMC calcification while use of calcimimetics can ameliorate calcification [146].

Influence of Uremic Toxins

Uremia upregulates the expression of RUNX2 and its target protein, osteopontin (OPN), independent of serum phosphate concentration. Bone morphogenic protein-2 (BMP-2), crucial in signaling related to transcriptional activity of RUNX2 and osteoblastic transformation of VSMCs, is also increased under uremic conditions. Thus, compared to non-uremic individuals, the uremic serum promotes mineralization of VSMCs [147, 148].

Inhibitors of Ectopic Osteochondrogenic Mineralization

In addition to ectopic osteogenesis, the lack of inhibitors of calcification play an important role behind vascular calcification. Matrix γ-Carboxyglutamic Acid Protein (MGP) is a mineral-binding protein that is dependent on vitamin K for γ-carboxylation for it to be fully functional [149]. MGP binds BMP-2 to mediate the osteoblastic differentiation of VSMCs and inhibits the activity of BMP-2 in the differentiation of mesenchymal cells [150]. MGP also binds to calcium crystals and inhibits crystal growth [151]. Hence MGP has a role in maintaining the normal phenotype of VSMCs and in preventing their osteoblastic differentiation. The consequence of warfarin treatment to increase the risk of calcific uremic arteriolopathy could be related to disturbance of MGP functions [129].

Osteopontin

Normally found in bones and teeth, acts by inhibiting apatite crystals and promoting osteoclast function [152]. *In vivo* animal studies with OPN null mice did not spontaneously calcify, but calcification seemed to be synergistically enhanced when these mice were bred with MGP null mice [153]. OPN is normally not found within vasculature, but observed in high concentration in calcified arteries potentially to counteract the calcification process [154].

Osteoprotegerin (OPG)

Produced by osteoblasts and other cell types, including arterial cell wall, acts a potent inhibitor of osteoclast differentiation. OPG serves as a decoy receptor and binds to RANKL preventing this ligand from binding to its receptor, RANK [155]. Numerous mouse models deficient in OPG has shown progressive vascular calcification [156, 157].

Fetuin-A

Produced primarily in the liver is a glycoprotein that binds calcium ions and hydroxyapatite. Unlike MGP, OPN, and OPG, which are all local factors, fetuin-A is a circulating inhibitor of vascular calcification. As previously mentioned, matrix vesicles from VSMCs become the nidus of mineral nucleation. VSMCs can take up the serum fetuin-A into its matrix vesicles and repeal the ability of the vesicles to form hydroxyapatite crystals [137].

Pyrophosphate (PPi)

Another important inhibitor of hydroxyapatite formation, is normally produced in the VSMCs by hydrolysis of nucleotide triphosphates by nucleotide pyrophosphatase phosphodiesterase family (NPP), especially by NPP-1. Inactivation of NPP-1 can lead to medial layer calcification due to lack of PPi, seen in idiopathic infantile arterial calcification [158, 159].

Role of FGF 23-Klotho

As previously discussed, FGF-23 regulates phosphate homeostasis and suppresses 1,25-dihydroxyvitamin D synthesis in the kidney acting via klotho. In animal studies, lack of FGF-23 or klotho caused medial vascular calcification [160]. It has been shown that FGF-23 and Klotho are present on VSMCs [161]. Increased expression of the sodium-phosphate co-transporters, Pit1/2 and Runx2 were noted in Klotho deficient animals. This suggests that absence of Klotho promotes phosphate uptake by VSMCs and progression of osteochondrocytic differentiation [161].

Role of Vitamin D

VDRAs are widely used for treatment of secondary hyperparathyroidism; however, there is conflicting data regarding their effects on the vasculature. VSMCs express the VDR and also possess CYP27A1 (25-hydroxylase) and CYP27B1, hence vitamin D can be utilized in an autocrine/paracrine fashion [162]. 1,25-dihydroxyvitamin D upregulates VDR expression in VSMCs and VDR activation is known to modulate cellular proliferation and differentiation. VDRAs encourage calcification by upregulation of RUNX2, osterix, and osteocalcin, and by increasing calcium influx into the VSMCs [163-165]. In contrast, several studies have also demonstrated the increase in calcification inhibitory factors like MGP and osteopontin by vitamin D [166]. FGF-23, as previously mentioned, also plays a vital role in vitamin D regulation since it can downregulate the renal CYP27B1, thereby reducing 1,25-dihydroxyvitamin D production as well as increases CYP24, resulting in inactivation of 1,25-dihydroxyvitamin D [17, 18].

The animal models of CKD in which calcitriol administration resulted in vascular calcification were performed with supra-therapeutic doses [163, 164]. Hence it's been suggested that with the usage of therapeutic doses, in order to suppress PTH without systemic hypercalcemia and hyperphosphatemia, vascular calcification might not occur [167]. However, in uremic animal models, VDRAs had differential effects on calcification. Compared to paricalcitol, doxercalciferol induced substantial vascular calcification, possibly due to the effects of doxercalciferol on increasing calcium phosphate product and induction of RUNX2 and osteocalcin, promoting osteoblastic differentiation [164, 168]. In the general population, low serum 1,25-dihydroxyvitamin D has been associated with increased risk of vascular calcification [169]. Several observational studies have noted a survival benefit in CKD with the use of vitamin D analogs, which is independent of serum calcium, phosphate, and PTH concentrations [170-174]. Clinical and *in vitro* studies have also shown that low and high vitamin D concentrations have abnormal vascular effects suggesting a bimodal association between vitamin D and vascular measures [175, 176]. Further investigation is required to determine the optimal VDRA and dosing for CKD patients.

Calciphylaxis

Calciphylaxis or calcific uremic arteriolopathy (CUA) is characterized by vascular calcification causing occlusion of microvessels in the subcutaneous adipose and dermis that results in intensely painful ischemic lesions [177]. Typically seen in ESRD, it has an annual incidence rate of 35 cases per 10,000 patients undergoing dialysis in the US [178]. This disorder can also been seen in early stages of CKD, acute kidney injury or post kidney transplant [179-181].

Clinical manifestations include severe painful skin lesions including livedo reticularis, reticulate purpura, violaceous plaques, or indurated nodules, which show poor healing and are complicated by ulcerations with secondary infections [182]. Sepsis from the resultant wounds is considered a common cause of death apart from progressive renal failure, myocardial infarction, and multiorgan failure [183, 184]. Calciphylaxis can be classified as uremic (in patients with ESRD) or non-uremic (in patients with normal renal function or earlier stages of CKD); central (example in abdomen or thighs) or peripheral (limited to peripheral sites like digits); non-ulcerated or ulcerated (seen in later stages) [177]. Patients with uremic calciphylaxis have mostly central distribution of lesions and also a worse prognosis compared to non-uremic calciphylaxis, possibly due to differences in co-existing conditions [178, 185].

The exact mechanism of pathogenesis remains unclear. Elevated calcium and phosphate product is associated with increased risk along with obesity, diabetes mellitus, hyperparathyroidism, and warfarin use [177]. It was observed that approximately 45% of patients on dialysis who presented with CUA had PTH concentrations below recommended target range. This suggested the overzealous use of calcium and vitamin D analogues, leading to adynamic bone disease, which can exacerbate extraskeletal calcium deposition [90, 179]. Warfarin, or vitamin K antagonist, use has been attributed to be a major risk factor for CUA with about 40-50% of patients with CUA who had been treated with warfarin [179, 186]. This is likely from inhibition of carboxylation of MGP, a vitamin K dependent process [149].

Diagnosis is primarily made clinically, and even though biopsy is the standard method of confirmation, its utility is up for significant debate in routine clinical practice due to concern for development of non-healing ulcers and infections [187]. Supportive care includes pain control and wound care. Wound debridement is useful in removing necrotic tissues and preventing infections. However, not all patients can tolerate wound debridement due to pain and concerns of wound healing. Hence the decision for debridement should be made on a case-by-case basis. In a retrospective study involving 64 patients with CUA, operative debridement suggested improved survival among patients [184]. Hyperbaric oxygen therapy can be used as an adjunct to aid wound healing. In a retrospective study with 34 patients, mainly with peripheral lesions, who underwent treatment with hyperbaric oxygen therapy, 58% showed improved wound scores with more than half of these patients showing complete wound healing [188]. Correction of hypercalcemia and hyperphosphatemia is of vital importance. In ESRD patients, increasing the length or frequency of dialysis sessions might help in controlling both phosphorus and calcium as well as with wound healing [189].

The primary pharmacological modality used in treatment of CUA is sodium thiosulfate, and a typical dose is 25 g in 100 ml of solution given intravenously thrice weekly during the last 30 to 60 minutes of hemodialysis. The beneficial effects of this medication has been attributed to its antioxidant, vasodilatory properties along with inhibition of adipocyte calcification and blockage of the ability of adipocytes to induce calcification of vascular smooth muscle cells [190, 191]. Several retrospective studies have shown beneficial effect, but randomized control trials are still ongoing [192, 193]. Adverse effects include nausea, hypotension, volume overload, QT prolongation, hypocalcemia, and metabolic acidosis. An intralesional approach can potentially avoid the side effects and has been suggested via case reports for patients with early and limited disease [194].

Early intervention should be considered once the diagnosis of CUA is being suspected and supportive measures including discontinuing vitamin K antagonist should be considered. The treatment modalities should be considered on a case-by-case basis with a clear understanding of the limitations of the available data.

CONCLUSION

The hormonal systems (FGF-23, Vit D, PTH) are tightly regulated by several feedback mechanisms to maintain the bone and mineral homeostasis. There has been increasing awareness about the role played by mineral and bone disorder contributing to cardiovascular mortality. Goal of therapy should include early intervention in CKD patients in order to prevent progression of bone disease and complications attributed to extraskeletal and vascular calcification. Currently, the employed methods for achieving target goals include dietary modification, frequent laboratory monitoring, and pharmacological interventions. However, there is still a great deal of knowledge to acquire regarding the timely diagnosis of the mineral and bone disorders. The success of the current therapeutic interventions require further controlled clinical studies.

REFERENCES

[1] Moe S, Drueke T, Cunningham J, Goodman W, Martin K, Olgaard K, et al. Definition, evaluation, and classification of renal osteodystrophy: a position statement from Kidney Disease: Improving Global Outcomes (KDIGO). *Kidney Int.* 2006;69(11):1945-53.

[2] Blau JE, Collins MT. The PTH-Vitamin D-FGF23 axis. *Rev Endocr Metab Disord.* 2015;16(2):165-74.

[3] Slatopolsky E, Delmez JA. Pathogenesis of secondary hyperparathyroidism. *Nephrol Dial Transplant.* 1996;11 Suppl 3:130-5.

[4] Kalantar-Zadeh K, Shah A, Duong U, Hechter RC, Dukkipati R, Kovesdy CP. Kidney bone disease and mortality in CKD: revisiting the role of vitamin D, calcimimetics, alkaline phosphatase, and minerals. *Kidney Int Suppl.* 2010(117):S10-21.

[5] Naveh-Many T, Rahamimov R, Livni N, Silver J. Parathyroid cell proliferation in normal and chronic renal failure rats. The effects of calcium, phosphate, and vitamin D. *J Clin Invest.* 1995;96(4):1786-93.

[6] Bergwitz C, Juppner H. Regulation of phosphate homeostasis by PTH, vitamin D, and FGF23. *Annu Rev Med.* 2010;61:91-104.

[7] Esbrit P, Alcaraz MJ. Current perspectives on parathyroid hormone (PTH) and PTH-related protein (PTHrP) as bone anabolic therapies. *Biochem Pharmacol.* 2013;85 (10):1417-23.

[8] Andress DL, Coyne DW, Kalantar-Zadeh K, Molitch ME, Zangeneh F, Sprague SM. Management of secondary hyperparathyroidism in stages 3 and 4 chronic kidney disease. *Endocr Pract.* 2008;14(1):18-27.

[9] Brown EM, Hebert SC. A cloned Ca(2+)-sensing receptor: a mediator of direct effects of extracellular Ca2+ on renal function? *J Am Soc Nephrol.* 1995;6(6):1530-40.

[10] Hruska KA, Choi ET, Memon I, Davis TK, Mathew S. Cardiovascular risk in chronic kidney disease (CKD): the CKD-mineral bone disorder (CKD-MBD). *Pediatr Nephrol.* 2010;25(4):769-78.

[11] Nechama M, Ben-Dov IZ, Silver J, Naveh-Many T. Regulation of PTH mRNA stability by the calcimimetic R568 and the phosphorus binder lanthanum carbonate in CKD. *Am J Physiol Renal Physiol.* 2009;296(4):F795-800.

[12] Delmez JA, Tindira C, Grooms P, Dusso A, Windus DW, Slatopolsky E. Parathyroid hormone suppression by intravenous 1,25-dihydroxyvitamin D. A role for increased sensitivity to calcium. *J Clin Invest.* 1989;83(4):1349-55.

[13] Ritter CS, Brown AJ. Direct suppression of Pth gene expression by the vitamin D prohormones doxercalciferol and calcidiol requires the vitamin D receptor. *J Mol Endocrinol.* 2011;46(2):63-6.

[14] Ben-Dov IZ, Galitzer H, Lavi-Moshayoff V, Goetz R, Kuro-o M, Mohammadi M, et al. The parathyroid is a target organ for FGF23 in rats. *J Clin Invest.* 2007;117(12): 4003-8.

[15] Komaba H, Fukagawa M. FGF23-parathyroid interaction: implications in chronic kidney disease. *Kidney Int.* 2010;77(4):292-8.

[16] Yamashita T, Yoshioka M, Itoh N. Identification of a novel fibroblast growth factor, FGF-23, preferentially expressed in the ventrolateral thalamic nucleus of the brain. *Biochem Biophys Res Commun.* 2000;277(2):494-8.

[17] Shimada T, Hasegawa H, Yamazaki Y, Muto T, Hino R, Takeuchi Y, et al. FGF-23 is a potent regulator of vitamin D metabolism and phosphate homeostasis. *J Bone Miner Res.* 2004;19(3):429-35.

[18] Shimada T, Yamazaki Y, Takahashi M, Hasegawa H, Urakawa I, Oshima T, et al. Vitamin D receptor-independent FGF23 actions in regulating phosphate and vitamin D metabolism. *Am J Physiol Renal Physiol.* 2005;289(5):F1088-95.

[19] Yamazaki Y, Okazaki R, Shibata M, Hasegawa Y, Satoh K, Tajima T, et al. Increased circulatory level of biologically active full-length FGF-23 in patients with

hypophosphatemic rickets/osteomalacia. *J Clin Endocrinol Metab*. 2002;87(11):4957-60.

[20] Isakova T, Gutierrez OM, Wolf M. A blueprint for randomized trials targeting phosphorus metabolism in chronic kidney disease. *Kidney Int*. 2009;76(7):705-16.

[21] Consortium A. Autosomal dominant hypophosphataemic rickets is associated with mutations in FGF23. *Nat Genet*. 2000;26(3):345-8.

[22] Shimada T, Mizutani S, Muto T, Yoneya T, Hino R, Takeda S, et al. Cloning and characterization of FGF23 as a causative factor of tumor-induced osteomalacia. *Proc Natl Acad Sci USA*. 2001;98(11):6500-5.

[23] Larsson T, Marsell R, Schipani E, Ohlsson C, Ljunggren O, Tenenhouse HS, et al. Transgenic mice expressing fibroblast growth factor 23 under the control of the alpha1(I) collagen promoter exhibit growth retardation, osteomalacia, and disturbed phosphate homeostasis. *Endocrinology*. 2004;145(7):3087-94.

[24] Shimada T, Kakitani M, Yamazaki Y, Hasegawa H, Takeuchi Y, Fujita T, et al. Targeted ablation of Fgf23 demonstrates an essential physiological role of FGF23 in phosphate and vitamin D metabolism. *J Clin Invest*. 2004;113(4):561-8.

[25] Sitara D, Razzaque MS, Hesse M, Yoganathan S, Taguchi T, Erben RG, et al. Homozygous ablation of fibroblast growth factor-23 results in hyperphosphatemia and impaired skeletogenesis, and reverses hypophosphatemia in Phex-deficient mice. *Matrix Biol*. 2004;23(7):421-32.

[26] Benet-Pages A, Orlik P, Strom TM, Lorenz-Depiereux B. An FGF23 missense mutation causes familial tumoral calcinosis with hyperphosphatemia. *Hum Mol Genet*. 2005;14(3):385-90.

[27] Goetz R, Beenken A, Ibrahimi OA, Kalinina J, Olsen SK, Eliseenkova AV, et al. Molecular insights into the klotho-dependent, endocrine mode of action of fibroblast growth factor 19 subfamily members. *Mol Cell Biol*. 2007;27(9):3417-28.

[28] Yamazaki Y, Tamada T, Kasai N, Urakawa I, Aono Y, Hasegawa H, et al. Anti-FGF23 neutralizing antibodies show the physiological role and structural features of FGF23. *J Bone Miner Res*. 2008;23(9):1509-18.

[29] Leunissen EH, Nair AV, Bull C, Lefeber DJ, van Delft FL, Bindels RJ, et al. The epithelial calcium channel TRPV5 is regulated differentially by klotho and sialidase. *J Biol Chem*. 2013;288(41):29238-46.

[30] Chang Q, Hoefs S, van der Kemp AW, Topala CN, Bindels RJ, Hoenderop JG. The beta-glucuronidase klotho hydrolyzes and activates the TRPV5 channel. *Science*. 2005;310(5747):490-3.

[31] Hu MC, Kuro-o M, Moe OW. Klotho and chronic kidney disease. *Contrib Nephrol*. 2013;180:47-63.

[32] Gutierrez O, Isakova T, Rhee E, Shah A, Holmes J, Collerone G, et al. Fibroblast growth factor-23 mitigates hyperphosphatemia but accentuates calcitriol deficiency in chronic kidney disease. *J Am Soc Nephrol*. 2005;16(7):2205-15.

[33] Lavi-Moshayoff V, Wasserman G, Meir T, Silver J, Naveh-Many T. PTH increases FGF23 gene expression and mediates the high-FGF23 levels of experimental kidney failure: a bone parathyroid feedback loop. *Am J Physiol Renal Physiol*. 2010;299(4): F882-9.

[34] Burnett-Bowie SM, Henao MP, Dere ME, Lee H, Leder BZ. Effects of hPTH(1-34) infusion on circulating serum phosphate, 1,25-dihydroxyvitamin D, and FGF23 levels in healthy men. *J Bone Miner Res*. 2009;24(10):1681-5.

[35] Bhan I, Shah A, Holmes J, Isakova T, Gutierrez O, Burnett SM, et al. Post-transplant hypophosphatemia: Tertiary 'Hyper-Phosphatoninism'? *Kidney Int*. 2006;70(8):1486-94.

[36] Evenepoel P, Naesens M, Claes K, Kuypers D, Vanrenterghem Y. Tertiary 'hyperphosphatoninism' accentuates hypophosphatemia and suppresses calcitriol levels in renal transplant recipients. *Am J Transplant*. 2007;7(5):1193-200.

[37] Liu N, Nguyen L, Chun RF, Lagishetty V, Ren S, Wu S, et al. Altered endocrine and autocrine metabolism of vitamin D in a mouse model of gastrointestinal inflammation. *Endocrinology*. 2008;149(10):4799-808.

[38] Latus J, Lehmann R, Roesel M, Fritz P, Braun N, Ulmer C, et al. Analysis of alpha-klotho, fibroblast growth factor-, vitamin-D and calcium-sensing receptor in 70 patients with secondary hyperparathyroidism. *Kidney Blood Press Res*. 2013;37(1):84-94.

[39] Renkema KY, Velic A, Dijkman HB, Verkaart S, van der Kemp AW, Nowik M, et al. The calcium-sensing receptor promotes urinary acidification to prevent nephrolithiasis. *J Am Soc Nephrol*. 2009;20(8):1705-13.

[40] Xue Y, Xiao Y, Liu J, Karaplis AC, Pollak MR, Brown EM, et al. The calcium-sensing receptor complements parathyroid hormone-induced bone turnover in discrete skeletal compartments in mice. *Am J Physiol Endocrinol Metab*. 2012;302(7):E841-51.

[41] Slatopolsky E, Brown A, Dusso A. Pathogenesis of secondary hyperparathyroidism. *Kidney Int Suppl*. 1999;73:S14-9.

[42] Nakanishi S, Kazama JJ, Nii-Kono T, Omori K, Yamashita T, Fukumoto S, et al. Serum fibroblast growth factor-23 levels predict the future refractory hyperparathyroidism in dialysis patients. *Kidney Int*. 2005;67(3):1171-8.

[43] Kazama JJ, Sato F, Omori K, Hama H, Yamamoto S, Maruyama H, et al. Pretreatment serum FGF-23 levels predict the efficacy of calcitriol therapy in dialysis patients. *Kidney Int*. 2005;67(3):1120-5.

[44] Kates DM, Sherrard DJ, Andress DL. Evidence that serum phosphate is independently associated with serum PTH in patients with chronic renal failure. *Am J Kidney Dis*. 1997;30(6):809-13.

[45] Pitts TO, Piraino BH, Mitro R, Chen TC, Segre GV, Greenberg A, et al. Hyperparathyroidism and 1,25-dihydroxyvitamin D deficiency in mild, moderate, and severe renal failure. *J Clin Endocrinol Metab*. 1988;67(5):876-81.

[46] Reichel H, Deibert B, Schmidt-Gayk H, Ritz E. Calcium metabolism in early chronic renal failure: implications for the pathogenesis of hyperparathyroidism. *Nephrol Dial Transplant*. 1991;6(3):162-9.

[47] Levin A, Bakris GL, Molitch M, Smulders M, Tian J, Williams LA, et al. Prevalence of abnormal serum vitamin D, PTH, calcium, and phosphorus in patients with chronic kidney disease: results of the study to evaluate early kidney disease. *Kidney Int*. 2007;71(1):31-8.

[48] Galitzer H, Ben-Dov IZ, Silver J, Naveh-Many T. Parathyroid cell resistance to fibroblast growth factor 23 in secondary hyperparathyroidism of chronic kidney disease. *Kidney Int*. 2010;77(3):211-8.

[49] Canalejo R, Canalejo A, Martinez-Moreno JM, Rodriguez-Ortiz ME, Estepa JC, Mendoza FJ, et al. FGF23 fails to inhibit uremic parathyroid glands. *J Am Soc Nephrol.* 2010;21(7):1125-35.

[50] Komaba H, Goto S, Fujii H, Hamada Y, Kobayashi A, Shibuya K, et al. Depressed expression of Klotho and FGF receptor 1 in hyperplastic parathyroid glands from uremic patients. *Kidney Int.* 2010;77(3):232-8.

[51] Parfitt AM. The hyperparathyroidism of chronic renal failure: a disorder of growth. *Kidney Int*. 1997;52(1):3-9.

[52] Slatopolsky E, Finch J, Denda M, Ritter C, Zhong M, Dusso A, et al. Phosphorus restriction prevents parathyroid gland growth. High phosphorus directly stimulates PTH secretion in vitro. *J Clin Invest. 1996;97(11):2534-40.*

[53] *Cunningham J, Locatelli F,* Rodriguez M. Secondary hyperparathyroidism: pathogenesis, disease progression, and therapeutic options. *Clin J Am Soc Nephrol.* 2011;6(4):913-21.

[54] Block GA, Hulbert-Shearon TE, Levin NW, Port FK. Association of serum phosphorus and calcium x phosphate product with mortality risk in chronic hemodialysis patients: a national study. *Am J Kidney Dis*. 1998;31(4):607-17.

[55] Ganesh SK, Stack AG, Levin NW, Hulbert-Shearon T, Port FK. Association of elevated serum PO(4), Ca x PO(4) product, and parathyroid hormone with cardiac mortality risk in chronic hemodialysis patients. *J Am Soc Nephrol*. 2001;12(10):2131-8.

[56] Kidney Disease: Improving Global Outcomes CKDMBDUWG. KDIGO 2017 Clinical Practice Guideline Update for the Diagnosis, Evaluation, Prevention, and Treatment of Chronic Kidney Disease-Mineral and Bone Disorder (CKD-MBD). *Kidney Int Suppl* (2011). 2017;7(1):1-59.

[57] Cozzolino M, Lu Y, Finch J, Slatopolsky E, Dusso AS. p21WAF1 and TGF-alpha mediate parathyroid growth arrest by vitamin D and high calcium. *Kidney Int.* 2001;60(6):2109-17.

[58] Dusso A, Cozzolino M, Lu Y, Sato T, Slatopolsky E. 1,25-Dihydroxyvitamin D downregulation of TGFalpha/EGFR expression and growth signaling: a mechanism for the antiproliferative actions of the sterol in parathyroid hyperplasia of renal failure. *J Steroid Biochem Mol Biol*. 2004;89-90(1-5):507-11.

[59] Silver J, Naveh-Many T, Mayer H, Schmelzer HJ, Popovtzer MM. Regulation by vitamin D metabolites of parathyroid hormone gene transcription in vivo in the rat. *J Clin Invest*. 1986;78(5):1296-301.

[60] Brown AJ, Zhong M, Finch J, Ritter C, McCracken R, Morrissey J, et al. Rat calcium-sensing receptor is regulated by vitamin D but not by calcium. *Am J Physiol*. 1996;270(3 Pt 2):F454-60.

[61] Brown AJ, Dusso AS, Slatopolsky E. Vitamin D analogues for secondary hyperparathyroidism. *Nephrol Dial Transplant*. 2002;17 Suppl 10:10-9.

[62] Walling MW. Intestinal Ca and phosphate transport: differential responses to vitamin D3 metabolites. *Am J Physiol*. 1977;233(6):E488-94.

[63] Rodriguez M, Caravaca F, Fernandez E, Borrego MJ, Lorenzo V, Cubero J, et al. Parathyroid function as a determinant of the response to calcitriol treatment in the hemodialysis patient. *Kidney Int*. 1999;56(1):306-17.

[64] Fukagawa M, Kitaoka M, Yi H, Fukuda N, Matsumoto T, Ogata E, et al. Serial evaluation of parathyroid size by ultrasonography is another useful marker for the long-

term prognosis of calcitriol pulse therapy in chronic dialysis patients. *Nephron.* 1994;68(2):221-8.

[65] Tominaga Y, Kohara S, Namii Y, Nagasaka T, Haba T, Uchida K, et al. Clonal analysis of nodular parathyroid hyperplasia in renal hyperparathyroidism. *World J Surg.* 1996;20(7):744-50; discussion 50-2.

[66] Fukuda N, Tanaka H, Tominaga Y, Fukagawa M, Kurokawa K, Seino Y. Decreased 1,25-dihydroxyvitamin D3 receptor density is associated with a more severe form of parathyroid hyperplasia in chronic uremic patients. *J Clin Invest.* 1993;92(3):1436-43.

[67] Block GA, Raggi P, Bellasi A, Kooienga L, Spiegel DM. Mortality effect of coronary calcification and phosphate binder choice in incident hemodialysis patients. *Kidney Int.* 2007;71(5):438-41.

[68] Hou SH, Zhao J, Ellman CF, Hu J, Griffin Z, Spiegel DM, et al. Calcium and phosphorus fluxes during hemodialysis with low calcium dialysate. *Am J Kidney Dis.* 1991;18(2):217-24.

[69] Meric F, Yap P, Bia MJ. Etiology of hypercalcemia in hemodialysis patients on calcium carbonate therapy. *Am J Kidney Dis.* 1990;16(5):459-64.

[70] Bleyer AJ, Burke SK, Dillon M, Garrett B, Kant KS, Lynch D, et al. A comparison of the calcium-free phosphate binder sevelamer hydrochloride with calcium acetate in the treatment of hyperphosphatemia in hemodialysis patients. *Am J Kidney Dis.* 1999;33 (4):694-701.

[71] Cunningham J, Floege J, London G, Rodriguez M, Shanahan CM. Clinical outcomes in secondary hyperparathyroidism and the potential role of calcimimetics. *NDT Plus.* 2008;1(Suppl 1):i29-i35.

[72] Colloton M, Shatzen E, Miller G, Stehman-Breen C, Wada M, Lacey D, et al. Cinacalcet HCl attenuates parathyroid hyperplasia in a rat model of secondary hyperparathyroidism. *Kidney Int.* 2005;67(2):467-76.

[73] Block GA, Zeig S, Sugihara J, Chertow GM, Chi EM, Turner SA, et al. Combined therapy with cinacalcet and low doses of vitamin D sterols in patients with moderate to severe secondary hyperparathyroidism. *Nephrol Dial Transplant.* 2008;23(7):2311-8.

[74] Jamal SA, Miller PD. Secondary and tertiary hyperparathyroidism. *J Clin Densitom.* 2013;16(1):64-8.

[75] Gilat H, Feinmesser R, Vinkler Y, Morgenstern S, Shvero J, Bachar G, et al. Clinical and operative management of persistent hyperparathyroidism after renal transplantation: a single-center experience. *Head Neck.* 2007;29(11):996-1001.

[76] Schlosser K, Endres N, Celik I, Fendrich V, Rothmund M, Fernandez ED. Surgical treatment of tertiary hyperparathyroidism: the choice of procedure matters! *World J Surg.* 2007;31(10):1947-53.

[77] Hsieh TM, Sun CK, Chen YT, Chou FF. Total parathyroidectomy versus subtotal parathyroidectomy in the treatment of tertiary hyperparathyroidism. *Am Surg.* 2012;78(5):600-6.

[78] Sadideen HM, Taylor JD, Goldsmith DJ. Total parathyroidectomy without autotransplantation after renal transplantation for tertiary hyperparathyroidism: long-term follow-up. *Int Urol Nephrol.* 2012;44(1):275-81.

[79] Moe SM. Vascular calcification and renal osteodystrophy relationship in chronic kidney disease. *Eur J Clin Invest.* 2006;36 Suppl 2:51-62.

[80] Hruska KA, Teitelbaum SL. Renal osteodystrophy. *N Engl J Med.* 1995;333(3):166-74.

[81] Sprague SM. The role of the bone biopsy in the diagnosis of renal osteodystrophy. *Semin Dial.* 2000;13(3):152-5.

[82] Coen G, Mazzaferro S, Ballanti P, Sardella D, Chicca S, Manni M, et al. Renal bone disease in 76 patients with varying degrees of predialysis chronic renal failure: a cross-sectional study. *Nephrol Dial Transplant.* 1996;11(5):813-9.

[83] Pierides AM, Edwards WG, Jr., Cullum UX, Jr., McCall JT, Ellis HA. Hemodialysis encephalopathy with osteomalacic fractures and muscle weakness. *Kidney Int.* 1980; 18(1):115-24.

[84] Coen G, Manni M, Addari O, Ballanti P, Pasquali M, Chicca S, et al. Metabolic acidosis and osteodystrophic bone disease in predialysis chronic renal failure: effect of calcitriol treatment. *Miner Electrolyte Metab.* 1995;21(6):375-82.

[85] Elder G. Pathophysiology and recent advances in the management of renal osteodystrophy. *J Bone Miner Res.* 2002;17(12):2094-105.

[86] Dabbagh S. Renal osteodystrophy. *Curr Opin Pediatr.* 1998;10(2):190-6.

[87] Piraino B, Chen T, Cooperstein L, Segre G, Puschett J. Fractures and vertebral bone mineral density in patients with renal osteodystrophy. *Clin Nephrol.* 1988;30(2):57-62.

[88] Kurz P, Monier-Faugere MC, Bognar B, Werner E, Roth P, Vlachojannis J, et al. Evidence for abnormal calcium homeostasis in patients with adynamic bone disease. *Kidney Int.* 1994;46(3):855-61.

[89] Hutchison AJ, Whitehouse RW, Freemont AJ, Adams JE, Mawer EB, Gokal R. Histological, radiological, and biochemical features of the adynamic bone lesion in continuous ambulatory peritoneal dialysis patients. *Am J Nephrol.* 1994;14(1):19-29.

[90] Mawad HW, Sawaya BP, Sarin R, Malluche HH. Calcific uremic arteriolopathy in association with low turnover uremic bone disease. *Clin Nephrol.* 1999;52(3):160-6.

[91] Avram MM, Mittman N, Myint MM, Fein P. Importance of low serum intact parathyroid hormone as a predictor of mortality in hemodialysis and peritoneal dialysis patients: 14 years of prospective observation. *Am J Kidney Dis.* 2001;38(6):1351-7.

[92] Sprague SM, Bellorin-Font E, Jorgetti V, Carvalho AB, Malluche HH, Ferreira A, et al. Diagnostic Accuracy of Bone Turnover Markers and Bone Histology in Patients With CKD Treated by Dialysis. *Am J Kidney Dis.* 2016;67(4):559-66.

[93] Slatopolsky E, Weerts C, Norwood K, Giles K, Fryer P, Finch J, et al. Long-term effects of calcium carbonate and 2.5 mEq/liter calcium dialysate on mineral metabolism. *Kidney Int.* 1989;36(5):897-903.

[94] Hamdy NA, Kanis JA, Beneton MN, Brown CB, Juttmann JR, Jordans JG, et al. Effect of alfacalcidol on natural course of renal bone disease in mild to moderate renal failure. *BMJ.* 1995;310(6976):358-63.

[95] Zisman AL, Hristova M, Ho LT, Sprague SM. Impact of ergocalciferol treatment of vitamin D deficiency on serum parathyroid hormone concentrations in chronic kidney disease. *Am J Nephrol.* 2007;27(1):36-43.

[96] Sprague SM, Crawford PW, Melnick JZ, Strugnell SA, Ali S, Mangoo-Karim R, et al. Use of Extended-Release Calcifediol to Treat Secondary Hyperparathyroidism in Stages 3 and 4 Chronic Kidney Disease. *Am J Nephrol.* 2016;44(4):316-25.

[97] Ketteler M, Block GA, Evenepoel P, Fukagawa M, Herzog CA, McCann L, et al. Executive summary of the 2017 KDIGO Chronic Kidney Disease-Mineral and Bone Disorder (CKD-MBD) Guideline Update: what's changed and why it matters. *Kidney Int.* 2017;92(1):26-36.

[98] Atsumi K, Kushida K, Yamazaki K, Shimizu S, Ohmura A, Inoue T. Risk factors for vertebral fractures in renal osteodystrophy. *Am J Kidney Dis*. 1999;33(2):287-93.

[99] Coco M, Rush H. Increased incidence of hip fractures in dialysis patients with low serum parathyroid hormone. *Am J Kidney Dis*. 2000;36(6):1115-21.

[100] Stehman-Breen C. Osteoporosis and chronic kidney disease. *Semin Nephrol*. 2004;24(1):78-81.

[101] Stein MS, Packham DK, Ebeling PR, Wark JD, Becker GJ. Prevalence and risk factors for osteopenia in dialysis patients. *Am J Kidney Dis*. 1996;28(4):515-22.

[102] Alem AM, Sherrard DJ, Gillen DL, Weiss NS, Beresford SA, Heckbert SR, et al. Increased risk of hip fracture among patients with end-stage renal disease. *Kidney Int*. 2000;58(1):396-9.

[103] Yenchek RH, Ix JH, Shlipak MG, Bauer DC, Rianon NJ, Kritchevsky SB, et al. Bone mineral density and fracture risk in older individuals with CKD. *Clin J Am Soc Nephrol*. 2012;7(7):1130-6.

[104] Iimori S, Mori Y, Akita W, Kuyama T, Takada S, Asai T, et al. Diagnostic usefulness of bone mineral density and biochemical markers of bone turnover in predicting fracture in CKD stage 5D patients--a single-center cohort study. *Nephrol Dial Transplant*. 2012;27(1):345-51.

[105] West SL, Lok CE, Langsetmo L, Cheung AM, Szabo E, Pearce D, et al. Bone mineral density predicts fractures in chronic kidney disease. *J Bone Miner Res*. 2015;30(5): 913-9.

[106] Naylor KL, Garg AX, Zou G, Langsetmo L, Leslie WD, Fraser LA, et al. Comparison of fracture risk prediction among individuals with reduced and normal kidney function. *Clin J Am Soc Nephrol*. 2015;10(4):646-53.

[107] Coen G, Mantella D, Manni M, Balducci A, Nofroni I, Sardella D, et al. 25-hydroxyvitamin D levels and bone histomorphometry in hemodialysis renal osteodystrophy. *Kidney Int*. 2005;68(4):1840-8.

[108] Behets GJ, Spasovski G, Sterling LR, Goodman WG, Spiegel DM, De Broe ME, et al. Bone histomorphometry before and after long-term treatment with cinacalcet in dialysis patients with secondary hyperparathyroidism. *Kidney Int*. 2015;87(4):846-56.

[109] Khairallah P, Nickolas TL. Management of Osteoporosis in CKD. *Clin J Am Soc Nephrol*. 2018;13(6):962-9.

[110] Markowitz GS, Fine PL, Stack JI, Kunis CL, Radhakrishnan J, Palecki W, et al. Toxic acute tubular necrosis following treatment with zoledronate (Zometa). *Kidney Int*. 2003;64(1):281-9.

[111] Saad F, Gleason DM, Murray R, Tchekmedyian S, Venner P, Lacombe L, et al. A randomized, placebo-controlled trial of zoledronic acid in patients with hormone-refractory metastatic prostate carcinoma. *J Natl Cancer Inst*. 2002;94(19):1458-68.

[112] Miller PD. Bone disease in CKD: a focus on osteoporosis diagnosis and management. *Am J Kidney Dis*. 2014;64(2):290-304.

[113] Jamal SA, Bauer DC, Ensrud KE, Cauley JA, Hochberg M, Ishani A, et al. Alendronate treatment in women with normal to severely impaired renal function: an analysis of the fracture intervention trial. *J Bone Miner Res*. 2007;22(4):503-8.

[114] Block GA, Bone HG, Fang L, Lee E, Padhi D. A single-dose study of denosumab in patients with various degrees of renal impairment. *J Bone Miner Res*. 2012;27(7): 1471-9.

[115] Chen CL, Chen NC, Hsu CY, Chou KJ, Lee PT, Fang HC, et al. An open-label, prospective pilot clinical study of denosumab for severe hyperparathyroidism in patients with low bone mass undergoing dialysis. *J Clin Endocrinol Metab*. 2014;99(7):2426-32.

[116] Festuccia F, Jafari MT, Moioli A, Fofi C, Barberi S, Amendola S, et al. Safety and efficacy of denosumab in osteoporotic hemodialysed patients. *J Nephrol*. 2017; 30(2):271-9.

[117] Miller PD, Schwartz EN, Chen P, Misurski DA, Krege JH. Teriparatide in postmenopausal women with osteoporosis and mild or moderate renal impairment. *Osteoporos Int*. 2007;18(1):59-68.

[118] Cejka D, Kodras K, Bader T, Haas M. Treatment of Hemodialysis-Associated Adynamic Bone Disease with Teriparatide (PTH1-34): A Pilot Study. *Kidney Blood Press Res*. 2010;33(3):221-6.

[119] Sumida K, Ubara Y, Hoshino J, Mise K, Hayami N, Suwabe T, et al. Once-weekly teriparatide in hemodialysis patients with hypoparathyroidism and low bone mass: a prospective study. *Osteoporos Int*. 2016;27(4):1441-50.

[120] Foley RN, Parfrey PS. Cardiovascular disease and mortality in ESRD. *J Nephrol*. 1998;11(5):239-45.

[121] London GM, Guerin AP, Marchais SJ, Metivier F, Pannier B, Adda H. Arterial media calcification in end-stage renal disease: impact on all-cause and cardiovascular mortality. *Nephrol Dial Transplant*. 2003;18(9):1731-40.

[122] Wilson PW, Kauppila LI, O'Donnell CJ, Kiel DP, Hannan M, Polak JM, et al. Abdominal aortic calcific deposits are an important predictor of vascular morbidity and mortality. *Circulation*. 2001;103(11):1529-34.

[123] Blacher J, Guerin AP, Pannier B, Marchais SJ, London GM. Arterial calcifications, arterial stiffness, and cardiovascular risk in end-stage renal disease. *Hypertension*. 2001;38(4):938-42.

[124] Rodriguez Garcia M, Naves Diaz M, Cannata Andia JB. Bone metabolism, vascular calcifications and mortality: associations beyond mere coincidence. *J Nephrol*. 2005;18(4):458-63.

[125] Paloian NJ, Giachelli CM. A current understanding of vascular calcification in CKD. *Am J Physiol Renal Physiol*. 2014;307(8):F891-900.

[126] Goodman WG, London G, Amann K, Block GA, Giachelli C, Hruska KA, et al. Vascular calcification in chronic kidney disease. *Am J Kidney Dis*. 2004;43(3):572-9.

[127] Berliner JA, Navab M, Fogelman AM, Frank JS, Demer LL, Edwards PA, et al. Atherosclerosis: basic mechanisms. Oxidation, inflammation, and genetics. *Circulation*. 1995;91(9):2488-96.

[128] Schwarz U, Buzello M, Ritz E, Stein G, Raabe G, Wiest G, et al. Morphology of coronary atherosclerotic lesions in patients with end-stage renal failure. *Nephrol Dial Transplant*. 2000;15(2):218-23.

[129] Mizobuchi M, Towler D, Slatopolsky E. Vascular calcification: the killer of patients with chronic kidney disease. *J Am Soc Nephrol*. 2009;20(7):1453-64.

[130] London GM, Marchais SJ, Guerin AP, Metivier F, Adda H. Arterial structure and function in end-stage renal disease. *Nephrol Dial Transplant*. 2002;17(10):1713-24.

[131] Block GA, Klassen PS, Lazarus JM, Ofsthun N, Lowrie EG, Chertow GM. Mineral metabolism, mortality, and morbidity in maintenance hemodialysis. *J Am Soc Nephrol*. 2004;15(8):2208-18.

[132] Cozzolino M, Dusso AS, Slatopolsky E. Role of calcium-phosphate product and bone-associated proteins on vascular calcification in renal failure. *J Am Soc Nephrol.* 2001;12(11):2511-6.
[133] Shroff R, Long DA, Shanahan C. Mechanistic insights into vascular calcification in CKD. *J Am Soc Nephrol.* 2013;24(2):179-89.
[134] Shanahan CM, Cary NR, Salisbury JR, Proudfoot D, Weissberg PL, Edmonds ME. Medial localization of mineralization-regulating proteins in association with Monckeberg's sclerosis: evidence for smooth muscle cell-mediated vascular calcification. *Circulation.* 1999;100(21):2168-76.
[135] Tyson KL, Reynolds JL, McNair R, Zhang Q, Weissberg PL, Shanahan CM. Osteo/chondrocytic transcription factors and their target genes exhibit distinct patterns of expression in human arterial calcification. *Arterioscler Thromb Vasc Biol.* 2003; 23(3):489-94.
[136] Shanahan CM, Cary NR, Metcalfe JC, Weissberg PL. High expression of genes for calcification-regulating proteins in human atherosclerotic plaques. *J Clin Invest.* 1994; 93(6):2393-402.
[137] Reynolds JL, Skepper JN, McNair R, Kasama T, Gupta K, Weissberg PL, et al. Multifunctional roles for serum protein fetuin-a in inhibition of human vascular smooth muscle cell calcification. *J Am Soc Nephrol.* 2005;16(10):2920-30.
[138] Reynolds JL, Joannides AJ, Skepper JN, McNair R, Schurgers LJ, Proudfoot D, et al. Human vascular smooth muscle cells undergo vesicle-mediated calcification in response to changes in extracellular calcium and phosphate concentrations: a potential mechanism for accelerated vascular calcification in ESRD. *J Am Soc Nephrol.* 2004; 15(11):2857-67.
[139] Kapustin AN, Davies JD, Reynolds JL, McNair R, Jones GT, Sidibe A, et al. Calcium regulates key components of vascular smooth muscle cell-derived matrix vesicles to enhance mineralization. *Circ Res.* 2011;109(1):e1-12.
[140] Genge BR, Wu LN, Wuthier RE. In vitro modeling of matrix vesicle nucleation: synergistic stimulation of mineral formation by annexin A5 and phosphatidylserine. *J Biol Chem.* 2007;282(36):26035-45.
[141] Pai A, Leaf EM, El-Abbadi M, Giachelli CM. Elastin degradation and vascular smooth muscle cell phenotype change precede cell loss and arterial medial calcification in a uremic mouse model of chronic kidney disease. *Am J Pathol.* 2011;178(2):764-73.
[142] Lee JS, Basalyga DM, Simionescu A, Isenburg JC, Simionescu DT, Vyavahare NR. Elastin calcification in the rat subdermal model is accompanied by up-regulation of degradative and osteogenic cellular responses. *Am J Pathol.* 2006;168(2):490-8.
[143] Pai AS, Giachelli CM. Matrix remodeling in vascular calcification associated with chronic kidney disease. *J Am Soc Nephrol.* 2010;21(10):1637-40.
[144] Jono S, McKee MD, Murry CE, Shioi A, Nishizawa Y, Mori K, et al. Phosphate regulation of vascular smooth muscle cell calcification. *Circ Res.* 2000;87(7):E10-7.
[145] Molostvov G, James S, Fletcher S, Bennett J, Lehnert H, Bland R, et al. Extracellular calcium-sensing receptor is functionally expressed in human artery. *Am J Physiol Renal Physiol.* 2007;293(3):F946-55.
[146] Alam MU, Kirton JP, Wilkinson FL, Towers E, Sinha S, Rouhi M, et al. Calcification is associated with loss of functional calcium-sensing receptor in vascular smooth muscle cells. *Cardiovasc Res.* 2009;81(2):260-8.

[147] Moe SM, Duan D, Doehle BP, O'Neill KD, Chen NX. Uremia induces the osteoblast differentiation factor Cbfa1 in human blood vessels. *Kidney Int.* 2003;63(3):1003-11.

[148] Chen NX, Duan D, O'Neill KD, Wolisi GO, Koczman JJ, Laclair R, et al. The mechanisms of uremic serum-induced expression of bone matrix proteins in bovine vascular smooth muscle cells. *Kidney Int.* 2006;70(6):1046-53.

[149] Luo G, Ducy P, McKee MD, Pinero GJ, Loyer E, Behringer RR, et al. Spontaneous calcification of arteries and cartilage in mice lacking matrix GLA protein. *Nature.* 1997;386(6620):78-81.

[150] Yao Y, Shahbazian A, Bostrom KI. Proline and gamma-carboxylated glutamate residues in matrix Gla protein are critical for binding of bone morphogenetic protein-4. *Circ Res.* 2008;102(9):1065-74.

[151] Roy ME, Nishimoto SK. Matrix Gla protein binding to hydroxyapatite is dependent on the ionic environment: calcium enhances binding affinity but phosphate and magnesium decrease affinity. *Bone.* 2002;31(2):296-302.

[152] Scatena M, Liaw L, Giachelli CM. Osteopontin: a multifunctional molecule regulating chronic inflammation and vascular disease. *Arterioscler Thromb Vasc Biol.* 2007; 27(11):2302-9.

[153] Speer MY, McKee MD, Guldberg RE, Liaw L, Yang HY, Tung E, et al. Inactivation of the osteopontin gene enhances vascular calcification of matrix Gla protein-deficient mice: evidence for osteopontin as an inducible inhibitor of vascular calcification *in vivo*. *J Exp Med.* 2002;196(8):1047-55.

[154] Kaartinen MT, Murshed M, Karsenty G, McKee MD. Osteopontin upregulation and polymerization by transglutaminase 2 in calcified arteries of Matrix Gla protein-deficient mice. *J Histochem Cytochem.* 2007;55(4):375-86.

[155] Yasuda H, Shima N, Nakagawa N, Mochizuki SI, Yano K, Fujise N, et al. Identity of osteoclastogenesis inhibitory factor (OCIF) and osteoprotegerin (OPG): a mechanism by which OPG/OCIF inhibits osteoclastogenesis in vitro. *Endocrinology.* 1998;139(3):1329-37.

[156] Bennett BJ, Scatena M, Kirk EA, Rattazzi M, Varon RM, Averill M, et al. Osteoprotegerin inactivation accelerates advanced atherosclerotic lesion progression and calcification in older ApoE-/- mice. *Arterioscler Thromb Vasc Biol.* 2006;26(9): 2117-24.

[157] Orita Y, Yamamoto H, Kohno N, Sugihara M, Honda H, Kawamata S, et al. Role of osteoprotegerin in arterial calcification: development of new animal model. *Arterioscler Thromb Vasc Biol.* 2007;27(9):2058-64.

[158] Harmey D, Hessle L, Narisawa S, Johnson KA, Terkeltaub R, Millan JL. Concerted regulation of inorganic pyrophosphate and osteopontin by akp2, enpp1, and ank: an integrated model of the pathogenesis of mineralization disorders. *Am J Pathol.* 2004;164(4):1199-209.

[159] Rutsch F, Ruf N, Vaingankar S, Toliat MR, Suk A, Hohne W, et al. Mutations in ENPP1 are associated with 'idiopathic' infantile arterial calcification. *Nat Genet.* 2003;34(4):379-81.

[160] Razzaque MS, Sitara D, Taguchi T, St-Arnaud R, Lanske B. Premature aging-like phenotype in fibroblast growth factor 23 null mice is a vitamin D-mediated process. *FASEB J.* 2006;20(6):720-2.

[161] Hu MC, Shi M, Zhang J, Quinones H, Griffith C, Kuro-o M, et al. Klotho deficiency causes vascular calcification in chronic kidney disease. *J Am Soc Nephrol.* 2011;22(1):124-36.

[162] Holick MF. Vitamin D deficiency. *N Engl J Med.* 2007;357(3):266-81.

[163] Shalhoub V, Shatzen E, Henley C, Boedigheimer M, McNinch J, Manoukian R, et al. Calcification inhibitors and Wnt signaling proteins are implicated in bovine artery smooth muscle cell calcification in the presence of phosphate and vitamin D sterols. *Calcif Tissue Int.* 2006;79(6):431-42.

[164] Wu-Wong JR, Noonan W, Ma J, Dixon D, Nakane M, Bolin AL, et al. Role of phosphorus and vitamin D analogs in the pathogenesis of vascular calcification. *J Pharmacol Exp Ther.* 2006;318(1):90-8.

[165] Zebger-Gong H, Muller D, Diercke M, Haffner D, Hocher B, Verberckmoes S, et al. 1,25-Dihydroxyvitamin D3-induced aortic calcifications in experimental uremia: up-regulation of osteoblast markers, calcium-transporting proteins and osterix. *J Hypertens.* 2011;29(2):339-48.

[166] Rebsamen MC, Sun J, Norman AW, Liao JK. 1alpha,25-dihydroxyvitamin D3 induces vascular smooth muscle cell migration via activation of phosphatidylinositol 3-kinase. *Circ Res.* 2002;91(1):17-24.

[167] Mathew S, Lund RJ, Chaudhary LR, Geurs T, Hruska KA. Vitamin D receptor activators can protect against vascular calcification. *J Am Soc Nephrol.* 2008; 19(8):1509-19.

[168] Mizobuchi M, Finch JL, Martin DR, Slatopolsky E. Differential effects of vitamin D receptor activators on vascular calcification in uremic rats. *Kidney Int.* 2007;72(6):709-15.

[169] Watson KE, Abrolat ML, Malone LL, Hoeg JM, Doherty T, Detrano R, et al. Active serum vitamin D levels are inversely correlated with coronary calcification. *Circulation.* 1997;96(6):1755-60.

[170] Kalantar-Zadeh K, Kuwae N, Regidor DL, Kovesdy CP, Kilpatrick RD, Shinaberger CS, et al. Survival predictability of time-varying indicators of bone disease in maintenance hemodialysis patients. *Kidney Int.* 2006;70(4):771-80.

[171] Shoji T, Shinohara K, Kimoto E, Emoto M, Tahara H, Koyama H, et al. Lower risk for cardiovascular mortality in oral 1alpha-hydroxy vitamin D3 users in a haemodialysis population. *Nephrol Dial Transplant.* 2004;19(1):179-84.

[172] Teng M, Wolf M, Lowrie E, Ofsthun N, Lazarus JM, Thadhani R. Survival of patients undergoing hemodialysis with paricalcitol or calcitriol therapy. *N Engl J Med.* 2003;349(5):446-56.

[173] Teng M, Wolf M, Ofsthun MN, Lazarus JM, Hernan MA, Camargo CA, Jr., et al. Activated injectable vitamin D and hemodialysis survival: a historical cohort study. *J Am Soc Nephrol.* 2005;16(4):1115-25.

[174] Tentori F, Hunt WC, Stidley CA, Rohrscheib MR, Bedrick EJ, Meyer KB, et al. Mortality risk among hemodialysis patients receiving different vitamin D analogs. *Kidney Int.* 2006;70(10):1858-65.

[175] London GM, Guerin AP, Verbeke FH, Pannier B, Boutouyrie P, Marchais SJ, et al. Mineral metabolism and arterial functions in end-stage renal disease: potential role of 25-hydroxyvitamin D deficiency. *J Am Soc Nephrol.* 2007;18(2):613-20.

[176] Shroff R, Egerton M, Bridel M, Shah V, Donald AE, Cole TJ, et al. A bimodal association of vitamin D levels and vascular disease in children on dialysis. *J Am Soc Nephrol*. 2008;19(6):1239-46.

[177] Nigwekar SU, Thadhani R, Brandenburg VM. Calciphylaxis. *N Engl J Med*. 2018; 379(4):399-400.

[178] Nigwekar SU, Zhao S, Wenger J, Hymes JL, Maddux FW, Thadhani RI, et al. A Nationally Representative Study of Calcific Uremic Arteriolopathy Risk Factors. *J Am Soc Nephrol*. 2016;27(11):3421-9.

[179] Brandenburg VM, Kramann R, Rothe H, Kaesler N, Korbiel J, Specht P, et al. Calcific uraemic arteriolopathy (calciphylaxis): data from a large nationwide registry. *Nephrol Dial Transplant*. 2017;32(1):126-32.

[180] Honda Y, Endo Y, Tanizaki H, Fujisawa A, Kitoh A, Miyachi Y, et al. Calciphylaxis associated with acute renal failure in multicentric Castleman's disease. *Eur J Dermatol*. 2015;25(5):497-9.

[181] Vanparys J, Sprangers B, Sagaert X, Kuypers DR. Chronic wounds in a kidney transplant recipient with moderate renal impairment. *Acta Clin Belg*. 2013;68(2):128-31.

[182] Sprague SM. Painful skin ulcers in a hemodialysis patient. *Clin J Am Soc Nephrol*. 2014;9(1):166-73.

[183] Nigwekar SU, Wolf M, Sterns RH, Hix JK. Calciphylaxis from nonuremic causes: a systematic review. *Clin J Am Soc Nephrol*. 2008;3(4):1139-43.

[184] Weenig RH, Sewell LD, Davis MD, McCarthy JT, Pittelkow MR. Calciphylaxis: natural history, risk factor analysis, and outcome. *J Am Acad Dermatol*. 2007; 56(4):569-79.

[185] Fine A, Zacharias J. Calciphylaxis is usually non-ulcerating: risk factors, outcome and therapy. *Kidney Int*. 2002;61(6):2210-7.

[186] Santos PW, He J, Tuffaha A, Wetmore JB. Clinical characteristics and risk factors associated with mortality in calcific uremic arteriolopathy. *Int Urol Nephrol*. 2017; 49(12):2247-56.

[187] Brandenburg VM, Evenepoel P, Floege J, Goldsmith D, Kramann R, Massy Z, et al. Lack of evidence does not justify neglect: how can we address unmet medical needs in calciphylaxis? *Nephrol Dial Transplant*. 2016;31(8):1211-9.

[188] An J, Devaney B, Ooi KY, Ford S, Frawley G, Menahem S. Hyperbaric oxygen in the treatment of calciphylaxis: A case series and literature review. *Nephrology* (Carlton). 2015;20(7):444-50.

[189] Baldwin C, Farah M, Leung M, Taylor P, Werb R, Kiaii M, et al. Multi-intervention management of calciphylaxis: a report of 7 cases. *Am J Kidney Dis*. 2011;58(6):988-91.

[190] Sowers KM, Hayden MR. Calcific uremic arteriolopathy: pathophysiology, reactive oxygen species and therapeutic approaches. *Oxid Med Cell Longev*. 2010;3(2):109-21.

[191] Chen NX, O'Neill K, Akl NK, Moe SM. Adipocyte induced arterial calcification is prevented with sodium thiosulfate. *Biochem Biophys Res Commun*. 2014;449(1):151-6.

[192] Zitt E, Konig M, Vychytil A, Auinger M, Wallner M, Lingenhel G, et al. Use of sodium thiosulphate in a multi-interventional setting for the treatment of calciphylaxis in dialysis patients. *Nephrol Dial Transplant*. 2013;28(5):1232-40.

[193] Nigwekar SU, Brunelli SM, Meade D, Wang W, Hymes J, Lacson E, Jr. Sodium thiosulfate therapy for calcific uremic arteriolopathy. *Clin J Am Soc Nephrol.* 2013;8(7):1162-70.

[194] Strazzula L, Nigwekar SU, Steele D, Tsiaras W, Sise M, Bis S, et al. Intralesional sodium thiosulfate for the treatment of calciphylaxis. *JAMA Dermatol.* 2013;149(8):946-9.

In: Issues in Kidney Disease – Dialysis
Editors: Stephen Z. Fadem and José A. Moura-Neto
ISBN: 978-1-68507-000-7

Chapter 5

END-STAGE KIDNEY DISEASE AND MALIGNANCY

Harini Bejjanki, MD, Omar Mamlouk, MD, and Biruh T. Workeneh*, MD
The University of Texas MD Anderson Cancer Center, Houston, TX, USA

ABSTRACT

Cancer incidence is high in patients with end-stage kidney disease (ESKD) compared to the general population. Population-based studies show a significantly increased standardized incidence ratio (SIR) for all cancers in the United States dialysis population compared to the general population. Multiple studies have shown that cancer risk is highest in the first year of dialysis initiation, including among younger patients. There are significant demographic variations in cancer incidence and risk. The risk for kidney (SIR 3.6; CI 3.5 to 3.8) and bladder (SIR 1.5; CI 1.4 to 1.6) cancers were increased, relatively more in younger than older patients and more in female patients (kidney: SIR 4.6, CI 4.3 to 4.9; bladder: SIR 2.7, CI 2.4 to 2.9) than male patients (kidney: SIR 3.2, CI 3.0 to 3.4; bladder: SIR 1.3, CI 1.2 to 1.3). There is a significant variation in the SIR of cancer in dialysis patients, depending on the geographic areas. The risk was most elevated for cancers of the kidney/renal pelvis (SIR, 4.03; 95% CI, 3.88-4.19) and bladder (SIR, 1.57; 95% CI, 1.51-1.64) in US Medicare dialysis patients. Increased risk of incident cancer was observed in dialysis patients with previous transplant failure. SIR during dialysis after transplant failure remained significantly elevated for leukemia, lung cancer, cancers related to kidney, urinary tract, and thyroid cancers, with thyroid cancer incidence significantly higher. The prevalence of several oncogenic viruses, such as hepatitis B and C, is high in ESKD patients. When adjusted for age, sex, and comorbidities, ESKD patients had a 2.41 (95% CI; 1.83-3.16) times increased risk of any human papillomavirus-related cancer compared with population controls. Current recommendations advise against routine cancer screening in patients on dialysis with "limited life expectancy and without signs or symptoms." However, regular dialysis therapy is an exceptional opportunity for early detection of certain malignancies such as kidney cancer and of the thyroid, which is frequently investigated in the diagnostic program of hyperparathyroidism. Challenges to cancer screening in dialysis patients include vascular calcifications in dialysis patients,

* Corresponding Author's E-mail: btworkeneh@mdanderson.org

high false-positive rates, and mammography interpretation in women with ESKD, which may be more difficult. Tumor markers (TM) are simple and easily measurable tests in diagnosing and clinical management of patients with cancer. However, the kinetics of TM in renal impairment often leads to false positive results. There are no consistent clinical guidelines for pre-transplant cancer screening in potential kidney transplant recipients with no prior history of malignancy. It may be necessary to implement routine cancer screening protocols in dialysis units undergoing transplant evaluation. The emerging model of personalized cancer screening for the general population may also benefit patients receiving dialysis.

Keywords: End-Stage Kidney Disease (ESKD), Standardized incidence ratio, standardized incidence ratio, cancer screening, cancer mortality, geography, acquired cystic kidney disease, renal cell cancer, transplant waiting list, human papilloma virus, Hepatitis B, Hepatitis C, tumor markers, USPSTF, USRDS

INTRODUCTION

Several studies have shown that cancer incidence is decidedly higher in patients with End-Stage Kidney Disease (ESKD) compared to the general population [1-10]. The hypothesis stating that there is an *added* factor in patients with lower GFR that might result in cancer is supported by the findings of Lowrance et al., who found in a retrospective cohort study of 1,190,538 adults with no prior evidence of malignancy that eGFR was independently and incrementally associated with an increased risk of renal cancer (hazard ratio, 2.28; 95% CI, 1.78 to 2.92 for eGFR < 30) [11]. Population-based studies repeatedly show a significantly increased standardized incidence ratio (SIR), which indicates the ratio of observed vs. expected cancers for all cancers in the dialysis population compared to the general population [1, 12] (Table 1). Among US adult patients enrolled in Medicare's ESKD program, SIR for cancer was 1.42 (95% CI, 1.41-1.43) [3]. These findings were confirmed more broadly by studies in Australia and New Zealand [1, 13], Italy, Korea, Taiwan, Singapore, Hongkong, and Germany (Table 2). Several theories have been proposed to explain the discrepancy. Impaired function of the immune system and DNA repair mechanisms and reduced antioxidant defense, accumulation of carcinogens partly due to decreased renal elimination, chronic infections, and chronic inflammatory state are found more frequently in patients with ESKD than the general population. These effects may act in a coordinated manner to accelerate the malignant transformation and tumor formation [14].

While dialysis patients showed a higher risk of certain cancers, there is no significant difference for each cancer risk between dialysis modalities (hemodialysis or peritoneal dialysis) [1, 15]. Furthermore, factors associated with the dialysis treatment, such as bio-incompatibility reactions due to complement activating membranes and immunosuppressive medications used during prior unsuccessful renal transplantation, may also contribute to malignant transformation [16].

Table 1. The standard incidence ratio of selected cancers in ESKD patients in the United states based on USRDS and Medicare data

SIR >5	SIR 2-5	SIR 1-2	SIR<1
Multiple Myeloma	Cervix of the Uterus	Overall cancer SIR (1.2-1.4)	Breast (Medicare ESKD)
	Kidney	Tongue	body of the Uterus
	Thyroid	GI: Stomach, intestinal, liver, Colorectal, pancreas	prostate (Medicare ESKD)
		Anogenital: other female genital, penis scrotum	
		Hematological: Non-Hodgkin Lymphoma, Hodgkin Lymphoma, Leukemia	
		lung, bladder, Breast (USRDS Data), Prostate (USRDS ESKD)	

Table 2. SIR based on cancer site and Country

Cancer Site	Country	SIR [95% CI]	Number of ESKD Patients/Study Method
Kidney Cancer	Hong Kong [22]	12.28 [8.44-17.08]	6254 /Multicenter Cohort Study
	US Medicare patients [3]	4.03 [3.88-4.19]	482,510/Retrospective cohort study
	Germany [20]	3.60 (3.45–3.76)	521,404/retrospective USRDS Database cohort
Urinary Tract (Kidney and Bladder)	United States USRDS [1]	3.7 [3.5-3.9]	5,235/ Prospective observational cohort study
	Korea [25]	4.7[2.4-8.1]	
Breast Cancer	Australia and New Zealand [1]	1.5[1.1-2.0]	13,497/Retrospective Cohort-Dialysis Registry
	Europe [1]	1[0.9-1]	296,903/Retrospective cohort European dialysis registry
	United States USRDS [1]	0.8[0.8-0.9]	521,404/retrospective USRDS Database
	US Medicare patients [3]	1.42[1.38-1.47]	482,510/Retrospective cohort study
Bladder Cancer	Taiwan [22]	8.2[6.7-9.9]	92,348/Population based cohort study
	US Medicare [3]	1.57[1.51-1.64]	482,510/Retrospective cohort study
	United States USRDS [1]	1.4[1.3-1.5]	521,404/521,404/retrospective USRDS Database
Liver cancer	Taiwan [22]	1.4[1.2-1.5]	92,348/Population based cohort study
Vulval Cancer	Australia [29]	4.2 [0.4-11.9]	7605 Dialysis Patients/retrospective cohort Australian and New Zealand database
Cervical cancer	Australia and New Zealand [1]	4[2.4-6.6]	13,497/Retrospective Cohort-Dialysis Registry
	Europe [1]	1.6[1.3-1.8]	296,903/Retrospective cohort European dialysis registry
	United States USRDS [1]	2.5[2.2-2.8]	521,404/retrospective USRDS Database
Tongue	Singapore [6]	5.01(1.62-15.53)	6254/Multicenter cohort study
Prostate	Michigan, USA [12]	Increased SIR	4161/Michigan cancer registry cohort
	United States USRDS [1]	0.7[0.6-0.7]	521,404/retrospective USRDS Database
	US Medicare [3]	1.06[1.03-1.09]	482,510/Retrospective cohort study
	Italy [2]	0.89[0.62-1.23]	3,407/Population based cohort study
Lung/Bronchus	US Medicare patients [3]	1.28[1.25-1.32]	482,510/Retrospective cohort study
	Australia/New Zealand [1]	1.4[1.1-1.8]	13,497/Retrospective Cohort-Dialysis Registry
	Europe [1]	0.9[0.8-0.9]	296,903/Retrospective cohort European dialysis registry
	United States USRDS [1]	1.1[1.1-1.2]	521,404/retrospective USRDS Database
	Italy [2]	1.09[0.74-1.55]	3,407/Population based cohort study
Colorectal cancer	US Medicare Patients [3]	1.27[1.23-1.30]	482,510/Retrospective cohort study
	Italy [2]	0.85[0.56-1.24]	3,407/Population based cohort study
Skin non melanoma	Italy [2]	1.81[1.46-2.22]	3,407/Population based cohort study

Table 3. Significance of tumor markers in ESKD

Tumor Marker	Molecular Mass	CKD	Hemodialysis	Peritoneal Dialysis	Indications
tPSA	33KdA	Decreased [84] No change [85] Increased [36, 86]	No change [85]	NA	Prostate Cancer-Screening, Diagnosis, treatment monitoring, recurrence [109]
fPSA	33kDa	Increased [87-89]	Increased [85]	NA	Prostate Cancer-Screening, Diagnosis, treatment monitoring, recurrence [109]
Chromogranin A	49kDa	Increased [90-93]	Increased [91, 93]	Increased [91, 93]	Neuroendocrine tumors- diagnosis, follow up [110]
Alpha-fetoprotein	65kDa	No change [94]	No change [104]	No change [94]	Diagnosis of liver cancer
Beta-2 microglobulin	11.8kDa	Increased [95]	Elevated in low flux HD. Decreased in high flux HD [105]	Increased but lower levels compared to HD [107]	Elevated in lymphoproliferative disorders
CA 15-3(MUC-1)	120-225kDa	No change [96, 97]	No change [96, 97] Increased [100,104]	NA	Metastatic breast cancer treatment surveillance [111]
CA 125	90kDa	No change [98, 99]	No change [99]	Increased [99, 108]	Ovarian Cancer [112]
CA 19-9	72.2 kDa	No change [97, 100] Increased [101, 102]	NA	NA	Colorectal cancer
hCG	36.7 kDa	Elevated [103]	Elevated [106]	Elevated [106]	Gestational trophoblastic disease-diagnosis, staging, follow up, recurrence [113]

INCIDENCE AND RISK FACTORS FOR CANCER IN ESKD PATIENTS

Age

A deeper analysis shows that a number of determinants are important to the development of cancer in the ESKD population and epidemiologic analysis show age as a significant factor. The most extensive United States study of 482,510 Medicare dialysis patients showed a 5-year cumulative incidence of any cancer was 9.48% (95% CI, 9.39%-9.57%) and was higher for older age dialysis patients [3]. This finding was supported by a few other studies, where being older was associated with a higher risk of new cancer in ESKD patients [17-20]. One study [21] found that the highest SIR scores were for middle-aged (ages 35-50) patients. Interestingly, the majority of the studies have confirmed that young dialysis patients (age <35) are at exceptionally high risk for incident cancer in ESKD, and the risk decreased with age [1, 2, 4-6, 10, 21-23]. Heidland et al. [24] postulated that the increased risk of cancer in younger dialysis patients may be attributed to a faster course of tumor promotion and progression and decreased predisposition to develop antibodies due to oncogenic viral infections in older dialysis patients. The expected survival of the elderly dialysis patients is less than 10 years and could be significantly reduced by the presence of ESKD, cardiovascular comorbidities, and frailty. As a result, these patients may die earlier, before the development of cancers. Due to the lower life expectancy and comorbidities, the elderly dialysis patients are less likely to receive cancer screening or invasive diagnostic procedures than the elderly in the general population. The consequence is that cancers could be underestimated in the elderly patients suffering from ESKD, especially those with low functional status.

Dialysis vintage, which reflects the time on dialysis, surprisingly, is not directly correlated with cancer incidence. Cancer incidence was the highest within the first year of dialysis based on several surveys [2, 6, 10, 22, 23]. This may be due to increased surveillance during the early years of dialysis. Patients are typically younger when dialysis is initiated, and the cumulative incidence of dialysis initiation is lower at older ages [25, 26]. Although cancer incidence is highest in the first year, some studies show long-term dialysis emerges as a risk factor for all cancers [17].

Race/Ethnicity

Race and ethnicity reflect genetic coding and, in many societies, impact socioeconomic status. The most extensive United States study showed a 5-year cumulative incidence of any cancer was 9.48% (95% CI, 9.39%-9.57%) and was higher for specific subgroups: nonwhites, non-Hispanics [3]. Other studies that provide insight about the impact of race limited to ESKD are intertwined with geography, which will be explored.

Geography

Geography impacts the incidence and pattern of cancer that develops in ESKD patients. In regions with similarly high rates of cancer, the frequency and pattern of distribution of the tumors vary [3, 6, 21-23, 27] (See Table 2). This may account for differences in the rates of particular cancer types; some studies showed kidney cancer carried the highest risk [2, 22] (SIR 12.28, 95% CI 8.44-17.08); others showed bladder cancer had the highest SIR (SIR: 8.2, 95% CI: 6.7-9.9) and frequency (21.2%), with liver cancer being the second highest (SIR: 1.4, 95% CI: 1.2-1.5) [23]. In the United States, the risk was most elevated for cancers of the kidney/renal pelvis (SIR, 4.03; 95% CI, 3.88-4.19) and bladder (SIR, 1.57; 95% CI, 1.51-1.64) in US Medicare dialysis patients [3]. High SIR was observed for cancer of the kidney (3.70 [3.5-3.9]), cervix (2.5 [2.2-2.8]), multiple myeloma (5.2[5-5.3]), and thyroid and other endocrine organs (2.4 [2.1-2.8]) [1].

A multicenter cohort study in over 6000 Asian dialysis patients between 1994 and 2014 in Hong Kong compared cancer incidence in dialysis patients with the general population. The standardized incidence ratio (SIR) was the highest for kidney cancer, followed by tongue and cancer of the cervix [22]. The three sites with the most increased cancer risks among dialysis patients in Hongkong compared to the general population are kidney, tongue, and multiple myeloma in another study [6]. Another population-based study analyzed data of 92,348 chronic dialysis patients in Taiwan between 1997-2008. In this study, bladder cancer carried the highest SIR, followed by liver cancer [23]. Dialysis patients in Japan were found to have an excess of liver, colorectal, bladder, and kidney cancers [10]. A Korean study of 14,382 patients shows colorectal cancer as the most common primary cancer site in both men and women. Compared to patients from Australia and New Zealand, the incidence of renal cell carcinoma (RCC) was higher, and that of transitional cell cancer (TCC) was lower in Japanese patients ($p < 0.001$) [28]. In ESKD patients in Korea, the most common cancer site was the gastrointestinal tract (GIT) (51%), followed by the urinary tract (20%), lung (8%), and thyroid (7%) [19]. Malignancies of the digestive organs were frequent and constituted 56% of all malignancies in Japanese ESKD patients [10].

A population-based European cohort study observed elevated risk for cancers of the kidney, skin non-melanoma, oral cavity, and Kaposi's sarcoma in younger dialysis patients within the first year of dialysis initiation [2]. Increased risk of liver and kidney cancer, thyroid, lymphoma, and multiple myeloma were noted in Italian patients in a small study [29]. An enhanced risk for cancer of the kidney, bladder, prostate, liver, oral cavity, and the pharynx and larynx, as well as of the lymphatic and hemopoietic systems, was found in North Bavaria ESKD patients [21]. In dialysis patients in Australia and New Zealand, vulval cancer occurred more commonly than expected (2 observed, 0.48 expected), giving a SIR of 4.2 (95% confidence interval = 0.4-11.9) [30]. Additional investigation is required to assess the risk of cancer in ESKD patients in the various regions of Africa and the Middle East.

Etiology of ESKD

There does not appear to be any particular association between excess cancer risk and the underlying etiology of ESKD, with a few exceptions [29]. In the Japanese population on dialysis, RCC is more common than TCC. The primary renal disease was chronic glomerulonephritis in patients with RCC (68.4%) and diabetic nephropathy in patients with TCC (43.8%, $p = 0.002$) [28]. Other etiologies of ESKD, such as Balkan nephropathy and the excess of kidney cancer in these conditions, were urothelial in origin [1].

Acquired Cystic Disease

The pattern of increased risk for renal parenchymal cancer in dialysis patients is consistent with causation through acquired renal cystic disease [1]. Acquired renal cystic disease is a known risk factor for RCC, with visible cysts noticed on imaging studies after 3 years of being on dialysis [31]. The development of acquired kidney cysts corresponds with the duration of dialysis, and approximately 2-7% of dialysis patients with acquired cysts develop RCC [32, 33]. Further, RCC arising in native kidneys of transplant patients seems to exhibit many favorable clinical, pathological, and outcome features compared with those diagnosed in dialysis-only patients [32]. While some clinicians suggest routine screening with imaging studies for patients with dialysis vintage > 3 years, this approach has not shown to be cost-effective due to low life expectancy [34, 35]. The North American and European professional transplantation societies recommend screening kidney transplant candidates for acquired cystic kidney disease, but the guidelines on whom should be screened are unclear. The American Society of Transplantation (AST) guideline recommends screening patients who are at high risk for renal cell carcinoma but does not define "high-risk" [36].

Comorbidities

Chronic liver disease is a significant risk factor for hepatoma and other malignancies [17]. Diabetes mellitus (DM) is a risk factor for cancer in the general population and the most common cause of ESKD. However, whether DM specifically is independently associated with higher incidence in ESKD patients is not fully characterized. However, some studies suggested lower incidence for non-diabetics compared to diabetics [27]. Ultimately, appears that underlying CKD may be an independent risk factor for malignancy [20, 37].

High SIR for urothelial cancers occurs in toxic nephropathies (chiefly analgesic nephropathy) [1]. Prolonged analgesic abuse is a risk factor for TCC of the bladder, ureter, kidney, and renal pelvis [38]. Prolonged oral cyclophosphamide, often used for certain primary renal diseases and rheumatic diseases is a known risk factor for bladder cancer [39]. There are similar concerns with the use of biologic agents, such as rituximab.

Previous Transplant History

Increased risk of incident cancer was observed in dialysis patients with previous transplant failure [7]. SIR during dialysis after transplant failure remained significantly elevated for leukemia, lung cancer, cancers related to kidney, urinary tract, and thyroid cancers, with thyroid cancer incidence substantially higher incidence rate ratio 6.77 (2.64 to 17.39) [40]. SIRs for most cancer types were not increased pretransplant, suggesting immune suppression may be responsible for the increased risk [13]. Excess cancer risk in patients occurred after transplantation and not during dialysis in a cohort of 4178 patients undergoing renal replacement therapy, of whom 3592 were treated with dialysis alone, and 1821 later had transplants [41].

Oncogenic Viruses

When adjusted for age, sex, and comorbidities, ESKD patients had a 2.41 (95% CI; 1.83-3.16) times increased risk of any potentially vaccine-preventable human papillomavirus-related cancer compared with population controls [42]. The prevalence of HPV DNA in cervical specimens in dialysis-dependent women is significantly higher (20%) compared to normal controls (4.5%) [43].

Recently, reactivation of EBV infection during long-term hemodialysis therapy has been described [44]. Susceptibility to oncogenic viruses in the dialysis patient has been linked to uremic immunodeficiency, characterized by an impaired monocyte function with a T-cell activation defect resulting in reduced immunosurveillance [45].

The Centers for Disease Control (CDC) recommend Hepatitis B vaccination for all susceptible chronic hemodialysis patients [46]. In the United States, the HBV infection incidence among hemodialysis patients has declined by approximately 95 percent since the initiation of hepatitis B vaccination. The annual incidence rate of HBV among dialysis patients has been stable since 1995 (0.12 percent in 2002). The prevalence for HBV in the United States has been estimated to be approximately 0.4% in the general population [47], with a prevalence rate (by HBsAg seropositivity) of 1 percent in dialysis patients [48]. The prevalence of HCV in the hemodialysis population exceeds that of the general population, with approximately 10% of patients in the recent DOPPS (Dialysis Outcomes and Practice Patterns Study) [49]. It is known that HCV Infection and chronic hepatitis B infections have been associated with hepatocellular cancer (HCC) [50]. Kidney Disease Improving Global Outcomes (KDIGO) recommends screening all patients for HCV infection upon initiation of in-center hemodialysis or upon transfer from another dialysis facility or modality (Grade 1A) and upon initiation of peritoneal dialysis or home hemodialysis (Grade 2D). KDIGO recommends testing for HBV infection before dialysis (Not Graded). If hepatitis B surface antigen (HbsAg) is present, the patient should undergo assessment for HBV therapy (Not Graded) [51].

Cancer Screening in ESKD

Recommendations regarding screening for ESKD and transplanted patients are published from three United States Organizations: the United States Preventative Services Task Force (USPSTF), KDIGO and AST [52, 53]. In 2012, as part of Choosing Wisely: An initiative of the American Board of Internal Medicine Foundation, the American Society of Nephrology recommended against routine cancer screening in patients on dialysis with "limited life expectancy and without signs or symptoms" [54]. Routine cancer screening seems to be excessive in the ESKD population due to lack of an individual patient centric approach and lack of guidelines [55, 56]. Previous studies suggested that cancer screening in the dialysis population is not cost-effective [57]. However, subgroups of dialysis patients such as renal transplant candidates may benefit from screening [58].

Regular dialysis therapy is a unique opportunity for early detection of certain malignancies such as kidney cancer and the thyroid, which is frequently investigated in the diagnostic program of hyperparathyroidism. Therefore, better surveillance may be the reason for the excess elevation of SIR, at least in part. However, numerous studies show that uremia per se is a vital promoting factor of malignancies [14].

Limitations of Routine Screening

Women receiving dialysis have a risk of acquiring breast cancer similar to other women, but a greater all-cause mortality rate due to competing comorbidities [59, 60]. It is uncertain whether routine screening is cost-effective in women receiving dialysis therapy. The presence of vascular calcifications in dialysis patients leads to high false-positive rates, and mammography interpretation in women with ESKD may be more difficult. The analysis by Wong et al. demonstrated the cost-effectiveness of screening for breast cancer in Australian women on maintenance dialysis therapy between the ages 50 and 69 [61]. A difference of 1 breast cancer was averted by screening, with an estimated incremental cost of $109,852/actual life-years saved. Disappointingly, the absolute reduction in breast cancer mortality was 0.1%, with a net gain in life expectancy of 1.3 days [61]. An international collaborative study that looked at 372,000 women on dialysis found no increase in breast cancer risk among women in the US and European registries but saw a SIR 1.5 (50% increase) among women in the Australian registry [1]. Targeting screening mammography according to life expectancy among women undergoing dialysis may be beneficial [62].

The observation complicates colorectal cancer screening that patients receiving dialysis have an increased rate of occult bleeding, which may be attributed to uremic solutes, development of angiodysplasia, and use of anticoagulation. The higher rates of gastrointestinal bleeding in ESKD may result in higher fecal occult blood tests than the general population. This may result in earlier detection of colorectal cancer in ESKD patients than in the general population [18, 63]. According to the age-based recommendations of the USPSTF, dialysis patients between the ages of 50-75 qualify for screening based on age alone. However, the life expectancy of dialysis patients over the age of 50 is less than 10 years per USRDS data [64]. Because of this, the ABIM's Choosing Wisely campaign, the American Society of Nephrology (ASN) in 2012, recommended against routine cancer screening among patients receiving maintenance dialysis "with limited life expectancy and without signs or symptoms [54]." Therefore, the decision to screen for colorectal cancer should be individualized as it may be appropriate in patients with prolonged expected survival and transplant potential [56].

The SIR for cervical cancer in ESKD patients is high regardless of the region (Table 2). The other Human Papillomavirus (HPV) related cancers such as tongue cancer are also high in the ESKD population [6]. Immunogenicity of HPV Recombinant vaccine in children and young adults with CKD and dialysis showed a 100% antibody response to all four HPV genotypes in a cohort study. The antibody response was excellent and sustained [65]. However, no specific Advisory Committee on Immunization Practices (ACIP) recommendation for this vaccine exists for dialysis patients or patients with chronic kidney disease [46]. Studies that evaluated pap smear findings in chronic renal failure patients compared with the normal population showed that CKD was not a predictive factor for cervical cancer [66].

Tumor markers (TM) are simple and easily measurable tests in the diagnosis and clinical management of patients with cancer. However, the kinetics of TM in renal impairment often leads to false-positive results [67] (Table 3). For molecular mass, indications for measurement and variations in levels of TM in chronic dialysis patients. Therefore, the utility of measuring TM in dialysis patients is unclear.

Total prostate-specific antigen (PSA) is probably valid in ESKD patients [19–21]. Still, free PSA and free/total PSA ratios are less useful, as free PSA rises with hemoconcentration, and high-flux dialysis membranes affect its clearance [68]. While some studies showed significantly increased SIR for prostate cancer [12], others showed no consistent increase in the ESKD population [1]. The American Cancer Society (ACS) recommends screening with the PSA for men aged more than 50 with average risk and expected to live at least 10 more years, which rules out most dialysis patients based on age alone. The ACS recommends earlier screening for younger men with high risk [69]. The ACS recommendations may be applicable for younger dialysis patients or patients with an expected life expectancy of greater than 10 years or transplant eligbile. This is particularly important as the SEER database suggested that colorectal cancers were significantly more likely to be diagnosed earlier in the ESKD group stratifying by cancer site. In contrast, prostate cancers were substantially more likely to be diagnosed at a later stage [18]. The routine screening of prostate cancer screening in the ESKD population is not cost-effective and does not seem sensitive enough in the early detection of prostate cancer [57, 70].

While some studies showed a significantly reduced risk of lung cancer in dialysis patients [23], others showed an increased SIR [3, 13] (Table 2). As with other cancer screening, individual patient risks and benefits of screening should be used to guide screening.

Cancer Screening in ESKD Patients Awaiting Transplant

Clinical guidelines suggest a 2–5-year cancer recurrence-free waiting period depending on the type of malignancy before kidney transplantation [39, 71-73]. However, there are no consistent clinical guidelines for pre-transplant cancer screening in potential kidney transplant recipients with no prior history of malignancy. Clinical practice guidelines from Australia, Europe, Canada, and the USA recommend screening per general population recommendations [74-77]. Effective screening and treatment of cancer before transplantation could reduce the risk of graft failure and post-transplant malignancy. It is generally accepted that immunosuppression increases the morbidity and mortality associated with cancer [77].

Prognosis and Clinical Outcomes

Frequent medical encounters in dialysis patients may provide an opportunity for early detection of malignancies despite low rates of cancer screening in this population, particularly in young dialysis patients. It is therefore ambiguous if dialysis patients are disadvantaged in terms of a cancer diagnosis. The likelihood of nonlocalized stage at diagnosis was similar for ESKD patients versus the standardized Surveillance, Epidemiology, and End Results (SEER) general population or matched Medicare control subjects. Stratifying by cancer site, colorectal cancers were significantly more likely to be diagnosed earlier in the ESKD group, whereas prostate cancers were substantially more likely to be diagnosed at a later stage [18]. The increased access and interaction with medical personnel might be offset by the inertia created by the diverging recommendations and outcomes in ESKD patients that is difficult to measure accurately.

In the United States, the average life expectancy of dialysis patients aged >50 years is less than 10 years, and among diabetic patients less than 6 years (USRDS Data). Studies have shown a significantly higher incidence of malignancies in the younger dialysis populations, suggesting screening should be individualized. The analysis of USRDS data from 2015-2017, taking into account primary cause of mortality, age, sex, race, ethnicity, and the primary cause of ESKD showed the highest mortality (37.2%) was due to cardiac arrest, while death attributable to malignancy was 3.8% [78]. The mortality rate was higher in men (4.1 vs. 3.4), age >75, and white Americans. Survival of patients with cancer was not different from that of non-cancer dialysis patients matched for age and sex, except in patients with hematological malignancies who had significant reduction in survival. Therefore, the data suggests for most cancers a survival advantage might not exist among patients with a history of cancer than matched patients without malignancy.

However, other international studies outside the US found contrasting findings to USRDS data. Using the standard mortality rate (SMR) in the general population, which was obtained for each sex and age class, the relative risk of death from cancer in dialysis patients was calculated. The risk ratio in dialysis patients was significantly increased, being 2.48 ($P < 0.05$) for males and 3.99 ($P < 0.05$) for females in Japan [79]. Mortality from malignancies was 2.9 times higher in dialysis patients and 1.7 times higher in transplant recipients than in Taiwan's general population [5]. The prevalence of RCC in dialysis patients is 41 times higher than that in the general population [34]. RCC arising in native kidneys of transplant patients seems to exhibit many favorable clinical, pathological, and outcome features compared with those diagnosed in dialysis-only patients [35].

Mortality can be estimated by a 6-month mortality life expectancy tool. This prognostic tool was developed by Cohen et al. in response to the need for prognostic information on survival in patients receiving chronic hemodialysis care [80]. This tool combines actuarial factors and the clinician's prediction of survival to create a validated model that estimates the 6-month mortality of patients receiving hemodialysis [81]. The prognosis for ESKD patients can be calculated using the Charlson Comorbidity Index (CCI) and the serum albumin [82, 83]. Based on the medical literature referenced, the CCI is as good as or better than other prognostic tools for ESKD patients and is easier to use in the non-research setting than the Index of Coexistent Diseases (ICED) [82].

ESKD patients will need to be assessed on an individual basis, considering cancer risk factors, transplant status, costs per unit of survival benefit, an absolute reduction in mortality, the net gain in life expectancy, costs per unit of survival benefit and, importantly, expected survival to proceed with cancer screening cost-effectively.

Conclusion

ESKD patients are vulnerable and are no strangers to serious complications, the development of cancer representing a grave threat. The published clinical evidence does not provide a robust guide on cost-effective screening and identifying cancer at early stages where the odds of survival are greatest. The general recommendations are vague, leaving it to the provider to best implement routine cancer screening protocols in dialysis units. ESKD patients undergoing transplant evaluation have a more uniform and comprehensive approach to cancer screening. As cancer screening adopts a personalized cancer screening model incorporating precision medicine, it appears that ESKD patients have much to benefit, given the inconsistent approach to cancer in this population.

Clinical Pearls

- Incidence of cancer is high in patients with ESKD compared to the general population.
- Cancer incidence may be highest during the first year of dialysis.
- In the US ESKD Population, the highest incidence observed were cancers of the kidney, bladder, cervix, thyroid and multiple myeloma.
- Acquired cystic kidney disease is a known risk factor for renal cell carcinoma. The American Society of Transplantation recommends screening patients who are at high risk for renal cell carcinoma for acquired cystic kidney disease.
- Increased risk of incident cancer was observed in dialysis patients with previous transplant failure, with thyroid cancer incidence significantly higher.
- ESKD patients are at an increased risk for oncogenic virus-related cancers such as HPV related cancers.
- The prevalence of hepatitis B and hepatitis C infection, which are known to cause hepatocellular carcinoma, is high in ESKD patients and should be screened for prior to initiating dialysis.
- Regular dialysis therapy and the transplant evaluation process represents an opportunity for early detection of certain malignancies.
- The presence of vascular calcifications in dialysis patients leads to high false positive rates and mammography interpretation in women with ESKD.
- The higher rates of gastrointestinal bleeding in ESKD may result in higher fecal occult blood tests than the general population. This may result in earlier detection of colorectal cancer in ESKD patients compared to the general population.
- Free PSA and free/total PSA ratios are less useful, as free PSA rises with hemoconcentration and high-flux dialysis membranes affect its clearance, which may be the reason why prostate cancers were significantly more likely to be diagnosed at a later stage.
- Tumor markers (TM) are simple and easily measurable tests in diagnosis and clinical management of patients with cancer. However, the kinetics of TM in renal impairment often leads to false positive results.
- The emerging model of personalized cancer screening for the general population is an encouraging development, but will need to be validated for dialysis patients.

REFERENCES

[1] Maisonneuve P, Agodoa L, Gellert R, Stewart JH, Buccianti G, Lowenfels AB, et al. Cancer in patients on dialysis for end-stage renal disease: an international collaborative study. *Lancet.* 1999;354(9173):93-9.

[2] Taborelli M, Toffolutti F, Del Zotto S, Clagnan E, Furian L, Piselli P, et al. Increased cancer risk in patients undergoing dialysis: a population-based cohort study in North-Eastern Italy. *BMC Nephrol.* 2019;20(1):107.

[3] Butler AM, Olshan AF, Kshirsagar AV, Edwards JK, Nielsen ME, Wheeler SB, et al. Cancer incidence among US Medicare ESKD patients receiving hemodialysis, 1996-2009. *Am J Kidney Dis.* 2015;65(5):763-72.

[4] Pan HC, Sun CY, Wu IW, Tsai TL, Sun CC, Lee CC. Higher risk of malignant neoplasms in young adults with end-stage renal disease receiving haemodialysis: A nationwide population-based study. *Nephrology* (Carlton). 2019;24(11):1165-71.

[5] Lin MY, Kuo MC, Hung CC, Wu WJ, Chen LT, Yu ML, et al. Association of dialysis with the risks of cancers. *PLoS One.* 2015;10(4):e0122856.

[6] Loy EY, Choong HL, Chow KY. Cancer among end-stage renal disease patients on dialysis. *Ann Acad Med Singap.* 2013;42(12):640-5.

[7] Chung CJ, Huang CY, Tsai HB, Muo CH, Chung MC, Chang CH, et al. Sex differences in the development of malignancies among end-stage renal disease patients: a nationwide population-based follow-up study in Taiwan. *PLoS One.* 2012;7(9):e44675.

[8] Janus N, Launay-Vacher V, Ferrero JM, Thariat J. [Risk of cancer in patients following chronic dialysis and kidney graft]. *Bull Cancer.* 2012;99(3):285-93.

[9] Stewart JH, Vajdic CM, van Leeuwen MT, Amin J, Webster AC, Chapman JR, et al. The pattern of excess cancer in dialysis and transplantation. *Nephrol Dial Transplant.* 2009;24(10):3225-31.

[10] Inamoto H, Ozaki R, Matsuzaki T, Wakui M, Saruta T, Osawa A. Incidence and mortality patterns of malignancy and factors affecting the risk of malignancy in dialysis patients. *Nephron.* 1991;59(4):611-7.

[11] Lowrance WT, Ordoñez J, Udaltsova N, Russo P, Go AS. CKD and the risk of incident cancer. *J Am Soc Nephrol.* 2014 Oct;25(10):2327-34.

[12] Port FK, Ragheb NE, Schwartz AG, Hawthorne VM. Neoplasms in dialysis patients: a population-based study. *Am J Kidney Dis.* 1989;14(2):119-23.

[13] Vajdic CM, McDonald SP, McCredie MR, van Leeuwen MT, Stewart JH, Law M, et al. Cancer incidence before and after kidney transplantation. *JAMA.* 2006;296(23):2823-31.

[14] Vamvakas S, Bahner U, Heidland A. Cancer in end-stage renal disease: potential factors involved. *Am J Nephrol.* 1998;18(2):89-95.

[15] Lee YC, Hung SY, Wang HK, Lin CW, Wang HH, Chang MY, et al. Is there different risk of cancer among end-stage renal disease patients undergoing hemodialysis and peritoneal dialysis? *Cancer Med.* 2018;7(2):485-98.

[16] Vamvakas S, Bahner U, Heidland A. [Increased cancer incidence in terminal kidney failure: potential pathogenetic mechanisms]. *Schweiz Med Wochenschr.* 1997;127(14):597-604.

[17] Chien CC, Han MM, Chiu YH, Wang JJ, Chu CC, Hung CY, et al. Epidemiology of cancer in end-stage renal disease dialysis patients: a national cohort study in Taiwan. *J Cancer.* 2017;8(1):9-18.

[18] Taneja S, Mandayam S, Kayani ZZ, Kuo YF, Shahinian VB. Comparison of stage at diagnosis of cancer in patients who are on dialysis versus the general population. *Clin J Am Soc Nephrol.* 2007;2(5):1008-13.

[19] Lee JE, Han SH, Cho BC, Park JT, Yoo TH, Kim BS, et al. Cancer in patients on chronic dialysis in Korea. *J Korean Med Sci.* 2009;24 Suppl:S95-S101.

[20] Wong G, Hayen A, Chapman JR, Webster AC, Wang JJ, Mitchell P, et al. Association of CKD and cancer risk in older people. *J Am Soc Nephrol.* 2009;20(6):1341-50.

[21] Teschner M, Garte C, Rückle-Lanz H, Mäder U, Stopper H, Klassen A, et al. [Incidence and spectrum of malignant disease among dialysis patients in North Bavaria]. *Dtsch Med Wochenschr.* 2002;127(47):2497-502.

[22] Cheung CY, Chan GC, Chan SK, Ng F, Lam MF, Wong SS, et al. Cancer Incidence and Mortality in Chronic Dialysis Population: A Multicenter Cohort Study. *Am J Nephrol.* 2016;43(3):153-9.

[23] Lin HF, Li YH, Wang CH, Chou CL, Kuo DJ, Fang TC. Increased risk of cancer in chronic dialysis patients: a population-based cohort study in Taiwan. *Nephrol Dial Transplant.* 2012;27(4):1585-90.

[24] Heidland A, Bahner U, Vamvakas S. Incidence and spectrum of dialysis-associated cancer in three continents. *Am J Kidney Dis.* 2000;35(2):347-51; discussion 52-3.

[25] Liu Y, Wang L, Han X, Wang Y, Sun X, Jiang H, et al. The Profile of Timing Dialysis Initiation in Patients with End-stage Renal Disease in China: A Cohort Study. *Kidney Blood Press Res.* 2020;45(2):180-93.

[26] Kurella Tamura M, Desai M, Kapphahn KI, Thomas IC, Asch SM, Chertow GM. Dialysis versus Medical Management at Different Ages and Levels of Kidney Function in Veterans with Advanced CKD. *J Am Soc Nephrol.* 2018;29(8):2169-77.

[27] Yoo KD, Lee JP, Lee SM, Park JY, Lee H, Kim DK, et al. Cancer in Korean patients with end-stage renal disease: A 7-year follow-up. *PLoS One.* 2017;12(7):e0178649.

[28] Satoh S, Tsuchiya N, Habuchi T, Ishiyama T, Seimo K, Kato T. Renal cell and transitional cell carcinoma in a Japanese population undergoing maintenance dialysis. *J Urol.* 2005;174(5):1749-53.

[29] Buccianti G, Maisonneuve P, Ravasi B, Cresseri D, Locatelli F, Boyle P. Cancer among patients on renal replacement therapy: a population-based survey in Lombardy, Italy. *Int J Cancer.* 1996;66(5):591-3.

[30] Fairley CK, Sheil AG, McNeil JJ, Ugoni AM, Disney AP, Giles GG, et al. The risk of ano-genital malignancies in dialysis and transplant patients. *Clin Nephrol.* 1994;41(2):101-5.

[31] Ishikawa I. Renal cell carcinoma in chronic hemodialysis patients--a 1990 questionnaire study in Japan. *Kidney Int Suppl.* 1993;41:S167-9.

[32] Gigante M, Neuzillet Y, Patard JJ, Tillou X, Thuret R, Branchereau J, et al. Renal cell carcinoma (RCC) arising in native kidneys of dialyzed and transplant patients: are they different entities? *BJU Int.* 2012;110(11 Pt B):E570-3.

[33] Levine E, Slusher SL, Grantham JJ, Wetzel LH. Natural history of acquired renal cystic disease in dialysis patients: a prospective longitudinal CT study. *AJR Am J Roentgenol.* 1991;156(3):501-6.

[34] Grantham JJ. Acquired cystic kidney disease. *Kidney Int*. 1991;40(1):143-52.

[35] Fick GM, Gabow PA. Hereditary and acquired cystic disease of the kidney. *Kidney Int*. 1994;46(4):951-64.

[36] Kasiske BL, Ramos EL, Gaston RS, Bia MJ, Danovitch GM, Bowen PA, et al. The evaluation of renal transplant candidates: clinical practice guidelines. Patient Care and Education Committee of the American Society of Transplant Physicians. *J Am Soc* Nephrol. 1995;6(1):1-34.

[37] Cengiz K. Increased incidence of neoplasia in chronic renal failure (20-year experience). *Int Urol Nephrol*. 2002;33(1):121-6.

[38] Stewart JH, Buccianti G, Agodoa L, Gellert R, McCredie MR, Lowenfels AB, et al. Cancers of the kidney and urinary tract in patients on dialysis for end-stage renal disease: analysis of data from the United States, Europe, and Australia and New Zealand. *J Am Soc Nephrol*. 2003;14(1):197-207.

[39] van den Brand JA, van Dijk PR, Hofstra JM, Wetzels JF. Cancer risk after cyclophosphamide treatment in idiopathic membranous nephropathy. *Clin J Am Soc Nephrol*. 2014;9(6):1066-73.

[40] van Leeuwen MT, Webster AC, McCredie MR, Stewart JH, McDonald SP, Amin J, et al. Effect of reduced immunosuppression after kidney transplant failure on risk of cancer: population based retrospective cohort study. *BMJ*. 2010;340:c570.

[41] Birkeland SA, Løkkegaard H, Storm HH. Cancer risk in patients on dialysis and after renal transplantation. *Lancet*. 2000;355(9218):1886-7.

[42] Skov Dalgaard L, Fassel U, Østergaard LJ, Jespersen B, Schmeltz Søgaard O, Jensen-Fangel S. Risk of human papillomavirus-related cancers among kidney transplant recipients and patients receiving chronic dialysis--an observational cohort study. *BMC Nephrol*. 2013;14:137.

[43] Fairley CK, Chen S, Tabrizi SN, McNeil J, Becker G, Walker R, et al. Prevalence of HPV DNA in cervical specimens in women with renal transplants: a comparison with dialysis-dependent patients and patients with renal impairment. *Nephrol Dial Transplant*. 1994;9(4):416-20.

[44] Winkelspecht B, Mueller-Lantzsch N, Köhler H. Serological evidence for reactivation of EBV infection due to uraemic immunodeficiency. *Nephrol Dial Transplant*. 1997;12(10):2099-104.

[45] Köhler H, Girndt M, Dumann H, Klingel R. [The immune defect in kidney failure. II. The mechanisms of the "uremic" immune defect]. *Dtsch Med Wochenschr*. 1993;118(21):790-5.

[46] B.S. CC, Priti Patel MD, M.P.H., Tamara Pilishvili MPH, Matt Moore MD, Trudy Murphy MD, Ray Strikas MD, M.P.H. *Guideline for Vaccinating Dialysis and Chronic Kidney Disease Patients* (updated Dec 2012) 2015 [Available from: https://www.cdc.gov/vaccines/pubs/downloads/dialysis-guide-2012.pdf.

[47] Kim WR. Epidemiology of hepatitis B in the United States. *Hepatology*. 2009;49(5 Suppl):S28-34.

[48] Finelli L, Miller JT, Tokars JI, Alter MJ, Arduino MJ. National surveillance of dialysis-associated diseases in the United States, 2002. *Semin Dial*. 2005;18(1):52-61.

[49] Jadoul M, Bieber BA, Martin P, Akiba T, Nwankwo C, Arduino JM, et al. Prevalence, incidence, and risk factors for hepatitis C virus infection in hemodialysis patients. *Kidney Int*. 2019;95(4):939-47.

[50] Tsukuma H, Hiyama T, Tanaka S, Nakao M, Yabuuchi T, Kitamura T, et al. Risk factors for hepatocellular carcinoma among patients with chronic liver disease. *N Engl J Med.* 1993;328(25):1797-801.

[51] Gordon CE, Berenguer MC, Doss W, Fabrizi F, Izopet J, Jha V, et al. Prevention, Diagnosis, Evaluation, and Treatment of Hepatitis C Virus Infection in Chronic Kidney Disease: Synopsis of the Kidney Disease: Improving Global Outcomes 2018 Clinical Practice Guideline. *Ann Intern Med.* 2019;171(7):496-504.

[52] Kasiske BL, Cangro CB, Hariharan S, Hricik DE, Kerman RH, Roth D, et al. The evaluation of renal transplantation candidates: clinical practice guidelines. *Am J Transplant.* 2001;1 Suppl 2:3-95.

[53] Chadban SJ, Ahn C, Axelrod DA, Foster BJ, Kasiske BL, Kher V, et al. KDIGO Clinical Practice Guideline on the Evaluation and Management of Candidates for Kidney Transplantation. *Transplantation.* 2020;104(4S1 Suppl 1):S11-S103.

[54] American Society of Nephrology. *ASN – Routine cancer screening for dialysis patients.* https://www.choosingwisely.org/clinician-lists/american-society-nephrology-routine-cancer-screening-for-dialysis-patients/. 2012.

[55] Thorsteinsdottir B, Hickson LJ, Ramar P, Reinalda M, Krueger NW, Crowson CS, et al. High rates of cancer screening among dialysis patients seen in primary care a cohort study. *Prev Med Rep.* 2018;10:176-83.

[56] Carlos CA, McCulloch CE, Hsu CY, Grimes B, Pavkov ME, Burrows NR, et al. Colon Cancer Screening among Patients Receiving Dialysis in the United States: Are We Choosing Wisely? *J Am Soc Nephrol.* 2017;28(8):2521-8.

[57] Chertow GM, Paltiel AD, Owen WF, Lazarus JM. Cost-effectiveness of cancer screening in end-stage renal disease. *Arch Intern Med.* 1996;156(12):1345-50.

[58] LeBrun CJ, Diehl LF, Abbott KC, Welch PG, Yuan CM. Life expectancy benefits of cancer screening in the end-stage renal disease population. *Am J Kidney Dis.* 2000;35(2):237-43.

[59] Castellanos MR, Paramanathan K, El-Sayegh S, Forte F, Buchbinder S, Kleiner M. Breast cancer screening in women with chronic kidney disease: the unrecognized effects of metastatic soft-tissue calcification. *Nat Clin Pract Nephrol.* 2008;4(6):337-41.

[60] Castellanos M, Varma S, Ahern K, Grosso SJ, Buchbinder S, D'Angelo D, et al. Increased breast calcifications in women with ESKD on dialysis: implications for breast cancer screening. *Am J Kidney Dis.* 2006;48(2):301-6.

[61] Wong G, Howard K, Chapman JR, Craig JC. Cost-effectiveness of breast cancer screening in women on dialysis. *Am J Kidney Dis.* 2008;52(5):916-29.

[62] Walter LC, Lindquist K, O'Hare AM, Johansen KL. Targeting screening mammography according to life expectancy among women undergoing dialysis. *Arch Intern Med.* 2006;166(11):1203-8.

[63] Bini EJ, Kinkhabwala A, Goldfarb DS. Predictive value of a positive fecal occult blood test increases as the severity of CKD worsens. *Am J Kidney Dis.* 2006;48(4):580-6.

[64] *United States Renal Data System.* USRDS Mortality 2018 report.

[65] Nelson DR, Neu AM, Abraham A, Amaral S, Batisky D, Fadrowski JJ. Immunogenicity of Human Papillomavirus Recombinant Vaccine in Children with CKD. *Clin J Am Soc Nephrol.* 2016;11(5):776-84.

[66] Haberal AN, Bilezikçi B, Ozen O, Yalçinkaya C, Arat Z, Kuşçu E, et al. Pap smear findings in chronic renal failure patients compared with the normal population according to Bethesda 2001. *Diagn Cytopathol.* 2008;36(11):776-9.
[67] Coppolino G, Bolignano D, Rivoli L, Mazza G, Presta P, Fuiano G. Tumour markers and kidney function: a systematic review. *Biomed Res Int.* 2014;2014:647541.
[68] Djavan B, Shariat S, Ghawidel K, Güven-Marberger K, Remzi M, Kovarik J, et al. Impact of chronic dialysis on serum PSA, free PSA, and free/total PSA ratio: is prostate cancer detection compromised in patients receiving long-term dialysis? *Urology.* 1999;53(6):1169-74.
[69] ACS. *American Cancer Society Recommendations for Prostate Cancer Early Detection.* https://www.cancer.org/cancer/prostate-cancer/detection-diagnosis-staging/acs-recommendations.html.
[70] Khairullah QT, Pamatmat SD, Chatha M, Provenzano R, Telang D, Temple M. Early detection of prostate cancer in the ESKD population. *Clin Nephrol.* 2004;61(5):308-15.
[71] Knoll G, Cockfield S, Blydt-Hansen T, Baran D, Kiberd B, Landsberg D, et al. Canadian Society of Transplantation consensus guidelines on eligibility for kidney transplantation. *CMAJ.* 2005;173(10):1181-4.
[72] Batabyal P, Chapman JR, Wong G, Craig JC, Tong A. Clinical practice guidelines on wait-listing for kidney transplantation: consistent and equitable? *Transplantation.* 2012;94(7):703-13.
[73] Campbell S, Pilmore H, Gracey D, Mulley W, Russell C, McTaggart S. KHA-CARI guideline: recipient assessment for transplantation. *Nephrology* (Carlton). 2013;18(6):455-62.
[74] Group ERBPTGD. ERBP Guideline on the Management and Evaluation of the Kidney Donor and Recipient. *Nephrol Dial Transplant.* 2013;28 Suppl 2:ii1-71.
[75] Abbud-Filho M, Adams PL, Alberú J, Cardella C, Chapman J, Cochat P, et al. A report of the Lisbon Conference on the care of the kidney transplant recipient. *Transplantation.* 2007;83(8 Suppl):S1-22.
[76] Pham PT, Pham PA, Pham PC, Parikh S, Danovitch G. Evaluation of adult kidney transplant candidates. *Semin Dial.* 2010;23(6):595-605.
[77] Penn I. Evaluation of transplant candidates with pre-existing malignancies. *Ann Transplant.* 1997;2(4):14-7.
[78] USRDS. *USRDS Mortality 2018 report.* https://www.ajkd.org/article/S0272-6386(18)31131-4/pdf.
[79] Iseki K, Osawa A, Fukiyama K. Evidence for increased cancer deaths in chronic dialysis patients. *Am J Kidney Dis.* 1993;22(2):308-13.
[80] Cohen LM, Ruthazer R, Moss AH, Germain MJ. Predicting six-month mortality for patients who are on maintenance hemodialysis. *Clin J Am Soc Nephrol.* 2010;5(1):72-9.
[81] Cohen. Hemodialysis mortality tool - 6 month. https://qxmd.com/calculate/calculator_135/6-month-mortality-on-hd.
[82] Beddhu S, Bruns FJ, Saul M, Seddon P, Zeidel ML. A simple comorbidity scale predicts clinical outcomes and costs in dialysis patients. *Am J Med.* 2000;108(8):609-13.
[83] Goldwasser P, Mittman N, Antignani A, Burrell D, Michel MA, Collier J, et al. Predictors of mortality in hemodialysis patients. *J Am Soc Nephrol.* 1993;3(9):1613-22.

[84] Tzanakis I, Kazoulis S, Girousis N, Kagia S, Spandidakis V, Karefillakis N, et al. Prostate-specific antigen in hemodialysis patients and the influence of dialysis in its levels. *Nephron.* 2002 Feb;90(2):230–3.

[85] Bruun L, Björk T, Lilja H, Becker C, Gustafsson O, Christensson A. Percent-free prostate specific antigen is elevated in men on haemodialysis or peritoneal dialysis treatment. *Nephrol Dial Transplant.* 2003 Mar;18(3):598–603.

[86] Wada Y, Nakanishi J, Takahashi W, Kai N, Nakayama Y, Yamashita Y, et al. Mass screening for prostate cancer in patients with end-stage renal disease: a comparative study. *BJU Int.* 2006 Oct;98(4):794–7.

[87] Bruun L, Savage C, Cronin AM, Hugosson J, Lilja H, Christensson A. Increase in percent free prostate-specific antigen in men with chronic kidney disease. *Nephrol Dial Transplant.* 2009 Apr;24(4):1238–41.

[88] Joseph DA, Thompson T, Saraiya M, Werny DM. Association between glomerular filtration rate, free, total, and percent free prostate-specific antigen. *Urology.* 2010 Nov;76(5):1042–6.

[89] Tarhan F, Orçun A, Küçükercan I, Camursoy N, Kuyumcuoglu U. Effect of hemodialysis on serum complexed prostate-specific antigen levels. *Scand J Urol Nephrol.* 2007;41(5):382–6.

[90] Takiyyuddin MA, Cervenka JH, Hsiao RJ, Barbosa JA, Parmer RJ, O'Connor DT. Chromogranin A. Storage and release in hypertension. *Hypertension.* 1990 Mar;15(3):237–46.

[91] Tramonti G, Ferdeghini M, Annichiarico C, Norpoth M, Donadio C, Bianchi R, et al. Relationship between renal function and blood level of chromogranin A. *Ren Fail.* 2001 Jul;23(3–4):449–57.

[92] Hsiao RJ, Mezger MS, O'Connor DT. Chromogranin A in uremia: progressive retention of immunoreactive fragments. *Kidney Int.* 1990 Mar;37(3):955–64.

[93] Castoldi G, Antolini L, Bombardi C, Perego L, Mariani P, Viganò MR, et al. Oxidative stress biomarkers and chromogranin A in uremic patients: effects of dialytic treatment. *Clin Biochem.* 2010 Dec;43(18):1387–92.

[94] Lye WC, Tambyah P, Leong SO, Lee EJ. Serum tumor markers in patients on dialysis and kidney transplantation. *Adv Perit Dial Conf Perit Dial.* 1994;10:109–11.

[95] Acchiardo S, Kraus AP, Jennings BR. Beta 2-microglobulin levels in patients with renal insufficiency. *Am J Kidney Dis.* 1989 Jan;13(1):70–4.

[96] Cases A, Filella X, Molina R, Ballesta AM, Lopez-Pedret J, Revert L. Tumor markers in chronic renal failure and hemodialysis patients. *Nephron.* 1991;57(2):183–6.

[97] Filella X, Cases A, Molina R, Jo J, Bedini JL, Revert L, et al. Tumor markers in patients with chronic renal failure. *Int J Biol Markers.* 1990 Jun;5(2):85–8.

[98] Menzin AW, Kobrin S, Pollak E, Goodman DB, Rubin SC. The effect of renal function on serum levels of CA 125. *Gynecol Oncol.* 1995 Sep;58(3):375–7.

[99] Buys SS, Partridge E, Black A, Johnson CC, Lamerato L, Isaacs C, et al. Effect of screening on ovarian cancer mortality: the Prostate, Lung, Colorectal and Ovarian (PLCO) Cancer Screening Randomized Controlled Trial. *JAMA.* 2011 Jun 8;305(22):2295–303.

[100] Zeferos N, Digenis GE, Christophoraki M, Alexopoulos I, Kostakis A, Gyftaki H, et al. Tumor markers in patients undergoing hemodialysis or kidney transplantation. *Nephron.* 1991;59(4):618–20.

[101] Xiaofang Y, Yue Z, Xialian X, Zhibin Y. Serum tumour markers in patients with chronic kidney disease. *Scand J Clin Lab Invest.* 2007;67(6):661–7.

[102] Arik N, Adam B, Akpolat T, Haşil K, Tabak S. Serum tumour markers in renal failure. *Int Urol Nephrol.* 1996;28(4):601–4.

[103] Soni S, Menon MC, Bhaskaran M, Jhaveri KD, Molmenti E, Muoio V. Elevated human chorionic gonadotropin levels in patients with chronic kidney disease: Case series and review of literature. *Indian J Nephrol.* 2013 Nov;23(6):424–7.

[104] Tzitzikos G, Saridi M, Filippopoulou T, Makri A, Goulioti A, Stavropoulos T, et al. Measurement of tumor markers in chronic hemodialysis patients. *Saudi J Kidney Dis Transplant.* 2010 Jan;21(1):50–3.

[105] Küchle C, Fricke H, Held E, Schiffl H. High-flux hemodialysis postpones clinical manifestation of dialysis-related amyloidosis. *Am J Nephrol.* 1996;16(6):484–8.

[106] Haninger-Vacariu N, Herkner H, Lorenz M, Säemann M, Vychytil A, Jansen M, et al. Exclusion of pregnancy in dialysis patients: diagnostic performance of human chorionic gonadotropin. *BMC Nephrol.* 2020 Feb 28;21(1):70.

[107] Scalamogna A, Imbasciati E, De Vecchi A, Castelnovo C, Pagliari B, De Cristofaro V, et al. Beta-2 microglobulin in patients on peritoneal dialysis and hemodialysis. Perit Dial *Int J Int Soc Perit Dial.* 1989;9(1):37–40.

[108] Mojahedi MJ, Hami M, Shakeri M-T, Hekmat R. Influence of dialysis duration, peritoneal transport parameters, and gender on effluent CA125 concentration in patients on peritoneal dialysis. *Iran J Kidney Dis.* 2007 Oct;1(2):78–81.

[109] Botchorishvili G, Matikainen MP, Lilja H. Early prostate-specific antigen changes and the diagnosis and prognosis of prostate cancer. *Curr Opin Urol.* 2009 May;19(3):221–6.

[110] Dayer-Métroz MD, Wollheim CB, Seckinger P, Dayer JM. A natural interleukin 1 (IL-1) inhibitor counteracts the inhibitory effect of IL-1 on insulin production in cultured rat pancreatic islets. *J Autoimmun.* 1989 Apr;2(2):163–71.

[111] Al-azawi D, Kelly G, Myers E, McDermott EW, Hill ADK, Duffy MJ, et al. CA 15-3 is predictive of response and disease recurrence following treatment in locally advanced breast cancer. *BMC Cancer.* 2006 Sep 5;6:220.

[112] Singh AP, Senapati S, Ponnusamy MP, Jain M, Lele SM, Davis JS, et al. Clinical potential of mucins in diagnosis, prognosis, and therapy of ovarian cancer. *Lancet Oncol.* 2008 Nov;9(11):1076–85.

[113] Kohorn EI. The new FIGO 2000 staging and risk factor scoring system for gestational trophoblastic disease: description and critical assessment. *Int J Gynecol.* 2001 Feb;11(1):73–7.

In: Issues in Kidney Disease – Dialysis
Editors: Stephen Z. Fadem and José A. Moura-Neto
ISBN: 978-1-68507-000-7

Chapter 6

DIALYSIS UREA CLEARANCE AND CLEARANCE TARGETS

Andrew Davenport*, MD
UCL Department of Renal Medicine, Royal Free Hospital,
University College London, London, UK

ABSTRACT

Urea, a small nitrogenous molecule, is retained in patients with chronic kidney disease, and has been used for many years as a biomarker of chronic kidney disease. As urea production is dependent upon protein turnover, urea is used in dialysis patients, both as a biomarker of dialytic clearance and also as a nutritional marker as a surrogate for dietary protein intake. There are accepted clinical targets for haemodialysis sessional urea clearance, which have now been adapted for patients using both incremental and more frequent haemodialysis schedules and also for peritoneal dialysis, However, it must be appreciated that whereas failing to achieve adequate urea clearance increases the risk of patients becoming unwell due to inadequate dialysis clearance, simply achieving a clinical urea target clearance does not guarantee that patients will be adequately dialysed, as other solutes which accumulate in chronic kidney failure do not have the same distribution and dialysis clearance as urea.

Keywords: dialysis, haemodialysis, peritoneal dialysis, urea, clearance, dialysis adequacy

INTRODUCTION

The waste products of cellular metabolism accumulate in patients with chronic kidney disease. Urea is the most recognised product of cell metabolism, being generated from the breakdown of proteins into amino acids, and subsequent recycling of amino acids in the urea cycle. Although there is debate as to the absolute toxicity of urea, urea is used in clinical

* Corresponding Author's E-mail: andrewdavenport@nhs.net.

practice as a surrogate measurement of retained azotaemic molecules, and urea removal by dialysis is used as an estimate of azotaemic molecule clearance.

Urea Clearance by Dialysis

Urea is a small uncharged molecule that is generated by intracellular metabolism. In plasma water, urea is rapidly cleared by diffusion during dialysis treatments. Diffusive clearance is made more efficient by the concentration gradient generated by counter-current blood and dialysate flows, increasing dialyzer surface area, dialyzer design to maximise blood and dialysate contact area, narrower diameter capillary fibres, and capillary fibre composition designed to minimise the resistance to passage of solutes. Each dialyzer comes with a manufacturer's measurements of ex-vivo urea clearance (Ko) at different blood pump and dialysate speeds for dialyzers of different surface area (A), but this laboratory clearance (KoA) is greater than that achievable in clinical practice, as it is not derived from experiments using human blood. For peritoneal dialysis (PD), urea diffusion depends upon the effective surface area, which is dependent upon peritoneal and intestinal capillary blood flow, and cycle fill volume and dwell time.

Although urea rapidly diffuses from plasma water during passage through the dialyzer, urea concentrations rapidly fall in the plasma during the first 30 minutes of the haemodialysis session and then plateau, as most urea is intracellular, and moves from the intracellular to extracellular compartments through urea transporters; and as this transport is slower than urea dialyzer clearance, serum urea concentrations fall. Thus, at slower blood pump speeds (< 300 ml/min), urea clearance is blood flow dependent, and then at blood pump speeds > 300 ml/min urea clearance can be increased with increasing dialyzer surface area, until clearance then becomes limited by urea transfer from intra- to extracellular compartments.

Sessional Dialyzer Clearance

The National Cooperative Dialysis Study (NCDS) was the first prospective haemodialysis study to examine the effect of urea clearance, randomising patients to a lower and higher time averaged blood urea nitrogen (BUN) target for 12 months. This was a relatively small study of around 150 patients, who were younger than contemporary dialysis cohorts, with minimal comorbidity, which reviewed patient study drop out due to physician decision or hospital admission. Although there was no difference in mortality, more patients in the higher time averaged urea group dropped out of the study. Time averaged BUN required a minimum of three blood samples, and Gotch and Sargent subsequently developed the concept of dialyzer urea clearance (KoA which became shortened to K), based on two blood samples, taken pre- and post-dialysis, and the time of the dialysis session (t). To allow comparison between patients, dialyzer urea clearance was adjusted to body water volume (V), with body water being estimated from anthropometric measurements derived from healthy subjects.

Kt/Vurea Targets

Gotch and Sargent initially reported that patients with a sessional Kt/Vurea of 0.9 or less were most at risk of dropping out of the NCDS study. Over time, by consensus, sessional Kt/Vurea targets were steadily increased to 1.2 and then to 1.4.

A second prospective trial, the Haemodialysis (HEMO) study compared the outcome of 1,850 patients randomised to an average single pool sessional Kt/Vurea of 1.32 versus 1.53, and reported no obvious benefit with the higher sessional Kt/Vurea, and as such most centres aim for a target of 1.4 to ensure that most patients achieve a sessional Kt/V > 1.3.

Kt/Vurea Models for Haemodialysis

The simplest model of dialyzer urea clearance is to calculate the urea reduction ratio (URR), comparing the fall in pre- to post-dialysis urea concentrations (See equations). URR does not take into account any additional urea clearance from the additional fluid removed by ultrafiltration. This led to the development of a series of Kt/Vurea models. The simplest model is the single pool Kt/V (spKt/V), which assumes that urea is distributed equally throughout the body, and that urea is removed equally from all body compartments during the dialysis session. However, blood flow distribution changes during dialysis, as the blood supply to muscle and skin, and internal organs falls, as blood preferentially pools in the larger venous capacitance vessels, and thus at the end of the dialysis session the blood urea concentration starts to rapidly rise as blood supply to muscle and internal organs is restored, and urea redistributes between body compartments. To compensate for this urea rebound effect, a number of techniques have been developed to standardise how blood samples should be taken at the end of the dialysis session. The stop-flow and slow-flow methods reduce blood and dialysate flows to allow a re-equilibration of urea, and so minimise the effect of the urea rebound phenomenon. To overcome the urea rebound effect, a second generation of Kt/V models were developed, termed equilibrated Kt/V (eKt/V) - designed to compensate for the differential removal of urea from different body compartments.

URR = (Pre-urea concentration – Post-urea concentration) x 100/Pre-urea concentration

Single pool Kt/V (spKt/V)

spKt/V = - natural logarithm (1-URR)

First Generation Equation

spKt/V = -Ln((Urea concentration post/Urea concentration pre) - 0.008 x t – 1 x UF/W),
t - dialysis session time hours
UF – ultrafiltration volume, L
W – post-dialysis weight, Kg

Second Generation Kt/V Equation

spKt/V = -Ln((Urea concentration post/Urea concentration pre) - 0.008 x t) + (4-3.5 x R) x UF/W.

R= URR

Equilibrated Kt/V

Rate adjustment method

eKt/V = spKt/V – 0.6 (spKt/V)/time hours + 0.03

Kt/Vurea Models to Adjust Haemodialysis Frequency

The sessional spKt/V and eKt/V equations are based on the premise that patients are dialysing thrice weekly, and blood samples are taken prior to and at the end of the mid-week dialysis session. However, clinical practice has changed over time, with some patients now dialysing less frequently, whereas other patients may be dialysing four or more times per week, with varying dialysis session times. So to allow for Kt/V dialysis targets to be set and comparison between patients dialysing with varying schedules, the concept of a standardised Kt/V (stdKt/V) was introduced, where stdKt/V is calculated from stdK multiplied by time (10,080 minutes per week) and adjusted by V.

Standardised Kt/V

$$stdKt/V = \frac{10{,}080 \times \frac{1-e^{-eKt/V}}{t}}{\frac{1-e^{-eKt/V}}{eKt/V} + \frac{10{,}080}{Ft} - 1}$$

t = treatment time, min; V = modeled two-pool post-dialysis volume, mL; F = frequency of treatment per week;

Urinary Urea Clearance (Kr)

$$Urinary\ urea\ clearance\ (Kr) = \frac{U \times V}{P}$$

U = Urinary urea nitrogen concentration of interdialytic urine sample (mg/dL)

V = Urine volume excretion rate during interdialytic collection (ml/min)

P = Time-averaged serum urea nitrogen concentration during interdialytic collection (mg/dL)

Variable Volume Model, with Kr

$$stdKt/V = \frac{Eq.6}{1 - \frac{0.74}{F}\left[\frac{Uf}{V}\right]} + Kr\frac{10{,}080}{V}$$

Uf = weekly fluid gain between dialyses, mL
F = frequency of treatment per week

Using the Dialysis Machine to Estimate Urea Clearance

Different dialysis machine manufacturers have adapted different technologies to estimate dialyzer urea clearance, termed online clearance. At body temperature, sodium and urea have very similar diffusion coefficients (Na+: 1.94 x 10 –5 cm2/s, Urea: 2.20 x 10 –5 cm2/s), despite differing in molecular weight and electrical charge. Dialysis machines measure dialysate conductivity, so by detecting changes in conductivity of fresh and spent dialysate in response to a pulse of increased fresh dialysate sodium, the machine can make an estimate of sodium diffusion, and by inference urea clearance. Repeating measurements during dialysis at intervals then allows an estimate of dialyzer urea clearance. To prevent sodium gain, the pulses of a change in fresh dialysate sodium alternate between an increased and then decreased sodium concentration. An alternative strategy has been to measure urea in the spent dialysate by the absorbance of ultraviolet light (UV) using optical sensors designed to detect absorbance from UV-C band: light emitting diodes at 280 nm -100 nm.

Estimating Clearance in Peritoneal Dialysis Patients

Whereas urea and creatinine fall with haemodialysis, serum urea and creatinine concentrations tend to remain relatively constant during therapy with peritoneal dialysis. As the majority of peritoneal dialysis patients pass urine, traditionally clearance in peritoneal dialysis patients is calculated as a combined weekly peritoneal and urinary clearance. Unlike haemodialysis, there has been no equivalent randomised prospective study to compare different urea or creatinine clearance targets. As such, different clinical guideline committees have suggested different targets; Kidney Disease Improving Global Outcomes (KDIGO) provide no weekly creatinine clearance target, but advise a weekly Kt/Vurea target of > 1.7; the European Renal Best Practice Group (ERBP) recommend a weekly creatinine clearance target of > 45L/1.73m2 for patients treated by automated peritoneal cyclers, and weekly Kt/Vurea > 1.7 for all modes of peritoneal dialysis; and the United Kingdom Renal Association recommend a weekly creatinine clearance of > 50 L/1.73m2 and weekly Kt/Vurea > 1.7.

However, it is important to remember that peritoneal clearance of urea and creatinine are not equivalent to the clearance of residual renal function. Observational studies have emphasised the importance of residual renal function, rather than peritoneal clearances, in maintaining the clinical care of patients treated by peritoneal dialysis.

Equations for Peritoneal Dialysis

Urine

Weekly litres of creatinine cleared (weekly LCrU) = ((24 hr Ur x 7/SeUr) + (24 hr UCr x 7/SeCr))/2

Weekly Urinary Kt/Vurea = Weekly litres creatinine cleared/V

Peritoneal

Weekly Peritoneal litres of creatinine cleared (weekly LCrP) = 24hr PCr x 7/SeCr

Weekly peritoneal Kt/Vurea = (PUr x 7)/(SeUr x V)

Combined clearances

Total weekly L creatinine cleared/1.73m^2 = ((weekly LCrP) + (weekly LCrU)) x 1.73/BSA

Total weekly Kt/Vurea = (weekly Urine Kt/Vurea) + (weekly Peritoneal Kt/Vurea)

Urine urea	UUr
Urine creatinine	UCr
Serum urea	SeUr
Serum creatinine	SeCr
Peritoneal dialysate urea	PUr
Peritoneal dialysate creatinine	PCr
Body surface urea	BSA

Incremental Dialysis for Solute Clearances

As many patients now start dialysis with residual renal function, this has led to the practice of incremental dialysis for both peritoneal and haemodialysis patients. Whereas urinary clearances have traditionally been used to estimate total clearance in peritoneal dialysis clearances, only a limited number of haemodialysis centres request patients to collect 24-hour urine collections. Whereas the combined urinary urea and creatinine clearance is used to estimate clearance for peritoneal dialysis patients, as dialyzer clearance is assessed in terms of urea clearance, then urinary collections are used to calculate urinary urea clearance (Kr) for haemodialysis patients. Kr is then adjusted to the volume of urea distribution to estimate the equivalent urinary renal clearance (EKRc), which is referred to as residual renal function (KRU).

The 2006 KDOQI adequacy guideline advised against reducing the dose of haemodialysis delivered to patients with a KRU of < 2 ml/min/1.73m2, equally one has to consider volume status and cardiovascular reserve when considering incremental dialysis, and thus less frequent dialysis schedules are not advised for patients with a residual urine output of < 600 ml/day, or those with reduced cardiac function or have large inter-dialytic weight gains of ≥ 3.5%. KDOQI suggested that for those with KRU > 2 ml/min/1.73m2, then for twice weekly schedules, then a sessional spKt/Vurea target of 1.93 for a 3.5 hour session and 1.68 for a 4.0 hour session, and for a KRU > 3 ml/min/1.73m2 then equivalent stdKt/Vurea of 1.2 for a 3.5-hour.

As 1 ml/min of dialyser urea clearance is not biologically equivalent to 1 ml/min of residual renal clearance, one cannot simply add the time-averaged residual urea clearance (KRU) to the time-averaged dialysis urea clearance (Kdurea) as this would underestimate the contribution of KRU to overall clearance. There have been proposed methods to add Kdurea to KRU by converting intermittent Kdurea to an equivalent continuous KRU or vice versa. One such method proposed has been to convert Kdurea to an equivalent continuous clearance and then combining with KRU.

Equivalent Renal Urea Clearance

Equivalent Renal Urea Clearance (EKRurea, ml/min) is the ratio of the net urea generation rate to the time-averaged urea concentration (TACurea, mg/ml). To compare averaged renal urea clearance and dialysis urea clearance between patients, then the EKRurea should be standardised to a urea volume (V, L) of 40 L, and is then termed corrected EKR (EKRc, ml/min/40 L). The same adjustment can be used to standardise KRU to a urea volume of 40 L, deriving corrected Kr (Krc, ml/min/40 L).

To prescribe Kt/Vurea corresponding to Krc and adjusting for the number of dialysis sessions per week, European clinical guidelines advise using the Casino and Lopez normogram (Figure) or an estimate using:

Thrice-weekly EKRc=1+ (10 × eKt/Vurea + Krc)

Twice-weekly EKRc=1+ (6 × eKt/Vurea + Krc)

This target EKRc was derived from achieving a thrice-weekly eKt/Vurea of 1.2 (taken from an eKt/Vurea 1.16 which was the standard dose used in the HEMO study), and approximates to 13 ml/min/40 L. This target is slightly higher than the target EKRc of 11 ml/min/40 L obtained from earlier studies.

Augmented Dialysis

Although patients initiating dialysis may start with less haemodialysis than the standard thrice weekly 4-hour schedule paradigm, as residual renal function is lost, then dialyzer clearance needs to be appropriately increased. This increase in dialysis is termed augmented dialysis, and when patients become anuric then augmented dialysis includes increasing the frequency of dialysis schedules, increasing session length, and introducing other techniques to improve the clearance of other azotaemic solutes, such as haemodiafiltration, higher permeability dialyzers, adsorption or displacement techniques designed to increase clearance of middle sized solutes and protein bound solutes to compensate for the loss of residual renal function.

Errors in Calculating Kt/V

Failure to allow for sufficient time for urea to re-equilibrate when taking the post-dialysis blood sample will result in a lower post-dialysis urea concentration, and thus an inflated estimate of dialyzer Kt/Vurea.

V is traditionally estimated using anthropometric equations which are based on healthy subjects. Body composition naturally changes with age, gender and ethnicity, and as muscle contains more water than fat, this leads to an over- estimation of V in large obese patients, and under estimation of V in small patients, and women. Thus, if all patients were to achieve the same target Kt/V, then not all patients would receive the same amount of dialyzer clearance. Small men would receive relatively less dialyzer clearance than larger men, and women would receive less dialyzer clearance that men. In the general population, morbidly obese patients are at greater risk of mortality, and women outsurvive men, but in the hemodialysis population morbidly obese patients outsurvive those patients with a normal body mass index, and women have similar or lower survival than men. Analysis of the HEMO study did show that women randomised to the higher sessional Kt/Vurea target had greater survival.

Online clearance methods tend to overestimate dialyzer clearances, as methods based on detecting changes in sodium diffusion are intermittent, so can potentially miss falls in blood pump speed or dialysate flow in between measurements, and the UV absorbance method tends to measure other nitrogen containing molecules in addition to urea.

Not all patients can provide, or are willing to provide, a 24-hour urine collection due to various reasons including incontinence and inconvenience. Similarly, not all urine may be accurately collected and may vary with fluid intake and physical activity. In addition, for haemodialysis patients the urine output and urinary urea excretion falls in the 24 hours immediately post a haemodialysis session and then starts to increase. As such, urine collections made after a dialysis session will under-estimate residual renal function, and timing of the urine collection in relation to dialysis sessions needs to be standardised. Although there have been attempts to derive equations measuring serum β2-microglobulin, β-trace protein and Cystatin C alone or in combinations, to provide an estimate of residual renal function rather than depending upon urinary collections, as of yet they have not been proven for clinical practice.

Convective Dialyzer Clearance

Dialysis is predominantly a diffusive technique, and as such is more effective in clearing small solutes. As small solutes may not be the most toxic of the waste products of cellular metabolism, then other techniques are required to remove larger solutes. This can be achieved by using dialyzers with larger pores, but as the pore size increases, then patients are at risk of losing small proteins and albumin. An alternative is to introduce convective clearance by applying an external hydrostatic pressure that drives water across the dialyzer membrane, according to the hydraulic permeability of the dialyzer, which differs with dialyzer membrane composition and structure. Whereas urea (molecular weight= 64 daltons) moves 18 times faster than β2-microglobulin (molecular weight= 11,800 daltons) by diffusion, convective clearance will be equal provided that both urea and β2-microglobulin can pass through the dialyzer membrane. Dialyzer flux is now defined according to clearance of β2-microglobulin, so high flux dialyzers allow greater β2-microglobulin than low flux.

During a standard haemodialysis treatment there will be some convective exchange if there has been ultrafiltration. In addition, depending upon the hydraulic permeability of the dialyzer, there may be internal diafiltration, which can be as much as 6-9 L during a 4-hour dialysis session. It may be because of this internal diafiltraton that studies comparing high-flux haemodiafiltration and high flux haemodialysis have not shown a major survival advantage for haemodiafiltration. Although the one trial designed to investigate high-volume convective exchange, aiming for 23 L/session, did show a survival benefit for high-volume haemodiafiltration.

Interpreting Adequacy in Haemodialysis Patients

It must be remembered that Kt/V is a measure of dialyzer urea clearance, and as such is only component of the dialysis prescription. Over time, the target has increased by consensus from 0.9 to 1.2 to 1.4. Urea is a small uncharged molecule that is readily removed by diffusion. As other waste products of metabolism are larger, may be charged and transfer from the intracellular compartment to the extracellular compartment at a slower rate, protein bound in plasma water then the clearance of these other solutes by dialysis will be much less efficient when compared to urea clearance. As such, simply achieving a sessional dialyser urea or peritoneal dialysis urea clearance target does not necessarily imply that the patient has received an adequate clearance of azotaemic waste products, whereas on the other hand, failure to achieve a urea clearance target would provide even lower clearance of other azotaemic solutes.

Alternative Methods of Assessing Adequacy of Dialyzer Clearance

The generation of waste products of metabolism depend upon total energy expenditure (TEE), which includes both the basal metabolic rate (BMR) and also active energy expenditure (AEE). BMR depends on the physical size of patients, and is closely aligned with body surface area (BSA). Re-analysis of the HEMO study showed that when the delivered dialysis dose (Kt) was adjusted for BSA, the patients who received a greater Kt/BSA had greater survival. The majority of dialysis patients in North America and Europe are elderly and have additional morbidity, so AEE is often only marginally greater than BMR. However, for younger, fitter, healthier patients, AEE is much greater. Studies have reported that when Kt is adjusted for TEE, then patients receiving the greater dose of dialysis have increased survival compared to those with lower Kt/TEE. Body composition studies show that AEE is closely aligned with appendicular muscle mass, which is also associated with BSA.

Thus, ideally, TEE would potentially be a better scaling adjustment for Kt, but if not available then BSA would be an improvement on the traditional V.

SUMMARY ADJUSTING KT/V TARGETS FOR INDIVIDUAL PATIENTS

Although the concept of a target Kt/V was to provide an equivalent dose of dialysis for all patients, there are several major confounders, and as such some patient groups receive a greater dialysis dose than others. As such it is important to recognise that some patient groups require a greater dose of dialysis above the standard target sessional Kt/V to guard against delivering a lower effective dialysis dose. The groups most at risk of receiving less dialysis, and as such require a delivered Kt/V above target include women, small men, patients who have less comorbidity, and those who are physically active and at work.

REFERENCES

Casino FG, Lopez T. The equivalent renal urea clearance: a new parameter to assess dialysis dose. *Nephrol Dial Transplant.* 1996 Aug;11(8):1574-81.

Daugirdas JT, Greene T, Rocco MV, Kaysen GA, Depner TA, Levin NW, et al. Effect of frequent hemodialysis on residual kidney function. *Kidney Int.* 2013 May;83(5):949-58.

European Best Practice Guidelines Expert Group on Hemodialysis ERA. Section I. Measurement of renal function, when to refer and when to start dialysis. *Nephrol Dial Transplant.* 2002;17 Suppl 7:7-15.

Gotch FA, Sargent JA. A mechanistic analysis of the National Cooperative Dialysis Study (NCDS). *Kidney Int.* 1985; 28: 526-534.

Hanson JA, Hulbert-Shearon TE, Ojo AO, Port F K, Wolfe RA, Agodoa LY, et al. Prescription of twice-weekly hemodialysis in the USA. *Am J Nephrol.* 1999;19(6):625-33.

Hemodialysis Adequacy Work G. Clinical practice guidelines for hemodialysis adequacy, update 2006. *Am J Kidney Dis*. 2006 Jul; 48 Suppl 1:S2-90.

Lin X, Yan Y, Ni Z, Gu L, Zhu M, Dai H, et al. Clinical outcome of twice-weekly hemodialysis patients in shanghai. *Blood Purif.* 2012;33(1-3):66-72.

Lowrie EG, Laird NM, Parker TF, Sargent JA. Effect of the hemodialysis prescription of patient morbidity: report from the National Cooperative Dialysis Study. *N Engl J Med.* 1981 Nov 12;305(20):1176-81.

Maduell F, Moreso F, Pons M, et al. High-efficiency postdilution online hemodiafiltration reduces all-cause mortality in hemodialysis patients. *J Am Soc Nephrol.* 2013;24:487–97.

Meyer TW, Sirich TL, Fong KD, et al. Kt/Vurea and Nonurea Small Solute Levels in the Hemodialysis Study. *J Am Soc Nephrol.* 2016; 27(11):3469-3478.

National Kidney Foundation. KDOQI Clinical Practice Guideline for Hemodialysis Adequacy: 2015 update. *Am. J Kidney Dis.* 2015 Nov;66(5):884-930.

Obi Y, Rhee CM, Mathew AT, Shah G, Streja E, Brunelli SM, et al. Residual Kidney Function Decline and Mortality in Incident Hemodialysis Patients. *J Am Soc Nephrol.* 2016 Dec;27(12):3758-3768.

Obi Y, Streja E, Rhee CM, Ravel V, Amin AN, Cupisti A, et al. Incremental Hemodialysis, Residual Kidney Function, and Mortality Risk in Incident Dialysis Patients: A Cohort Study. *Am. J Kidney Dis.* 2016 Aug;68(2):256-265.

Rocco MV, Lockridge RS, Jr., Beck GJ, Eggers PW, Gassman JJ, Greene T, et al. The effects of frequent nocturnal home hemodialysis: the Frequent Hemodialysis Network Nocturnal Trial. *Kidney Int.* 2011 Nov;80(10):1080-91.

Shafi T, Jaar BG, Plantinga LC, Fink NE, Sadler JH, Parekh RS, et al. Association of residual urine output with mortality, quality of life, and inflammation in incident hemodialysis patients: the Choices for Healthy Outcomes in Caring for End-Stage Renal Disease (CHOICE) Study. *Am J Kidney Dis.* 2010 Aug;56(2):348-58.

Tangvoraphonkchai K, Davenport A. Incremental Haemodialysis - A European Perspective. *Semin Dial.* 2017 May; 30(3):270-276.

Tangvoraphonkchai K, Davenport A. Increasing Haemodialytic Clearances as Residual Renal Function Declines: An Incremental Approach. *Blood Purif.* 2017;44(3):217-226.

Tattersall JE, DeTakats D, Chamney P, Greenwood RN, Farrington K. The post-hemodialysis rebound: predicting and quantifying its effect on Kt/V. *Kidney Int.* 1996 Dec;50(6):2094-102.

Termorshuizen F, Dekker FW, van Manen JG, Korevaar JC, Boeschoten EW, Krediet RT, et al. Relative contribution of residual renal function and different measures of adequacy to survival in hemodialysis patients: an analysis of the Netherlands Cooperative Study on the Adequacy of Dialysis (NECOSAD)-2. *J Am Soc Nephrol.* 2004 Apr;15(4):1061-70.

Wang AY, Lai KN. The importance of residual renal function in dialysis patients. *Kidney Int.* 2006 May;69(10):1726-32.

Watson PE, Watson ID, Batt RD. Total body water volumes for adult males and females estimated from simple anthropometric measurements. *Am J Clin Nutr.* 1980 Jan;33 (1):27-39.

In: Issues in Kidney Disease – Dialysis
Editors: Stephen Z. Fadem and José A. Moura-Neto
ISBN: 978-1-68507-000-7

Chapter 7

Fatigue in People Treated with Dialysis

Federica Picariello[1], PhD, Hugh Rayner[2], MD, Andrew Mooney[3], MD, Joseph Chilcot[1], PhD and James Tattersall[3,*], MD

[1]Institute of Psychiatry, Psychology, and Neuroscience, King's College, London, UK
[2]University Hospitals Birmingham NHS Foundation Trust, Birmingham, UK
[3]Leeds Teaching Hospitals, Leeds, UK

Abstract

The majority of people treated with dialysis experience fatigue, which is defined as a subjective feeling of extreme tiredness, exhaustion, and weakness that is unrelated to activity and exertion and is not relieved by rest and recuperation. Patients and their caregivers consider fatigue to be one of the most important symptoms affecting their quality of life. It is more common in patients treated with dialysis than with other long-term conditions, such as cancer and heart disease; however, the fatigue experienced is otherwise similar. Patients who suffer from fatigue are likely to have worse clinical outcomes, including being admitted to hospital and dying. Fatigue is a complex and multifactorial symptom. Factors linked directly to the disease (precipitants) are likely to trigger it, while psychological factors (perpetuators) can maintain it over time. Patients with chronic kidney disease are uraemic, even when treated with dialysis. Uraemia results in neuropathy and malnutrition and is associated with inflammation and vascular disease. These, in turn, are associated with functional and structural abnormalities of muscle that result in weakness and contribute to fatigue. People treated with dialysis often are elderly and have comorbidities, such as diabetes or heart disease, where fatigue is more likely. Age and comorbidities are associated with psychological distress which also predisposes to fatigue. The dialysis process itself can contribute to fatigue through inflammation and loss of amino acids in haemodialysis and loss of albumin in peritoneal dialysis; all of these can cause muscle wasting (sarcopenia). Solute and fluid disequilibrium affecting the brain is another possible cause of fatigue after a haemodialysis session. Dialysis is time-consuming and can require travelling and an early start to the day. The reduction in time available for

* Corresponding Author's E-mail: jamestattersall@doctors.org.uk.

rest, recreation, and essential activities can in itself be fatiguing, independent of patho-physiological or patho-psychological mechanisms. The way people think about their symptoms and their kidney disease more generally can amplify negative emotions and determine how they cope with fatigue. Excessive rest, avoidance, or inconsistent patterns of activity and rest, and withdrawal from social and favored activities can worsen fatigue. These behaviors can lead to deconditioning, increased physiological arousal, and a disrupted sleeping pattern, contributing to a cycle of worsening fatigue. Because fatigue has many interrelated causes, it is unlikely to respond to any single intervention. Different approaches should be considered, addressing both precipitants and perpetuators of fatigue. An individualized approach based on multiple interventions and guided by an understanding of the causes can significantly improve the quality of life of patients treated with dialysis.

Keywords: fatigue, dialysis, psychological, adverse effects, peritoneal dialysis, hemodialysis, behavior therapy, cognitive

INTRODUCTION

Fatigue is defined as a subjective feeling of extreme tiredness, exhaustion, and weakness, which is not related to activity and not relieved by rest and recuperation. Dialysis patients describe their fatigue in terms such as "I've got no energy whatsoever…I feel like I've got a big, heavy load on me and I'm just so tired" [1]. It may be constant or limited to the period after dialysis. The former is similar to the fatigue reported by people with other long-term conditions. Post-dialysis fatigue is somewhat different, being related to the dialysis treatment. A person may experience both forms, their constant fatigue being worse in the hours after hemodialysis.

There are currently no published guidelines for the management of fatigue in patients treated with dialysis. Furthermore, there are no recommended methods for diagnosing or quantifying fatigue and relatively few randomized controlled trials (RCTs) of interventions in this patient group. The trials that have been done are small in size or inconclusive in outcome. Multiple different ways have been used to quantify fatigue, which makes it difficult to compare or aggregate results.

Fatigue in patients treated with dialysis often persists after causes such as anemia, depression, and heart failure have been adequately managed. A combination of factors may be responsible, making it hard to determine priorities for treatment. Treatment of one cause may exacerbate another; for example, removal of excess fluid to relieve heart failure may result in dehydration and hypotension at the end of dialysis.

Fatigue is perpetuated by a cycle of negative emotional and physiological consequences [2]. It is associated with depression, frustration, sleep disorders, and loss of motivation to engage in health-promoting behaviors. These psychological effects can have negative physical consequences that, in turn, increase fatigue. Interventions to disrupt this cycle may reduce the impact of fatigue.

We will explore these aspects in more detail in this chapter.

THE IMPORTANCE OF FATIGUE

In a recent Standardized Outcomes in Nephrology (SONG) study, more than 1000 participants ranked 34 outcomes of haemodialysis in order of importance [3, 4]. Participants included patients, caregivers/family members, nephrologists, surgeons, nurses, social workers, psychologists, dieticians, pharmacists, policy makers, researchers, and industry representatives with experience or interest in haemodialysis. A formal Delphi methodology was used to achieve consensus among the participants. Fatigue, defined as "Feeling tired with no energy for weeks, for most of the time," was one of the five most important outcomes to be used in future clinical trials.

In the Hemodialysis (HEMO) Study, 1,798 prevalent haemodialysis patients were studied for up to six years. Fatigue, as assessed by repeated questionnaires, was strongly associated with mortality [5]. A more recent observational study of 174 dialysis patients also found that fatigue was associated with an increased risk of mortality and reduced likelihood of transplantation [6].

The impact of fatigue on the quality of life of patients treated with dialysis was recently reviewed [7]. Patients describe fatigue as highly unpleasant, debilitating, and destructive of normal life experiences in the following ways:

- Fatigue symptom is unpleasant in itself
- Post-dialysis recovery time increases the burden of disease and reduces time to enjoy life
- Unable to take part in normal activities
- Reduces ability to take part in family life and sustain relationships
- Fear of being perceived as lazy
- Failure to meet expectations

THE PREVALENCE OF FATIGUE IN PATIENTS TREATED WITH DIALYSIS

In two recent studies, a total of over 1,400 people treated with haemodialysis returned questionnaires reporting their symptoms [8]. Fatigue was reported by 89% and 77% of the participants and was the most commonly reported symptom in both studies. In an earlier systematic review of 59 studies, fatigue was the most common symptom, reported by a mean of 71% of patients treated with dialysis across all studies [9]. The prevalence varied between 12% and 97%, probably due to differences in how fatigue was defined and measured in the individual studies. In a study of patients with chronic kidney disease that used structured interviews and questionnaires, fatigue was the most commonly reported symptom [10]. 56% of participants reported fatigue without being asked specifically, with a further 28% reporting it when prompted.

In studies specifically asking about fatigue after the dialysis treatment, 66% of patients reported post-dialysis fatigue [11]. The median time taken to recover from the treatment was 3 hours, with 10% of patients taking over 12 hours. The length of the recovery time correlated with the severity of fatigue.

FACTORS ASSOCIATED WITH FATIGUE IN THE GENERAL POPULATION

Fatigue is reported by about 10% of the population. The majority of these people have long-term conditions such as multiple sclerosis, cancer, rheumatoid arthritis, inflammatory bowel disease, systemic lupus erythematosus, and chronic kidney disease. A minority have no associated condition and are diagnosed with chronic fatigue syndrome/myalgic encephalomyelitis (CFS/ME). Features common to the fatigue associated with all these conditions include inflammation, disorders of muscle function, and specific unhelpful thoughts and behaviors.

Inflammation

Markers of inflammation are associated with the prevalence and severity of fatigue. Healthy animals administered pro-inflammatory cytokines enter into a state of reduced activity and appetite, and avoid contact with other animals [12]. Fatigue may be triggered by inflammation and have evolved to conserve energy, avoid risk of injury, and reduce the spread of infection between animals.

There is evidence that the behavioral and psychological changes resulting from fatigue (lack of exercise [13], social isolation [14], psychological distress [15]) may induce inflammation. So, inflammation may be part of a cycle where it is both a cause and consequence, amplifying and perpetuating fatigue.

Muscular Dysfunction

Fatigue is almost always associated with morphological abnormalities of muscles that are typical of disuse. These include reduced muscle mass (sarcopenia), fat infiltration, and a relative reduction in the number of type II, fast twitch muscle fibers. Muscle strength and the ability to perform sustained or repeated exercise are correspondingly reduced. These abnormalities occur normally with ageing but are more advanced compared to non-fatigued individuals of a similar age. It is usually not clear whether they precede and cause the fatigue, but they certainly contribute to it and are exacerbated by the resulting lack of exercise [16].

Depression and Anxiety

Fatigue is associated with depression and anxiety, which could be a cause and/or a consequence of fatigue. Low mood and withdrawal from social interactions and favored activities can be physically and mentally draining, while the restrictions imposed by fatigue on day-to-day activities may contribute to low mood and anxiety.

Depression is associated with an increased risk of hospitalization [17], thereby adding to the burden of disease. Both depression and fatigue are associated with all-cause mortality in patients treated with dialysis [5]. Social isolation and poverty are risk factors for fatigue, depression, and anxiety.

Treatment with antidepressants is not helpful for fatigue unless depression is also present. Similarly, psychological treatments aimed at depression are insufficient to address fatigue; larger improvements are made following psychological treatments specifically aimed at fatigue [18].

Sleep Disorders

Patients' perception of their sleep quality is strongly associated with fatigue [19]. People with fatigue typically have interrupted sleep at night and tend to sleep for periods during the day. Sleeping during the day may be a consequence of reduced activity and may reduce the need for sleep at night. The resulting loss of normal sleep quality and rhythm contributes to fatigue.

Depression, anxiety, and potentially unhelpful thought processes contribute to the sleep disorders. Taking daytime naps, having irregular bedtime habits, and mental stimulation at bedtime such as watching TV can worsen fatigue. Physical conditions likely to interrupt sleep include sleep apnea, pain, shortness of breath, and the restless legs syndrome.

Cognitive-Behavioral Factors

Wessely et al. have proposed a bio-psychosocial cognitive-behavioral model to explain the fatigue associated with long-term conditions [20]. Precipitants related to the underlying disease, such as anemia and dialysis, may trigger fatigue; how patients then react cognitively, emotionally, and behaviorally to the initial symptoms may worsen and perpetuate fatigue over time.

For example, a person may believe that fatigue is doing damage to his or her body, these thoughts leading to anxiety and low mood. The person may rest to try to reduce the damage being done to the body, but excessive rest may in turn evoke thoughts of being unable to be active and of never getting better.

Deconditioning, an insidious complication of rest, may decrease stamina and increase the feeling of fatigue. Poor sleep and physiological arousal related to anxiety may continue the vicious cycle of fatigue.

Cognitive Responses to Fatigue Include [21]

- Catastrophizing - obsessive and irrational thoughts anticipating the worst possible outcome
- Damage beliefs - the perception that fatigue is damaging the body
- Fear avoidance - activity is believed to be causing physical damage
- Embarrassment avoidance - the patient is ashamed of his or her symptoms
- Symptom focus - the patient is constantly thinking about associated symptoms

Unhelpful Behaviors in Response to Fatigue Include [21]

- Resting and avoidance of physical activity and exercise, contributing to muscle deconditioning and dysfunction
- All-or-nothing behavior - inconsistent patterns of activity and rest with episodes of over-exertion followed by excessive rest
- Avoiding social contact

Psychological factors in fatigue are likely to be common to most long-term conditions [22, 23, 24]. The type of chronic illness explains only 11% of the variance in the severity of fatigue, whereas female sex, age, motivational and concentration problems, pain, sleep disturbance, physical functioning, reduced activity, and lower self-efficacy concerning fatigue explain 55%. Interaction between the type of chronic illness and the transdiagnostic factors explains a further 6% [25].

In patients treated with haemodialysis, cognitive and behavioral factors play a dominant role in fatigue severity and functional impairment. Patients' negative beliefs related to mood and unhelpful behaviors are associated with the severity of fatigue and explain 36% of the variance in the severity of fatigue [26]. Similarly, mood, damage beliefs, avoidance behaviors, and fatigue severity explain 44% of variance in fatigue-related functional impairment. Damage beliefs predict increasing fatigue-related functional impairment over time [2].

Beliefs that patients have about their kidney disease can also play a role [27]. These include:

- identity - how symptoms are experienced and attributed to the illness
- cause - beliefs about the causes of the illness
- timeline - beliefs about the duration of the illness, whether is cyclical, acute or chronic
- consequence - beliefs about the impact of the illness
- control/cure - beliefs regarding the controllability or curability of the illness

Patients who hold a severe illness identity and have stronger consequence beliefs are more likely to suffer with fatigue [28, 29].

Fatigue in Patients Treated with Dialysis

In a survey of 87 patients with chronic kidney disease not receiving dialysis (eGFR $\leq$45 ml/min/1.73 m^2) and 86 treated with dialysis, the prevalence and severity of fatigue was similar in both groups [19]. The prevalence and severity of fatigue are similar in patients treated with peritoneal and haemodialysis. In the HEMO study, patients receiving dialysis with longer treatment times had a lower severity of fatigue. This suggests that dialysis is not the only trigger of fatigue and that pathophysiological triggers may be affected by kidney replacement therapy. Fatigue may also persist following kidney transplantation, with fatigue affecting about half of recipients with stable function [30].

Severe uraemia causes motor neuropathy and protein malnutrition. However, no uremia biomarker has been found that correlates with fatigue in patients who are adequately treated with dialysis. Fatigue is more common and more severe in dialysis patients with lower urea and creatinine levels, due to their relationship with malnutrition and muscle wasting [31]. Fatigue is also common in patients treated by successful kidney transplant [26], despite the absence of uremia.

Factors linked to fatigue in the general population, such a long-term conditions, inflammation and muscle dysfunction, apply equally to patients treated with dialysis. In addition, uremia-related comorbidities such as fluid overload, anemia, hyperparathyroidism, and neuropathy can contribute to fatigue.

Uremia induces muscle wasting, especially when there is also malnutrition and/or inflammation [32, 33]. Muscle total mass and mitochondrial mass are reduced [34]. Type II, fast twitch fibers are lost, as found with disuse [35]. Neuropathy is often present, sometimes independent of muscle abnormalities, especially in patients with diabetes.

Fatigue is associated with subjectively poor sleep quality and sleepiness during the day but not to objectively measured sleep quality [19]. Poor sleep quality may not necessarily be a trigger of fatigue, but likely to contribute to the vicious cycle of fatigue in patients treated with dialysis.

POST-DIALYSIS FATIGUE

Many patients treated with haemodialysis experience an increase in fatigue following a dialysis session [36]. This symptom can be measured simply by asking the question: "How long does it take you to recover from a dialysis session?"

The Dialysis Outcomes and Practice Patterns Study has investigated dialysis recovery time [37]. 68% of patients reported a recovery time of at least 2 hours, and 10% took more than 12 hours. Patients with older age, longer dialysis vintage, higher body mass index, diabetes, and psychiatric disorder were likely to have a longer recovery time. Of treatment related factors, greater interdialytic weight gain, longer dialysis session length, and lower dialysate sodium concentration were associated with longer recovery time. Recovery time was correlated with increased symptoms of kidney failure and the kidney disease burden score, and with worse scores on both mental and physical components of the health-related quality of life questionnaire. In another recent study, recovery time was associated with measures of psychological distress [38].

Longer recovery time was also associated with greater risks of hospitalization and mortality. Patients reporting a recovery time >12 hours had a 22% higher rate of first hospitalization and a 47% higher mortality rate than those with a recovery time between 2 and 6 hours.

Because recovery time is so simple to measure and strongly linked to major outcomes, it should be used as an important measure of dialysis outcomes in research studies and routine clinical care.

It might be expected that fatigue after dialysis would be caused by fluid and solute disequilibrium during the dialysis process. However, this has not been confirmed by clinical studies. High ultrafiltration rate was associated with shorter recovery times in one study [39] whilst the opposite was shown in another [40]. Similarly, in a randomized controlled trial, reducing solute disequilibrium by reducing blood flow rate did not reduce recovery time [41].

Daily and nocturnal dialysis [42] have been shown to reduce dialysis recovery time compared to conventional three times weekly dialysis. Both techniques reduce the peak levels of uraemic toxins and fluid overload, and nocturnal dialysis reduces solute and fluid disequilibrium.

Having a dialysate sodium concentration <140 mmol/L was associated with longer recovery time, even after allowing for differences in interdialytic weight gain. This association was stronger when comparing dialysis units that used the same dialysate sodium concentration for all their patients. Patients in these units are allocated a sodium concentration mainly according to where they live rather than for any clinical reasons, making the association with recovery time more convincing.

Higher dialyzate sodium concentration reduces the osmotic shifts across the blood–brain barrier that cause cerebral disequilibrium. The association of longer recovery times with lower concentrations suggests that the symptoms may be partly a manifestation of the effects of dialysis on the brain. A controlled trial of the effect of different dialysate sodium concentrations on fatigue after dialysis has not yet been performed.

Diagnosis and Measurement of Fatigue

Fatigue experienced by patients treated with dialysis is typically assessed using measures that have been evaluated in the general population [24]. Measurement of fatigue is challenging, as it is complex and subjective in nature. To date, there is no objective "gold standard" measure of fatigue; instead, different self-report questionnaires are available to capture patients' perceptions of fatigue and its impact [43, 4].

An ideal measurement of fatigue needs to be simple, concise, and have a recall period of under four weeks. It should focus on the impact of fatigue on the person's life and capture the idiosyncratic features of fatigue related to dialysis. Currently, such a measure does not exist, making it difficult to distinguish factors associated with general fatigue from those specific to dialysis-related fatigue [4].

A systematic review of 123 studies of patients with kidney failure found 43 different ways of measuring fatigue. The most widely used instrument in patients treated with dialysis is the vitality subscale of the SF-36 [44]. Other validated questionnaires [45] include the 9-question Fatigue Severity Scale [46], the 12-question EORTC QLQ-FA12 scale [47], and the 11-question Chalder Fatigue Questionnaire [48].

Potentially unhelpful beliefs and behaviors in response to fatigue can be captured by the Cognitive and Behavioral Responses to Symptoms Questionnaire (CBSQ) [49].

Neuromuscular Measurements

Muscle mass as a proportion of total body mass can be measured using bioimpedance spectroscopy (BIS). This technique analyzes the impedance to an electric current at a range of frequencies flowing between electrodes at the wrist and ankle. A body composition model is required in dialysis patients to account for variations in fluid content. BIS can be performed at the bedside and is suitable for routine clinical care. In addition, it provides a measure of the volume of any fluid overload or depletion.

Ultrasound can be used to measure the cross-sectional area of the femoral rectus muscle. This has been shown to correlate strongly with muscle mass calculated by BIS [50].

Handgrip strength can easily be measured at the bedside and reflects more general neuromuscular function. Reduced handgrip strength is associated with increased mortality [51].

If muscle wasting or weakness is detected, protein intake should be assessed. Intake is calculated from the urea nitrogen appearance rate. In peritoneal dialysis this is measured from timed collections of urine and PD fluid; in haemodialysis the rate of rise in serum urea concentration between hemodialysis sessions is used. In an anuric patient treated by dialysis, an adequate protein intake results in the serum urea concentration rising by about 10 mmol/L/day.

Neuropathy is detected and quantified by nerve conduction studies.

Approach to a Person Complaining of Fatigue

Clinicians tend to neglect fatigue. In a study of kidney transplant recipients, 59% of patients experienced fatigue but this was only documented in the medical records of 13% [52].

Fatigue is best thought of as a complex multifactorial biopsychosocial phenomenon. Factors that trigger fatigue differ from those that maintain it over time. The complexity of the condition and the management plan designed to address these factors need to be explained carefully.

The patient should be assessed for potentially modifiable underlying conditions such as malnutrition, inflammation, depression, inadequate dialysis dose, hyperparathyroidism, heart failure, anemia, hyper- or hypothyroidism, hypo- or hypertension, fluid overload, dehydration, and poor diabetic control.

The patient should also be assessed to discover as much as possible about their symptoms, priorities, and expectations. An empathetic process of trying to understand the problem from the patient's point of view is likely, of itself, to have psychological benefit [53].

It is important not to make value judgements about the results of objective and subjective assessments of fatigue. In most cases, it will not be possible to establish the cause of the fatigue with any certainty. Even when psychological or behavioral factors are strongly suspected, it will not be possible to rule out effects of the underlying disease or its treatment. Treatment needs to be tailored to the patient's own aspirations and priorities, not to universal clinical benchmarks. For example, attempting to increase muscle strength by an exercise program is unlikely to be effective if the patient does not see muscle weakness as a problem.

Ideally, the patient will identify activities or functions which they would like to undertake but which are prevented by their fatigue. The results of subjective and objective tests can then be used to inform the patient, which are the relevant physical and psychological barriers to be overcome.

It is important to help the patient develop coping strategies to minimize the negative consequences of fatigue on their function and quality of life. In a survey of patients with cancer and fatigue, the most common advice provided by healthcare professionals was to rest and relax

[54]. Far from helping, this may lead to further deconditioning, and worsen and perpetuate fatigue.

With most patients, it should be possible to plan interventions to help them overcome the barriers they have identified. Even if this is not possible, interventions that are a pleasurable distraction are still worthwhile (Figure 1).

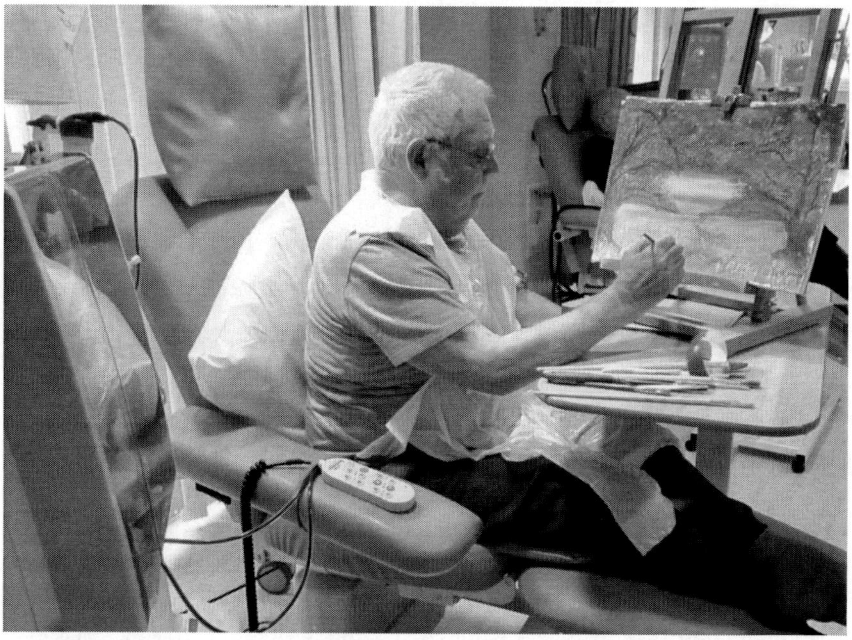

Figure 1. Creating artwork during the hemodialysis is a pleasurable distraction from the treatment and can restore a sense of achievement.

POTENTIAL TREATMENTS FOR CHRONIC FATIGUE IN PATIENTS TREATED WITH DIALYSIS

Changes in Dialysis Modality

Since its prevalence and severity are similar in patients treated with haemodialysis and peritoneal dialysis, there is no consistent benefit from changing modality if the patient is otherwise stable. A change to enhanced hemodialysis, such as long nocturnal and/or daily dialysis, may reduce the time needed to recover after dialysis and may help reduce the tendency for symptomatic hypotension during dialysis. However, nocturnal dialysis should be avoided in patients who still pass significant amounts of urine as it can hasten the loss of residual kidney function.

If the psychological burden of hospital hemodialysis is considered to be contributing to fatigue, it may be worth considering a switch to home dialysis.

Dialyzing at home places different demands on the patient compared to hospital treatment. Home dialysis avoids travel and gives patients more control over their treatment. Hospital dialysis facilitates social interaction, support and help with the treatment. Each will have a different potential to influence fatigue, depending on the patient's personality and relationships.

Inadequate dialysis results in anorexia, malnutrition, neuropathy and muscle loss, all causes of fatigue. With modern hemodialysis machines and dialyzers, it is relatively easy to achieve the recommended dialysis dose. With conventional thrice weekly dialysis, there is no benefit from increasing the dose above the recommended targets ($Kt/V > 1.2$; blood volume processed = ideal body weight). An adequate dose may be harder to achieve with peritoneal dialysis in an anuric patient.

Correction of Anemia

In patients with anemia, raising the hemoglobin concentration to 100 g/L improves fatigue. Small further improvements may be gained by increasing the concentration above 100 g/L in younger, more active patients. Fatigue is not improved by increasing hemoglobin above 120 g/L [55].

Even if the patient is not anemic, actual and functional iron deficiency should still be corrected. Iron deficiency is associated with fatigue in dialysis patients who are not anemic [56] and, in people with heart disease, correcting iron deficiency improves fatigue.

Adjustments to diet or nutritional supplements may be required to correct nutritional deficiencies. However, non-specific supplementation in the absence of proven deficiency does not improve fatigue [57].

Pharmacological Agents

A review of pharmacological treatments, including l-carnitine, growth hormone, nandrolone decanoate, and vitamin C, among dialysis patients concluded that these medications cannot be recommended for the prevention of fatigue, and complete and prolonged relief from fatigue is rare [58].

Physical Exercise

Dialysis patients are commonly less physically active than normal, and the degree of inactivity correlates with objective measurements of muscular strength and function. Structured interviews of dialysis patients reveal multiple barriers to increasing physical activity other than reduced muscle strength [59]. These include fatigue, fear of falling, lack of motivation, and fear that exercise will worsen their condition.

Patients treated with peritoneal dialysis have similarly reduced physical activity to those treated with hemodialysis [60]. Patients treated with peritoneal dialysis may be more likely to believe that exercise is harmful to their health, including that it may cause peritoneal leaks.

Exercise training can improve muscle strength and mass [61] but may be unsuitable for patients with multi-morbidities, disabilities, and other contraindications. To maintain the benefit, exercise needs to be part of normal lifestyle; hence, it must be appealing and not dependent upon inaccessible facilities or resources [62].

It can be hard to start exercising, even more so with a chronic and progressive condition. Exercise needs to be selected according to personal needs and resources to make it more appealing and sustainable in the long term. Where motivation is an issue, a combined approach of exercise and psychological therapy can be offered [59].

Despite a lack of strong evidence that exercise improves objective measures of muscle function, a meta-analysis of the literature concluded that interventions to increase physical activity did reduce subjective symptoms, including restless legs syndrome, depression, and fatigue, in people treated by haemodialysis and peritoneal dialysis [63]. A suggested regimen might be 20–60 minutes per day of continuous aerobic exercise, on three to five days a week, and resistance exercises of moderate intensity two to three days per week. The literature on fatigue in patients with multiple sclerosis indicates that the mechanisms through which exercise improves fatigue may vary by type of exercise and the choice needs to be informed by the patient's needs and preferences [64].

Treatment of Sleep Disorders

A Cochrane review has identified 67 studies of the treatment of sleep disorders in patients treated with dialysis [65]. Treatments included relaxation techniques, exercise, acupressure, cognitive behavioral therapy (CBT), sleep hygiene or health behavior education, telephone support, reflexology, light therapy, music, aromatherapy and massage. Medications included benzodiazepines, dopaminergic agonist therapy and melatonin. While some of the studies reported benefits, the evidence was weak or inconsistent. An earlier review and meta-analysis [66] concluded that CBT was effective and that acupressure or exercise may be helpful in improving sleep quality. In two pilot trials, CBT for sleep quality led to small but significant improvements in fatigue among patients treated with dialysis [67, 68].

Obstructive sleep apnea is common in patients treated with dialysis; it might be expected that its correction would have multiple benefits, including fatigue. However, evidence is limited to a single case report [69] and a study of oxygen therapy in 40 patients treated by peritoneal dialysis [70]. More studies are needed in this area.

Mind-Body Exercise

Mind-body exercise techniques combine body movement with mental concentration. These include dance, Tai Chi, yoga, and Qigong [71]. Meta-analyses of their use in cancer and multiple sclerosis found that these were safe and moderately effective at reducing symptoms, including fatigue [72, 73]. However, they have not yet been studied in kidney patients.

Cognitive Behavioral Therapy

Cognitive behavioral therapy (CBT) was originally developed for the treatment of mood disorders [74]. It is a tailored and time-limited talking therapy founded on the premise that it is the interpretation of events and subsequent coping attempts that matter, rather than the events themselves. The CBT protocol aimed at fatigue differs from that for mood disorders, the focus being on unhelpful thoughts in relation to fatigue, addressing inconsistent activity routines, and gradually increasing daily activity.

CBT is effective across a range of conditions, particularly auto-immune and inflammatory conditions, where pharmacological interventions do not consistently demonstrate benefit [75]. CBT protocols may need to be adapted for patients with cognitive impairment. CBT combined with graded exercises is more effective than CBT or exercise alone in patients with cancer [76, 77], although the benefits on fatigue over the long term remain unclear.

There have been few studies [78] of psychological interventions for fatigue, and specifically CBT, in people with kidney failure. A systematic review found promising evidence of benefit particularly in patients who met diagnostic thresholds for fatigue [65], supported by a small feasibility randomized-controlled trial of CBT-based fatigue intervention in patients treated with haemodialysis [79]. Mediation analyses of CBT support the theory that cognitive-behavioral factors perpetuate fatigue [80, 81]. Changes in negative perceptions of fatigue were key mediators of the reduction in fatigue, rather than changes in anxiety and depression [79].

Patients treated with haemodialysis already have a high burden of treatment, so it is important to deliver these interventions flexibly and in an appealing way.

Potential Treatments for Post-Hemodialysis Fatigue

Switching from conventional thrice-weekly dialysis to nocturnal or daily dialysis can shorten recovery time, from a mean of 4 hours to 30 minutes. Thrice-weekly haemodialysis at home has shorter recovery times than treatment in a dialysis unit, a median of 30 versus 55 minutes. Psychological distress caused by dialysis may be reduced by self-care at home. The impact of post-dialysis fatigue may be reduced by scheduling dialysis later in the day [82]. A switch from hemodialysis to peritoneal dialysis would eliminate any distress due to the hemodialysis procedure including the post-dialysis recovery time.

Having more residual kidney function is associated with a shorter recovery time [83]. This can be achieved by avoiding hypotensive events during dialysis, post-dialysis dehydration, intensive dialysis, and nephrotoxic medications. Incremental dialysis, which includes residual kidney function in the total dose of dialysis and reduces the amount of dialysis required, is associated with shorter recovery times. Increasing dialysis time may be helpful for anuric patients, whereas longer dialysis may be counterproductive for those still passing urine [84].

Hypotensive events during dialysis can be avoided through accurate targeting of dry weight and reducing the need for ultrafiltration, such as by dietary salt restriction. Bioimpedance spectroscopy can be helpful in determining the correct target weight [85].

Conclusion

Despite its high prevalence and impact on the quality and duration of the life of dialysis patients, fatigue is often neglected. Nephrologists may be reluctant to discuss fatigue with patients due to a lack of confidence in its diagnosis or knowledge of effective treatments. This needs to change.

Management of fatigue is made challenging by the lack of regular fatigue assessments using a measure validated in patients treated with dialysis, and by the interaction of a multitude of possible precipitants and perpetuators that differ between patients. There is unlikely to be a single effective intervention; each patient needs an individualized assessment and treatment regimen.

Simply focusing attention on fatigue is an important first step for improving the quality of life of patients treated with dialysis.

REFERENCES

[1] Picariello F, Moss-Morris R, Macdougall IC, Chilcot J. 'It's when you're not doing too much you feel tired': A qualitative exploration of fatigue in end-stage kidney disease. *Br J Health Psychol*. 2018 May;23(2):311-333.

[2] Picariello F, Norton S, Moss-Morris R, Macdougall IC, Chilcot J. A prospective study of fatigue trajectories among in-centre haemodialysis patients. *Br J Health Psychol*. 2020 Feb;25(1):61-88.

[3] Evangelidis N, Tong A, Manns B, Hemmelgarn B, Wheeler DC, Tugwell P, Crowe S, Harris T, Van Biesen W, Winkelmayer WC, Sautenet B, O'Donoghue D, Tam-Tham H, Youssouf S, Mandayam S, Ju A, Hawley C, Pollock C, Harris DC, Johnson DW, Rifkin DE, Tentori F, Agar J, Polkinghorne KR, Gallagher M, Kerr PG, McDonald SP, Howard K, Howell M, Craig JC; Standardized Outcomes in Nephrology–Hemodialysis (SONG-HD) Initiative. Developing a Set of Core Outcomes for Trials in Hemodialysis: An International Delphi Survey. *Am J Kidney Dis*. 2017 Oct;70(4):464-475.

[4] Ju A, Unruh M, Davison S, Dapueto J, Dew MA, Fluck R, Germain M, Jassal SV, Obrador G, O'Donoghue D, Josephson MA, Craig JC, Viecelli A, O'Lone E, Hanson CS, Manns B, Sautenet B, Howell M, Reddy B, Wilkie C, Rutherford C, Tong A; SONG-HD Fatigue Workshop Collaborators. Establishing a Core Outcome Measure for Fatigue in Patients on Hemodialysis: A Standardized Outcomes in Nephrology-Hemodialysis (SONG-HD) Consensus Workshop Report. *Am J Kidney Dis*. 2018 Jul;72(1):104-112.

[5] Jhamb M, Pike F, Ramer S, Argyropoulos C, Steel J, Dew MA, Weisbord SD, Weissfeld L, Unruh M. Impact of fatigue on outcomes in the hemodialysis (HEMO) study. *Am J Nephrol*. 2011;33(6):515-23.

[6] Picariello F, Norton S, Moss-Morris R, Macdougall IC, Chilcot J. Fatigue in Prevalent Haemodialysis Patients Predicts All-cause Mortality and Kidney Transplantation. *Ann Behav Med*. 2019 May 3;53(6):501-514.

[7] Jacobson J, Ju A, Baumgart A, Unruh M, O'Donoghue D, Obrador G, Craig JC, Dapueto JM, Dew MA, Germain M, Fluck R, Davison SN, Jassal SV, Manera K, Smith AC, Tong A. Patient Perspectives on the Meaning and Impact of Fatigue in Hemodialysis: A Systematic Review and Thematic Analysis of Qualitative Studies. *Am J Kidney Dis*. 2019 Aug;74(2):179-192.

[8] Rhee EP, Guallar E, Hwang S, Kim N, Tonelli M, Moe SM, Himmelfarb J, Thadhani RI, Powe NR, Shafi T. Prevalence and Persistence of Uremic Symptoms in Incident Dialysis Patients. *Kidney360*. 2020 Feb;1(2):86-92.

[9] Murtagh FE, Addington-Hall J, Higginson IJ. The prevalence of symptoms in end-stage renal disease: a systematic review. *Adv Chronic Kidney Dis*. 2007;14(1):82-99.

[10] James G, Nyman E, Fitz-Randolph M, Niklasson A, Hedman K, Hedberg J, Wittbrodt ET, Medin J, Moreno Quinn C, Allum AM, Emmas C. Characteristics, Symptom Severity, and Experiences of Patients Reporting Chronic Kidney Disease in the PatientsLikeMe Online Health Community: Retrospective and Qualitative Study. *J Med Internet Res*. 2020 Jul 15;22(7):e18548.

[11] Bossola M, Di Stasio E, Monteburini T, Parodi E, Ippoliti F, Bonomini M, Santarelli S, Eugenio Nebiolo P, Sirolli V, Cenerelli S. Intensity, Duration, and Frequency of Post-Dialysis Fatigue in Patients on Chronic Haemodialysis. *J Ren Care*. 2020 Jun;46(2):115-123.

[12] Munshi S, Parrilli V, Rosenkranz JA. Peripheral anti-inflammatory cytokine Interleukin-10 treatment mitigates interleukin-1β - induced anxiety and sickness behaviors in adult male rats. *Behav Brain Res*. 2019 Oct 17;372:112024.

[13] Cabral-Santos C, de Lima Junior EA, Fernandes IMDC, Pinto RZ, Rosa-Neto JC, Bishop NC, Lira FS. Interleukin-10 responses from acute exercise in healthy subjects: A systematic review. *J Cell Physiol*. 2019 Jul;234(7):9956-9965.

[14] Ahmadian AJ, Lin JE, Neylan TC, Woolley JD, O'Donovan A, Cohen BE. Social integration and inflammation in individuals with and without posttraumatic stress disorder. *Brain Behav Immun*. 2020 Oct;89:168-174.

[15] Slavich GM, Irwin MR. From stress to inflammation and major depressive disorder: a social signal transduction theory of depression. *Psychol Bull*. 2014 May;140(3):774-815.

[16] McCormick R, Vasilaki A. Age-related changes in skeletal muscle: changes to life-style as a therapy. *Biogerontology*. 2018;19(6):519-536. doi:10.1007/s10522-018-9775-3.

[17] Lacson E Jr, Bruce L, Li NC, Mooney A, Maddux FW. Depressive affect and hospitalization risk in incident hemodialysis patients. *Clin J Am Soc Nephrol*. 2014 Oct 7;9(10):1713-9.

[18] Kangas M, Bovbjerg DH, Montgomery GH. Cancer-related fatigue: a systematic and meta-analytic review of non-pharmacological therapies for cancer patients. *Psychol Bull*. 2008 Sep;134(5):700-741.

[19] Jhamb M, Liang K, Yabes J, Steel JL, Dew MA, Shah N, Unruh M. Prevalence and correlates of fatigue in chronic kidney disease and end-stage renal disease: are sleep disorders a key to understanding fatigue? *Am J Nephrol*. 2013;38(6):489-95.

[20] Wessely, S., Butler, S., Chalder, T., & David, A. The cognitive behavioural management of the post-viral fatigue syndrome. In J. R. & J. Mowbrey (Eds.), *Postviral fatigue syndrome* (pp. 305 – 334). Chichester: John Wiley & Sons. 1991.

[21] Moss-Morris R. Symptom perceptions, illness beliefs and coping in chronic fatigue syndrome, *Journal of Mental Health*. 2005;14:3:223-235.

[22] van Kessel K, Moss-Morris R. Understanding multiple sclerosis fatigue: a synthesis of biological and psychological factors. *J Psychosom Res*. 2006 Nov;61(5):583-5.

[23] Hewlett S, Chalder T, Choy E, Cramp F, Davis B, Dures E, Nicholls C, Kirwan J. Fatigue in rheumatoid arthritis: time for a conceptual model. *Rheumatology (Oxford)*. 2011 Jun;50(6):1004-6.

[24] Bower JE. Cancer-related fatigue-mechanisms, risk factors, and treatments. *Nat Rev Clin Oncol*. 2014 Oct;11(10):597-609.

[25] Menting J, Tack CJ, Bleijenberg G, Donders R, Droogleever Fortuyn HA, Fransen J, Goedendorp MM, Kalkman JS, Strik-Albers R, van Alfen N, van der Werf SP, Voermans NC, van Engelen BG, Knoop H. Is fatigue a disease-specific or generic symptom in chronic medical conditions? *Health Psychol.* 2018 Jun;37(6):530-543.

[26] Chilcot J, Moss-Morris R, Artom M, Harden L, Picariello F, Hughes H, Bates S, Macdougall IC. Psychosocial and Clinical Correlates of Fatigue in Haemodialysis Patients: the Importance of Patients' Illness Cognitions and Behaviours. *Int J Behav Med.* 2016 Jun;23(3):271-281.

[27] Leventhal, H., Nerenz, D. R., & Purse, J. Illness representations and coping with health threats. In A. Baum, S. E. Taylor & J. E. Singer (Eds.), *Handbook of psychology and health* (pp. 219-252). Hillsdale, NJ: Lawrence Erlbaum Associates, Inc. 1984.

[28] Picariello F, Moss-Morris R, Macdougall IC, Chilcot AJ. The role of psychological factors in fatigue among end-stage kidney disease patients: a critical review. *Clin Kidney J.* 2017 Feb;10(1):79-88.

[29] Timmers L, Thong M, Dekker FW, Boeschoten EW, Heijmans M, Rijken M, Weinman J, Kaptein A; Netherlands Cooperative Study on the Adequacy of Dialysis (NECOSAD) Study Group. Illness perceptions in dialysis patients and their association with quality of life. *Psychol Health.* 2008;23(6):679-90.

[30] Bossola M, Pepe G, Vulpio C. Fatigue in kidney transplant recipients. *Clin Transplant.* 2016 Nov;30(11):1387-1393.

[31] Jhamb M, Argyropoulos C, Steel JL, Plantinga L, Wu AW, Fink NE, Powe NR, Meyer KB, Unruh ML; Choices for Healthy Outcomes in Caring for End-Stage Renal Disease (CHOICE) Study. Correlates and outcomes of fatigue among incident dialysis patients. *Clin J Am Soc Nephrol.* 2009 Nov;4(11):1779-86.

[32] Cheema B, Abas H, Smith B, O'Sullivan AJ, Chan M, Patwardhan A, Kelly J, Gillin A, Pang G, Lloyd B, Berger K, Baune BT, Singh MF. Investigation of skeletal muscle quantity and quality in end-stage renal disease. *Nephrology (Carlton).* 2010 Jun;15(4):454-63.

[33] Johansen KL, Shubert T, Doyle J, Soher B, Sakkas GK, Kent-Braun JA. Muscle atrophy in patients receiving hemodialysis: effects on muscle strength, muscle quality, and physical function. *Kidney Int.* 2003;63(1):291-297.

[34] Watson EL, Baker LA, Wilkinson TJ, Gould DW, Graham-Brown MPM, Major RW, Ashford RU, Philp A, Smith AC. Reductions in skeletal muscle mitochondrial mass are not restored following exercise training in patients with chronic kidney disease. *FASEB J.* 2020 Jan;34(1):1755-1767.

[35] Sawant, A., Garland, S. J., House, A. A., & Overend, T. J. (2011). Morphological, electrophysiological, and metabolic characteristics of skeletal muscle in people with end-stage renal disease: a critical review. *Physiotherapie Canada*, 63(3), 355–376.

[36] Alvarez L, Brown D, Hu D, Chertow GM, Vassalotti JA, Prichard S. Intradialytic Symptoms and Recovery Time in Patients on Thrice-Weekly In-Center Hemodialysis: A Cross-sectional Online Survey. *Kidney Med.* 2019;2(2):125-130.

[37] Rayner HC, Zepel L, Fuller DS, Morgenstern H, Karaboyas A, Culleton BF, Mapes DL, Lopes AA, Gillespie BW, Hasegawa T, Saran R, Tentori F, Hecking M, Pisoni RL, Robinson BM. Recovery time, quality of life, and mortality in hemodialysis patients: the Dialysis Outcomes and Practice Patterns Study (DOPPS). *Am J Kidney Dis.* 2014 Jul;64(1):86-94.

[38] Yoowannakul, S., Tangvoraphonkchai, K. & Davenport, A. Patient-reported intradialytic symptoms and post-dialysis recovery times are influenced by psychological distress rather than dialysis prescription. *Ren Replace Ther* .2019;5:14.

[39] Bossola M, Di Stasio E, Monteburini T, Parodi E, Ippoliti F, Cenerelli S, Santarelli S, Nebiolo PE, Sirolli V, Bonomini M, Antocicco M, Zuccalà G, Laudisio A. Recovery Time after Hemodialysis Is Inversely Associated with the Ultrafiltration Rate. *Blood Purif.* 2019;47(1-3):45-51.

[40] Hussein WF, Arramreddy R, Sun SJ, Reiterman M, Schiller B. Higher Ultrafiltration Rate Is Associated with Longer Dialysis Recovery Time in Patients Undergoing Conventional Hemodialysis. *Am J Nephrol.* 2017;46(1):3-10.

[41] Duggal V, Hussein WF, Reiterman M, Sun SJ, Abra GE, Schiller B. The effect of blood flow rate on dialysis recovery time in patients undergoing maintenance hemodialysis: A prospective, parallel-group, randomized controlled trial. *Hemodial Int.* 2019;23(2):223-229.

[42] Ok E, Duman S, Asci G, et al. Comparison of 4- and 8-h dialysis sessions in thrice-weekly in-centre haemodialysis: a prospective, case-controlled study. *Nephrol Dial Transplant.* 2011;26(4):1287-1296.

[43] Whitehead L. The measurement of fatigue in chronic illness: a systematic review of unidimensional and multidimensional fatigue measures. *J Pain Symptom Manage.* 2009 Jan;37(1):107-28.

[44] Ju A, Unruh ML, Davison SN, Dapueto J, Dew MA, Fluck R, Germain M, Jassal SV, Obrador G, O'Donoghue D, Tugwell P, Craig JC, Ralph AF, Howell M, Tong A. Patient-Reported Outcome Measures for Fatigue in Patients on Hemodialysis: A Systematic Review. *Am J Kidney Dis.* 2018 Mar;71(3):327-343.

[45] Hewlett S, Dures E, Almeida C. Measures of fatigue: Bristol Rheumatoid Arthritis Fatigue Multi-Dimensional Questionnaire (BRAF MDQ), Bristol Rheumatoid Arthritis Fatigue Numerical Rating Scales (BRAF NRS) for severity, effect, and coping, Chalder Fatigue Questionnaire (CFQ), Checklist Individual Strength (CIS20R and CIS8R), Fatigue Severity Scale (FSS), Functional Assessment Chronic Illness Therapy (Fatigue) (FACIT-F), Multi-Dimensional Assessment of Fatigue (MAF), Multi-Dimensional Fatigue Inventory (MFI), Pediatric Quality Of Life (PedsQL) Multi-Dimensional Fatigue Scale, Profile of Fatigue (ProF), Short Form 36 Vitality Subscale (SF-36 VT), and Visual Analog Scales (VAS). *Arthritis Care Res (Hoboken).* 2011 Nov;63 Suppl 11:S263-86.

[46] Krupp LB, LaRocca NG, Muir-Nash J, Steinberg AD: The fatigue severity scale. Application to patients with multiple sclerosis and systemic lupus erythematosus. *Arch Neurol* 1989;46:1121-1123.

[47] Kecke S, Ernst J, Einenkel J, Singer S, Hinz A. Psychometric Properties of the Fatigue Questionnaire EORTC QLQ-FA12 in a Sample of Female Cancer Patients. *J Pain Symptom Manage.* 2017;54(6):922-928.

[48] Chalder T, Berelowitz G, Pawlikowska T, Watts L, Wessely S, Wright D, et al. Development of a fatigue scale. *J Psychosom Res* 1993; 37: 147– 53.

[49] Ryan EG, Vitoratou S, Goldsmith KA, Chalder T. Psychometric Properties and Factor Structure of a Long and Shortened Version of the Cognitive and Behavioural Responses Questionnaire. *Psychosom Med.* 2018 Feb/Mar;80(2):230-237.

[50] Matsuzawa R, Yamamoto S, Suzuki Y, Imamura K, Harada M, Matsunaga A, Tamaki A, Fukui T, Shimokado K. The clinical applicability of ultrasound technique for diagnosis of sarcopenia in hemodialysis patients. *Clin Nutr*. 2020 Aug 1:S0261-5614(20)30390-3.

[51] Hwang SH, Lee DH, Min J, Jeon JY. Handgrip Strength as a Predictor of All-Cause Mortality in Patients With Chronic Kidney Disease Undergoing Dialysis: A Meta-Analysis of Prospective Cohort Studies. *J Ren Nutr*. 2019;29(6):471-479.

[52] Chan W, Bosch JA, Jones D, Kaur O, Inston N, Moore S, McClean A, McTernan PG, Harper L, Phillips AC, Borrows R. Predictors and consequences of fatigue in prevalent kidney transplant recipients. *Transplantation*. 2013 Dec 15;96(11):987-94.

[53] Riess H. The Science of Empathy. *J Patient Exp*. 2017 Jun;4(2):74-77.

[54] Stone P, Ream E, Richardson A, Thomas H, Andrews P, Campbell P, Dawson T, Edwards J, Goldie T, Hammick M, Kearney N, Lean M, Rapley D, Smith AG, Teague C, Young A. Cancer-related fatigue--a difference of opinion? Results of a multicentre survey of healthcare professionals, patients and caregivers. *Eur J Cancer Care (Engl)*. 2003 Mar;12(1):20-7.

[55] Johansen KL, Finkelstein FO, Revicki DA, Evans C, Wan S, Gitlin M, Agodoa IL. Systematic review of the impact of erythropoiesis-stimulating agents on fatigue in dialysis patients. *Nephrol Dial Transplant*. 2012 Jun;27(6):2418-25.

[56] Motonishi S, Tanaka K, Ozawa T. Iron deficiency associates with deterioration in several symptoms independently from hemoglobin level among chronic hemodialysis patients. *PLoS One*. 2018 Aug 2;13(8):e0201662.

[57] Fukuda S, Koyama H, Kondo K, Fujii H, Hirayama Y, Tabata T, Okamura M, Yamakawa T, Okada S, Hirata S, Kiyama H, Kajimoto O, Watanabe Y, Inaba M, Nishizawa Y. Effects of nutritional supplementation on fatigue, and autonomic and immune dysfunction in patients with end-stage renal disease: a randomized, double-blind, placebo-controlled, multicenter trial. *PLoS One*. 2015 Mar 6;10(3):e0119578.

[58] Bossola M, Vulpio C, Tazza L. Fatigue in chronic dialysis patients. *Semin Dial*. 2011 Sep-Oct;24(5):550-5.

[59] Sutherland S, Penfold R, Doherty A, Milne Z, Dawes H, Pugh C, Boulton M, Newton JL. A cross-sectional study exploring levels of physical activity and motivators and barriers towards physical activity in haemodialysis patients to inform intervention development. *Disabil Rehabil*. 2019 Oct 24:1-7.

[60] Painter PL, Agarwal A, Drummond M. Physical Function and Physical Activity in Peritoneal Dialysis Patients. *Perit Dial Int*. 2017 Nov-Dec;37(6):598-604.

[61] Regolisti G, Sabatino A, Fiaccadori E. Exercise in patients on chronic hemodialysis: current evidence, knowledge gaps and future perspectives. *Curr Opin Clin Nutr Metab Care*. 2020 May;23(3):181-189.

[62] Sherwood NE, Jeffery RW. The behavioral determinants of exercise: implications for physical activity interventions. *Annu Rev Nutr*. 2000;20:21-44.

[63] Thangarasa T, Imtiaz R, Hiremath S, Zimmerman D. Physical Activity in Patients Treated With Peritoneal Dialysis: A Systematic Review and Meta-analysis. *Can J Kidney Health Dis*. 2018 Jun 18;5:2054358118779821.

[64] Langeskov-Christensen M, Bisson EJ, Finlayson ML, Dalgas U. Potential pathophysiological pathways that can explain the positive effects of exercise on fatigue in multiple sclerosis: A scoping review. *J Neurol Sci*. 2017 Feb 15;373:307-320.

[65] Natale P, Ruospo M, Saglimbene VM, Palmer SC, Strippoli GF. Interventions for improving sleep quality in people with chronic kidney disease. *Cochrane Database Syst Rev*. 2019 May 26;5(5):CD012625.

[66] Yang B, Xu J, Xue Q, Wei T, Xu J, Ye C, Mei C, Mao Z. Non-pharmacological interventions for improving sleep quality in patients on dialysis: systematic review and meta-analysis. *Sleep Med Rev*. 2015 Oct;23:68-82.

[67] Chen HY, Cheng IC, Pan YJ, Chiu YL, Hsu SP, Pai MF, Yang JY, Peng YS, Tsai TJ, Wu KD. Cognitive-behavioral therapy for sleep disturbance decreases inflammatory cytokines and oxidative stress in hemodialysis patients. *Kidney Int*. 2011 Aug;80(4):415-22.

[68] Chen HY, Chiang CK, Wang HH, Hung KY, Lee YJ, Peng YS, Wu KD, Tsai TJ. Cognitive-behavioral therapy for sleep disturbance in patients undergoing peritoneal dialysis: a pilot randomized controlled trial. *Am J Kidney Dis*. 2008 Aug;52(2):314-23.

[69] Park KS, Chang JH, Kang EW. Effects of 12 months of continuous positive airway pressure therapy on cognitive function, sleep, mood, and health-related quality of life in a peritoneal dialysis patient with obstructive sleep apnea. *Kidney Res Clin Pract*. 2018;37(1):89-93.

[70] Kumagai T, Ishibashi Y, Kawarazaki H, Kawarazaki W, Shimizu H, Kaname S, Fujita T. Effects of nocturnal oxygen therapy on sleep apnea syndrome in peritoneal dialysis patients. *Clin Nephrol*. 2008 Oct;70(4):332-9.

[71] Boehm K, Ostermann T, Milazzo S, Büssing A. Effects of yoga interventions on fatigue: a meta-analysis. *Evid Based Complement Alternat Med*. 2012;2012:124703.

[72] Duan L, Xu Y, Li M. Effects of Mind-Body Exercise in Cancer Survivors: A Systematic Review and Meta-Analysis. *Evid Based Complement Alternat Med*. 2020;2020:7607161.

[73] Senders A, Wahbeh H, Spain R, Shinto L. Mind-body medicine for multiple sclerosis: a systematic review. *Autoimmune Dis*. 2012;2012:567324.

[74] Beck, J. S. *Cognitive behavior therapy: Basics and beyond* (2nd edition). New York, NY: Guilford Press. 2011.

[75] Hulme K, Safari R, Thomas S, Mercer T, White C, Van der Linden M, Moss-Morris R. Fatigue interventions in long term, physical health conditions: A scoping review of systematic reviews. *PLoS One*. 2018 Oct 12;13(10):e0203367.

[76] Abrahams HJG, Gielissen MFM, Braamse AMJ, Bleijenberg G, Buffart LM, Knoop H. Graded activity is an important component in cognitive behavioral therapy to reduce severe fatigue: results of a pragmatic crossover trial in cancer survivors. *Acta Oncol*. 2019 Dec;58(12):1692-1698.

[77] Bernard P, Romain AJ, Caudroit J, Chevance G, Carayol M, Gourlan M, Needham Dancause K, Moullec G. Cognitive behavior therapy combined with exercise for adults with chronic diseases: Systematic review and meta-analysis. *Health Psychol*. 2018 May;37(5):433-450.

[78] Picariello F, Hudson JL, Moss-Morris R, Macdougall IC, Chilcot J. Examining the efficacy of social-psychological interventions for the management of fatigue in end-stage kidney disease (ESKD): a systematic review with meta-analysis. *Health Psychol Rev*. 2017 Jun;11(2):197-216.

[79] Picariello F, Moss-Morris R, Norton S, Macdougall IC, Da Silva-Gane M, Farrington K, Clayton H, Chilcot J. Feasibility Trial of Cognitive Behavioral Therapy for Fatigue in

Hemodialysis (BReF Intervention). *J Pain Symptom Manage*. 2020 Oct 14:S0885-3924(20)30800-9.

[80] Knoop H, van Kessel K, Moss-Morris R. Which cognitions and behaviours mediate the positive effect of cognitive behavioural therapy on fatigue in patients with multiple sclerosis? *Psychol Med*. 2012 Jan;42(1):205-13.

[81] van den Akker LE, Beckerman H, Collette EH, Knoop H, Bleijenberg G, Twisk JW, Dekker J, de Groot V; TREFAMS-ACE study group. Cognitive behavioural therapy for MS-related fatigue explained: A longitudinal mediation analysis. *J Psychosom Res*. 2018 Mar;106:13-24.

[82] Rayner HC. How Do We Improve the Quality of Life of Haemodialysis Patients? Now That's a Good Question. *Am J Nephrol*. 2017;46(1):1-2.

[83] Jayanti A, Foden P, Morris J, Brenchley P, Mitra S; BASIC-HHD study group. Time to recovery from haemodialysis: location, intensity and beyond. *Nephrology (Carlton)*. 2016 Dec;21(12):1017-1026.

[84] Kraus MA, Kansal S, Copland M, Komenda P, Weinhandl ED, Bakris GL, Chan CT, Fluck RJ, Burkart JM. Intensive Hemodialysis and Potential Risks with Increasing Treatment. *Am J Kidney Dis*. 2016 Nov;68(5S1):S51-S58.

[85] Keane DF, Baxter P, Lindley E, Rhodes L, Pavitt S. Time to Reconsider the Role of Relative Blood Volume Monitoring for Fluid Management in Hemodialysis. *ASAIO J*. 2018 Nov/Dec;64(6):812-818.

In: Issues in Kidney Disease – Dialysis
Editors: Stephen Z. Fadem and José A. Moura-Neto
ISBN: 978-1-68507-000-7

Chapter 8

Reducing Hospitalizations and Readmissions in End-Stage Kidney Disease Patients

Fahad Aziz[1], MD and Madhukar Misra[2,*], MD

[1]Department of Medicine, Division of Nephrology,
University of Wisconsin School of Medicine and Public Health, Madison, WI, USA
[2]Department of Medicine, Division of Nephrology,
University of Missouri-Columbia, Columbia, MO, USA

Abstract

Patients with end-stage kidney disease (ESKD) have a high risk of frequent hospitalizations and readmissions. These frequent admissions are associated with poor quality of life, increased mortality and morbidity, and a considerable cost burden on the healthcare system. Numerous factors are associated with these admissions, including chronic volume overload, underlying cardiac conditions, nutritional deficiencies, anemia, and depression. A multidisciplinary approach is needed to reduce admissions. In the outpatient setting, both the primary nephrologists and the dialysis units can play a crucial role in the identification of these risk factors, which can lead to a reduction in admissions. Furthermore, meticulous care coordination after discharge from the hospital can further reduce hospitalizations in dialysis patients.

Keywords: end-stage kidney disease, hospitalizations and readmissions, factors, prevention

Introduction

Hospitalizations and 30-day readmission among patients with end-stage kidney disease (ESKD) remain a significant healthcare burden and are associated with poor quality of life [1]. Patients on dialysis have significantly higher mortality and hospitalization rates compared to the general population [2,3]. The coordinated and targeted management of complex

* Corresponding Author's E-mail: misram@health.missouri.edu.

comorbidities in patients on dialysis can significantly reduce their hospitalizations and can improve not only the quality of life but also their mortality.

Among dialysis patients, individuals just starting dialysis represent the most vulnerable group, with significantly increased healthcare utilization [4-9]. Multiple studies have shown that hospitalizations and readmissions are highest during the first three months, especially in the first week, after the initiation of dialysis [10-14]. Special attention should be paid to the proper education of patients who are new to dialysis. Further, excellent coordination between nephrologists, primary care physicians, and dialysis units can prevent many unnecessary hospitalizations. Premature discharges, suboptimal management during hospitalization, or improper post-hospital discharge follow-ups may be responsible for such frequent readmissions in ESKD patients [15,16].

The utilization of dialysis by the elderly has also been gradually increasing over the last two decades [8,17]. Chan et al. showed that approximately 80% of new ESKD patients were over 65 years old [13]. These elderly patients on dialysis have much higher mortality rates when compared to the age-matched population [18,19]. With increased pre-existing morbidity and mortality in elderly patients, the initiation of dialysis is associated with even higher risks of hospitalizations and readmissions. It is crucial to identify the patients who are at the highest risk of hospitalizations and readmissions. Prevention of frequent hospitalizations in elderly patients not only improves their mortality but also increases their quality of life.

As per the United States Renal Data System (USRDS), ESKD care accounts for 6% of Medicare costs [1,20]. Thirty-eight percent of Medicare funds for ESKD are spent on inpatient services [1,19]. Understanding the factors associated with hospitalizations and recurrent admissions can reduce this considerable cost burden. The majority of factors associated with frequent hospitalizations can be managed in outpatient settings by improving communication and care coordination between all physicians taking care of ESKD patients. Further, these patients need close monitoring by their dialysis units.

The purpose of this chapter is to describe essential interventions and coordination planning necessary to reduce hospitalizations and readmissions in ESKD patients. Various factors associated with frequent hospitalizations will also be described.

The Magnitude of the Problem: Hospitalization in ESKD Patients

Patients with ESKD have a higher risk of hospitalization compared to other patients with chronic medical conditions, including congestive heart failure, pulmonary disease, or cancer [21]. As per the USRDS data, patients with ESKD are admitted to the hospital nearly twice a year, on average. Thirty-five percent of these patients are readmitted to the hospital within 30 days of the first discharge [22]. Hospitalization in ESKD patients has declined slightly over the last ten years. In 2015, the adjusted rates of admission for hemodialysis (HD) and peritoneal dialysis (PD) patients decreased to 1.7 per person per year as compared to 2.1 in 2006, which is a 19% reduction in the hospitalization rate [22]. However, it continues to be a significant burden due to additional healthcare costs.

Using the USDRS database, Lovasik et al. examined all US adult patients with an ESKD diagnosis from 2005 to 2011. Close to 800,000 patients started ESKD treatment during the study period. Approximately 70% of these patients had at least one emergency department visit during the study period. More than half (55%) of all patients with ESKD visited the emergency department during their first dialysis. Hyperkalemia and fluid overload were the two most preventable ESKD-related complications, which accounted for 1.2% of the emergency room visits. Nearly half of the ESKD patients who had an emergency department visit were admitted to the hospital. The three most common hospital admission diagnoses were hemodialysis access complications (12.6%), sepsis (7.8%), and congestive heart failure (2.2%) [23].

Using national registry data, Plantinga et al. analyzed the major reasons for 30-day admissions in patients with ESKD. They found that 23% of the hospital admissions were followed by readmission. Nearly half of these admissions were associated with pulmonary edema. Dialysis duration < 1 year (OR = 2.32, 95%Cl 1.14 - 1.22), chronic obstructive pulmonary disease (OR = 1.34, 95%Cl 1.29 - 1.38), dialysis non-compliance (OR = 1.53, 95%Cl 1.41 – 1.64) and congestive heart failure (OR = 1.85, 95%Cl 1.77 – 1.93) were found to be associated with the increased incidence of pulmonary edema in ESKD patients [24].

Hickson et al. examined the rates, causes, timing, and predictors of 30-day readmissions among adult dialysis patients. They found that 31% of patients had ≥ 1 hospitalization, and 15% had ≥ 2 readmissions. The readmission rate was 1.1% per person per day post-discharge, and the highest rates occurred ≤ 5 days after index admission. The overall cumulative readmission rate was 33.8% at day 30. The most common readmission diagnoses included cardiac issues (22%), vascular disorders (19%), and infections (13%). They also found that younger age at dialysis initiation, inability to ambulate, higher number of previous hospitalizations, and longer duration on dialysis were associated with higher readmission rates in multivariable analyses [25].

Quinn et al. looked at the hospitalization rates between the two primary dialysis modalities (i.e., hemodialysis vs. peritoneal dialysis). The hemodialysis group showed a trend in higher rates of hospitalizations. Cardiovascular disease, infectious complications, and elective surgeries were the most common reasons for hospital admissions. They concluded that peritoneal dialysis utilization is unlikely to result in an increased rate of hospitalizations [26].

In a recent study, Tanaka et al. compared patients on a combination of peritoneal dialysis and hemodialysis (PD + HD) to patients on hemodialysis (HD) alone, calculating the risk of hospitalization for each. After adjusting for baseline demographics, the cumulative incidence of hospitalization was not significantly different between the two groups (p = 0.36). However, PD + HD patients had a higher risk of dialysis access-related complications than HD patients [27].

Several studies have shown that such repeated hospitalizations in ESKD patients are associated with significantly increased morbidity and mortality. Shimizu et al. showed that a higher cumulative number of hospitalizations in ESKD patients is associated with an increase in post-discharge mortality. The cause-specific hospitalization category of "infectious disease" showed an impact on mortality similar to that of hospitalization for "cancer." They suggested that special attention should be paid to reduce preventable hospitalizations in these patients to reduce their mortality [28].

The studies mentioned above clearly demonstrate that the ESKD patient population is at increased risk for hospitalizations and readmissions. The frequent hospitalizations are not only a significant burden on healthcare costs but are also associated with increased mortality, morbidity, and poor quality of life. Identifying the factors associated with an increased incidence of hospitalization can reduce the number of admissions, therefore improving the mortality and quality of life in patients on any form of dialysis. Table 1 highlights the individual factors which may be responsible for the increased risk of hospitalizations and frequent readmissions in patients with ESKD.

Table 1. Factors associated with frequent hospitalizations and readmissions

A. Chronic fluid overload
B. Dialysis access issues
C. Anemia
D. Nutritional deficiencies
E. Cardiovascular diseases
F. Depression

Chronic Fluid Overload

Chronic Fluid Overload Is Associated with Increased Mortality and Hospitalization in the ESKD Population

Patients on maintenance HD are at significantly higher risk of premature coronary artery disease, sudden cardiac death from arrhythmias, and congestive heart failure (CHF) as compared to the general population [29-31]. Although CHF has multiple causes, chronic fluid overload (CFO) in ESKD patients plays a significant role in its causation. Multiple studies have shown that CFO in ESKD patients is associated with increased mortality [32, 33]. Inadequate assessment of the dry weight is associated not only with adverse cardiovascular outcomes but also with substantial increases in healthcare costs among dialysis patients [34-37]. According to one estimate, the average cost per episode for the treatment of CFO is around 6,372 US dollars [38]. A survey of practice patterns in dialysis units across Britain reported that only 22% of the units had any documented fluid management policy. Seventy-seven percent of the units that were surveyed felt there was a real need for evidence-based management of the volume and the estimation of the dry weight [39].

CFO starts in the early stages of chronic kidney disease (CKD). Hung et al. evaluated 338 patients with chronic kidney disease (CKD) stage III – V and found that only 48% of patients were euvolemic. Fifty-two percent of patients with volume overload were found to have difficulty controlling blood pressure and increased cardiovascular events [40]. Further, volume-dependent hypertension was found to be associated with much higher CV adverse events as compared to non-volume-dependent hypertension. Pre-dialysis fluid overload is very common in patients on maintenance HD [41, 42].

CFO is associated with higher mortality. In a cohort of 269 prevalent HD patients, the hazard ratio for CFO as an essential and independent predictor of mortality was found to be second only to diabetes [43]. More recently, an observational study of 39,566 incident HD patients in 26 countries examined the association of baseline and one-year cumulative fluid overload with all-cause mortality. CFO was present in 46% of patients, based on predefined criteria. Both baseline and cumulative exposure to CFO was associated with higher mortality risk across all strata of B.P. The authors reported that the mortality risk of CFO is comparable to the presence of coronary heart disease or an age increase of more than 12 years [44]. In short,

CFO is widely prevalent in ESKD patients and is associated with hypertension, LVH, and reduced arterial compliance. All of these factors may play a role in the higher mortality and frequent hospitalizations and readmissions seen in patients with CFO.

STRATEGIES TO MANAGE CFO

CFO-related hospitalizations may be preventable with better fluid management practices at dialysis units. Some relevant measures include:

Assessment and Adjustment of "Dry Weight"

The concept of "dry weight" is as old as dialysis itself. The definition of "dry weight" has evolved over the last five decades [45]. Initially, it was defined as the weight achieved by the reduction of blood pressure to hypotensive levels during ultrafiltration [46]. Later in the 1990s, "dry weight" was defined as the bodyweight at the end of dialysis at which a patient could remain normotensive until the next dialysis, ideally without the use of antihypertensive medications [47]. Finally, Sinha et al. defined "dry weight" as the lowest tolerated post-dialysis weight achieved via a gradual change in post-dialysis weight at which there are minimal signs or symptoms of hypovolemia or hypervolemia [48]. Physical examination is an inadequate assessment tool for the volume assessment. The presence of lung crackles, either alone or with pedal edema, has been reported to be a poor estimate of the interstitial lung edema [49].

Regardless of the above discussion, it is essential to realize that there are several advantages of achieving dry weight (and thus better volume control) in patients on HD, which include: better blood pressure control, improved left ventricular mass, and reduced admissions with CHF exacerbation (Table 2).

Table 2. Advantages of better volume control in ESKD patients

Better blood pressure control
Decreased CHF exacerbation episodes
Improved left ventricular hypertrophy
Reduced hospitalizations with volume overload
Improved quality of life
Decreased mortality

Optimization of Outpatient HD Prescription

There are numerous reasons why patients tend to have CFO. Potential barriers in preventing CFO include infrequent monitoring and adjustment of dialysis prescription and dry weight; lack of dietary counseling; short HD sessions due to hypotension and cramps; patient resistance to the adjustment of time, frequency of HD sessions, or both; and lack of reimbursement for additional HD sessions and other associated costs. Some possible strategies to improve fluid removal are given below (Table 3).

Table 3. Strategies to improve outpatient dialysis

More Frequent dialysis
Longer HD Session duration
Improving HD session tolerance

More Frequent Dialysis

CFO is a significant cause of left ventricular abnormalities in patients on H.D. Improvements in left ventricular mass and function lower the morbidity and mortality associated with left ventricular abnormalities. The FHN trial compared frequent HD to the conventional HD and reported clinically meaningful benefits for the co-primary composite endpoint of death or 12-month change in left ventricular mass [50].

Longer HD Session Duration

Many observational studies have shown that shorter dialysis sessions are associated with worse outcomes in terms of increased morbidity and mortality [51-53]. Flythe et al. compared patients with prescribed dialysis sessions greater and less than 240 minutes. They reported that shorter dialysis sessions were associated with higher adjusted mortality despite adequate urea clearance [54].

Improving HD Session Tolerance

Since intradialytic hypotension is a common complication of ultrafiltration and may lead to adverse clinical outcomes, any strategy to minimize hypotensive episodes should help the management of CFO. A study comparing high-efficiency online hemodiafiltration (OL-HDF) with the conventional high flux HD reported significantly fewer hypotensive episodes in the OL-HDF arm, thus highlighting its role in improving session tolerance. The OL-HDF group also showed a 30% reduction in all-cause mortality [55].

The evidence cited above reinforces the concept that close attention to fluid overload and "dry weight" at the end of each dialysis treatment, as well as counseling about salt restriction, can prevent many volume-related hospitalizations and readmissions. Further, by reducing numerous cardiovascular complications associated with CFO, we can reduce the incidence of frequent hospitalizations and readmissions in these patients.

Dialysis Access Issues

Appropriate access to chronic dialysis is critical to the survival of patients with ESKD. Issues with dialysis access are often associated with frequent hospitalizations and readmissions (Table 4).

Table 4. Access issues associated with frequent hospitalizations

Temporary tunneled dialysis catheters	**Arteriovenous Fistula (AVF) and Arterio-venous Grafts (AVG)**
Bloodstream infections	AVF Stenosis
Tunnel infections	AVF Thrombosis
Exit site infections	AVF delayed maturation
Misplacement of the catheters	AVG stenosis
Non-functional catheters	AVG thrombosis
	AVG infections

As per one estimate, more than 20% of hospitalizations in hemodialysis patients in the United States are related to access issues [56], which constitutes a considerable financial burden on the healthcare system. The tendency towards a late referral to nephrologists is not only associated with an increased cost but also with the short-term hospitalization for the initiation of dialysis by establishing temporary access [57].

Xue et al. found that one-year crude death rates were 24.9%, 27.2%, 28.2%, and 41.5% for patients with simple fistulae, autologous vein grafts, synthetic grafts, and hemodialysis catheters, respectively. Interestingly, patients with fistulae had the lowest likelihood of death ($p < 0.0001$) compared with grafts (HR = 1.160, 95% Cl 1.084 to 1.241) or catheters (HR = 1.696, 95% Cl 1.593 to 1.806) [58]. Roubicek et al. found that late referrals to nephrologists resulted in 73% of patients starting dialysis through a temporary catheter [59].

Issues with Tunneled Dialysis Catheters

Tunneled dialysis catheters are often used for the initiation of dialysis while waiting for the fistula to be placed or waiting for the fistulas to be matured; however, the catheters cause a two- to three-fold increased risk of hospitalization for infection and death as compared to patients who have grafts or a fistula [60]. The tunneled dialysis catheter includes bloodstream infections, tunnel infections, and exit site infections. Multiple studies have shown that the incidence of catheter-related bloodstream infections is 1.1 to 5.5 episodes per 1,000 catheter days, and these infections are not only associated with increased risk for hospitalization, but also with increased mortality [61-64]. Metastatic infectious complications related to these bloodstream infections include endocarditis, osteomyelitis, spinal epidural abscess, septic arthritis, and pulmonary emboli [65].

Several factors are associated with catheter infections, including the site of catheter insertion, duration of use, and poor hygiene practices [66-68]. Special attention should be paid to take all measures to reduce the risk of infection, including the selection of the catheter site, proper hand hygiene practices, and education for the patients and caregivers [69, 70]. By reducing catheter-related infections, many hospitalizations and readmissions can be prevented.

Issues with Arteriovenous Fistula (AVF) and the Grafts (AVG)

Multiple studies have shown that AVF has superior outcomes over AVG and tunneled catheters [71-74]. AVF and AVG should be monitored regularly for early detection of stenosis and thrombosis. Multiple studies suggest that prophylactic repair of the AVF or AVG stenosis can prevent thrombosis, which significantly prolongs the life of the access point and reduces the need for further interventions [75-77]. Prevention of stenosis is the ultimate goal, which eliminates access issue-related hospitalizations. Several studies have shown that the use of antiplatelet in specific patient groups can reduce stenosis and thrombosis in AVF and AVG [78-80]. By using a longitudinal health insurance database of Taiwan, Hsu et al. reviewed 34,354 patients with first vascular access failure. Age $\geq$ 65 years, diabetes, hyperlipidemia, cerebral vascular disease, congestive heart failure, peripheral vascular disease, and sepsis were found to important risk factors associated with early vascular access failure. They found that antiplatelet therapy increased the AVF and AVG patency times with adjusted odds ratios of 0.78 (95% Cl 0.703 – 0.796, p = 0.0001) and 0.810 (95% Cl 0.728-0.901, p = 0.0001) respectively. Further, a significant decrease in vascular access failure risk was observed with an increase in the cumulative defined daily dose of antiplatelet agents [81].

The above discussion demonstrates that early referrals should be made to nephrologists for the timely placement of AVF and to avoid tunneled catheters. If tunneled catheters need to be placed, special attention should be paid to prevent infection related to the access. Further, in patients with AVF and AVG, the access should be monitored carefully for the development of stenosis. By taking care of these issues, unnecessary hospitalizations related to vascular access can be avoided. Further, by reducing problems with the vascular access, the mortality and morbidity of these ESKD patients can be improved.

ANEMIA IN ESKD PATIENTS

Anemia is common in ESKD patients and is associated with several poor outcome measures, as shown in Table 5.

Ma et al. examined a Medicare hemodialysis cohort to find the association between anemia and mortality. They found that after adjusting for medical diseases, patients with a hematocrit of less than 30% had a significantly higher risk of all-cause (12 to 33%) and cause-specific mortality, compared to patients who had a hematocrit of more than 30%. Their findings suggest that by treating the anemia, the mortality in ESKD patients can be improved [82].

Table 5. Problems associated with anemia in ESKD patients

Increased fatigue
Shortness of breath
Increased mortality
Increased cardiovascular events
Increased incidence of hospitalizations and readmissions

Table 6. Strategies to manage anemia in ESKD patients

Regular screening of hemoglobin and hematocrit
Iron deficiency and supplementation
Erythropoietic agents (ESAs)

Using Medicare data, Xia et al. examined the association between hematocrit and future hospitalization risks in ESKD patients. Five hematocrit groups were defined: hematocrit < 27%, 27 to < 30%, 30 to < 33%, 33 to < 36%, and ≥36%. Compared to the baseline group of 30 to < 33%, patients with hematocrit levels < 30% had a 14 to 30% increased risk of hospitalization without disease severity adjustment ($p = 0.0001$), and 7 to 18% increased risk with disease severity adjustment ($p = 0.0001$). The patients in the 33 to < 36% group had the lowest risk, at 0.93 and 0.88 ($p = 0.0001$) with and without adjustment for disease severity, respectively. They concluded that ESKD patients on dialysis should be maintained on a hematocrit of 33 to 36% to reduce the incidence of hospitalization [83]. Many other studies showed the same results: the treatment of anemia is associated not only with improved morbidity and mortality but also with reduced subsequent hospitalizations [84, 85]. Strategies to effectively manage anemia in ESKD patients are highlighted in Table 6.

World Health Organization (WHO) defined anemia as hemoglobin <13 g/dl in adult males and hemoglobin <12 g/dl for premenopausal women [86]. The following strategies should be adopted to manage anemia in ESKD patients to minimize their frequent hospitalizations and readmissions:

Regular Screening of Hemoglobin and Hematocrit

All patients should be screened for anemia at the initiation of dialysis. If found anemic, other causes of anemia should be ruled out. The evaluation of anemia includes 1. Red cell indices; 2. Reticulocytes; 3. Serum iron panel including ferritin, total iron-binding capacity, and percent transferrin saturation (TSAT); and 4. Vitamin B12 and folate [87].

As per the guidelines in Kidney Disease: Improving Global Outcomes (KDIGO), hemoglobin should be monitored every three months. If anemia is found, iron studies should be done, and the decision should be made between iron replacement and initiation of erythropoiesis-stimulating agents (ESA) [87, 88].

Iron Deficiency and Supplementation

In ESKD patients, chronic inflammation leads to increased hepcidin production, which in turn inhibits both the uptake of dietary iron and the mobilization of stored iron from the reticuloendothelial system to circulating transferrin [89]. The combination of insufficient dietary iron uptake and intestinal bleeding also contributes to severe iron deficiency in these patients [90-92]. Further, the use of ESA leads to increased demand for iron to support erythropoiesis [93, 94].

In a meta-analysis, Shepshelovich et al. assessed data from 24 randomized clinical trials: 13 patients with non-dialysis chronic kidney disease, and 11 patients on dialysis. They found that the patients treated with intravenous (IV) iron were more likely to achieve a hemoglobin increase of more than 1 gm/dl than patients treated with oral iron alone. The rates of mortality and serious adverse events were found to be similar for the IV and oral iron groups. However, IV iron was associated with a higher risk of hypotension but fewer gastrointestinal symptoms [95].

Brookhart et al. examined Medicare patients dialyzing at a large dialysis organization. They found that the bolus dosing of iron was associated with a small increase in the relative risk of infection-related hospitalizations compared with maintenance dosing [96].

Erythropoiesis-Stimulating Agents (ESAs)

ESAs are administered to anemic ESKD patients who are not iron deficient and have hemoglobin < 10 gm/dl [87]. ESAs are useful in the management of anemia in dialysis patients.

Besarab et al. studied patients with heart failure or ischemic heart disease who were undergoing hemodialysis. The patients were assigned to either receiving doses of Epogen to achieve a hematocrit of 42%or receiving Epogen to achieve a hematocrit of 30%. They found that mortality rates significantly decreased with the increasing hematocrit values in both groups [97, 98].

Multiple studies have recently shown that ESAs not only reduces the requirement for blood transfusions but also improve exercise tolerance and left ventricular hypertrophy [99-102]. By improving the cardiovascular morbidity and quality of life, hospitalizations and readmissions can be effectively reduced.

The implementation of anemia protocols in dialysis units can prevent multiple hospitalizations besides reducing admissions due to cardiovascular issues.

Nutritional Deficiencies in ESKD Patients

Multiple studies have shown that malnutrition in ESKD patients is associated with a significant increase in morbidity and mortality in both adults and pediatric patients [103-105]. Causes of nutritional deficiencies in ESKD patients are highlighted in Table 7.

Table 7. Causes of nutritional deficiencies in ESKD patients

Hormonal imbalances
Decreased appetite
Uremia
Generalized inflammation
Increased catabolism
Metabolic derangements
Depression
Poor socioeconomic status
Inadequate dialysis
Chronic volume overload
Dietary restrictions
Use of phosphorous binders

In the general population, malnutrition is usually secondary to decreased dietary intake. However, in ESKD patients, malnutrition is due to multiple factors such as hormonal imbalances, decreased appetite, generalized inflammation, increased catabolism, nutrient losses in dialysate, metabolic derangements, and uremia [106-110]. Uremic anorexia leads to protein-energy malnutrition in ESKD patients due to inadequate dietary protein and energy intake [111, 112]. Further, depression and poor socioeconomic status are also associated with nutritional deficiencies [113, 114]. The data from a randomized clinical trial in patients receiving maintenance HD (HEMO Study) indicated that despite an adequate dose of dialysis, patients on dialysis lose weight over time [115]. The flux of the dialyzer and duration of dialysis was also found to have no impact on the nutritional Status of ESKD patients [50, 116].

Due to insulin resistance and insulin deprivation, patients with diabetes and ESKD have a higher incidence of protein-energy malnutrition compared to patients without diabetes [117-120]. Gastrointestinal disturbances like diabetic gastroparesis, nausea, vomiting, pancreatic insufficiency, and bacterial overgrowth in the gut can also lead to protein-energy malnutrition in ESKD patients [121]. Depression is also ubiquitous in ESKD patients and is linked with weight loss and a lack of appetite [122, 123]. Similarly, dietary restrictions and fluid restrictions can lead to a decrease in caloric intake in these patients [124]. Further, several medications, like phosphorus binders, can impair nutrient absorption in ESKD patients.

Malnutrition in ESKD Patients Is Associated with High Mortality and Hospitalizations

Approximately one-third of all ESKD patients have mild to moderate malnutrition. Six to eight percent of these patients have severe malnutrition, which is associated with increased morbidity and mortality [125]. Moderate to severe malnutrition is a preventable cause of hospitalization, readmissions, and mortality in ESKD patients.

Several studies have shown that malnutrition and low serum albumin are associated with a significantly increased risk of total and cardiovascular-specific mortality in the dialysis population [126-128]. Using Dialysis Outcomes and Practice Patterns Study (DOPPS) data, Pifer et al. found that lower baseline BMI, serum albumin, serum creatinine, and lymphocyte counts were independently associated with a higher risk of mortality. At a six-month follow-up, a decrease in BMI, serum albumin, and serum creatinine were also associated with higher mortality [129].

Several studies showed that nutritional deficiencies also lead to prolonged hospitalization in ESKD patients. Aziz et al. described a case of severe phosphorous and trace element deficiency in a dialysis patient, which lead to intubation, mechanical ventilation, and a very prolonged hospital course. By merely supplementing her with phosphorous and trace elements, her condition recovered very quickly [130].

Effective Management of Malnutrition in ESKD Patients to Reduce Mortality and Hospitalizations

All ESKD patients' protein-energy malnutrition should be evaluated carefully. Multidisciplinary team efforts are required to address the underlying potential reasons for malnutrition, including the presence of chronic medical conditions, concurrent infections, psychosocial issues, and depression. High-risk patients like patients with diabetes and underlying cardiac problems should be evaluated for nutritional deficiencies in dialysis units at regular intervals.

If malnutrition is identified in a dialysis patient, special attention should be paid to the dialysis adequacy (Table 8). Nephrologists on their routine dialysis rounds should also evaluate other underlying medical conditions. These patients should be provided with nutritional supplements. Nutritionists usually determine the exact ingredients of the nutrition supplements. If the patients continue to lose weight, intradialytic parenteral nutrition (IDPN) can be considered. Many studies have shown that IDPN is convenient and beneficial in many patients [131, 132].

Table 8. Management of nutritional deficiencies in ESKD patients

Frequent evaluation for nutritional deficiencies
Adequate dialysis
Nutritional supplement when required
Mood assessment for the presence of depression
Consider TPN if continuing to lose weight
Rule out underlying conditions

The above information shows that nutritional deficiencies are common in ESKD patients. The appropriate management of these nutritional disturbances is critical to improving morbidity and mortality, and decreasing incidences of hospitalization and readmissions, in ESKD patients. ESKD patients should be evaluated at regular intervals for these deficiencies.

Cardiovascular Disease in ESKD Patients

Cardiovascular disease (CVD) is 10-20 times higher in ESKD patients as compared to people with normal kidney function [133]. Multiple studies have shown that coronary artery disease is much more common in ESKD patients [134, 135].

Dialysis is a Risk for CVD

Rostland et al. reviewed the records of 44 dialysis patients who had undergone one or more coronary angiograms to determine the incidence of coronary artery disease in this patient population. They found that 73% of the ESKD patients had significant coronary artery disease, with more than 50% stenosis [136]. Similar results were reported by the Hemodialysis study, which found that 40% of dialysis patients had CVD at the start of dialysis, and 63% of the CVD admissions in this patient population were due to coronary artery disease [137]. Multiple studies have shown that hemodialysis is associated with myocardial stunning, which is associated with reduced survival [138, 139]. Management of multiple risk factors of CVD in dialysis patients not only improves the mortality in dialysis patients but also reduces their rate of hospitalizations and readmissions (Table 9).

Table 9. Cardiovascular risk factors in ESKD patients

Hypertension
Electrolytes disturbances
Uremia
Acidosis
Vascular calcification
Vascular access
Chronic volume overload
Myocardial stunning
Volume shifts

Hypertension Management

Hypertension in the general population is associated with a significantly increased risk of cardiovascular mortality and morbidity [140]. In patients with advanced CKD, both high and low blood pressure, be detrimental in determining patient outcomes [141, 142]. The prevalence of hypertension in hemodialysis patients is 86% [143]. Despite the well-known prevalence of hypertension in these patients, only 30% of dialysis patients have controlled blood pressures [144]. Almost 12% of dialysis patients have uncontrolled hypertension [144].

The high prevalence of uncontrolled blood pressure in dialysis patients leads to an increased risk of cardiovascular events. By effectively controlling the blood pressure in these patients, we can not only reduce the incidence of cardiovascular disease, but also reduce hospitalizations and readmissions associated with uncontrolled blood pressures, hypertensive urgencies, and cardiovascular events.

Electrolyte Disturbances

Poor calcium metabolism leads to cardiovascular calcification in dialysis patients, which is a well-known cardiovascular risk factor. In these patients, cardiovascular calcifications lead to an increased incidence of arrhythmias, sudden cardiac death, stroke, ischemic coronary artery disease, increased pulse pressure, and aortic stenosis [145, 146]. Wang et al., in their metanalysis, showed that a higher degree of cardiovascular calcifications is associated with increased mortality [147]. Particular attention should be paid to the electrolyte management in patients on dialysis to reduce not only their mortality but also cardiovascular-related admissions and readmissions.

Acidosis

Metabolic acidosis is common among patients with advanced chronic kidney disease. It not only increases the risk of malnutrition, inflammation, and bone disease disorder, but it also increases mortality [148]. Raikou et al. analyzed the effect of metabolic acidosis in 52 patients. Kaplan-Meier analyses showed that lower serum bicarbonate status was strongly associated with both peripheral vascular disease and diastolic dysfunction [149]. Djamali et al. reviewed 2,128 kidney transplant recipients for CVE and found that metabolic acidosis was an independent risk factor for ischemic cardiac disease after kidney transplantation [150].

Considering that metabolic acidosis plays a vital role in increasing the incidence of cardiovascular disease in patients on dialysis and advanced CKD., protocols should be adopted in dialysis units to check bicarbonate levels and keep serum bicarbonate levels routinely >22 mEq/L to not only reduce associated cardiovascular mortality but also to reduce hospitalizations from cardiovascular diseases.

Uremia

The accumulation of uremic toxins in patients with advanced CKD is a well-known risk factor for cardiovascular diseases [151, 152]. Multiple studies have shown that the high concentration of certain uremic compounds like p-cresol in serum is not only associated with increased cardiovascular risk but also with increased mortality [153-155]. Studies have shown that specific phosphorus binders can bind p-cresol and reduce cardiovascular mortality associated with its high levels [156-158]. Similarly, another uremic toxin, indoxyl sulfate, is also shown to be associated with an increased incidence of thrombosis and vascular damage [159-161]. This highlights the importance of providing adequate dialysis to get better clearance of multiple uremic toxins. Achieving adequate KT/V goals can prevent hospital admissions associated with cardiovascular issues in patients on dialysis.

Depression in ESKD Patients

Different psychiatric illnesses are common among patients on dialysis. As per Kimmel et al., in dialysis patients, psychiatric disorders are responsible for 1.5 to 3 times higher rates of admissions as compared to those with other chronic illnesses [162]. Fukunishi et al. looked at the various psychiatric disorders in patients undergoing hemodialysis. They found that the one-year incidence rate of these psychiatric disorders was 10.6%, the one-year incidence of the rate of dementia in aged patients was 4.2%, and the one-year incidence rate of multi-infarct dementia was 7.4% higher as compared to the general population [163].

Depression in Dialysis Patients Is Common and Is Associated with Increased Mortality and Morbidity

In a meta-analysis, Palmer et al. looked at the prevalence of depression among ESKD patients. They found that the prevalence of interview-based depression in CKD stage V was 21.4% (Cl 11.1 – 37.2), and when clinician-administered rating scales were used, the prevalence of depression was found to be 39.3% (Cl 36.8 – 42). These findings suggest that self-reporting may underestimate the prevalence of depression in patients with advanced CKD [164].

Peterson et al. found that depression was an important early indicator of worse prognoses in patients on dialysis [165]. Similar results were found by many other studies [166, 167]. In a meta-analysis of 14 studies, Palmer et al. found that the incidence of all-cause mortality was much higher in the depressed dialysis patients as compared to the non-depressed dialysis patients (RR = 1.4, 95% Cl 1.2 to 1.5) [168].

Depression and the Increased Risk of Hospitalization in ESKD Patients

By using the Centralized Veterans Affairs (V.A.) database, Hedayati et al. analyzed close to 1,600 dialysis patients. They found that the presence of depression was not only associated with prolonged hospitalizations (HR = 1.31, 95% Cl 1.04 to 1.66) but also with more frequent hospitalizations (HR = 1.30, 95% Cl 1.11 to 1.52) [169]. In another study, Lacson et al. found that depression was associated with a significantly increased risk of hospitalizations (HR = 1.12, 95% Cl 1.04 to 1.20). Depression was also found to be associated with an increase in the number of days in the hospital (HR = 1.20, 95% Cl 1.07 to 1.35) [170]. Kurella et al. found that the crude rate of suicide was 24.2 suicides per 100,000 patient-years in ESKD patients, and the multivariable model noted that ESKD was a significant predictor of suicide [171]. This high suicide risk due to depression also leads to high admissions rates in these patients.

Diagnosis and Treatment of Depression Can Reduce Hospitalizations in ESKD Patients

As per KDOQI guidelines, every patient on dialysis should be evaluated regularly for the signs and symptoms of depression [172]. Further, patients who are showing changes in their behavior, refusal to get full dialysis treatments, non-compliance with medications, and non-compliance with prescribed dialysis treatments, and problems with memory should be evaluated for possible underlying depression. Depression can be challenging to diagnose, as many patients do not even realize that they are depressed.

Durate et al. assessed the effectiveness of cognitive-behavioral therapy (CBT) on patients on chronic dialysis diagnosed with major depressive disorder. It was a randomized clinical trial in which the patients were divided into either the control group or intervention group. Patients in the intervention group received weekly sessions of CBT by a trained psychologist for three months, while the patients in the control group received the usual treatment offered in the dialysis unit. They found that the patients in the intervention arm had significant improvement in depression scores on the Beck Depression Inventory. They concluded that CBT is an effective treatment for depression in patients on chronic dialysis [173].

Later, Cukor et al. also demonstrated that the administration of CBT in dialysis patients with depression was not only associated with improvement in depression symptoms but also with an improvement in the quality of life and compliance with dialysis treatments [174].

The combination of CBT with anti-depressant medications can be used to treat dialysis patients with depression. Surveys have shown that depression is often undertreated in patients on dialysis [175]. When these patients need treatment with anti-depressant medications, special attention should be paid to the proper dosing of these medications, and the medications should be adjusted based on the dialysis clearance of the medications.

Management of Depression Improves the Quality of Life and Decreases Frequent Hospitalizations

Depression is a common cause for frequent and prolonged hospitalization in dialysis patients, but it is easy to miss. All patients on dialysis should be assessed regularly for the presence of depression. When depression is suspected, referrals to psychiatrists should be made promptly for CBT and initiation of anti-depressant therapies. Depression symptoms should be assessed frequently to make sure patients are on adequate therapy for their depression. By effectively managing depression in this patient population, frequent hospitalizations can be reduced.

Intervention Model to Reduce Frequent Hospitalizations and Readmissions

A three-pronged intervention model to reduce frequent hospitalizations and readmissions in patients on dialysis is shown in Figure 1.

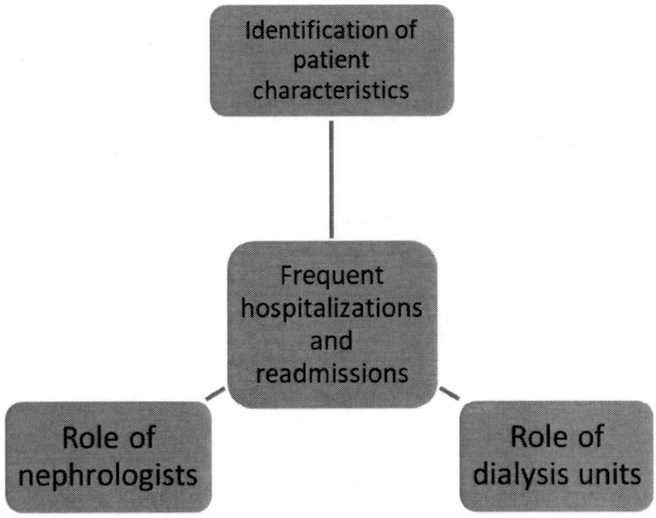

Figure 1. Intervention model to reduce frequent hospitalizations and readmissions.

Identification of Patient Characteristics

The three fundamental determinants to avoid frequent hospitalizations and readmissions are the ESKD patients, the nephrologists, and the dialysis units. Their relationship needs to be carefully evaluated to avoid frequent admissions and readmissions of dialysis patients.

It is essential to understand that specific patient characteristics may be associated with an increased risk of hospitalization in ESKD patients. Understanding these factors is crucial in preventing hospitalization in ESKD patients (Table 10).

It is important to understand that specific patient characteristics may be associated with an increased risk of hospitalization in ESKD patients. Understanding these factors is essential to preventing hospitalization in ESKD patients.

Table 10. Patient characteristics associated with frequent hospitalizations

Low socioeconomic status
Unemployment
Male gender
Older age
Previous hospitalizations
Chronic medical conditions
Lack of physical activity

Multiple studies have shown that low socioeconomic demographics, unemployment status, male gender, older age, and chronic medical conditions are associated with not only an increased risk of frequent admissions but also with readmissions after hospitalization [176-181]. Further studies have shown that previous hospitalizations and lack of physical activity are associated with readmissions in patients [177].

The ability of patients to engage in their complicated dialysis care is also an essential factor that plays a vital role in preventing frequent hospitalizations. Similarly, the role of caregivers is crucial in this group of patients.

These factors should be documented at the initiation of dialysis and should be assessed regularly. By identifying these patients, special attention should be paid to prevent frequent admission and readmission.

Role of Primary Nephrologists in Preventing Readmissions

Misky et al. looked into the factors associated with 30-day readmissions in hospitalized patients. They found that patients lacking timely follow-up by primary care physicians were ten times more likely to be readmitted (OR = 9.9, p = 0.04) [182]. Similarly, the role of follow-up with the primary nephrologist after any hospitalization in ESKD patients is vital.

After every hospitalization, the nephrologist needs to assess the following factors: changes in weight, need to establish new dry weight, nutritional status, medication adjustments for creatinine clearance, adjustments in antihypertensive medications, and ensuring that all the necessary specialist follow-ups are set up for the patient.

As per one study, the follow-up with the primary nephrologist is often delayed after a hospitalization due to the busy schedule of outpatient nephrologists [176]. The lack of timely re-assessment of these patients leads to frequent readmissions.

Role of Dialysis Units in Preventing Readmissions

In dialysis units, patients are taken care of by a team, which includes dialysis nurses, technicians, dietitians, social workers, and the nephrologist. After every hospitalization, patients should be assessed by the dialysis nurses and technicians to make sure that they are at their adequate dry weight, have reasonable control of their blood pressure, and all their medications are appropriately adjusted. These patients should also be assessed by nutritionists to make sure their nutritional needs are well adjusted. Further, social workers need to evaluate patients for any depressive symptoms and provide adequate support. If team members identify any of these issues, the primary nephrologist should be alerted, and an attempt should be made to resolve all matters when the patient is receiving follow-up care in the dialysis unit. This multidisciplinary care approach can prevent many potential readmissions. This will not only reduce the cost burden on the health system but may also be associated with improved patient mortality and morbidity.

Conclusion

Frequent hospitalizations and readmissions are common among patients on chronic dialysis and are associated with increased mortality and morbidity in these chronically ill patients. It also poses a considerable cost burden on our health system. There are multiple factors associated with hospitalizations and readmissions, such as issues with the volume overload, multiple cardiac risk factors, depression, vascular access issues, and poor nutritional status of the patients. By adequately addressing these issues, many hospitalizations can be prevented, and mortality and morbidity in this complicated group of patients can be improved. A multidisciplinary approach is needed to address all of these issues adequately.

REFERENCES

[1] *United States Renal Data System 2014 Annual Data Report: Atlas of Chronic Kidney Disease and End-Stage Renal Disease in the United States, National Institutes of Health, National Institute of Diabetes and Digestive and Kidney Diseases.* Bethesda, MD2014 [Available from: https://www.usrds.org/2014/view/.

[2] Sarnak MJ, Levey AS, Schoolwerth AC, Coresh J, Culleton B, Hamm LL, et al. Kidney disease as a risk factor for development of cardiovascular disease: a statement from the American Heart Association Councils on Kidney in Cardiovascular Disease, High Blood Pressure Research, *Clinical Cardiology, and Epidemiology and Prevention. Circulation.* 2003;108(17):2154-69.

[3] Pippias M, Kramer A, Noordzij M, Afentakis N, Alonso de la Torre R, Ambuhl PM, et al. The European Renal Association - European Dialysis and Transplant Association Registry Annual Report 2014: a summary. *Clin Kidney J.* 2017;10(2):154-69.

[4] Collins AJ, Foley RN, Gilbertson DT, Chen SC. The state of chronic kidney disease, ESRD, and morbidity and mortality in the first year of dialysis. *Clin J Am Soc Nephrol.* 2009;4 Suppl 1:S5-11.

[5] Schoonover KL, Hickson LJ, Norby SM, Hogan MC, Chaudhary S, Albright RC, Jr., et al. Risk factors for hospitalization among older, incident haemodialysis patients. *Nephrology* (Carlton). 2013;18(11):712-7.

[6] Kassam H, Sun Y, Adeniyi M, Agaba EI, Martinez M, Servilla KS, et al. Hospitalizations before and after initiation of chronic hemodialysis. *Hemodial Int.* 2011;15(3):341-9.

[7] Quinn MP, Cardwell CR, Rainey A, McNamee PT, Kee F, Maxwell AP, et al. Patterns of hospitalisation before and following initiation of haemodialysis: a 5 year single centre study. *Postgrad Med J.* 2011;87(1028):389-93.

[8] Kurella M, Covinsky KE, Collins AJ, Chertow GM. Octogenarians and nonagenarians starting dialysis in the United States. *Ann Intern Med.* 2007;146(3):177-83.

[9] Kurella Tamura M, Covinsky KE, Chertow GM, Yaffe K, Landefeld CS, McCulloch CE. Functional status of elderly adults before and after initiation of dialysis. *N Engl J Med.* 2009;361(16):1539-47.

[10] Plantinga LC, King L, Patzer RE, Lea JP, Burkart JM, Hockenberry JM, et al. Early hospital readmission among hemodialysis patients in the United States is associated with subsequent mortality. *Kidney Int.* 2017;92(4):934-41.

[11] Foley RN, Chen SC, Collins AJ. Hemodialysis access at initiation in the United States, 2005 to 2007: still "catheter first." *Hemodial Int.* 2009;13(4):533-42.

[12] Knauf F, Aronson PS. ESRD as a window into America's cost crisis in health care. *J Am Soc Nephrol.* 2009;20(10):2093-7.

[13] Chan KE, Maddux FW, Tolkoff-Rubin N, Karumanchi SA, Thadhani R, Hakim RM. Early outcomes among those initiating chronic dialysis in the United States. *Clin J Am Soc Nephrol.* 2011;6(11):2642-9.

[14] Mix TC, St Peter WL, Ebben J, Xue J, Pereira BJ, Kausz AT, et al. Hospitalization during advancing chronic kidney disease. *Am J Kidney Dis.* 2003;42(5):972-81.

[15] Lopes AA, Leavey SF, McCullough K, Gillespie B, Bommer J, Canaud BJ, et al. Early readmission and length of hospitalization practices in the Dialysis Outcomes and Practice Patterns Study (DOPPS). *Hemodial Int.* 2004;8(3):287-94.

[16] Leppin AL, Gionfriddo MR, Kessler M, Brito JP, Mair FS, Gallacher K, et al. Preventing 30-day hospital readmissions: a systematic review and meta-analysis of randomized trials. *JAMA Intern Med.* 2014;174(7):1095-107.

[17] Verdalles U, Abad S, Aragoncillo I, Villaverde M, Jofre R, Verde E, et al. Factors predicting mortality in elderly patients on dialysis. *Nephron Clin Pract.* 2010;115(1):c28-34.

[18] Behl M, Sun Y, Agaba EI, Martinez M, Servilla KS, Raj DS, et al. Death during hospitalization in patients on chronic hemodialysis. *Hemodial Int.* 2010;14 Suppl 1:S14-21.

[19] Collins AJ, Foley RN, Herzog C, Chavers B, Gilbertson D, Ishani A, et al. US Renal Data System 2010 Annual Data Report. *Am J Kidney Dis.* 2011;57(1 Suppl 1):A8, e1-526.

[20] Kutner NG, Johansen KL, Zhang R, Huang Y, Amaral S. Perspectives on the new kidney disease education benefit: early awareness, race and kidney transplant access in a USRDS study. *Am J Transplant.* 2012;12(4):1017-23.

[21] Morris JN, Howard EP, Steel K, Schreiber R, Fries BE, Lipsitz LA, et al. Predicting risk of hospital and emergency department use for home care elderly persons through a secondary analysis of cross-national data. *BMC Health Serv Res.* 2014;14:519.

[22] 2017 USRDS Annual Data Report 2017 [Available from: https://www.usrds.org/2017.

[23] Lovasik BP, Zhang R, Hockenberry JM, Schrager JD, Pastan SO, Mohan S, et al. Emergency Department Use and Hospital Admissions Among Patients With End-Stage Renal Disease in the United States. *JAMA Intern Med.* 2016;176(10):1563-5.

[24] Plantinga LC, King LM, Masud T, Shafi T, Burkart JM, Lea JP, et al. Burden and correlates of readmissions related to pulmonary edema in US hemodialysis patients: a cohort study. *Nephrol Dial Transplant.* 2018;33(7):1215-23.

[25] Hickson LJ, Thorsteinsdottir B, Ramar P, Reinalda MS, Crowson CS, Williams AW, et al. Hospital Readmission among New Dialysis Patients Associated with Young Age and Poor Functional Status. *Nephron.* 2018;139(1):1-12.

[26] Quinn RR, Ravani P, Zhang X, Garg AX, Blake PG, Austin PC, et al. Impact of modality choice on rates of hospitalization in patients eligible for both peritoneal dialysis and hemodialysis. *Perit Dial Int.* 2014;34(1):41-8.

[27] Tanaka M, Ishibashi Y, Hamasaki Y, Kamijo Y, Idei M, Kawahara T, et al. Health-related quality of life on combination therapy with peritoneal dialysis and hemodialysis in comparison with hemodialysis and peritoneal dialysis: A cross-sectional study. *Perit Dial Int.* 2020:896860819894066.

[28] Shimizu S, Fukuma S, Ikenoue T, Akizawa T, Fukuhara S. Increased Mortality Rate after Hospitalization Among Chronic Hemodialysis Patients: A Prospective Cohort Study. *Nephron.* 2018;140(3):194-202.

[29] Holdaas H, Fellstrom B, Jardine AG, Holme I, Nyberg G, Fauchald P, et al. Effect of fluvastatin on cardiac outcomes in renal transplant recipients: a multicentre, randomised, placebo-controlled trial. *Lancet*. 2003;361(9374):2024-31.

[30] Baigent C, Burbury K, Wheeler D. Premature cardiovascular disease in chronic renal failure. *Lancet*. 2000;356(9224):147-52.

[31] Sarnak MJ Cardiovascular complications in chronic kidney disease. *Am J Kidney Dis*. 2003;41(5 Suppl):11-7.

[32] Chazot C, Wabel P, Chamney P, Moissl U, Wieskotten S, Wizemann V. Importance of normohydration for the long-term survival of haemodialysis patients. *Nephrol Dial Transplant*. 2012;27(6):2404-10.

[33] Agarwal R. Hypervolemia is associated with increased mortality among hemodialysis patients. *Hypertension*. 2010;56(3):512-7.

[34] Cabrera C, Brunelli SM, Rosenbaum D, Anum E, Ramakrishnan K, Jensen DE, et al. A retrospective, longitudinal study estimating the association between interdialytic weight gain and cardiovascular events and death in hemodialysis patients. *BMC Nephrol*. 2015;16:113.

[35] Flythe JE, Kshirsagar AV, Falk RJ, Brunelli SM. Associations of Posthemodialysis Weights above and below Target Weight with All-Cause and Cardiovascular Mortality. *Clin J Am Soc Nephrol*. 2015;10(5):808-16.

[36] Kalantar-Zadeh K, Regidor DL, Kovesdy CP, Van Wyck D, Bunnapradist S, Horwich TB, et al. Fluid retention is associated with cardiovascular mortality in patients undergoing long-term hemodialysis. *Circulation*. 2009;119(5):671-9.

[37] Saran R, Li Y, Robinson B, Abbott KC, Agodoa LY, Ayanian J, ct al. US Rcnal Data System 2015 Annual Data Report: Epidemiology of Kidney Disease in the United States. *Am J Kidney Di*s. 2016;67(3 Suppl 1):Svii, S1-305.

[38] Arneson TJ, Liu J, Qiu Y, Gilbertson DT, Foley RN, Collins AJ. Hospital treatment for fluid overload in the Medicare hemodialysis population. *Clin J Am Soc Nephrol*. 2010;5(6):1054-63.

[39] Dasgupta I, Farrington K, Davies SJ, Davenport A, Mitra S. UK National Survey of Practice Patterns of Fluid Volume Management in Haemodialysis Patients: A Need for Evidence. *Blood Purif*. 2016;41(4):324-31.

[40] Hung SC, Kuo KL, Peng CH, Wu CH, Lien YC, Wang YC, et al. Volume overload correlates with cardiovascular risk factors in patients with chronic kidney disease. *Kidney Int*. 2014;85(3):703-9.

[41] Passauer J, Petrov H, Schleser A, Leicht J, Pucalka K. Evaluation of clinical dry weight assessment in haemodialysis patients using bioimpedance spectroscopy: a cross-sectional study. *Nephrol Dial Transplant*. 2010;25(2):545-51.

[42] Antlanger M, Hecking M, Haidinger M, Werzowa J, Kovarik JJ, Paul G, et al. Fluid overload in hemodialysis patients: a cross-sectional study to determine its association with cardiac biomarkers and nutritional status. *BMC Nephrol*. 2013;14:266.

[43] Wizemann V, Wabel P, Chamney P, Zaluska W, Moissl U, Rode C, et al. The mortality risk of overhydration in haemodialysis patients. *Nephrol Dial Transplant*. 2009;24(5):1574-9.

[44] Zoccali C, Moissl U, Chazot C, Mallamaci F, Tripepi G, Arkossy O, et al. Chronic Fluid Overload and Mortality in ESRD. *J Am Soc Nephrol*. 2017;28(8):2491-7.

[45] Agarwal R, Weir MR. Dry-weight: a concept revisited in an effort to avoid medication-directed approaches for blood pressure control in hemodialysis patients. *Clin J Am Soc Nephrol.* 2010;5(7):1255-60.
[46] Thomson GE, Waterhouse K, McDonald HP, Jr., Friedman EA. Hemodialysis for chronic renal failure. Clinical observations. *Arch Intern Med.* 1967;120(2):153-67.
[47] Charra B, Laurent G, Chazot C, Calemard E, Terrat JC, Vanel T, et al. Clinical assessment of dry weight. *Nephrol Dial Transplant.* 1996;11 Suppl 2:16-9.
[48] Sinha AD, Agarwal R. Can chronic volume overload be recognized and prevented in hemodialysis patients? The pitfalls of the clinical examination in assessing volume status. *Semin Dial.* 2009;22(5):480-2.
[49] Torino C, Gargani L, Sicari R, Letachowicz K, Ekart R, Fliser D, et al. The Agreement between Auscultation and Lung Ultrasound in Hemodialysis Patients: The LUST Study. *Clin J Am Soc Nephrol.* 2016;11(11):2005-11.
[50] Group FHNT, Chertow GM, Levin NW, Beck GJ, Depner TA, Eggers PW, et al. In-center hemodialysis six times per week versus three times per week. *N Engl J Med.* 2010;363(24):2287-300.
[51] Miller JE, Kovesdy CP, Nissenson AR, Mehrotra R, Streja E, Van Wyck D, et al. Association of hemodialysis treatment time and dose with mortality and the role of race and sex. *Am J Kidney Dis.* 2010;55(1):100-12.
[52] Lowrie EG, Li Z, Ofsthun N, Lazarus JM. Measurement of dialyzer clearance, dialysis time, and body size: death risk relationships among patients. *Kidney Int.* 2004;66(5):2077-84.
[53] Saran R, Bragg-Gresham JL, Levin NW, Twardowski ZJ, Wizemann V, Saito A, et al. Longer treatment time and slower ultrafiltration in hemodialysis: associations with reduced mortality in the DOPPS. *Kidney Int.* 2006;69(7):1222-8.
[54] Flythe JE, Curhan GC, Brunelli SM. Shorter length dialysis sessions are associated with increased mortality, independent of body weight. *Kidney Int.* 2013;83(1):104-13.
[55] Maduell F, Moreso F, Pons M, Ramos R, Mora-Macia J, Carreras J, et al. High-efficiency postdilution online hemodiafiltration reduces all-cause mortality in hemodialysis patients. *J Am Soc Nephrol.* 2013;24(3):487-97.
[56] Feldman HI, Held PJ, Hutchinson JT, Stoiber E, Hartigan MF, Berlin JA. Hemodialysis vascular access morbidity in the United States. *Kidney Int.* 1993;43(5):1091-6.
[57] Joseph S, Adler S. Vascular access problems in dialysis patients: pathogenesis and strategies for management. *Heart Dis.* 2001;3(4):242-7.
[58] Xue JL, Dahl D, Ebben JP, Collins AJ. The association of initial hemodialysis access type with mortality outcomes in elderly Medicare ESRD patients. *Am J Kidney Dis.* 2003;42(5):1013-9.
[59] Roubicek C, Brunet P, Huiart L, Thirion X, Leonetti F, Dussol B, et al. timing of nephrology referral: influence on mortality and morbidity. *Am J Kidney Dis.* 2000;36(1):35-41.
[60] Dhingra RK, Young EW, Hulbert-Shearon TE, Leavey SF, Port FK Type of vascular access and mortality in U.S. hemodialysis patients. *Kidney Int.* 2001;60(4):1443-51.
[61] Lee T, Barker J, Allon M. Tunneled catheters in hemodialysis patients: reasons and subsequent outcomes. *Am J Kidney Dis.* 2005;46(3):501-8.
[62] Lok CE, Stanley KE, Hux JE, Richardson R, Tobe SW, Conly J. Hemodialysis infection prevention with polysporin ointment. *J Am Soc Nephrol.* 2003;14(1):169-79.

[63] Weijmer MC, ter Wee PM. Temporary vascular access for hemodialysis treatment. Current guidelines and future directions. *Contrib Nephrol.* 2004;142:94-111.

[64] Weijmer MC, van den Dorpel MA, Van de Ven PJ, ter Wee PM, van Geelen JA, Groeneveld JO, et al. Randomized, clinical trial comparison of trisodium citrate 30% and heparin as catheter-locking solution in hemodialysis patients. *J Am Soc Nephrol.* 2005;16(9):2769-77.

[65] Miller LM, Clark E, Dipchand C, Hiremath S, Kappel J, Kiaii M, et al. Hemodialysis Tunneled Catheter-Related Infections. *Can J Kidney Health Dis.* 2016;3:205 4358116669129.

[66] Tokars JI, Light P, Anderson J, Miller ER, Parrish J, Armistead N, et al. A prospective study of vascular access infections at seven outpatient hemodialysis centers. *Am J Kidney Dis.* 2001;37(6):1232-40.

[67] Lata C, Girard L, Parkins M, James MT. Catheter-related bloodstream infection in end-stage kidney disease: a Canadian narrative review. *Can J Kidney Health Dis.* 2016;3:24.

[68] Lok CE, Mokrzycki MH. Prevention and management of catheter-related infection in hemodialysis patients. *Kidney Int.* 2011;79(6):587-98.

[69] Costello JM, Morrow DF, Graham DA, Potter-Bynoe G, Sandora TJ, Laussen PC. Systematic intervention to reduce central line-associated bloodstream infection rates in a pediatric cardiac intensive care unit. *Pediatrics.* 2008;121(5):915-23.

[70] Guerin K, Wagner J, Rains K, Bessesen M. Reduction in central line-associated bloodstream infections by implementation of a postinsertion care bundle. *Am J Infect* Control. 2010;38(6):430-3.

[71] Miller PE, Tolwani A, Luscy CP, Deierhoi MH, Bailey R, Redden DT, et al. Predictors of adequacy of arteriovenous fistulas in hemodialysis patients. *Kidney Int.* 1999;56(1):275-80.

[72] Palder SB, Kirkman RL, Whittemore AD, Hakim RM, Lazarus JM, Tilney NL. Vascular access for hemodialysis. Patency rates and results of revision. *Ann Surg.* 1985;202(2):235-9.

[73] Woods JD, Turenne MN, Strawderman RL, Young EW, Hirth RA, Port FK, et al. Vascular access survival among incident hemodialysis patients in the United States. *Am J Kidney Dis.* 1997;30(1):50-7.

[74] Fan PY, Schwab SJ. Vascular access: concepts for the 1990s. *J Am Soc Nephrol.* 1992;3(1):1-11.

[75] Besarab A, Sullivan KL, Ross RP, Moritz MJ. Utility of intra-access pressure monitoring in detecting and correcting venous outlet stenoses prior to thrombosis. *Kidney Int.* 1995;47(5):1364-73.

[76] Sands JJ, Miranda CL. Prolongation of hemodialysis access survival with elective revision. *Clin Nephrol.* 1995;44(5):329-33.

[77] Windus DW. Permanent vascular access: a nephrologist's view. *Am J Kidney Dis.* 1993;21(5):457-71.

[78] Windus DW, Santoro SA, Atkinson R, Royal HD. Effects of antiplatelet drugs on dialysis-associated platelet deposition in polytetrafluoroethylene grafts. *Am J Kidney* Dis. 1997;29(4):560-4.

[79] Himmelfarb J, Couper L. Dipyridamole inhibits PDGF- and bFGF-induced vascular smooth muscle cell proliferation. *Kidney Int.* 1997;52(6):1671-7.

[80] Sreedhara R, Himmelfarb J, Lazarus JM, Hakim RM. Antiplatelet therapy in graft thrombosis: results of a prospective, randomized, double-blind study. *Kidney Int.* 1994;45(5):1477-83.

[81] Hsu YH, Yen YC, Lin YC, Sung LC. Antiplatelet agents maintain arteriovenous fistula and graft function in patients receiving hemodialysis: A nationwide case-control study. *PLoS One.* 2018;13(10):e0206011.

[82] Ma JZ, Ebben J, Xia H, Collins AJ. Hematocrit level and associated mortality in hemodialysis patients. *J Am Soc Nephrol.* 1999;10(3):610-9.

[83] Xia H, Ebben J, Ma JZ, Collins AJ. Hematocrit levels and hospitalization risks in hemodialysis patients. *J Am Soc Nephrol.* 1999;10(6):1309-16.

[84] Collins A, Ellefson J. Association between hematocrit level and mortality in hemodialysis patients. Case study of the anemic patient. *Nephrol Nurs J.* 2000;27(2):233-6.

[85] Collins AJ, Li S, St Peter W, Ebben J, Roberts T, Ma JZ, et al. Death, hospitalization, and economic associations among incident hemodialysis patients with hematocrit values of 36 to 39%. *J Am Soc Nephrol.* 2001;12(11):2465-73.

[86] World Health Organization. Nutritional Anaemias: Report of a WHO Scientific Group Geneva, Switzerland [Available from: https://apps.who.int/iris/handle/10665/40707.

[87] Berns JS. *Treatment of anemia in hemodialysis patients* Waltham, MA 2020 [

[88] *KDIGO Guidelines* [Available from: https://kdigo.org/wp-content/uploads/2017/02/2017-KDIGO-CKD-MBD-GL-Update.pdf.

[89] Wish JB. Assessing iron status: beyond serum ferritin and transferrin saturation. *Clin J Am Soc Nephrol.* 2006;1 Suppl 1:S4-8.

[90] Fishbane S, Pollack S, Feldman HI, Joffe MM. Iron indices in chronic kidney disease in the National Health and Nutritional Examination Survey 1988-2004. *Clin J Am Soc Nephrol.* 2009;4(1):57-61.

[91] Gotloib L, Silverberg D, Fudin R, Shostak A. Iron deficiency is a common cause of anemia in chronic kidney disease and can often be corrected with intravenous iron. *J Nephrol.* 2006;19(2):161-7.

[92] Silverberg DS, Blum M, Agbaria Z, Deutsch V, Irony M, Schwartz D, et al. The effect of i.v. iron alone or in combination with low-dose erythropoietin in the rapid correction of anemia of chronic renal failure in the pre-dialysis period. *Clin Nephrol.* 2001;55(3):212-9.

[93] Horl WH. Non-erythropoietin-based anaemia management in chronic kidney disease. *Nephrol Dial Transplant.* 2002;17 Suppl 11:35-8.

[94] Li S, Foley RN, Gilbertson DT, Liu J, Collins AJ. Clinical factors associated with achieving K/DOQI hemoglobin targets in hemodialysis patients. *Int Urol Nephrol.* 2003;35(3):399-405.

[95] Shepshelovich D, Rozen-Zvi B, Avni T, Gafter U, Gafter-Gvili A. Intravenous Versus Oral Iron Supplementation for the Treatment of Anemia in CKD: An Updated Systematic Review and Meta-analysis. *Am J Kidney Dis.* 2016;68(5):677-90.

[96] Brookhart MA, Freburger JK, Ellis AR, Wang L, Winkelmayer WC, Kshirsagar AV. Infection risk with bolus versus maintenance iron supplementation in hemodialysis patients. *J Am Soc Nephrol.* 2013;24(7):1151-8.

[97] Besarab A, Bolton WK, Browne JK, Egrie JC, Nissenson AR, Okamoto DM, et al. The effects of normal as compared with low hematocrit values in patients with cardiac

disease who are receiving hemodialysis and epoetin. *N Engl J Med.* 1998;339(9):584-90.

[98] Besarab A, Goodkin DA, Nissenson AR, Normal Hematocrit Cardiac Trial A. The normal hematocrit study--follow-up. *N Engl J Med.* 2008;358(4):433-4.

[99] Zehnder C, Zuber M, Sulzer M, Meyer B, Straumann E, Jenzer HR, et al. Influence of long-term amelioration of anemia and blood pressure control on left ventricular hypertrophy in hemodialyzed patients. *Nephron.* 1992;61(1):21-5.

[100] Levin NW, Lazarus JM, Nissenson AR. National Cooperative rHu Erythropoietin Study in patients with chronic renal failure--an interim report. The National Cooperative rHu Erythropoietin Study Group. *Am J Kidney Dis.* 1993;22(2 Suppl 1):3-12.

[101] Benz RL, Pressman MR, Hovick ET, Peterson DD. A preliminary study of the effects of correction of anemia with recombinant human erythropoietin therapy on sleep, sleep disorders, and daytime sleepiness in hemodialysis patients (The SLEEPO study). *Am J Kidney Dis.* 1999;34(6):1089-95.

[102] Parfrey PS, Lauve M, Latremouille-Viau D, Lefebvre P. Erythropoietin therapy and left ventricular mass index in CKD and ESRD patients: a meta-analysis. *Clin J Am Soc Nephrol.* 2009;4(4):755-62.

[103] Kang SS, Chang JW, Park Y. Nutritional status Predicts 10-Year Mortality in Patients with End-Stage Renal Disease on Hemodialysis. *Nutrients.* 2017;9(4).

[104] Wong CS, Hingorani S, Gillen DL, Sherrard DJ, Watkins SL, Brandt JR, et al. Hypoalbuminemia and risk of death in pediatric patients with end-stage renal disease. *Kidney Int.* 2002;61(2):630-7.

[105] Canpolat N, Caliskan S, Sever L, Tasdemir M, Ekmekci OB, Pehlivan G, et al. Malnutrition and its association with inflammation and vascular disease in children on maintenance dialysis. *Pediatr Nephrol.* 2013;28(11):2149-56.

[106] Mastrangelo A, Paglialonga F, Edefonti A. Assessment of nutritional Status in children with chronic kidney disease and on dialysis. *Pediatr Nephrol.* 2014;29(8):1349-58.

[107] Zha Y, Qian Q. Protein Nutrition and Malnutrition in CKD and ESRD. *Nutrients.* 2017;9(3).

[108] Kohaut EC. Chronic renal disease and growth in childhood. *Curr Opin Pediatr.* 1995;7(2):171-5.

[109] Mak RH. Cachexia in children with chronic kidney disease: challenges in diagnosis and treatment. *Curr Opin Support Palliat Care.* 2016;10(4):293-7.

[110] Tu J, Cheung WW, Mak RH. Inflammation and nutrition in children with chronic kidney disease. *World J Nephrol.* 2016;5(3):274-82.

[111] Rocco MV, Paranandi L, Burrowes JD, Cockram DB, Dwyer JT, Kusek JW, et al. Nutritional Status in the HEMO Study cohort at baseline. Hemodialysis. *Am J Kidney Dis.* 2002;39(2):245-56.

[112] Wang AY, Sanderson J, Sea MM, Wang M, Lam CW, Li PK, et al. Important factors other than dialysis adequacy associated with inadequate dietary protein and energy intakes in patients receiving maintenance peritoneal dialysis. *Am J Clin Nutr.* 2003;77(4):834-41.

[113] Wright M, Woodrow G, O'Brien S, King N, Dye L, Blundell J, et al. Disturbed appetite patterns and nutrient intake in peritoneal dialysis patients. *Perit Dial Int.* 2003;23(6):550-6.

[114] Mamoun AH, Anderstam B, Sodersten P, Lindholm B, Bergstrom J. Influence of peritoneal dialysis solutions with glucose and amino acids on ingestive behavior in rats. *Kidney Int*. 1996;49(5):1276-82.

[115] Rocco MV, Dwyer JT, Larive B, Greene T, Cockram DB, Chumlea WC, et al. The effect of dialysis dose and membrane flux on nutritional parameters in hemodialysis patients: results of the HEMO Study. *Kidney Int.* 2004;65(6):2321-34.

[116] Locatelli F, Martin-Malo A, Hannedouche T, Loureiro A, Papadimitriou M, Wizemann V, et al. Effect of membrane permeability on survival of hemodialysis patients. *J Am Soc Nephrol*. 2009;20(3):645-54.

[117] Cano NJ, Roth H, Aparicio M, Azar R, Canaud B, Chauveau P, et al. malnutrition in hemodialysis diabetic patients: evaluation and prognostic influence. *Kidney Int.* 2002;62(2):593-601.

[118] Deger SM, Sundell MB, Siew ED, Egbert P, Ellis CD, Sha F, et al. Insulin resistance and protein metabolism in chronic hemodialysis patients. *J Ren Nutr*. 2013;23(3):e59-66.

[119] Siew ED, Ikizler TA. Determinants of insulin resistance and its effects on protein metabolism in patients with advanced chronic kidney disease. *Contrib Nephrol.* 2008;161:138-44.

[120] Siew ED, Pupim LB, Majchrzak KM, Shintani A, Flakoll PJ, Ikizler TA. Insulin resistance is associated with skeletal muscle protein breakdown in non-diabetic chronic hemodialysis patients. *Kidney Int.* 2007;71(2):146-52.

[121] Ikizler TA. A patient with CKD and poor nutritional status. *Clin J Am Soc Nephrol.* 2013;8(12):2174-82.

[122] Nagler EV, Webster AC, Vanholder R, Zoccali C. Antidepressants for depression in stage 3-5 chronic kidney disease: a systematic review of pharmacokinetics, efficacy and safety with recommendations by European Renal Best Practice (ERBP). *Nephrol Dial Transplant.* 2012;27(10):3736-45.

[123] Carrero JJ. Identification of patients with eating disorders: clinical and biochemical signs of appetite loss in dialysis patients. *J Ren Nutr*. 2009;19(1):10-5.

[124] Sherman RA, Cody RP, Rogers ME, Solanchick JC. Interdialytic weight gain and nutritional parameters in chronic hemodialysis patients. *Am J Kidney Dis.* 1995;25(4):579-83.

[125] Holland DC, Lam M. Predictors of hospitalization and death among pre-dialysis patients: a retrospective cohort study. *Nephrol Dial Transplant*. 2000;15(5):650-8.

[126] Avram MM, Sreedhara R, Fein P, Oo KK, Chattopadhyay J, Mittman N. Survival on hemodialysis and peritoneal dialysis over 12 years with emphasis on nutritional parameters. *Am J Kidney Dis.* 2001;37(1 Suppl 2):S77-80.

[127] Combe C, Chauveau P, Laville M, Fouque D, Azar R, Cano N, et al. Influence of nutritional factors and hemodialysis adequacy on the survival of 1,610 French patients. *Am J Kidney Dis*. 2001;37(1 Suppl 2):S81-8.

[128] Fung F, Sherrard DJ, Gillen DL, Wong C, Kestenbaum B, Seliger S, et al. Increased risk for cardiovascular mortality among malnourished end-stage renal disease patients. *Am J Kidney Dis*. 2002;40(2):307-14.

[129] Pifer TB, McCullough KP, Port FK, Goodkin DA, Maroni BJ, Held PJ, et al. *Mortality risk in hemodialysis patients and changes in nutritional indicators*: DOPPS. Kidney Int. 2002;62(6):2238-45.

[130] Aziz F, Chaudhary K. Life threatening nutritional deficiencies in a dialysis patient. *Hemodial Int.* 2017;21(3):E50-E3.

[131] Pupim LB, Flakoll PJ, Brouillette JR, Levenhagen DK, Hakim RM, Ikizler TA. Intradialytic parenteral nutrition improves protein and energy homeostasis in chronic hemodialysis patients. *J Clin Invest.* 2002;110(4):483-92.

[132] Foulks CJ. Intradialytic parenteral nutrition treatment. *Am J Kidney Dis.* 1999;33(6):1202.

[133] Foley RN, Parfrey PS, Sarnak MJ. Epidemiology of cardiovascular disease in chronic renal disease. *J Am Soc Nephrol.* 1998;9(12 Suppl):S16-23.

[134] Stack AG, Bloembergen WE. Prevalence and clinical correlates of coronary artery disease among new dialysis patients in the United States: a cross-sectional study. *J Am Soc Nephrol.* 2001;12(7):1516-23.

[135] Collins AJ, Kasiske B, Herzog C, Chavers B, Foley R, Gilbertson D, et al. Excerpts from the United States Renal Data System 2004 annual data report: atlas of end-stage renal disease in the United States. *Am J Kidney Dis.* 2005;45(1 Suppl 1):A5-7, S1-280.

[136] Rostand SG, Kirk KA, Rutsky EA. Dialysis-associated ischemic heart disease: insights from coronary angiography. *Kidney Int.* 1984;25(4):653-9.

[137] Cheung AK, Sarnak MJ, Yan G, Berkoben M, Heyka R, Kaufman A, et al. Cardiac diseases in maintenance hemodialysis patients: results of the HEMO Study. *Kidney Int.* 2004;65(6):2380-9.

[138] Burton JO, Jefferies HJ, Selby NM, McIntyre CW. Hemodialysis-induced cardiac injury: determinants and associated outcomes. *Clin J Am Soc Nephrol.* 2009;4(5):914-20.

[139] Assa S, Hummel YM, Voors AA, Kuipers J, Westerhuis R, de Jong PE, et al. Hemodialysis-induced regional left ventricular systolic dysfunction: prevalence, patient and dialysis treatment-related factors, and prognostic significance. *Clin J Am Soc Nephrol.* 2012;7(10):1615-23.

[140] Lewington S, Clarke R, Qizilbash N, Peto R, Collins R, Prospective Studies C. Age-specific relevance of usual blood pressure to vascular mortality: a meta-analysis of individual data for one million adults in 61 prospective studies. *Lancet.* 2002;360(9349):1903-13.

[141] Kalantar-Zadeh K, Kilpatrick RD, McAllister CJ, Greenland S, Kopple JD. Reverse epidemiology of hypertension and cardiovascular death in the hemodialysis population: the 58th annual fall conference and scientific sessions. *Hypertension.* 2005;45(4):811-7.

[142] Zager PG, Nikolic J, Brown RH, Campbell MA, Hunt WC, Peterson D, et al. *"U" curve association of blood pressure and mortality in hemodialysis patients.* Medical Directors of Dialysis Clinic, Inc. Kidney Int. 1998;54(2):561-9.

[143] Agarwal R. Hypertension and survival in chronic hemodialysis patients--past lessons and future opportunities. *Kidney Int.* 2005;67(1):1-13.

[144] Malliara M. The management of hypertension in hemodialysis and CAPD patients. *Hippokratia.* 2007;11(4):171-4.

[145] Cozzolino M, Mangano M, Stucchi A, Ciceri P, Conte F, Galassi A. Cardiovascular disease in dialysis patients. *Nephrol Dial Transplan*t. 2018;33(suppl_3):iii28-iii34.

[146] Bover J, Evenepoel P, Urena-Torres P, Vervloet MG, Brandenburg V, Mazzaferro S, et al. Pro: cardiovascular calcifications are clinically relevant. *Nephrol Dial Transplant.* 2015;30(3):345-51.

[147] Wang Z, Jiang A, Wei F, Chen H. Cardiac valve calcification and risk of cardiovascular or all-cause mortality in dialysis patients: a meta-analysis. *BMC Cardiovasc Disord.* 2018;18(1):12.

[148] Vashistha T, Kalantar-Zadeh K, Molnar MZ, Torlen K, Mehrotra R. Dialysis modality and correction of uremic metabolic acidosis: relationship with all-cause and cause-specific mortality. *Clin J Am Soc Nephrol.* 2013;8(2):254-64.

[149] Raikou VD, Kyriaki D. Association between Low Serum Bicarbonate Concentrations and Cardiovascular Disease in Patients in the End-Stage of Renal Disease. *Diseases.* 2016;4(4): 36.

[150] Djamali A, Singh T, Melamed ML, Stein JH, Aziz F, Parajuli S, et al. Metabolic Acidosis 1 Year Following Kidney Transplantation and Subsequent Cardiovascular Events and Mortality: An Observational Cohort Study. *Am J Kidney Dis.* 2019;73(4):476-85.

[151] Cozzolino M, Galassi A, Pivari F, Ciceri P, Conte F. The Cardiovascular Burden in End-Stage Renal Disease. *Contrib Nephrol.* 2017;191:44-57.

[152] Moradi H, Sica DA, Kalantar-Zadeh K. Cardiovascular burden associated with uremic toxins in patients with chronic kidney disease. *Am J Nephrol.* 2013;38(2):136-48.

[153] Meijers BK, Bammens B, De Moor B, Verbeke K, Vanrenterghem Y, Evenepoel P. Free p-cresol is associated with cardiovascular disease in hemodialysis patients. *Kidney Int.* 2008;73(10):1174-80.

[154] Meijers BK, Claes K, Bammens B, de Loor H, Viaene L, Verbeke K, et al. p-Cresol and cardiovascular risk in mild-to-moderate kidney disease. *Clin J Am Soc Nephrol.* 2010;5(7):1182-9.

[155] Cerini C, Dou L, Anfosso F, Sabatier F, Moal V, Glorieux G, et al. P-cresol, a uremic retention solute, alters the endothelial barrier function in vitro. *Thromb Haemost.* 2004;92(1):140-50.

[156] Lin CJ, Pan CF, Chuang CK, Liu HL, Huang SF, Chen HH, et al. Effects of Sevelamer Hydrochloride on Uremic Toxins Serum Indoxyl Sulfate and P-Cresyl Sulfate in Hemodialysis Patients. *J Clin Med Res.* 2017;9(9):765-70.

[157] Bennis Y, Cluet Y, Titeca-Beauport D, El Esper N, Urena P, Bodeau S, et al. The Effect of Sevelamer on Serum Levels of Gut-Derived Uremic Toxins: Results from In Vitro Experiments and A Multicenter, Double-Blind, Placebo-Controlled, Randomized Clinical Trial. *Toxins* (Basel). 2019;11(5).

[158] Guida B, Cataldi M, Riccio E, Grumetto L, Pota A, Borrelli S, et al. Plasma p-cresol lowering effect of sevelamer in peritoneal dialysis patients: evidence from a Cross-Sectional Observational Study. *PLoS One.* 2013;8(8):e73558.

[159] Shivanna S, Kolandaivelu K, Shashar M, Belghasim M, Al-Rabadi L, Balcells M, et al. The Aryl Hydrocarbon Receptor is a Critical Regulator of Tissue Factor Stability and an Antithrombotic Target in Uremia. *J Am Soc Nephrol.* 2016;27(1):189-201.

[160] Chitalia VC, Shivanna S, Martorell J, Balcells M, Bosch I, Kolandaivelu K, et al. Uremic serum and solutes increase post-vascular interventional thrombotic risk through altered stability of smooth muscle cell tissue factor. *Circulation.* 2013;127(3):365-76.

[161] Kaminski TW, Pawlak K, Karbowska M, Mysliwiec M, Pawlak D. Indoxyl sulfate - the uremic toxin linking hemostatic system disturbances with the prevalence of cardiovascular disease in patients with chronic kidney disease. *BMC Nephrol.* 2017;18(1):35.

[162] Kimmel PL, Thamer M, Richard CM, Ray NF. Psychiatric illness in patients with end-stage renal disease. *Am J Med.* 1998;105(3):214-21.

[163] Fukunishi I, Kitaoka T, Shirai T, Kino K, Kanematsu E, Sato Y. Psychiatric disorders among patients undergoing hemodialysis therapy. *Nephron.* 2002;91(2):344-7.

[164] Palmer S, Vecchio M, Craig JC, Tonelli M, Johnson DW, Nicolucci A, et al. Prevalence of depression in chronic kidney disease: systematic review and meta-analysis of observational studies. *Kidney Int.* 2013;84(1):179-91.

[165] Peterson RA, Kimmel PL, Sacks CR, Mesquita ML, Simmens SJ, Reiss D. Depression, perception of illness and mortality in patients with end-stage renal disease. *Int J Psychiatry Med.* 1991;21(4):343-54.

[166] Kimmel PL, Weihs K, Peterson RA. Survival in hemodialysis patients: the role of depression. *J Am Soc Nephrol.* 1993;4(1):12-27.

[167] Kimmel PL, Peterson RA, Weihs KL, Simmens SJ, Alleyne S, Cruz I, et al. Psychosocial factors, behavioral compliance and survival in urban hemodialysis patients. *Kidney Int.* 1998;54(1):245-54.

[168] Palmer SC, Vecchio M, Craig JC, Tonelli M, Johnson DW, Nicolucci A, et al. Association between depression and death in people with CKD: a meta-analysis of cohort studies. *Am J Kidney Dis.* 2013;62(3):493-505.

[169] Hedayati SS, Grambow SC, Szczech LA, Stechuchak KM, Allen AS, Bosworth HB. Physician-diagnosed depression as a correlate of hospitalizations in patients receiving long-term hemodialysis. *Am J Kidney Dis.* 2005;46(4):642-9.

[170] Lacson E, Jr., Bruce L, Li NC, Mooney A, Maddux FW. Depressive affect and hospitalization risk in incident hemodialysis patients. *Clin J Am Soc Nephrol.* 2014;9(10):1713-9.

[171] Kurella M, Kimmel PL, Young BS, Chertow GM. Suicide in the United States end-stage renal disease program. *J Am Soc Nephrol.* 2005;16(3):774-81.

[172] Workgroup KD. K/DOQI clinical practice guidelines for cardiovascular disease in dialysis patients. *Am J Kidney Dis.* 2005;45(4 Suppl 3):S1-153.

[173] Duarte PS, Miyazaki MC, Blay SL, Sesso R. Cognitive-behavioral group therapy is an effective treatment for major depression in hemodialysis patients. *Kidney Int.* 2009;76(4):414-21.

[174] Cukor D, Ver Halen N, Asher DR, Coplan JD, Weedon J, Wyka KE, et al. Psychosocial intervention improves depression, quality of life, and fluid adherence in hemodialysis. *J Am Soc Nephrol.* 2014;25(1):196-206.

[175] Andreucci VE, Fissell RB, Bragg-Gresham JL, Ethier J, Greenwood R, Pauly M, et al. Dialysis Outcomes and Practice Patterns Study (DOPPS) data on medications in hemodialysis patients. *Am J Kidney Dis.* 2004;44(5 Suppl 2):61-7.

[176] Mathew AT, Strippoli GF, Ruospo M, Fishbane S. Reducing hospital readmissions in patients with end-stage kidney disease. *Kidney Int.* 2015;88(6):1250-60.

[177] Shipton S. Risk factors associated with multiple hospital readmissions. *Home Care Provid.* 1996;1(2):83-5.

[178] Tsuchihashi M, Tsutsui H, Kodama K, Kasagi F, Setoguchi S, Mohr M, et al. Medical and socioenvironmental predictors of hospital readmission in patients with congestive heart failure. *Am Heart J.* 2001;142(4):E7.

[179] Crews DC, Gutierrez OM, Fedewa SA, Luthi JC, Shoham D, Judd SE, et al. Low income, community poverty and risk of end stage renal disease. *BMC Nephrol.* 2014;15:192.

[180] Ward MM. Socioeconomic status and the incidence of ESRD. *Am J Kidney Dis.* 2008;51(4):563-72.

[181] Norris K, Nissenson AR. Race, gender, and socioeconomic disparities in CKD in the United States. *J Am Soc Nephrol.* 2008;19(7):1261-70.

[182] Misky GJ, Wald HL, Coleman EA. Post-hospitalization transitions: Examining the effects of timing of primary care provider follow-up. *J Hosp Med.* 2010;5(7):392-7.

In: Issues in Kidney Disease – Dialysis
Editors: Stephen Z. Fadem and José A. Moura-Neto
ISBN: 978-1-68507-000-7

Chapter 9

LEFT VENTRICULAR HYPERTROPHY IN DIALYSIS PATIENTS

Viviane Calice-Silva[1,*], MD, PhD, Silvio Barberato[2], MD, PhD and Roberto Pecoits-Filho[2,3], MD, PhD

[1]Research Department, Pro-Rim Foundation, Joinville, Brazil and Department of Medicine, UNIVILLE, Joinville, Brazil
[2]School of Medicine, Pontifical Catholic University of Parana, Curitiba, Brazil
[3]DOPPS Program, Arbor Research Collaborative for Health, Ann Arbor, MI, USA

ABSTRACT

Left ventricular hypertrophy (LVH) is a maladaptive response to chronic pressure load, mainly induced by systolic blood pressure, but exacerbated by diabetes, anemia, and mineral metabolism disorders. There is a wide spectrum of LVH with clinical implications in risk stratification, from a purely physiological adaptation to exercise in athletes to a complex remodeled and fibrotic heart present in patients with multiple comorbidities, including chronic kidney disease. The differentiation in heart structure and function using current tools is challenging and studies designed to address the cause-effect relationship between LVH and poor clinical outcomes are lacking especially in patients with renal disease. In this chapter, we aim to discuss the potential mechanisms involved in LVH, especially those associated with chronic kidney disease and dialysis, as well as to review its current diagnostic methods.

Keywords: cardiovascular disease, left ventricular hypertrophy, end-stage renal disease, dialysis

* Corresponding Author's E-mail: viviane.silva@prorim.org.br.

INTRODUCTION

Cardiovascular disease (CVD) morbidity and mortality are very high in chronic kidney disease (CKD), particularly in patients with end stage renal disease (ESRD) treated with renal replacement therapies (RRT) [1, 2]. Based on observations from the HEMO study [3], approximately 80% of hemodialysis (HD) patients presented cardiovascular diseases at the study baseline. Coronary artery disease (CAD, 22 to 39%), congestive heart failure (CHF, 20 to 40%), atrial fibrillation (AF, 11-27%), and left ventricular hypertrophy (LVH, 29-75%) are highly prevalent in ESRD patients. Although atherosclerotic CAD, peripheral and cerebral vascular disease represent a major burden to ESRD patients, there is emerging evidence that non-atherosclerotic heart disease, particularly heart failure (CHF) and LVH, play a major role in determining poor outcomes in this group of patients [4-6]. LVH is one of the most common findings in the cardiovascular evaluation of patients starting dialysis and its presence has been associated with poor patient prognosis. In this chapter will focus on the pathophysiology and diagnostic methods for LVH in dialysis patients.

LVH DEFINITION

Left ventricular hypertrophy is defined as an increase in the left ventricle (LV) mass of that can be secondary to an increase in wall thickness, cavity size or both; its presentation can vary depending upon the underlying pathology [7]. In addition to long-term pressure, volume overload status, or their combination are responsible for LVH, infiltrative cardiac processes also lead to LV wall thickness. Examples of infiltrative cardiac processes include amyloidosis and sarcoidosis. Fibrotic infiltration is caused by distinct pathological processes, such as chronic inflammatory injury, metabolic disorders, and uremic toxicity. These processes frequently coexist with LVH, particularly in CKD. LVH per se does not have specific signs and symptoms. Associated signs and symptoms are those of its pathologic causes (e.g., systemic hypertension, aortic stenosis, aortic or mitral regurgitation, hypertrophic cardiomyopathy, etc.) [8].

NATURAL HISTORY OF LVH IN CKD AND ESRD

Basic Concepts

Longitudinal and cross-sectional studies have demonstrated that LV mass in CKD increases as renal dysfunction develops and progresses during the pre-dialysis stages of CKD [9, 10]. Approximately 70 to 80% of patients with stage 4 to 5 CKD have some manifestation of LVH before the initiation of dialysis. Systolic arterial hypertension and elevated pulse pressure are strongly associated with LVH in those patients with advanced CKD, suggesting that fluid overload and increased arterial stiffness play a role in LVH well before the start of dialysis therapy [10].

As CKD progresses, its complications, such as anemia, bone-mineral disease, hyperparathyroidism and hypervolemia, are more prevalent. An increase in the uremic toxins levels is also expected. All these factors have an important effect in the pathophysiology of LVH in this population. Additionally, there are some peculiarities of certain kidney diseases that could contribute to the evolution of this hypertrophy such as autosomal dominant polycystic kidney disease (ADPKD).

Cardiovascular manifestations occur in a high percentage of patients with ADPKD, including hypertension, LVH, cardiac valvular abnormalities, and intracranial aneurysms, being the cardiovascular complications the leading cause of morbidity and mortality in this group of patients [11]. With the use of echocardiographic analyses, many studies have demonstrated a significantly higher left ventricular mass index in groups of young individuals with ADPKD as compared to control groups [12]. Generalized connective tissue dysfunction, manifested by a deficiency or complete absence of type III collagen or, a defect in the extracellular matrix, may be responsible for the myxomatous degeneration, fragmentation, and wasting of collagen demonstrated within the heart valves in ADPKD patients [12-14]. Also, ADPKD cardiac manifestations could be due to a component of an insertion-deletion (I/D) polymorphism of the angiotensin-converting enzyme gene I (ACE) which would be responsible for arterial hypertension, kidney failure and for the effects of individual genotypes on the disease evolution in this group of patients [12].

Considering the hemodynamic factors related to renal replacement therapies (RRT), more frequent and/or longer dialysis sessions were suggested as the ideal therapy. An RCT published in 2007, applying frequent nocturnal hemodialysis versus 3 times weekly - conventional HD showed improved left ventricular mass, reduced the need for blood pressure medications, improved some measures of mineral metabolism, and improved selected measures of quality of life in patients undergoing frequent nocturnal HD [15]. These findings were not corroborated by other later trial performed in its nocturnal arm [16]. In Frequent Hemodialysis Network Daily Trial (FHN), frequent HD resulted in a significant reduction in LV mass - (LVM 13.1 g; 95% CI, 5.0-21.3 g; $p = 0.002$), LVM index (6.9 g/m^2; 95% CI, 2.4-11.3 g/m^2; $p = 0.003$), and percent change in geometric mean of LVM (7.0%; 95% CI, 1.0%-12.6; $p = 0.02$), being the more pronounced effect of frequent HD on LVM evident among patients with previous LVH at study baseline [16]. In this group, changes in LVM were associated with changes in blood pressure (conventional hemodialysis: $R = 0.28$, $p = 0.01$, daily hemodialysis: $R = 0.54$, $p = 0.001$) and the magnitude of reduction in left and right ventricular end diastolic volumes with frequent hemodialysis was accentuated among patients with residual urine output (at least 100 ml/d (p- value interaction = 0.02), indicating effects on blood pressure and volume control may mediate this improvement, which may be the responsible factors for the improvements on hard outcomes in the HD population [16, 17].

There are also data to support the concept that a reduction in the degree of LVH (but not reversion to normal) can be achieved by aggressive fluid and BP control and perhaps by treatment of anemia, at least in certain circumstances [15].

Regarding kidney transplantation, supposed to be the RRT modality which offers an interesting opportunity for improvement/regression of the uremic cardiomyopathy, LVH is still observed in nearly half of patients after kidney transplantation, certainly, as a consequence of previous exposure to the uremic milieu during the progression of CKD and the time spent in dialysis before transplantation [18, 19]. However, even though some studies have reported an improvement in cardiomyopathy after successful kidney transplantation [20, 21], more recent clinical reports showed that LVH may not regress, particularly in the subgroup of patients in which renal function was not fully recovered after the transplantation [22].

LVH Determinants on CKD - Mechanisms (Observation and Interaction)

The mechanisms underlying left ventricular abnormalities in CKD are diverse and involve many aspects: 1) preload-related factors: volume overload, anemia, arterial-venous fistula which results in myocardial cell lengthening and eccentric LV remodeling; 2) afterload-related factors: systemic arterial resistance (systolic and diastolic hypertension) and vascular compliance disturbances (vascular calcification) resulting in myocardial cell thickening and concentric LV remodeling and; 3) hemodynamic-independent factors such as oxidative stress, and inflammation; hyperphosphatemia; hyperparathyroidism; and hypovitaminosis D, which play an important role starting in the earlier stages and increasing in the more advanced stages of CKD [9, 23, 24]. LVH has been widely taken as a surrogate end-point for mortality in randomized trials, as several studies of HD patients have shown LV mass as a good predictor of cardiovascular outcomes and death [9, 25, 26].

A general assumption that interventions which trigger LVH regression may well reduce cardiovascular risk in HD patients emerged from the results of these studies. However, a recent meta-analysis questioned the role of LVH as an effective surrogate in CKD patients because no clear association was found between intervention-induced LV mass regression and mortality [27]. Perhaps confounding factors related to the diagnosis of LVH by cardiovascular imaging may have contributed to the contradictory results of this meta-analysis. Several imaging biomarkers have been used to reliably diagnose LVH in HD patients, but we know that there are a number of intrinsic pitfalls in all of them. The clinician should bear in mind a critical view of the strengths and limitations regarding the usefulness of noninvasive imaging methods for the LV mass assessment in this group of patients.

Among CKD patients who develop LVH, serum levels of inflammatory biomarkers are significantly higher than those values observed among those without LVH [28]. The same relationship has been noted for C-reactive protein and N-terminal pro-B-type, natriuretic peptide [29], suggesting a link between LV filling pressure and inflammation. It is also well known that CKD patients frequently have excessive activation of the renin–angiotensin–aldosterone system (RAS), potentially inducing myocardial fibrosis and hypertrophy. Activation of the intra-cardiac RAS seems to be critically involved in overload status observed in CKD, but angiotensin II and aldosterone can also be involved in myocardial cell hypertrophy and fibrosis independent of afterload [9]. Angiotensin II promotes growth in both fibroblasts and cardiac myocytes, contributing to the cardiomyopathy of dialysis patients [30], and high aldosterone levels seem to be correlated with LVH independent of hypertension in hemodialysis patients [31].

Also, some novel cellular mediator systems that translate hemodynamic and circulatory alterations to an increase in ventricular mass have brought attention to other pathways to produce or aggravate LVH. These potential cellular systems include vitamin D receptor activation, calcineurin/nuclear factor of activated T cells, G-protein coupled receptor to angiotensin II and endothelin 1 and the mammalian target of rapamycin (mTOR) paths [9]. The development of new efficient therapeutic strategies may be possible once these systems actions are bettered explained and comprehended.

Systemic Arterial Hypertension

Left ventricular hypertrophy (LVH) is a common complication even in mild hypertension, found in up to 30% of patients [32, 33]. Chronic systemic hypertension leads to structural and functional changes in the heart. These changes include LVH, fibrosis of the myocardial interstitium and coronary angiopathy. Chronic arterial hypertension leads to increased wall stress both in the systemic arteries and in the LV [34]. Increased wall stress impairs LV systolic performance and induces compensatory cardiomyocyte hypertrophy and increased LV wall thickness to reduce wall stress, following Laplace's law. As a consequence, the ratio between wall thickness and internal chamber diameter (relative wall thickness) increases, and LV geometry becomes more concentric [35, 36].

Other mechanisms related to LVH secondary to hypertension are: a) the increased sympathetic nervous system activity, which leads to neuroendocrine activation in hypertension, including stimulation of the renin-angiotensin system (RAS), the natriuretic peptide family and the adrenoceptor-signaling cascade [37], b) the RAS system as a major regulator of blood pressure and hypertrophic response in hypertension and c) angiotensin II that stimulates sympathetic activity and aldosterone production, d) aldosterone promotes endothelial dysfunction, vascular remodeling, oxidative stress and inflammation through the mineralocorticoid receptor [38]. Other main pathways and signaling molecules of importance for the hypertrophic response to arterial hypertension include endothelin-1 and G proteins, micro ribonucleic acids (miRNAs), oxidative stress, heat shock proteins, calcium and some kinases [39].

In obese subjects, a number of non-hemodynamic determinants of LVH have been identified including altered renal sodium handling, increased blood volume, insulin resistance, stimulation of the sympathetic nervous system, visceral fat production of angiotensinogen, adipokines, pro-inflammatory cytokines (mainly belonging to the tumor necrosis factor alpha and interleukin 6 families) and mineralocorticoid-releasing factors [40]. Co-presence of hypertension increases in parallel with degree of obesity, and 75% of subjects with body mass index >35 kg/m^2 have hypertension, exposing the LV for hemodynamic as well as non-hemodynamic stimulators of hypertrophy [35].

Anemia

Presence of anemia during the first year of renal replacement therapy was also associated with an increase in the prevalence of LVH (10 g/m^2 per 1.0 g of decline in hemoglobin) [41]. The impact of anemia on cardiomyopathy among CKD patients was recently evaluated in a clinical study including serial echocardiograms. In this study, anemia was an independent risk factor for diastolic heart failure even after adjustment for age, diabetes, and ischemic heart disease [41]. The treatment of severe anemia with erythropoietin and iron to increase hemoglobin levels seems to be beneficial for LVH, but treatment of lesser degrees of anemia to even higher targets has not been proven to be beneficial for LVH [9].

Phosphate, Vitamin D and PTH

Mineral metabolism disorders, including hyperphosphatemia, elevated parathyroid hormone (PTH) levels and hypovitaminosis D are common in CKD patients and have been associated to LVH and myocardial hypertrophy [42], with early cardiovascular mortality and sudden cardiac death in dialysis patients [43]. Secondary to this evidence, there has been recognition that phosphate adequate control, vitamin D therapy and prevention of hyperparathyroidism are very important. However, the benefits of these aspects of CKD treatment on LVH and its consequences, such as hospitalization due to heart failure (HF), progression of CKD and cardiovascular (CV) mortality, remain uncertain [9].

Two randomized trials approaching mineral bone disease treatment have been published: The EVOLVE study (EValuation of Cinacalcet Hydrochloride Therapy to Lower Cardiovascular Events) and the PRIMO (Paricalcitol Capsule Benefits in Renal Failure Induced Cardiac Morbidity) studies. In the EVOLVE study, cinacalcet was compared to placebo in 3883 hemodialysis patients with secondary hyperparathyroidism, the primary end point (death, myocardial infarction, unstable angina, heart failure, or peripheral vascular disease) in an unadjusted intention to treat analysis was not significant (HR 0.93; 95% CI 0.85-1.02, $p = 0.11$) in contrast to the a priori defined secondary end points of an adjusted intention to treat analysis (HR 0.88; 95% CI 0.79-0.97, $p = 0.008$) [5, 44]. In the PRIMO study, 227 patients with CKD stage 3-4 and left ventricular hypertrophy were assessed by echocardiography and randomized to paricalcitol or placebo. The primary end point evaluated was change in left ventricular mass index by CMRI after 12 months, which was not different between the two groups, but the pre-specified end point of cardiovascular related hospitalizations were reduced in the paricalcitol treated group ($p = 0.04$) [44, 45].

Other studies evaluated the effects of vitamin D on the heart and it has been well established that vitamin D has several biological effects on the heart, including cardiac cell contraction, proliferation, hypertrophy, protein and collagen expression of cardiomyocyte, and potentially play a role in the maintenance of vascular tone and cardiac output [46], presenting a potential role of hypovitaminosis D in the development of heart failure in CKD patients [9, 47].

There are many reasons for the negative results of those trials; maybe the main one is that the CKD-MBD has different paths needing treatment and all of these proposed medications effects should be studied combined and in a different profiles of patients, for example, with a greater LVH or followed for longer periods of time to then being able to demonstrate in real life the effects found in animal models, and also may help to clarify if there is any role of LVH in CKD/ESRD patients outcomes.

FGF-23 and LVH

FGF-23 is a hormone secreted by osteocytes and osteoblasts that has been established as a regulator of circulating phosphate and 1,25-dihydroxyvitamin D (1,25(OH)2D) concentrations [48]. It promotes the urinary excretion of phosphorus and decreased its intestinal absorption through 1,25(OH)2D synthesis inhibition [48]. In patients with CKD, FGF-23 is a key regulator of phosphorus that maintains serum phosphorus within the normal range. It increases since the earlier stages of CKD and by the time patients reach end stage renal disease, FGF-23 concentrations are often 100 times above the normal range [49].

Recently, elevated FGF-23 concentrations were found to be associated with death, cardiovascular events and kidney disease progression in patients with CKD. FGF receptors have been implicated in the pathogenesis of LVH, which predisposes to left ventricular (LV) dysfunction, and is an important predictor of mortality in patients with CKD [50].

Chronic dialysis patients' participants of the Homocysteine in Kidney and End Stage Renal Disease (HOST) Study with FGF-23 in the highest tertile had an 8% decrease in the ejection fraction (EF) compared to participants in the lowest tertile (β -8.0, 95% CI -15.5 to -0.53; p = 0.04), demonstrating higher FGF-23 concentration was an independently predictor of LV systolic dysfunction in that population [51].

Also, in a subset study as part of the prospective Chronic Renal Insufficiency Cohort (CRIC) study, FGF-23 levels were assessed in the baseline plasma samples from 3,070 individuals who underwent echocardiography 1 year later. Multivariable analyses adjusted for many confounder factors demonstrated that elevated FGF-23 was independently associated with increased LV mass index (LVMI-1.5 g m-2.7 greater LVMI per unit increase in FGF-23, 95% CI, 0.8-2.2; P < 0.001) and conferred greater risk of eccentric and concentric LVH (RR 1.5 per unit increase in lnFGF23; 95% CI, 1.3 1.9; P < 0.001). The authors also found that elevated FGF-23 levels at baseline were associated with increased future risk of new-onset LVH when it was expressed on a continuous scale (N = 411 CRIC participants, prospectively evaluated, 20% developed new-onset LVH 2.9 ± 0.5 years later - RR 2.4 per unit increase in FGF-23; 95% CI, 1.6-3.6; P < 0.001) [52].

A direct causal role for elevated FGF-23 in the pathogenesis of LVH has been demonstrated in animal models, with findings such as FGF-23 directly inducing pathological hypertrophy of isolated cardiomyocytes, developing LVH after intraventricular or intravenous injection of FGF23 in mice [52]. Thus, FGF-23 receptors blockers may be a potential way to ameliorate LVH and dysfunction in CKD patients.

LVH Diagnostic Methods

Electrocardiography was the first test used to diagnose LVH, but nowadays echocardiography (ECHO) is in general, considered to be more accurate than electrocardiogram for that purpose [53]. On the other hand, cardiac magnetic resonance imaging (CMRI) is currently considered the gold standard technique for measurement of LV mass, volume and function, independently of geometric assumptions [54].

CMRI offers very high spatial resolution and tissue contrast therefore being able to assess myocardial fibrosis [47]. Native T1 mapping is a novel non-contrast CMRI technique that can quantify increased extracellular volume, i.e., fibrosis, and may be an interesting alternative method of measuring myocardial fibrosis. In advanced CKD or ESKD population, CMRI has been largely avoided due to the need for intravenous gadolinium contrast to detect myocardial fibrosis during the procedure. Rarely, Gadolinium can cause nephrogenic systemic fibrosis [55-57] in CKD and CMRI benefits should outweigh the risk of this complication. CMRI reduced availability, high costs, and the contraindications of claustrophobia or cardiac implantable devices, also limit its use in clinical practice [9]. Contrast enhanced cardiac tomography (CT) also precisely measures LV mass, and quantifies coronary calcium and coronary arterial stenosis. However, it involves ionizing radiation and the use of iodinated contrast agents, which may affect renal function.

Table 1. Normal values for LV mass and thresholds for diagnosis of mild, moderate and severe increases in LV mass in men and women by M-Mode ECHO, 2D ECHO and CMRI

	Women				Men			
	Upper Limit	Mildly abnormal	Moderately abnormal	Severely abnormal	Upper Limit	Mildly abnormal	Moderately abnormal	Severely abnormal
M-Mode method								
Mass/BSA, g/m²	95	96-108	109-121	≥122	115	116-131	132-148	≥149
Mass/height, g/m	99	100-115	116-128	≥129	126	127-144	145-162	≥163
Mass/height^{2,7}, g/m^{2,7}	44	45-51	52-58	≥59	48	49-55	56-63	≥64
2D method								
Mass/BSA, g/m²	88	89-100	101-112	≥113	102	103-116	117-130	≥131
CMRI								
Mass/BSA, g/m²	75				95			
Mass/height, g/m	82				114			

ECHO, echocardiography; 2D, two-dimensional; CMRI, cardiac magnetic resonance imaging; BSA, body surface area. Adapted from Lang et al. and Salton et al.

Because of the issues concerning CMRI and CT, ECHO is well established as the main tool for the LV mass assessment both in clinical practice and in many research protocols. The accuracy of assessment of LVH by ECHO in CKD patients depends on which technique is used, the timing of test relative to dialysis session, and the index used for "normalization" of the data generated [58]. LV mass estimates can be derived from M-mode ECHO, two-dimensional (2D) ECHO, and real-time three-dimensional (3D) ECHO. Each method for LV mass measurement has advantages, disadvantages, and value in specific situations. The serial monitoring of LV mass by ECHO is potentially useful clinical tool in the evaluation of prognosis and success of interventions that may result in regression of LVH (Table 1 shows LVM reference values in men and women by M-Mode ECHO, 2D ECHO and CMRI).

Conclusion

Left ventricular hypertrophy is associated with poor outcomes in CKD and ESRD patients. Currently, there is a lack of studies able to provide sufficient information about the chronology of LVH installation. Is LVH per se the greater burden to these patients' hearts? What manifestation comes first? Would all those aforementioned variables combined be responsible for the worse outcomes our patients have along their lives? The evidence clearly states an association between many factors related to CKD which lead to LVH such as hypervolemia, hypertension, anemia, phosphate, vitamin D and PTH, FGF-23 and many others. These CKD related risk factors associated with patients' comorbidities and traditional cardiovascular risk factors play an important role in the LVH development and cardiovascular morbidity and mortality especially in dialysis population. The more the comprehension of those mechanisms becomes clear, the greater our capability will be to develop the strategies to prevent and treat LVH and cardiovascular disease in dialysis patients.

REFERENCES

[1] Saran R, Li Y, Robinson B, Ayanian J, Balkrishnan R, Bragg-Gresham J, et al. US Renal Data System 2014 Annual Data Report: Epidemiology of Kidney Disease in the United States. *Am J Kidney Dis*. 2015;66(1 Suppl 1):Svii, S1-305.

[2] Herzog CA, Asinger RW, Berger AK, Charytan DM, Diez J, Hart RG, et al. Cardiovascular disease in chronic kidney disease. A clinical update from Kidney Disease: Improving Global Outcomes (KDIGO). *Kidney Int*. 2011;80(6):572-86.

[3] Cheung AK, Sarnak MJ, Yan G, Berkoben M, Heyka R, Kaufman A, et al. Cardiac diseases in maintenance hemodialysis patients: results of the HEMO Study. *Kidney Int*. 2004;65(6):2380-9.

[4] Wanner C, Krane V, Marz W, Olschewski M, Asmus HG, Kramer W, et al. Randomized controlled trial on the efficacy and safety of atorvastatin in patients with type 2 diabetes on hemodialysis (4D study): demographic and baseline characteristics. *Kidney Blood Press Res*. 2004;27(4):259-66.

[5] Investigators ET, Chertow GM, Block GA, Correa-Rotter R, Drueke TB, Floege J, et al. Effect of cinacalcet on cardiovascular disease in patients undergoing dialysis. *N Engl J Med*. 2012;367(26):2482-94.

[6] Sharp Collaborative G. Study of Heart and Renal Protection (SHARP): randomized trial to assess the effects of lowering low-density lipoprotein cholesterol among 9,438 patients with chronic kidney disease. *Am Heart J*. 2010;160(5):785-94 e10.

[7] Lazzeroni D, Rimoldi O, Camici PG. From Left Ventricular Hypertrophy to Dysfunction and Failure. *Circ J*. 2016;80(3):555-64.

[8] Gersh BJ, Maron BJ, Bonow RO, Dearani JA, Fifer MA, Link MS, et al. 2011 ACCF/AHA guideline for the diagnosis and treatment of hypertrophic cardiomyopathy: executive summary: a report of the American College of Cardiology Foundation/American Heart Association Task Force on Practice Guidelines. *J Am Coll Cardiol*. 2011;58(25):2703-38.

[9] Glassock RJ, Pecoits-Filho R, Barberato SH. Left ventricular mass in chronic kidney disease and ESRD. *Clin J Am Soc Nephrol*. 2009;4 Suppl 1:S79-91.

[10] Paoletti E, Bellino D, Cassottana P, Rolla D, Cannella G. Left ventricular hypertrophy in nondiabetic predialysis CKD. *Am J Kidney* Dis. 2005;46(2):320-7.

[11] Liut F, Izzi C, Dallera N, Scolari F. [ADPKD and Heart]. *G Ital Nefrol*. 2017;34(Suppl 69):119-30.

[12] Wanic-Kossowska M, Posnik B, Kobelski M, Pawliczak E, Pawlaczyk K, Hoppe K, et al. The polymorphism of the ACE gene affects left ventricular hypertrophy and causes

disturbances in left ventricular systolic/diastolic function in patients with autosomal dominant polycystic kidney disease. *Sci World J*. 2014;2014:707658.

[13] Leier CV, Baker PB, Kilman JW, Wooley CF. Cardiovascular abnormalities associated with adult polycystic kidney disease. *Ann Intern Med*. 1984;100(5):683-8.

[14] Ubara Y, Tagami T, Hoshino J, Takaichi K, Takei R. [ADPKD patients on dialysis]. *Nihon Rinsho*. 2004;62 Suppl 6:20-30.

[15] Culleton BF, Walsh M, Klarenbach SW, Mortis G, Scott-Douglas N, Quinn RR, et al. Effect of frequent nocturnal hemodialysis vs conventional hemodialysis on left ventricular mass and quality of life: a randomized controlled trial. *JAMA*. 2007;298(11):1291-9.

[16] Chan CT, Greene T, Chertow GM, Kliger AS, Stokes JB, Beck GJ, et al. Determinants of left ventricular mass in patients on hemodialysis: Frequent Hemodialysis Network (FHN) Trials. *Circ Cardiovasc Imaging*. 2012;5(2):251-61.

[17] Chan CT, Greene T, Chertow GM, Kliger AS, Stokes JB, Beck GJ, et al. Effects of frequent hemodialysis on ventricular volumes and left ventricular remodeling. *Clin J Am Soc Nephrol*. 2013;8(12):2106-16.

[18] Rigatto C, Parfrey P. Therapy insight: management of cardiovascular disease in the renal transplant recipient. *Nat Clin Pract Nephrol*. 2006;2(9):514-26.

[19] Pecoits-Filho R, Calice-Silva V. Unchain the heart: impact of left ventricular myocardial hypertrophy regression in kidney transplant outcomes. *Nephrol Dial Transplant*. 2016;31(7):1025-6.

[20] Parfrey PS, Harnett JD, Foley RN, Kent GM, Murray DC, Barre PE, et al. Impact of renal transplantation on uremic cardiomyopathy. *Transplantation*. 1995;60(9):908-14.

[21] Rigatto C, Foley RN, Kent GM, Guttmann R, Parfrey PS. Long-term changes in left ventricular hypertrophy after renal transplantation. *Transplantation*. 2000;70(4):570-5.

[22] Patel RK, Mark PB, Johnston N, McGregor E, Dargie HJ, Jardine AG. Renal transplantation is not associated with regression of left ventricular hypertrophy: a magnetic resonance study. *Clin J Am Soc Nephrol*. 2008;3(6):1807-11.

[23] Diez J, Laviades C. [Hypertensive heart disease in the patient with chronic kidney disease]. *Nefrologia*. 2008;28(2):135-42.

[24] Lopez B, Gonzalez A, Hermida N, Laviades C, Diez J. Myocardial fibrosis in chronic kidney disease: potential benefits of torasemide. *Kidney Int Suppl*. 2008(111):S19-23.

[25] McCullough PA, Chan CT, Weinhandl ED, Burkart JM, Bakris GL. Intensive Hemodialysis, Left Ventricular Hypertrophy, and Cardiovascular Disease. *Am J Kidney Dis*. 2016;68(5S1):S5-S14.

[26] Barberato SH, Bucharles SG, Barberato MF, Pecoits-Filho R. Association between Clinical and Doppler Echocardiographic Parameters with Sudden Death in Hemodialysis Patients. *Arq Bras Cardiol*. 2016;107(2):124-30.

[27] Badve SV, Palmer SC, Strippoli GFM, Roberts MA, Teixeira-Pinto A, Boudville N, et al. The Validity of Left Ventricular Mass as a Surrogate End Point for All-Cause and Cardiovascular Mortality Outcomes in People With CKD: A Systematic Review and Meta-analysis. *Am J Kidney Dis*. 2016;68(4):554-63.

[28] Cottone S, Nardi E, Mule G, Vadala A, Lorito MC, Riccobene R, et al. Association between biomarkers of inflammation and left ventricular hypertrophy in moderate chronic kidney disease. *Clin Nephrol*. 2007;67(4):209-16.

[29] Ortega O, Gallar P, Munoz M, Rodriguez I, Carreno A, Ortiz M, et al. Association between C-reactive protein levels and N-terminal pro-B-type natriuretic peptide in pre-dialysis patients. *Nephron Clin Pract.* 2004;97(4):c125-30.

[30] Vlahakos DV, Hahalis G, Vassilakos P, Marathias KP, Geroulanos S. Relationship between left ventricular hypertrophy and plasma renin activity in chronic hemodialysis patients. *J Am Soc Nephrol.* 1997;8(11):1764-70.

[31] Sato A, Funder JW, Saruta T. Involvement of aldosterone in left ventricular hypertrophy of patients with end-stage renal failure treated with hemodialysis. *Am J Hypertens.* 1999;12(9 Pt 1):867-73.

[32] Koren MJ, Devereux RB, Casale PN, Savage DD, Laragh JH. Relation of left ventricular mass and geometry to morbidity and mortality in uncomplicated essential hypertension. *Ann Intern Med.* 1991;114(5):345-52.

[33] Levy D, Garrison RJ, Savage DD, Kannel WB, Castelli WP. Prognostic implications of echocardiographically determined left ventricular mass in the Framingham Heart Study. *N Engl J Med.* 1990;322(22):1561-6.

[34] Devereux RB, de Simone G, Ganau A, Roman MJ. Left ventricular hypertrophy and geometric remodeling in hypertension: stimuli, functional consequences and prognostic implications. *J Hypertens Suppl.* 1994;12(10):S117-27.

[35] Cramariuc D, Gerdts E. Epidemiology of left ventricular hypertrophy in hypertension: implications for the clinic. *Expert Rev Cardiovasc Ther.* 2016;14(8):915-26.

[36] Aurigemma GP, Silver KH, Priest MA, Gaasch WH. Geometric changes allow normal ejection fraction despite depressed myocardial shortening in hypertensive left ventricular hypertrophy. *J Am Coll Cardiol.* 1995;26(1):195-202.

[37] Diamond JA, Phillips RA. Hypertensive heart disease. *Hypertens Res.* 2005;28(3):191-202.

[38] Briet M, Barhoumi T, Mian MOR, Coelho SC, Ouerd S, Rautureau Y, et al. Aldosterone-Induced Vascular Remodeling and Endothelial Dysfunction Require Functional Angiotensin Type 1a Receptors. *Hypertension.* 2016;67(5):897-905.

[39] Cacciapuoti F. Molecular mechanisms of left ventricular hypertrophy (LVH) in systemic hypertension (SH)-possible therapeutic perspectives. *J Am Soc Hypertens.* 2011;5(6):449-55.

[40] de Simone G, Izzo R, De Luca N, Gerdts E. Left ventricular geometry in obesity: Is it what we expect? *Nutr Metab Cardiovasc Dis.* 2013;23(10):905-12.

[41] Foley RN, Parfrey PS, Harnett JD, Kent GM, Murray DC, Barre PE. The impact of anemia on cardiomyopathy, morbidity, and and mortality in end-stage renal disease. *Am J Kidney Dis.* 1996;28(1):53-61.

[42] Bucharles S, Barberato SH, Stinghen AE, Gruber B, Meister H, Mehl A, et al. Hypovitaminosis D is associated with systemic inflammation and concentric myocardial geometric pattern in hemodialysis patients with low iPTH levels. *Nephron Clin Pract.* 2011;118(4):c384-91.

[43] Wolf M, Shah A, Gutierrez O, Ankers E, Monroy M, Tamez H, et al. Vitamin D levels and early mortality among incident hemodialysis patients. *Kidney Int.* 2007;72(8):1004-13.

[44] Moe SM, Thadhani R. What have we learned about chronic kidney disease-mineral bone disorder from the EVOLVE and PRIMO trials? *Curr Opin Nephrol Hypertens.* 2013;22(6):651-5.

[45] Pritchett Y, Jemiai Y, Chang Y, Bhan I, Agarwal R, Zoccali C, et al. The use of group sequential, information-based sample size re-estimation in the design of the PRIMO study of chronic kidney disease. *Clin Trials*. 2011,8(2).165-74.

[46] Achinger SG, Ayus JC. The role of vitamin D in left ventricular hypertrophy and cardiac function. *Kidney Int Suppl*. 2005(95):S37-42.

[47] Pecoits-Filho R, Bucharles S, Barberato SH. Diastolic heart failure in dialysis patients: mechanisms, diagnostic approach, and treatment. *Semin. Dial.* 2012;25(1):35-41.

[48] Stubbs J, Liu S, Quarles LD. Role of fibroblast growth factor 23 in phosphate homeostasis and pathogenesis of disordered mineral metabolism in chronic kidney disease. *Semin Dial*. 2007;20(4):302-8.

[49] Gutierrez OM, Mannstadt M, Isakova T, Rauh-Hain JA, Tamez H, Shah A, et al. Fibroblast growth factor 23 and mortality among patients undergoing hemodialysis. *N Engl J Med*. 2008;359(6):584-92.

[50] Kendrick J, Cheung AK, Kaufman JS, Greene T, Roberts WL, Smits G, et al. FGF-23 associates with death, cardiovascular events, and initiation of chronic dialysis. *J Am Soc Nephrol*. 2011;22(10):1913-22.

[51] Sharma S, Joseph J, Chonchol M, Kaufman JS, Cheung AK, Rafeq Z, et al. Higher fibroblast growth factor-23 concentrations associate with left ventricular systolic dysfunction in dialysis patients. *Clin Nephrol*. 2013;80(5):313-21.

[52] Faul C, Amaral AP, Oskouei B, Hu MC, Sloan A, Isakova T, et al. FGF23 induces left ventricular hypertrophy. *J Clin Invest*. 2011;121(11):4393-408.

[53] Perrone-Filardi P, Coca A, Galderisi M, Paolillo S, Alpendurada F, de Simone G, et al. Non-invasive cardiovascular imaging for evaluating subclinical target organ damage in hypertensive patients: A consensus paper from the European Association of Cardiovascular Imaging (EACVI), the European Society of Cardiology Council on Hypertension, and the European Society of Hypertension (ESH). *Eur Heart J Cardiovasc Imaging*. 2017;18(9):945-60.

[54] Marwick TH, Gillebert TC, Aurigemma G, Chirinos J, Derumeaux G, Galderisi M, et al. Recommendations on the Use of Echocardiography in Adult Hypertension: A Report from the European Association of Cardiovascular Imaging (EACVI) and the American Society of Echocardiography (ASE). *J Am Soc Echocardiogr*. 2015;28(7):727-54.

[55] Graham-Brown MP, March DS, Churchward DR, Stensel DJ, Singh A, Arnold R, et al. Novel cardiac nuclear magnetic resonance method for noninvasive assessment of myocardial fibrosis in hemodialysis patients. *Kidney Int*. 2016;90(4):835-44.

[56] Rutherford E, Talle MA, Mangion K, Bell E, Rauhalammi SM, Roditi G, et al. Defining myocardial tissue abnormalities in end-stage renal failure with cardiac magnetic resonance imaging using native T1 mapping. *Kidney Int*. 2016;90(4):845-52.

[57] Woolen SA, Shankar PR, Gagnier JJ, MacEachern MP, Singer L, Davenport MS. Risk of Nephrogenic Systemic Fibrosis in Patients With Stage 4 or 5 Chronic Kidney Disease Receiving a Group II Gadolinium-Based Contrast Agent: A Systematic Review and Meta-analysis. *JAMA Intern Med*. 2020 Feb 1;180(2):223-230.

[58] Barberato SH, Pecoits-Filho R. [Echocardiographic alterations in patients with chronic kidney failure undergoing hemodialysis]. *Arq Bras Cardiol*. 2010;94(1):140-6.

In: Issues in Kidney Disease – Dialysis
Editors: Stephen Z. Fadem and José A. Moura-Neto
ISBN: 978-1-68507-000-7

Chapter 10

BASICS IN HEMODIALYSIS ARTERIOVENOUS FISTULA

Vo Nguyen**, *MD

Memorial Nephrology Associates, Olympia, WA, USA

ABSTRACT

There are three main types of permanent vascular access currently in use for patients undergoing hemodialysis: (1) native arteriovenous fistulas (AVF), (2) polytetrafluoroethylene (PTFE) arteriovenous grafts, and (3) tunneled dialysis catheters. Multiple studies have demonstrated that the fistulas have superior patency rate, lower infectious risks, and require fewer interventions compared to grafts and catheters. A successful AVF program depends greatly on the nephrologist's skills as the leader of a vascular access multidisciplinary team in the early preservation of arm veins, selection of suitable vessels, early referral to AVF surgery, monitoring and management of AVF function, and its potential complications to ensure optimal use of AVF and to reduce the use of arteriovenous grafts and catheters.

Keywords: AV fistula, selection of suitable vessels for AV fistula surgery, pre-op mapping, preservation of arm veins for AV fistula, AV fistula remodeling, AV fistula primary failure, mature AV fistula, AV fistula stenosis, neo-intimal hyperplasia, AV fistula complications

INTRODUCTION

An AVF is created by connecting a native vein to an artery. Compared to an artery, the vein wall is more compliant and has lower resistance to blood flow. Hence, a fistula results in a significant drop in the resistance of the arterio-venous circuit, leading to an immediate rise in blood flow rate, according to a simplified Poiseuille's equation:

* Corresponding Author's E-mail: vdnguyen59@gmail.com.

$$R = \frac{P1\text{-}P2}{Q} \text{ or } Q = \frac{P1\text{-}P2}{R}$$

Q: blood flow rate
P1-P2: difference in blood pressure at the two ends of the tube
R: resistance

The increased blood flow results in flow-mediated vascular remodeling by generating an increase in shear stress on vessel wall. The higher shear stress causes dilation of both artery and vein. This dilation further reduces resistance to flow, and increases flow further, which in turn further raises the shear stress. Corpataux et al. [1] showed that the pre-AVF vein diameter of 2.37 mm increased to 6.62 mm (a 2.8 fold increase in diameter, equivalent to a 7.8 fold increase in the vessel's cross-section) twelve weeks after fistula creation. Flow increased to 750 mL/min. Of note, a mature (usable) AVF requires a minimum venous diameter of 4 mm or greater and flow volume of 500 mL/min or greater [2].

Types of AVF

Arm vessels are preferred for AVF creation, and leg vessels should be a last resort option since leg AVF has many complications. In most situations, distal AVF is preferable to the upper arm one to preserve upper arm veins for future use. Distal forearm radio-ccphalic AVF is typically created at the wrist level, although a snuffbox type is possible if vessels are optimal. Forearm basilic vein is usually better preserved from needle sticks due to its posterior position. Distal fistula using forearm basilic vein and ulnar artery usually requires vein transposition to the volar surface of forearm in a second phase to facilitate its cannulation and prevent uncomfortable arm position during dialysis. Of note, transposition itself is an invasive procedure and may create a swing segment, which can be a source of disturbed blood flow related neointimal hyperplasia and stenosis.

Unfortunately, as the dialysis population has become older with high level of co-morbid factors and poorer blood vessel quality, distal AVF creation has become more challenging with higher rate of primary failure. Upper arm AVF types, including brachio-cephalic AVF and brachio-basilic vein AVF, have become more prevalent. Of note, the basilic vein is located in deep layers near the mid-upper arm level where it joins the deep brachial vein. Thus, it will always require transposition to a more superficial position in a second surgical step, usually two months after initial surgery. Brachio-basilic AVF surgery, including transposition, may also be done in a single step. There is currently a debate on one- versus two-step basilic vein transposition. Doppler mapping will always be required pre-op to ensure that the basilic vein is long enough to allow transposition.

Multi-channel types of AVF can be created using the elbow perforating vein with anastomosis to either the brachial artery [3] or the proximal radial artery [4]. This type of anastomosis has the advantage of the arterialization of several veins in the forearm and the upper arm for dialysis use. Duplex scan is required in these types of AVF to locate elbow perforating vein and its anatomic relation to antecubital veins and brachial or proximal radial artery.

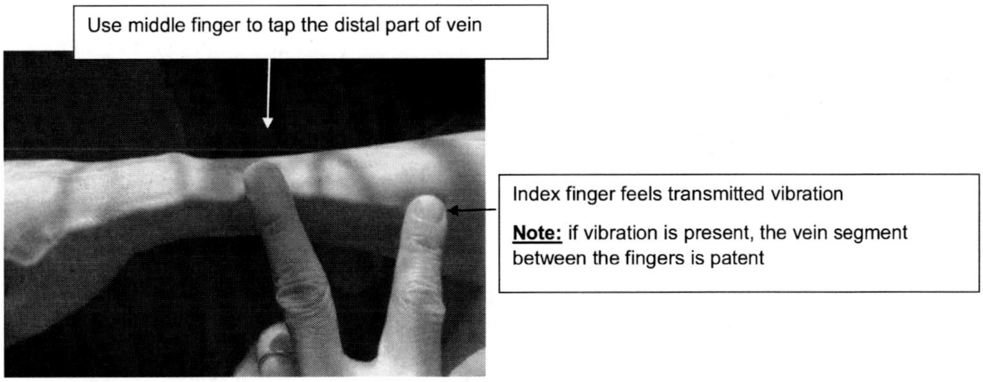

Figure 1. Checking vein patency.

SELECTION OF SUITABLE VESSELS

The selection of suitable vessels should include two parameters: 1) the measurement of the pre-op vessel diameter, and 2) the pre-op determination of the ability of both the artery and the vein to undergo pre-op dilatation, and to increase blood flow rate. These measurements simulate post-op AVF remodeling (arbitrarily defined as vessel function). Silva and coworkers defined two criteria for identifying suitable vessel size: arterial lumen diameter 2.0 mm or more and venous luminal diameter greater than or equal to 2.5 mm [5]. Using microsurgery techniques, groups like Pirozzi, et al. have been successful in creating mature AVF with smaller vessels. They reported the creation of mature AVF among elderly, diabetic, and ischemic patients with much smaller vessels. In their series, the mean distal radial artery and cephalic vein internal diameters, measured with ultrasound, were 1.3 mm and 1.9 mm, respectively [6]. The value of these studies suffers from the small patient size, lack of randomization, and lack of studies of vessel function. Furthermore, success of surgery is highly dependent on the surgeon's skills [7]. Hence, each surgeon in the community should define his/her own concept of adequacy with respect to pre-op vessel size.

Pre-op vessel assessment by physical examination should be done by nephrologists to define vessel suitability for future AVF. Vein patency (Figure 1) and the existence of a valid outflow, diameter, ability of vein dilation with a tourniquet, and wall thickness should be assessed. A thick muscular wall is more desirable.

However, as dialysis population has become older with a high incidence of co-morbid factors including atherosclerosis or obesity, Duplex mapping of arm vessels is now required in all patients. Duplex mapping can also detect anatomic variation in arm vessels [8]. Furthermore, Duplex scanning is the only imaging method that can measure the size, depth, and function of both arteries and veins. Venogram and arteriogram are invasive, usually requiring nephrotoxic dye, and cannot determine depth and function. They are no longer the methods of choice. However, venogram is still indicated in case of potential central vein stenosis.

A detailed discussion of Duplex scan is beyond the scope of this chapter. Nevertheless, nephrologists should be familiar with its salient features and be able to interpret the Duplex report. The readers are referred to the Olympia mapping protocol for more information: http://kidneyregistrylb.com/wp-content/uploads/2012/06/5duplexavf.pdf

A duplex report should include:

A. Vein study:
   1. Size, depth to skin, absence of thrombosis. Deep veins (more than 5 mm) may need transposition.
   2. Function: Can the vein dilate? Veins should dilate by at least 50% with use of tourniquet [9].

The Duplex study should include the integrity of central veins (if their integrity is doubtful, a venogram will be required), the length of upper arm basilic vein, the location of the elbow perforating vein in relation to antecubital veins, and the brachial and proximal radial artery, also important for upper arm AVF surgery planning.

B. Artery study: radial, ulnar, brachial arteries
   1. Size, presence or absence of stenosis or calcification. Of note, artery calcification does not necessarily preclude its use for successful AVF creation [9].
   2. Function: Can the artery dilate by inducing arterial reactive hyperemia?

A reactive hyperemic maneuver is done by having the patient clench the fist for about 60 seconds. This causes metabolic changes, mediated by nitric oxide, leading to arteriolar vasodilatation and lower resistance. Reactive hyperemia is induced with opening of the clenched fist. This maneuver should change a triphasic high resistance flow to a bi-phasic low resistance flow. The same reaction is expected after AVF creation when the peripheral resistance in the artery is suddenly decreased after arteriovenous (AV) anastomosis. A positive reactive hyperemia indicates good arterial function post-AVF placement. Alternatively, resistance index can be measured and should drop below 0.7 [9].

VEIN PRESERVATION

Ideally, vein preservation should start years before patients require dialysis. The nephrologist should educate referring providers to refer chronic kidney disease (CKD) patients at stage 3B (eGFR < 45 ml/min), especially among those with higher risks of progression to stage 5. These patient populations include those with poor compliance, with proteinuria more than 3 gm/day, uncontrolled hypertension requiring multiple medications, poorly controlled diabetes mellitus, unstable renal function, or severe cardio-vascular diseases [10]. Nephrologists should also educate patients to preserve their own veins by not allowing venipuncture on the most suitable arm veins for AVF.

A careful examination of all veins by physical exam will help the nephrologists to decide which veins to preserve:

- If both arms have suitable veins, both arm veins should be preserved and hand dorsal veins should be used for phlebotomy when possible. If hand dorsal veins are not usable, posterior forearm basilic veins should be used.

- If only one arm has suitable veins, that arm should be protected, even if this arm is the dominant one.
- If neither arm has suitable veins, protect the non-dominant arm. Of note, automatic vein preservation in non-dominant arm without a careful assessment is not recommended since veins in that arm may not necessarily be suitable for AVF.

Once the examination is complete, the nephrologist should provide the patient with a note to always be shown to the phlebotomist or IV therapist specifying the arm vein preservation process. In addition, education of hospital medical staff, IV therapists, interventional radiologists, and laboratory personnel about vein preservation will help enhance fistula rates. The nephrologist should help write hospital arm vein preservation protocols which should include the avoidance of subclavian catheters and peripherally inserted peripheral catheters (PICC lines) [11]. Patients that need a central vein catheter should have a small-bore (Fr 4 or 5) internal jugular catheter [12]. Furthermore, pacemaker guidewires that are usually placed through the subclavian vein should not be placed on the side chosen for future AVF. Transradial access should be preferred for angiogram procedures.

Timing of Surgery and Choice of AVF Types

The 2017 United States Renal Data System (USRDS) Annual report indicated that 80% of all new HD patients initiated dialysis with a central venous HD catheter. This high-incident HD catheter use partially reflected the failure of nephrologists to refer CKD patients for AVF surgery in a timely fashion. Timing of AVF surgery is challenging due to several variable and potentially unpredictable factors, including the time required for new AVF to mature, patients' clinical conditions, rate of CKD progression, and estimated time to needing dialysis. Nephrologists experienced in vein mapping by exam are in an ideal position to help guide their surgeon colleagues in making these decisions. For example, healthy young patients in stable CKD stage 3, who have excellent arm vessels allowing maturation of AVF within a few weeks, can be referred in advanced stage 4. Ideally, a distal AVF should be placed in these patients.

In contrast, subgroups of elderly CKD patients with more rapid rate of progression of kidney failure and multiple comorbid factors such as ischemic heart disease are at higher risk of an acute medical problem potentially leading to a sudden irreversible loss of renal function and need for initiation on chronic HD within days. Because of poorer vessel quality, primary failure rate may be higher, especially among distal AVF. Furthermore, AVF maturation may be slower. Therefore, access surgery should optimally be performed during CKD stage 3B or early stage 4. Upper arm AVF may be more frequently chosen in this group of patients if referred at CKD late stage 4 or at stage 5.

Patients with poor vessels should be advised to consider peritoneal dialysis if appropriate. Hence, all CKD patients with potential need of renal replacement therapy should be educated in all the options including home dialysis and transplant. Furthermore, patients who prefer the peritoneal option should consider an AVF placement as a backup in case of peritoneal catheter placement malfunction and avoid the need of hemodialysis catheter.

Selection of Vascular Surgeons

Nephrologists should select surgeons who are skilled, experienced in AVF creation, and willing to cooperate with the vascular access team [7]. The recent development of percutaneous fistula devices [13] may lead to an increased creation of AVF by interventional nephrologists.

Definition of a Usable New AVF

A mature AVF requires a minimum venous diameter of 4 mm or greater and flow volume of 500 mL/min or greater using Duplex scanning (2). However, most HD programs rely on physical examination to determine the timing of first cannulation of a new AVF. Per community standard, the rule of 6 applies; i.e., 6 mm in diameter, 6 cm in length. Vein should be superficial (less than 5 mm deep) to allow ease of cannulation [14], otherwise transposition closer to the surface will be required.

Adequacy of blood flow should be assessed by pulse augmentation test, which is performed by occluding the vein 4 cm above the anastomosis and by feeling the strength of the pulse created which is dependent on systolic arterial inflow.

Vein wall should be thick enough to prevent profuse bleeding at cannulation site [15]. Vein wall gets thicker after AVF surgery from medial hypertrophy, which is related to increased hoop stress during post-op vessel remodeling. This is a more gradual process than vein dilatation associated with increased shear stress. Therefore, timing of first cannulation should not be based solely on vein diameter or a fixed temporal factor, conventionally defined as 6 weeks, because it may take days, weeks, or even months, depending on the pre-op quality of the venous wall and the level of hoop stress. In practice, it may be best to rely on an experienced dialysis nurse or patient care technician to determine the maturation of a new AVF. Cannulation of new AVF should always be done by the most skilled dialysis staff, using small gauge needles. Buttonhole cannulation technique may be helpful in new AVF.

Primary Failure of AVF

Primary failure of AVF is defined as failure to mature within three months after its creation. Nephrologists should check AVF progress within two weeks post-op. Persistent poor flow and/or small size within four to six weeks may indicate the need for an early intervention [16]. A poorly constructed AVF will not improve over time without intervention.

Primary AVF failure is related to vein stenosis due to neointimal hyperplasia. After the fistula is created, vessel resistance drops, leading to increased blood flow. High flow in vulnerable areas of veins may result in disturbed flow. This turbulence leads to oscillatory shear stress forces that promote endothelial proliferation, apoptosis, vasocontriction, coagulation, platelet aggregation and ultimately neointimal hyperplasia.

The areas of disturbed flow tend to be in the supra-anastomotic area where the vein is connected to the artery at a non physiological angle [17]. Furthermore, at the wrist level, the anatomic position of cephalic vein in relation to radial artery tends to predispose to high rate of vein torsion during fistula placement, further increasing the risk of disturbed flow. These factors may account for a higher rate of inflow vein stenoses in the first 3-4 cm vein segment immediately above the anastomosis (distal swing segment) among distal radio-cephalic AVF. The piggyback straight line onlay technique (pSLOT) reduces the risk of torsion induced disturbed flow and the incidence of primary failure in distal AVF [18]. In upper arm fistulas, stenoses is more common in the upper venous outflow segment [19] partly due to the angle of transposition in a transposed brachial-basilic AV fistula.

Poor arterial inflow can be assessed by the pulse augmentation test (see section on definition of a usable new AVF). The presence of a venous outflow stenosis is indicated by vein pulsation below the stenosis and reduction of vein size and thrill above the stenosis.

Most stenosis in venous and arterial sides of AVF circuit will improve with percutaneous angioplasty. Supra-anastomotic stenosis in distal radio-cephalic AVF may also be revised surgically by placing a new anastomosis just above the stenosis.

Prevention of Primary Failure

Risk of AVF failure may be reduced by pre-op selection of suitable vessels by Duplex mapping [5]. Furthermore, suitable arm veins should be protected from injury by catheters years before the AVF is needed. Referral for surgery in earlier stages of CKD is important since neointimal hyperplasia and calcification have been documented in medium-sized arteries in adult patients with advanced CKD during AVF surgery [20]. Finally, the skills and experiences of surgeons may play an important part in AVF creation success [7].

Conversion of Graft into Secondary AVF

Pre-existing forearm grafts lead to the arterialization and dilatation of outflow veins in ipsilateral upper arm (Figure 2). One study showed that cephalic vein diameter averaged 6.4 mm (ranging 4-10 mm) and basilic vein diameter averaged 9.1 mm (6-14 mm) in the presence of forearm AV grafts [21]. The vein arterialization greatly facilitates the successful creation of secondary AV fistulas [22], since the required mature AVF diameter is only 4 mm [2].

Complications of AVF

Steal Syndrome

AVF creation in elderly patients with high co-morbid factors and atherosclerotic vascular disease can cause a reduction of blood flow to the distal extremity resulting from increased blood flow through the AV fistula. The risk of steal syndrome can be reduced by pre-op Duplex ultrasound detection of arterial disease and by privileging distal or proximal radial artery which may limit and prevent excessive blood flow rate [4]. If brachial artery is used in at-risk patients, the size of the arteriotomy should be kept at 4 to 6 mm, and continuous suture be used [23].

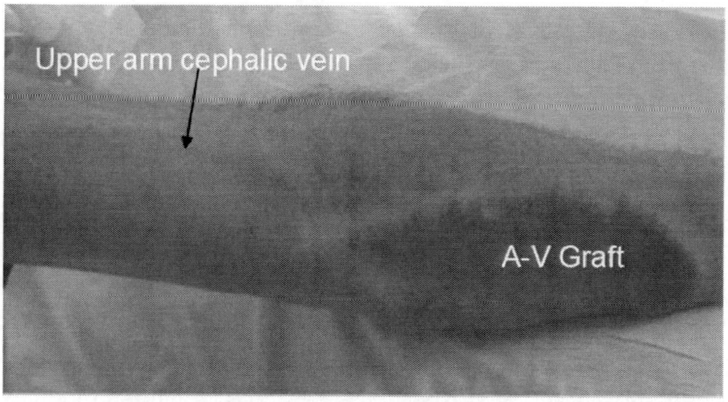

Figure 2. Arterialization of upper arm cephalic vein (diameter 8 mm) by forearm AV graft.

Steal syndrome presents with hand numbness, pain, or coolness associated with the reduction in sensation and/or motor function; digit cyanosis, discoloration, ulceration or necrosis; and reduced or absent pulses. Patient with steal symptoms should be promptly referred to the surgery service. Its presence can be confirmed using noninvasive vascular testing: digital photoplethysmography tracings and pressure measurements with and without fistula compression or Duplex sonography. Patients with only minor problems of cold hand and minor paresthesia should be closely monitored and encouraged to use gloves to keep their hands warm. In case of inflow arterial atherosclerosis, percutaneous angioplasty may be indicated. The surgical management depends on the AVF blood flow rate. High-flow AV access (>1500 mL/min) may need flow reduction by banding. Revascularization surgery may be indicated for a lower flow AVF (≤1500 mL/min) [24, 25]. If ischemia is severe and revascularization is not possible, the AVF will need ligation.

High Cardiac Output Heart Failure

AVF creation leads to reduction in vascular resistance and an augmentation in cardiac output. The increase in cardiac output is usually clinically insignificant and rarely causes high output congestive heart failure. Risk factors include patients with pre-existing severe heart disease and upper-arm AVF due to higher blood flow [26]. Management consists of excluding other etiologies of heart failure; reduction of volume excess through salt restriction, dialysis, or diuretics; correction of anemia; better control of hypertension; and the use of cardiac medication as indicated. If these measures fail, surgical reduction of AVF blood flow may be necessary [25].

Aneurysms of AVF

Aneurysms of the AVF, defined as an enlargement of the vein three times the diameter of the nearby normal arterialized vein, may be caused by high blood flow or venous outflow stenosis. Both conditions can cause higher intra-access pressure and vein dilatation. Pseudoaneurysm of AVF (a collection of blood outside the vessel wall contained by fibrous tissue) is usually caused by repeated cannulations at the same area. Complications of aneurysms and pseudoaneurysms include erosion of the overlying skin with rupture, catastrophic bleeding, and the loss of suitable vein area available for cannulation. Cannulation through a pseudoaneurysm must be avoided. Pseudoaneurysms can be prevented by proper rope ladder cannulation or buttonhole techniques. Surgical revision is required in case of rapid expansion in size with thinning of the aneurysm wall. However, an aneurysm presenting with skin necrosis, often associated with a blister filled with bloody fluid, is a true emergency, potentially associated with lethal rupture and bleeding (Figure 3). In this case, patient should be sent to the hospital by ambulance and immediate surgical repair be done. If venous outflow stenosis is present with high intra-access pressure, early percutaneous angioplasty may help to reduce the rate of progression of aneurysm.

AVF Related Infection

AVF related infection may be local, causing cellulitis or an abscess surrounding cannulation sites. AVF may also be a common source of bacteremia in dialysis patients, which frequently occurs during cannulation without a local AVF infection. Faulty cannulation technique is the usual cause of AVF related infection. The Buttonhole technique may also have higher risk of infection than the rope ladder method [27]. *Staphylococcus aureus* and *Staphylococcus epidermidis* are the predominant pathogens. The 2006 National Kidney Foundation (NKF)/Dialysis Outcomes Quality Initiative (K/DOQI) guidelines recommends intravenous antibiotics for 6 weeks for AVF-related bacteremia. Local infection with abscess should be surgically drained and the infected vein should be excised partially or totally as indicated.

AVF Failure

Most mature AVF will develop neointimal hyperplasia induced stenosis over time. Neointimal hyperplasia may be due to disturbed flow as discussed in primary failure of AVF section, or trauma from repeated vein cannulation. Although the thrombosis rate associated with stenosis induced reduction in blood flow rate is much lower in AVF compared with AV graft, it is still important to diagnose stenosis and intervene in a timely fashion. There are two methods for detecting AVF stenosis.

Clinical monitoring consists of physical examination of AVF and monitoring for problems with dialysis such as drop in dialysis clearance (Kt/V), prolonged bleeding, inability to cannulate, etc. The *National Kidney Foundation Kidney Disease Outcomes Quality Initiative (KDOQI) Clinical Practice Guideline for Vascular Access: 2019 Update* recommends that a physical assessment of the hemodialysis patient be done weekly.

Surveillance uses measurement of intra-access flow, duplex scan to evaluate intra-access flow, or by measuring static dialysis venous pressure. However, the effectiveness of clinical monitoring and surveillance for AVF remains in question [28]. Since the thrombosis rate is much lower in AV fistulas compared with AV grafts, it is more challenging for research investigators to show an improvement in the thrombosis or patency rates by early diagnosis of stenosis and preemptive intervention. Furthermore, percutaneous angioplasty potentially causes injury to vessel intima, leading to an increase in cellular proliferation, accelerated neointimal hyperplasia and more rapidly recurrent stenosis [29]. Hence, angioplasty of a non-clinically significant or stable stenosis may be potentially harmful and may negate the benefit of early detection of AVF stenosis by surveillance and interventions.

CONCLUSION

A successful AVF program depends greatly on the nephrologist's skills as a vascular access multidisciplinary team leader in the early preservation of arm veins, selection of suitable vessels, early referral to AVF surgery, monitoring and management of AVF primary and secondary function, and the rapid identification of its potential complications. Lower AVF use in the USA as compared to other developed countries is mostly related to differences in providers' practice [29]. Interventions within programs with low AVF rates helped improve their clinical outcomes by educating providers and by promoting the vascular access multidisciplinary team model [30]. These best vascular access practices may have helped many dialysis centers in the Pacific Northwest achieve 80-100% AV Fistula rates [31].

ACKNOWLEDGMENTS

The author wishes to thank Dr. Nicola Pirozzi, Interventional Nephrology Unit CdC Nuova ITOR, Rome, and Dr. Mai Lin Nguyen, my daughter for their helpful suggestions and editorial assistance.

REFERENCES

[1] Corpataux JM, Haesler E, Silacci P, et al. Low-pressure environment and remodelling of the forearm vein in Brescia-Cimino haemodialysis access. *Nephrol Dial Transplant*. 2002;17:1057-62.

[2] Robbin ML, Chamberlain NE, Lockhart ME, et al. Hemodialysis arteriovenous fistula maturity: US evaluation. *Radiology*. 2002;225(1):59-64.

[3] Bender MH, Bruyninckx CM, Gerlag PG. The Gracz arteriovenous fistula evaluated: results of the brachiocephalic elbowfistula in haemo-dialysis angio-access. *Eur J Vasc Endovasc Surg*. 1995;10:294-7.

[4] Bruns, S, Jennings, W. Proximal radial artery as inflow site for native arteriovenous fistula. *J Am Coll Surg*. 2003; 197(1): 58-63.

[5] Silva MB Jr, Hobson RW 2nd, Pappas PJ, et al. A strategy for increasing use of autogenous hemodialysis access procedures: impact of preoperative noninvasive evaluation. *J Vasc Surg*. 1998;27(2):302-308.

[6] Pirozzi N, Apponi F, Napoletano AM, Luciani R, Pirozzi V, Pugliese F. Microsurgery and preventive haemostasis for autogenous radial-cephalic direct wrist access in adult patients with radial artery internal diameter below 1.6 mm. *Nephrol Dial Transplant*. 2010;25(2):520-525.

[7] Huber TS. Surgeon Characteristics and Arteriovenous Fistula Maturation Success. *Am J Kidney Dis*. 2020;75(2):151-152.

[8] Kusztal M, Weyde W, Letachowicz K, Gołebiowski T, Letachowicz W. Anatomical vascular variations and practical implications for access creation on the upper limb. *J Vasc Access*. 2014;15 Suppl. 7:S70-S75.

[9] Malovrh M. Native Arteriovenous Fistulas for Hemodialysis: preoperative evaluation. *Am J Kidney Dis. 2002;* 39(6):1218-25.

[10] Ishani A, Grandits GA, Grimm RH et al. Association of single measurements of dipstick proteinuria, estimated glomerular filtration rate, and hematocrit with 25-year incidence of end-stage renal disease in the multiple risk factor intervention trial. *J Am Soc Nephrol*. 2006;17:1444-1452.

[11] Allen AW, Megargell JL, Brown DB, et al. Venous thrombosis associated with the placement of peripherally inserted central catheters. *J Vasc Interv Radiol*. 2000;11(10):1309-1314. doi: 10.1016/s1051-0443(07)61307-4.

[12] Sasadeusz KJ, Trerotola SO, Shah H, et al. Tunneled jugular small-bore central catheters as an alternative to peripherally inserted central catheters for intermediate-term venous access in patients with hemodialysis and chronic renal insufficiency. *Radiology*. 1999; 213(1):303-306.

[13] Wasse H. Place of Percutaneous Fistula Devices in Contemporary Management of Vascular Access. *Clin J Am Soc Nephrol*. 2019;14(6):938-940.

[14] Inkollu S, Wellen J, Beller Z, Zhang T, Vachharajani N, Shenoy S. Successful use of minimal incision superficialization technique for arteriovenous fistula maturation. *J Vasc Surg*. 2016;63(4):1018-1025.

[15] Donnelly SM, Marticorena RM. When is a new fistula mature? The emerging science of fistula cannulation. *Semin Nephrol*. 2012;32(6):564-571.

[16] Ferring M, Henderson J, Wilmink T. Accuracy of early postoperative clinical and ultrasound examination of arteriovenous fistulae to predict dialysis use. *J Vasc Access*. 2014; 15:291.

[17] Ene-Iordache B, Remuzzi A. Disturbed flow in radial-cephalic arteriovenous fistulae for haemodialysis: low and oscillating shear stress locates the sites of stenosis. *Nephrol Dial Transplant*. 2012;27(1):358-368.

[18] Bharat A, Jaenicke M, Shenoy S. A novel technique of vascular anastomosis to prevent juxtaanastomotic stenosis following arteriovenous fistula creation. *J Vasc Surg*. 2012; 55:274.

[19] Turmel-Rodrigues L, Pengloan J, Baudin S, et al. Treatment of stenosis and thrombosis in haemodialysis fistulas and grafts by interventional radiology. *Nephrol Dial. Transplant*. 2000;15(12):2029-2036.

[20] Chitalia N, Ross L, Krishnamoorthy M, et al. Neointimal hyperplasia and calcification in medium sized arteries in adult patients with chronic kidney disease. *Semin Dial*. 2015;28(3):E35-E40.

[21] Ash S, Beathard GA. American Society of Diagnostic and Interventional Nephrology: Interventionalist's Role in Identifying Candidates for Secondary Fistulas. *Semin Dial*. 2004;17 (3): 233-236.

[22] Nguyen VD, Treat L, Griffith C, Robinson K. Creation of secondary AV fistulas from failed hemodialysis grafts: the role of routine vein mapping. *J Vasc Access*. 2007;8(2):91-96.

[23] Sidawy AN, et al. The Society for Vascular Surgery: clinical practice guidelines for the surgical placement and maintenance of arteriovenous hemodialysis access. *J Vasc Surg*. 2008;48(5 Suppl):2S.

[24] Zanow J, et al. Diagnosis and differentiated treatment of ischemia in patients with arteriovenous vascular access. In: *Vascular Access for Hemodialysis VII*, Henry ML (Ed), Gore, Chicago 2001. p. 201.

[25] Maresca B, et al. Early echocardiographic modifications after flow reduction by proximal radial artery ligation in patients with high-output heart failure due to high-flow forearm arteriovenous fistula. *J Vasc Access*. 2020 Sep;21(5):753-759.

[26] Basile C, Lomonte C, Vernaglione L, Casucci F, Antonelli M, Losurdo N. The relationship between the flow of arteriovenous fistula and cardiac output in haemodialysis patients. *Nephrol Dial Transplant*. 2008;23(1):282-287.

[27] Wong B, Muneer M, Wiebe N, et al. Buttonhole versus rope-ladder cannulation of arteriovenous fistulas for hemodialysis: a systematic review. *Am J Kidney Dis*. 2014; 64:918.

[28] Ken Abreo et al. Is there a need to mandate access surveillance in the dialysis clinic? *Nephrol News Issues*. 2010;17 (7): 30-32.

[29] Chang CJ, Ko PJ, Hsu LA, et al. Highly increased cell proliferation activity in the restenotic hemodialysis vascular access after percutaneous transluminal angioplasty: implication in prevention of restenosis. *Am J Kidney Dis*. 2004;43:74-84.

[30] Nguyen VD, Lawson L, Ledeen M, et al. Successful multidisciplinary interventions for arterio-venous fistula creation by the Pacific Northwest Renal Network 16 vascular access quality improvement program. *J Vasc Access*. 2007;8(1):3-11.

[31] Nguyen V, Ball LK. Exceeding KDOQI AV Fistula Target at Northwest Renal Network 16. Is 80-90% AV Fistula rate achievable? *Semin Dial*. 2014;27 (6): E66-E70.

In: Issues in Kidney Disease – Dialysis
Editors: Stephen Z. Fadem and José A. Moura-Neto
ISBN: 978-1-68507-000-7

Chapter 11

INTENSIVE HEMODIALYSIS

Athanasios Roumeliotis[1], MD, PhD,
Stefanos Roumeliotis[1], MD, PhD and Andreas Pierratos[2,*], MD
[1]Division of Nephrology and Hypertension, 1st Department of Internal Medicine, AHEPA Hospital, Aristotle University of Thessaloniki, Thessaloniki, Greece
[2]Humber River Hospital, University of Toronto, Toronto, Canada

ABSTRACT

The need to improve outcomes of renal replacement therapy, decrease the cost and increase the utilization of home dialysis has led to a growing interest in 'intensive hemodialysis'. It includes long and/or more frequent dialysis done both in-center and especially at home. There is growing evidence in the literature, from both cohort as well as randomized controlled trials, that intensive hemodialysis improves cardiovascular outcomes, blood pressure control, solute removal, quality of life and possibly patient survival. Despite the advantages of home intensive hemodialysis, the utilization of home hemodialysis remains low. New home-friendly dialysis machines, financial incentives and political will, may hopefully increase the utilization of home hemodialysis, as mandated by the Advancing American Kidney Health Initiative in the US, which has set as a goal an incident rate of kidney transplantation and home dialysis of 80% by the year 2025.

Keywords: intensive hemodialysis, nocturnal hemodialysis, home hemodialysis, long and frequent hemodialysis, hemodialysis, daily hemodialysis, end-stage renal disease, end-stage kidney disease

INTRODUCTION

End-stage renal disease (ESRD) is a global epidemic with an increasing number of patients on renal replacement therapy dialyzed mostly in-center for 3-4 hours thrice weekly. There were 746,557 prevalent patients with ESRD in the US at the end of 2017, of which 124,500 were

* Corresponding Author's E-mail: a.pierratos@utoronto.ca.

new cases, translating to a crude incidence rate of 370.2/million/year [1]. Despite some recent improvements in patient outcomes, data from the United Stated Renal Data System (USRDS) show that patient mortality and hospitalization rates are still unacceptably high [2].

Home hemodialysis, when developed in the 1960s, was used by 32% of the patients in the US. Less than 15% of patients on dialysis were on home hemodialysis by 1978, falling to less than 5% by 1980 and to 1.9% in 2018. The changes may be related to the enactment of the Medicare entitlement act of 1972, the advent of peritoneal dialysis in the late 70s and misalignment of financial incentives [3]. There has been a recent increase in incident home HD in the US, but despite an increase by 120.8% since 2007, its overall use was only 0.4% of all incident ESRD patients receiving dialysis in 2018. Total utilization of either HHD or PD among incident dialysis patients reached its highest level since 1997. In the prevalent patient population, total utilization of either HHD or PD was 11.9% in 2017, also its highest level since 1997. By the end of 2017, there were more than 62,000 patients dialyzing at home in the United States.

Utilization of home HD is low in most other countries except those with strong HHD culture as New Zealand and Australia (14% and 8% respectively), while Canada and Europe have higher HHD rates than the US [3].

To improve poor dialysis outcomes and lighten the financial impact, several avenues have been pursued involving changes in the dialysis dose and schedules, support for home-based regimens, improvements in technology, focus on treatment of comorbidities, and change in public policy including financial incentives.

Dialysis Dose

The National Cooperative Dialysis Study (NCDS) introduced Kt/V_{urea} as the measure of the small molecule clearance, and the lowest adequate dose was later established at 1.2 by DOQI [4]. It found no beneficial effect of longer dialysis ($p = 0.06$) [5]. The Hemodialysis study (HEMO) [6] failed to show improvement in patient survival with increasing dialysis dose (Kt/V 1.4), while on the same regimen.

Dialysis Schedules

High patient survival rates and good blood pressure control on 8-hour hemodialysis thrice weekly were reported from Tassin, France, giving credence to the benefit of long dialysis [7]. Improved outcomes were reported on short daily hemodialysis mainly from Italy [8] and Daily Nocturnal Hemodialysis from Toronto, Canada [9]. These experiences rekindled interest in long and more frequent dialysis schedules [10]. Improved outcomes were published in observational studies and later on, in randomized control trials (RCTs) [11-13].

Technological Changes

These led to improvements in, for example, hemodialysis machines, membranes, and dialysate composition. More recently, machines were specifically made or were adapted for home dialysis use [14].

Treatment Location

This includes the hospital setting, freestanding units or at home. Support for home dialysis has grown for both clinical and financial reasons [15]. Different strategies have been used to promote home modalities. Among others, they include financial incentives for patients, physicians and dialysis providers. Other approaches include the 'PD first' or 'Home Dialysis First' policies [16, 17].

Dialysis Delivery

It is provided as full care in a dialysis unit by nurses and technicians, self-care or assisted-care at home by patients, by unpaid or paid helpers [18].

Focus on Comorbidities or Patient-Reported Outcome Measures

Among others, they include cardiovascular disease, diabetes and metabolic bone disease. Research has shifted towards patient-reported outcome measures [19, 20].

Public Policy/Financial Incentives

In the US, the Expanded ESRD Prospective Payment System (PPS) bundled injectable medications in the dialysis fee and added payments for home dialysis training [21, 22]. More recently there has been organized institutional support for home dialysis and dialysis-related innovations through the Advancing American Kidney Health Initiative [15].

In this review, we will examine the dialysis regimens lumped under the collective name of 'intensive hemodialysis' including more frequent HD and/or session duration within the wider perspective of home HD.

TECHNICAL ASPECTS

Several hemodialysis machines have been modified or designed *de novo* for daily or/and home HD. Fresenius 2008K@home, NxStage System One and One S and Tablo (Outset) [23] have been approved for home use in the US. Other machines are in development or in use in other countries [14].

Dialysate is produced via a reverse osmosis process or the use of a deionizer. Water softener treatment prior to the water purification system may occasionally be needed.

The NxStage System One, used by the majority of the patients in the U.S., uses Pureflow® SL to produce 40, 50 or 60L lactate-based dialysate to be used within 72 hours. It can last for up to 1-3 dialysis sessions depending on the prescription. Dialysate flow is adjusted so that the prescribed volume lasts for the prescribed duration, being as low as 63 for longer to up to 200 (300 for the One S model) ml/min for shorter sessions. Pre-made dialysate in 5L bags is available, mainly for traveling purposes. NxStage provides a dialysis dose prescription formula, available online: https://dosingcalculator.nxstage.com/ DosingCalculator/, for the desired weekly dialysis dose (stdKt/V).

Other optional features include telemonitoring [24, 25], smartphone applications, interactive videoconferencing, real-time data transmission, electronic health record patient portals, remote monitoring, leak sensors and on-line electrolyte measurements [26-35]. None of these is essential for the treatment. Dialyzer reuse, although initially practiced, has been abandoned due to decreasing dialyzer cost [36].

HD Prescription

Daily (quotidian) HD is provided 5-7 times a week, usually for 2-4 hours, in the dialysis facility or at home. A longer regimen is encouraged (e.g., >3 hours) as it is associated with better phosphate control [37].

High Dialysate Volume Approach

When using conventional machines or those modified for home use, dialysate composition is similar to thrice-weekly HD (600-800 ml/L). Blood and dialysate flow are kept at their highest to achieve the best clearances.

Low Dialysate Volume Approach

The NxStage System One uses low dialysate flow and total volume to contain cost [38, 39].

Low dialysate flow rate leads to higher dialysate solute saturation leading to more efficient use of dialysate. Blood flow is kept to the maximum possible. Flow fraction (FF), ratio of dialysate to blood flow, is an indirect measure of the dialysate urea saturation. An FF of 40% correlates to a 90% dialysate urea saturation. The total dialysate volume needed can be calculated from the desired daily Kt/V (typical 0.6) and the FF (typical 40%). If the blood flow changes during dialysis, and the FF is kept stable, the dialysate flow can be changed by the machine in parallel and dialysis duration be adjusted to achieve the desired Kt/V. If the desired Kt/V is not achievable, the FF can be increased (slower dialysate flow, same volume, higher saturation, longer dialysis) or dialysate volume can be increased (usually along with longer dialysis), with negative financial implications.

Nocturnal HD (NHD) is performed overnight, for 6-8 h per session, 3-7 days per week. Intermittent nocturnal HD is performed thrice weekly or on an alternate day schedule (3.5 weekly sessions) and daily nocturnal HD is usually performed 6 nights a week [12, 40, 41]. The intermittent nocturnal regimen takes place in a dialysis unit or at home, while daily nocturnal HD is done at home. The patient or a helper can perform both regimens, when at home, while the dialysis unit staff usually delivers the facility-based intermittent HD.

High Dialysate Volume Approach

The prescription for long HD includes low blood flow of 200-300 ml/min for adults and 100 ml/min for children and a dialysate flow of <100 to more than 500, usually 300 ml/min. Dialysate bicarbonate concentration on nocturnal HD is usually about 30 mEq/L for the daily and 35 mEq/L for the intermittent form. Calcium concentration is usually set at 2.5 to 3 mEq/L (1.25-1.5 mmol/L) [39]. If higher dialysate calcium is required (e.g., high alkaline phosphatase, post parathyroidectomy, pregnancy), calcium chloride powder can be added into the acid concentrate (7 ml of powder added to a ~4.5 L jug of acid concentrate raises the dialysate calcium by about 0.5 mEq/L or 0.25 mmol/L). To avoid negative calcium balance, post dialysis serum calcium should be maintained higher than predialysis calcium, unless the patient is on calcium-based phosphate binders. There is an improvement in phosphate control on intensive HD [41-43]. Daily nocturnal HD can even lead to hypophosphatemia even off phosphate binders. Sodium phosphate can be added into the acid or bicarbonate concentrate: 30-135mL of Fleet Enema® (sodium phosphate) per 4.5 L of dialysate, leads to a dialysate phosphate concentration of 1-3mg/dL (0.3-0.9mmoL/L) [41-43].

Low Dialysate Volume Approach

Dialysate flow using the NxStage HD machine is lower (63-130 ml/min) so that the prescribed volume (usually 30 or 60 L) lasts for the total length of dialysis. The NxStage system provides base in the form of lactate at 40 or 45 mmol/L dialysate calcium and is set at 3 mEq/L (1.5 mmol/L). No dialysate additives can be used in the NxStage system. Detailed prescription details are reviewed elsewhere [44].

Not enough data exists on dialyzer choice, but it is reasonable to suggest high flux dialyzers for intensive HD.

Anticoagulation

Anticoagulation includes unfractionated or low molecular weight heparin (LMWH) [45]. In the case of heparin-induced thrombocytopenia, either danaparoid or argatroban can be used [46]. The NxStage system does not have a pump so LMWH or an external pump for heparin can be used. Lack of blood air interface decreases the need for anticoagulation.

Dialysis Access

Permanent central venous catheters, AV fistulas, and grafts can be used for all forms of intensive HD, in-center or at home. Daily HD in the FHN study was associated with increased risk of vascular complications [47]. Closed connector devices (InterLink®, Tego™ needle-free catheter caps) are recommended during dialysis while asleep for prevention of air emboli and arterial limb bleeding if disconnection accidentally occurs [48]. Lower rates of catheter-related bloodstream infection have been also reported in patients who used these devices but adequate studies are missing [49].

The buttonhole technique for fistula [50], but not graft cannulation can be used for daily or nocturnal HD when a single operator (patient or helper) is involved, but not for in-center HD where it has been associated with a higher complication rate [51]. The buttonhole technique either at home or in-center has been associated with a significantly higher rate of bacteremia, which can be mostly prevented through the application of mupirocin cream on the puncture site after the completion of dialysis [48, 52, 53]. Careful adherence to the antiseptic technique is crucial. For the 'buttonhole' to be established, regular sharp needles are needed for the first week to form the cannulation canal. Theoretical buttonhole advantages include less pain, greater ease of cannulation, faster hemostasis and decreased risk for aneurysm creation, but have not been proven in large randomized control trials [48, 54-56]. A 'single needle system' is encouraged for NHD as it decreases the risk and complications of an accidental dislodgement (air alarm is triggered), while solute clearance is largely unaffected in view of the long duration of dialysis. Furthermore, it is associated with a smaller number of cannulations. Secure fastening of the dialysis needle for nocturnal HD is critical, as is the use of moisture sensors (easily available enuresis alarms or commercially available devices) [32, 34] on the puncture site and on the floor for blood or dialysate leaks. Significant attention should be given to safety issues during training for nocturnal HD [57, 58].

Solute Clearance

Small Molecule Removal-Urea

Weekly stdKt/V has been largely adopted as a measure of dialysis dose adequacy especially for frequent HD as well as for peritoneal dialysis despite lack of credible data. It uses the mid-week pre-dialysis rather than the time average concentration (TAC) of BUN for the calculation, and therefore it favors frequent dialysis. A stdKt/V of 2.3 per week and a minimum stdKt/V of 2.1 represent the current Kidney Disease Outcomes Quality Initiative (KDOQI) recommended dose guidelines for alternative dialysis schedules [59]. A weekly stdKt/V of 2.3 would be equivalent to daily equilibrated Kt/V of 0.38 for 6 sessions per week. Although the dialysate volume and flow prescribed for the NxStage system is usually lower, the weekly stdKt/V can usually be maintained above 2.1. Longer sessions (e.g., 3-8 hours daily) at a lower flow rate allow for higher dialysate solute saturation and are preferable [39]. Daily nocturnal HD, six times per week, using a conventional machine provides a stdKt/V at 4-6 [60]. We support achieving a stdKt/V of more than the recommended 2.3 per week for intensive HD, hoping for better outcomes than are associated with the current dialysis guidelines.

Middle Molecule Removal

Both middle and large molecule removal by HD is time dependent and possibly correlate with better clinical outcomes [61-63]. A four-fold increase in weekly dialysis time (daily nocturnal HD) leads to a four-fold increase in beta$_2$-microglobulin removal, leading to lower serum beta$_2$-microglobulin levels [64]. Other molecules such as advanced glycated products [65], indole-3-acetic and acid indoxyl sulfate [66] may be more efficiently removed through daily HD although data from the FHN trial did not confirm significant decrease in p-cresol sulfate or indoxyl sulfate levels on frequent dialysis [67]. Dialysis duration of more than 12 hours per week is advised even if the minimum stdKt/V is achieved in shorter time. Despite the lower dialysate flow, it is expected that nocturnal HD using the NxStage system is equally efficacious in removing middle molecules [68, 69].

Phosphate Removal

Vascular calcification (VC), cardiovascular disease (CVD), and renal osteodystrophy, significant risk factors contributing to patient mortality, are all closely correlated to phosphate levels in HD patients [70]. Phosphate is efficiently removed by dialysis. Slow phosphate movement between body compartments results in low plasma phosphate during HD and is the limiting factor in controlling hyperphosphatemia [71]. The effect of dialysis on phosphate removal is closely dependent on HD session length, as long as dialysis allows time for the intercompartmental movement of phosphate to take place.

Original cohort studies [72], the FHN [73], and the Alberta trials [11] showed an improvement in phosphate control in both daily and nocturnal regimens leading to decreasing dose or discontinuation of phosphate binders in the NHD group. Phosphate addition into the dialysate was needed to prevent hypophosphatemia in 75% of the patients [32, 72, 74]. Short daily HD has a modest effect on phosphate control, but it improved further when dialysis time was increased to 3 hours daily [37, 73]. As phosphate removal is time dependent, the NxStage system is similarly effective during long dialysis.

Patient Selection for an Intensive Dialysis Schedule

Patient education and preparation, starting dialysis, modality and resource availability, and local culture are variable in different countries. A KDIGO conference addressed some of these issues [75].

If available, the majority of the patients would benefit from daily/long HD. Indications are both medical and psychosocial. Cardiovascular instability, cardiomyopathy, uremic symptoms, uncontrolled hypertension, sleep apnea, intra- and inter-dialytic symptoms, persistent overhydration, ascites, and malnutrition have all improved with intensive HD, especially in large patients [76-78]. In these cases, transfer to either short daily HD or nocturnal HD in the dialysis unit or at home should be considered. Hemodynamic instability or low intradialytic blood pressure related to cardiomyopathy represent indications rather than contraindications to home nocturnal HD [77].

Psychosocial indications include the desire of patients to improve their quality of life and promote physical and vocational rehabilitation. Patients who are not eligible for transplantation, want to work [79], or live away from dialysis units and have difficulty adjusting to an in-center HD program. Those who need to transfer from CAPD to HD should be encouraged to choose home HD [80] as data may indicate better outcomes than transferring to in-center HD [81]. Caregiver or paid helper training should also be considered [18].

Patients who would benefit but cannot be on home HD should consider daily HD or nocturnal NHD at the dialysis center if available.

Contraindications for home hemodialysis include patient inability or lack of motivation to be trained, poor insight, unstable behavioral issues, untreated psychosis, inappropriate housing and if alone at home, communication difficulties [82], brittle diabetes prone to hypoglycemia and uncontrolled seizure disorder. A good alternative for these cases is the presence of a caregiver trained to perform dialysis. Dialysis at home without a partner present has been allowed by most centers in hemodynamically stable patients on frequent or nocturnal HD, but not while on conventional HD thrice weekly.

TRAINING FOR AN INTENSIVE HOME DIALYSIS SCHEDULE

A comprehensive evaluation of a patient-candidate for home HD and early education commencement remains the cornerstone for intensive regimens [83]. Ideally, incident patients who are candidates for home HD should dialyze separately from the prevalent HD patients until the training starts as they otherwise settle on conventional HD and do not transfer to home dialysis. Transitional Care Units (TCU) during the first few weeks of hemodialysis provide emotional support [84], education about modality selection and, by selecting the proper dialysis schedule, provide a smooth initiation to dialysis with proper fluid management, BP control and amelioration of uremic symptoms [85]. Trial dialysis runs simulating home hemodialysis regimens have also been advocated [86]. They also help encourage patients to choose home HD [87]. Dedicated staff including nurses, technologists, pharmacists, dieticians, social workers and physicians trains the patient or the caregiver. Training usually lasts for about 4-12 weeks depending on the patient's knowledge and skills. A European study reports a relatively rapid training for home HD of a median 2.5 weeks [88]. The training is typically performed on the dialysis days either thrice weekly or daily. Part of the training (mainly general knowledge and fistula cannulation) can be taught in the transitional dialysis unit prior to the initiation of formal training. Adjustment of training depending on the patient's type of learning ability has been suggested [89].

A home visit by the training nurse and technologist prior to the training to evaluate the house (room space, plumbing and electrical requirements) and on the first day of discharge are useful. In some centers, patients have performance re-assessment on a regular basis.

Patients on home HD are usually requested to do laboratory tests monthly and visit the dialysis clinic every 1-4 months depending on their clinical stability. Training and supplies are provided so that patients can collect water and blood samples for testing, blood cultures, centrifuge blood samples, and self-infuse intravenous antibiotics and iron. Thrombolytic tissue plasminogen activator (TPA) vials to be used for central venous catheter blood clot fibrinolysis are supplied, especially for patients residing far from the dialysis unit. Remote monitoring [90] as a 'virtual ward' [91] is a potential useful practice, but its utility needs to be confirmed.

Barriers to Home HD

Although intensive HD is associated with favorable outcomes, the adoption of these regimens remains unacceptably low as is adoption of home dialysis in general [92]. There are multiple barriers to home dialysis [93, 94].

Systemic Barriers

Home dialysis programs were unavailable; only 38% of dialysis facilities offered home dialysis services in 2006, though this did increase to 44% of facilities in 2013. In contrast, 98% of Australian programs offered PD and 92% offered home HD in 2009 [3]. Further barriers include inadequate dialysis center and physician reimbursement rates; financial burden to patients; and lack of culture supportive of home dialysis.

Facility Barriers

Such barriers include lack of proper culture promoting home dialysis; lack of financial incentives; inadequate local knowledge and experience; poor staff training and patient education, especially in the pre-dialysis stage; lack of a champion, especially during the early stages of the creation of a program; insufficient number of training staff; and small size of the home dialysis program with small cumulative experience.

Technological Barriers

These include lack of patient friendly dialysis machines. More user-friendly machines were created, and new creative approaches are being adopted, including manufacturing of wearable or implantable dialysis devices [14].

Patient Related Barriers

These barriers comprise medical contraindications, which are rare; inability or unwillingness to train; psychological reasons including fear of catastrophic events [95]; lack of appropriate housing including nursing home residence; lack of home support or lack of a helper; and financial disincentives, some related to increased utility costs related to dialysis. The cost of conventional home HD was calculated at $420 and for daily nocturnal HD $1269 Canadian dollars in 2017 [96]. Use of paid helpers has been helpful in overcoming some of the barriers in our center [18]. The barriers to home dialysis and possible solutions were addressed in an NKF-KDOQI sponsored conference [93, 97].

History of Financial Factors Affecting the Home HD Utilization in the US

A fee-for-service for physician payments for dialysis established in 2004 favoring in-center HD payments was associated with a decrease in the adoption of home dialysis by 12-16%. To improve quality of care and decrease cost, CMS as part of the ESRD Prospective Payment System (PPS) created in 2011, bundled the HD rate payment with profitable items previously paid extra, such as erythropoietic stimulating agents and more recently calcimimetics [98]. The expanded PPS in 2017 included payment for home training and relaxation of the maximum number of HHD treatments funded per week at home. The Medicare Administrative Contactors (MAC's), that implement the PPS locally through LCDs (local coverage decisions), have maintained the strict criteria for funding of extra HHD sessions [99]. Therefore, the CMS incentives were not passed on to the HD providers. Furthermore, possible financial benefits from the use of home dialysis, by possibly decreasing hospitalization rates, do not reward the facilities that promote home dialysis [100].

A major initiative for the promotion of home dialysis was established in 2018 in the form of The Kidney Health Initiative (KHI) — a public-private partnership between the American Society of Nephrology (ASN), the US Food & Drug Administration (FDA) and over 100 other organizations and companies. A roadmap [101] was published in October 2018, and in 2019 a patient-friendly summary of the KHI roadmap was published. The initiative includes funding for innovation (KidneyX - www.kidneyx.org), as well as financial incentives for home dialysis and potentially financial disincentives for in-center HD.

In July 2019, the US Department of Health and Human Services (HHS) launched a federal executive order-Advancing American Kidney Health Initiative (AAKH). HHS set three goals to improve kidney health in the United States: 1) reduce the number of Americans developing ESRD; 2) increase the number of new (incident) American patients on home dialysis or transplantation to 80% by 2025; and 3) double the number of organs available for transplantation by 2025 [102].

In July 2020, CMS issued a proposed rule for the ESRD PPS, which expands its transitional add-on payment adjustment in the form of add-on payment adjustments for new and innovative equipment and supplies (TPNIES), specifically for machines used for home dialysis.

The ESRD Treatment Choices (ETC) Model is being considered by CMS. It includes providing funding and other incentives to 50% of randomly selected ESRD facilities in all states for 5 years. It will give ESRD beneficiaries the freedom and choice of ESRD treatment that best works with their lifestyles including more frequent home HD.

In August of 2020, CMS announced an increase in the payments to physicians attending home dialysis patients by 30% as another incentive to promote utilization of home dialysis as part of the KHI initiative.

The issue of the financial incentive misalignment in the US, as well as the impact of the new initiatives, are discussed in several publications [3, 100, 102, 103].

OUTCOMES

Quality of Life

Quality of life (QOL) is seriously hampered in patients initiating dialysis [104]. Several observational studies report improved QOL on intensive regimens [105, 106]. Patients on intensive HD have reported improvements measured by the Kidney Disease QOL instrument (KDQOL) [107-110]. In addition, while on daily regimens, patients themselves report positive feedback [111, 112], higher feeling thermometer score, better general health, and shorter recovery time after a dialysis session [113]. Improved QOL measured by QALYs has also been documented in both short daily and nocturnal HD [114-116]. Conversion from conventional to in-center intermittent nocturnal HD was not associated with negative effects on QOL measurements despite the nighttime dialysis [116]. Daily nocturnal HD has been associated with an improvement in QOL along with a decreased cost [105, 114].

The main randomized control trials that assessed QOL of patients on intensive HD regimens are the Alberta and the FHN trials. Fifty-one patients in the Alberta study were randomized to either conventional or home nocturnal HD for 6 months. Evaluation of the EQ-5D index scores regarding QOL improvement on nocturnal HD just shy of statistical significance. Yet, kidney specific QOL sub-scores showed significant improvement on nocturnal HD [106, 117]. The FHN trial randomized 245 patients to conventional or short daily in-center HD. The daily HD arm of the FHN trial showed a significant improvement in the general health scale instrument, in self-reported mental health and physical performance [13]. Nevertheless, a similar improvement was not demonstrated in the nocturnal arm of the trial [12]. No change was observed in the adjusted mean Beck Depression Inventory Score with either daily or nocturnal HD [118]. Health related QOL improved on more frequent HD in the FHN trial [119]. In the ACTIVE trial, 200 patients on conventional HD in-center or at home were randomized to extended hemodialysis (>24 hours) by mainly increasing the length on dialysis or standard (12-15) hours dialysis for 12 months. There was no effect on the primary end point of EuroQoL-5 Dimension-3 Level (EQ-5D-3L) health utility but was associated with improvement in Short Form-36 (SF-36) Physical Component Summary (PCS) and Mental Component Summary (MCS) [120].

A Meta-Analysis in the 4 RCTs above was associated with a small but consistent improvement in physical and mental quality of life as measured by PCS (overall difference, 2.4; 95% CI, 1.2 to 3.6) and by MCS (overall difference, 3.0; 95% CI, 1.5 to 4.4) [121].

CARDIOVASCULAR BENEFITS

Left Ventricular (LV) Morphology and LV Function

Hypervolemia, hypertension, uremic molecule retention, and mineral metabolism disorders lead to LV hypertrophy (LVH) in conventional HD patients and eventually to congestive heart failure and adverse CV outcomes. LVH regression is significantly associated with a lower risk of clinical adverse outcomes [122]. Short daily and daily nocturnal HD have shown a regression of LV mass (LVM) and an improvement in LV ejection fraction (LVEF) [77, 123-125].

Conversion from conventional to intensive HD regimens reduced mean LVM, LV end-diastolic diameter (LVEDD), LV posterior wall (LVPW) thickness, septal wall thickness [13, 126, 127], mean LVM index (LVMi), whereas patients who remain on conventional HD demonstrated an increase in mean LVMi [123]. Beneficial effects on LV function are also exhibited by an improvement in global circumferential strain and decrease in torsion after conversion to nocturnal HD [128]. Transfer to intensive regimens and changes in LVM lead to improved blood pressure (BP) control [129]. Although lack of regression of LVH on long intermittent regimens was reported in older studies [130, 131], more recent studies confirmed the LVH regression [127, 132, 133].

These results are supported by observational RCTs [12, 126], as well as two meta-analyses [134, 135]. In the FHN RCT Trial, patients on 6 daily sessions per week compared to patients on 3 conventional sessions revealed LVM regression [12]. This significant outcome was not shown in patients on nocturnal HD, probably related to the underpowered nocturnal study arm. *Post hoc* analysis of the FHN trial showed that patients with baseline LVH experienced a more pronounced LVM regression on intensive HD [129]. These results confirmed the outcome of the earlier Alberta RCT on daily nocturnal HD patients [126].

Non-hemodynamic factors may also influence LVM in the HD population. These include the retention of molecules with possible effect on cardiac remodelling and mineral metabolism disorders [136]. Patients in the FHN group undergoing frequent dialysis regimens experienced LVH regression, which was associated to increased Klotho circulating levels [137]. In addition, conversion from conventional to nocturnal HD reduced fibroblast proliferation and activation of innate immunity, which in turn minimized cardiomyocyte apoptosis [138]. More detailed analysis of the CV effects of intensive HD is reviewed elsewhere [139].

BP Control

Sodium and fluid intake between conventional HD sessions leads to volume expansion and increased BP [140]. Elevated BP is also affected by increased sympathetic activation, endothelial dysfunction, and inappropriate renin-angiotensin system activity, and is strongly associated with LVH [141]. In addition, decreased session duration and increased ultrafiltration leads to augmentation of BP variability and hypertension [142].

Improved BP control has been shown in short daily [76, 109, 124, 143, 144], long intermittent [7, 145], and daily nocturnal HD [123, 146]. Systolic, diastolic [13, 123, 142, 147-151], and mean arterial BP [146, 152] are significantly reduced in nocturnal HD. Anti-hypertensive medication mean number and dosage are decreased and often discontinued in patients on intensive regimens [134, 135, 142, 153]. Furthermore, nocturnal HD decreases arterial stiffness measured by pulse wave velocity [154]. In short daily HD, this effect has been attributed to a decrease in intravascular volume expansion [124]. On the contrary, though, in daily nocturnal HD, the extracellular volume, assessed by bioelectrical impedance, remained unchanged [123, 146].

Both the Alberta [11] and FHN trials [12, 13, 150] have confirmed the beneficial effects of intensive HD on BP. Moreover, salt restriction advocated on conventional and intermittent nocturnal HD [155] is not as important on daily nocturnal HD [41].

Vascular Calcification

Vascular calcification (VC) significantly contributes to the increased CV risk and mortality of HD patients. Mineral bone disorders and the uremic milieu have been identified as potential contributors towards coronary calcification and CV mortality [156]. Nocturnal HD through increased dialysis time improves phosphate control and solute clearance, showing eventually a beneficial impact on coronary artery calcification. One year after patient conversion from conventional to nocturnal HD, CT scans showed a non-significant progress in coronary artery calcification scores [157]. Conversely, other studies of patients undergoing conventional HD reported an increase in coronary calcification rates [158]. Studies of patients on intermittent nocturnal HD also reported a decrease in VC [74].

Endothelial and Autonomous Nervous System Function

In the HD population, there is impairment of endothelial-dependent vasodilation (EDV) likely contributing to the CV risk [159]. It has been associated to uremia, hyperphosphatemia, hyperparathyroidism, hypertension and increased plasma concentrations of asymmetric dimethylarginine (ADMA) [160]. Conversion from conventional to nocturnal HD was associated with restoration of the impaired vasodilatory response to relief of ischemia caused by the inflation of a BP cuff, and to response to nitroglycerin, both measures of EDV. It was also associated with decrease in plasma norepinephrine levels and decrease in total peripheral resistance as measured by echocardiography [152]. This possibly implies an endothelial mechanism in BP reduction on nocturnal HD [152]. The endothelial and vasodilatory effects were possibly associated with improved phosphate and hyperparathyroidism control, but not with ADMA levels [160]. In addition, arterial baroreceptor function and arterial compliance improved after conversion to nocturnal HD [161].

Endothelial Progenitor Cells (EPCs)

Endothelial progenitor cells (EPCs) appear at the site of tissue damage in order to repair vascular injury and restore endothelial integrity [162]. The number of EPCs is inversely associated with CV risk [163, 164], and their number and function are reduced in patients on conventional HD [165, 166]. EPC number and migratory function were restored upon conversion from conventional to nocturnal HD [166] with implications in CV risk reduction.

Heart Rate Variability

Heart rate variability (HRV) is a non-invasive assessment of autonomic modulation of sino-atrial discharge and poses a risk factor for CV events in the dialysis population [167]. HRV independently predicts mortality in CKD patients [168]. Decreased HRV in ESRD patients is associated with significant fluid-overload between sessions, obstructive sleep apnea, myocardial ischemia, elevated norepinephrine levels, and sympathetic activation [169, 170]. These parameters lead to increased risk of death in this population [171-173].

The FHN trial confirmed previous smaller studies by demonstrating that the daily dialysis arm was associated with increased HRV compared to controls [174, 175]. It is suggested that more frequent HD by decreasing ultrafiltration rate, fluid volume removal and myocardial stunning, decreases myocardial ischemia, reduces central sympathetic activity and increases HRV [13, 173]. Conversion from conventional to nocturnal HD leads to decreased apnea-hypopnea index, nocturnal hypoxemia, and a decrease in heart rate and HRV during sleep [176].

Mineral Metabolism

Calcium-phosphate balance is important in the dialysis population, relevant to mineral bone metabolism and to the development of vascular calcifications [164, 177].

Patients on intensive dialysis may exhibit a negative calcium balance related to: a) decreased, or lack of need for calcium-based phosphate binders, b) increased calcium loss by high ultrafiltration volumes, while on a liberal diet and c) low gastrointestinal calcium absorption related to low serum vitamin D levels. This leads to a need for a calcium rich diet, oral calcium supplementation or higher dialysate calcium. In most patients on daily nocturnal HD, a dialysate calcium concentration of at least 3 mEq/L (1.5mmol) is necessary [178]. It should be noted that mild transient hypercalcemia can or needs to be observed post-dialysis in order to maintain or create positive calcium balance or help bone repair. Post parathyroidectomy state, pregnancy, and the presence of elevated bone-derived alkaline phosphatase levels indicate the need for further increase in dialysate calcium or oral calcium supplements [179]. In the presence of VC, hypercalcemia should probably be avoided, and hyperparathyroidism should be treated preferably with calcimimetics or parathyroidectomy. Calcium dialysate composition can be adjusted through addition of calcium chloride powder into the acid concentrate; 15 mL of powder increases dialysate calcium by 1 mEq/L (0.5mmol/L). The amount needed can be finely adjusted based on pre and post HD calcium levels, alkaline phosphatase and PTH.

Conventional HD is associated with hyperphosphatemia. Improving phosphate levels reduces the incidence of VC [180]. Strict dietary phosphate restriction, use of phosphate binders, and PTH control using vitamin D analogues or calcimimetics often do not succeed in reducing serum phosphate levels.

Several studies have examined the effect of intensive HD on phosphate balance [73, 123, 157, 181-184]. Longer dialysis time results in reduced calcium-phosphate product, diet liberalization, and reduction or discontinuation of phosphate binder use [73, 123, 157, 183, 185]. Initiation of nocturnal HD [157] also reduced VC in x-rays of hands and feet [182], resolved extraosseous calcifications [186], and stabilized coronary artery calcifications [157]. Furthermore, the majority of patients on daily nocturnal HD need phosphate addition into the dialysate in the form of sodium phosphate (usually Fleet Enema®) in bicarbonate or acid concentrate. The low pH in the latter prevents calcium and phosphate precipitation, even if both calcium and phosphate are added into the acid concentrate [43]. Unless the length of dialysis is increased to more than 3 hours, short daily dialysis results in lower phosphate removal as a result of slow phosphate mobilization from the tissues [37].

PTH levels can be mostly managed through dialysate calcium level adjustments and, as a result, both short and nocturnal HD regimens have been found to decrease PTH levels [37, 74, 187]. Rising serum alkaline phosphatase, along with high PTH levels, often suggest inadequate dialysate calcium levels or low oral calcium intake.

Sleep

Symptoms related to sleep such as sleep apnea, insomnia, restless leg syndrome, and daytime sleepiness are highly prevalent in HD patients and are associated with increased CV morbidity and mortality [188, 189]. Sleep apnea is associated with fluid overload, hypoxemia, hypercapnia, destabilization of central ventilatory control, and upper airway obstruction. It eventually leads to endothelial dysfunction, oxidative stress and inflammation [188, 190-193]. Untreated sleep apnea may result in CVD in HD patients [191, 193]. Conventional HD and CAPD do not appear to offer a significant benefit towards correction of sleep apnea [193]. Conversion from conventional to nocturnal HD leads to a significant reduction in the apnea-hypopnea index in dialysis patients with sleep apnea. Yet, daytime sleepiness and periodic limb movement are not affected [188]. Heart rate variability during sleep decreased on daily nocturnal HD [176].

This mechanism for the improvement of OSA on daily nocturnal HD has been mainly attributed to more efficient fluid removal, which prevents obstruction of the upper airway during sleep time [194]. Fluid shift towards the upper airway during the night, which is associated with sleep apnea severity [195], may be ameliorated by APD at night as compared to CAPD and nocturnal HD [188, 196]. Additionally, nocturnal HD may correct the dialysis-associated ventilatory instability and maintain oxygen and carbon dioxide levels within normal limits [197]. In patients with sleep apnea, periodic fluctuations in upper airway muscle activity lead to irregular or periodic breathing, especially during certain sleep stages. Conversion from conventional to nocturnal HD is associated with an improvement in irregular breathing and a decrease in ventilator sensitivity to hypercapnia [198].

EPO Dose and Anemia Management

Observational studies on the intensive regimens report an increase in hemoglobin and a decrease in EPO dose [76, 109, 199]. In the FHN Study, despite an increase in hemoglobin in the daily HD group, more frequent sessions did not reveal a clinically significant benefit on anemia management [200].

Nutrition

Amino acid loss in the dialysate during HD would suggest a higher loss rate on more frequent and longer HD [201]. Yet, conversion of patients from conventional to short daily HD in observational studies was associated with increased body weight, nPNA, cholesterol, serum albumin and pre-albumin levels, arm muscle area, and increase in appetite and well-being [145, 202-204]. Daily nocturnal HD reveals an improved serum amino acid profile [205]. Patients on intensive HD are on a more liberal, and depending on the regimen, quite unrestricted diet. Nutritional stability, not noted in conventional HD [206], is reported in long HD regimens [203]. Studies on the quotidian nocturnal regimen showing that post-HD serum albumin levels are lower than the pre-dialysis values were attributed to an increased vascular refilling when the patient lies in the recumbent position [207]. Bioimpedance measurements during the FHN trial did not reveal significant improvement in nutritional and body composition parameters in frequent modalities over one year [208]. Serum albumin levels and dietary nutrient intake changes did not reach statistically significant improvement in the Alberta study [209].

Pregnancy

Women on conventional HD suffer from decreased fertility and even when pregnancy occurs it is often associated with poor outcomes [210]. An increased dialysis frequency has been proposed to achieve increased fertility rates and pregnancy outcomes. Daily HD may lead to improved hormonal function [211]. In two small cohort studies, most women undergoing daily nocturnal HD had successful pregnancies that resulted in live infants [212, 213]. In a larger, comparative study, live birth rates were markedly higher in women receiving intensive HD regimens of at least 36 hours per week [214]. In addition, longer gestational age and greater infant birth weight was reported for women on more intensive schedules. Thus, intensive HD regimens are advocated prior to and during pregnancy.

During pregnancy, serum calcium, phosphorus, and PTH levels pre- and post-dialysis should be measured, and the dialysis prescription adjusted accordingly. Increased need for calcium and phosphate -usually added in the dialysate- are likely related to the growth of the fetal skeleton. Dialysate calcium levels should be generally higher than 3.5 mEq/L (1.75mmol/L) in order to prevent a significant rise in PTH. It is not unusual to add even 200 ml of Fleet enema® per dialysate jug in order to meet the phosphate needs. Anemia management through supplementation of erythropoietic agents and increased dose of intravenous iron is usually required during pregnancy.

If hypertension develops during pregnancy, both pharmacological treatments as well as ultrafiltration have been used. Acceptable medications include labetalol and alpha methyldopa. The role for increased ultrafiltration for blood pressure control remains unclear, as the effects on placental flow are largely unknown. Ultrafiltration, with caution in significant fluid overload and dyspnea, should be considered. When uncontrolled hypertension coexists with overhydration, higher ultrafiltration rate is reasonable. During the postpartum period, liberal ultrafiltration can improve BP control, with unknown effects on milk production.

Lastly, respiratory alkalosis with low serum bicarbonate, normally seen in pregnancy, can be simulated by decreasing dialysate bicarbonate concentration.

Residual Kidney Function

Peritoneal dialysis has been credited with longer maintenance of residual renal function than hemodialysis [215]. The effect of more frequent HD on residual renal function was addressed by the FHN trial. Although no conclusion can be drawn from the daily study as most of the patients were anuric, patients on nocturnal HD lost residual renal function faster than the controls on conventional home HD [216]. It is speculated that the cause is related to decreased extracellular volume more easily achieved on this schedule to improve BP control. Other potential contributing factors include chronic inflammation from long exposure to hemodialysis circuits, microbubbles, platelet activation and dialysis-induced tissue ischemia [217]. Loss of residual renal function is potentially compensated by the increased solute removal associated with the modality.

Patient Hospitalization and Survival

All-cause hospitalization and mortality rates remain high on HD. The mortality rate at 165 per 1,000 patient years has though decreased by 20% from 2001 to 2010 and by 7% from 2011 to 2017 [2].

Data on survival rates of patients on intensive compared to conventional schedules are conflicting [218-220]. In a long-standing HD center with experience in the nocturnal regimen, a median patient survival of 14.6 years, along with median technique survival of 7.8 years was reported [221]. In several studies, in-center intermittent nocturnal HD, when compared to conventional HD was associated with decreased hospitalization and increased patient survival rates [218, 222, 223]. In a retrospective analysis, a Canadian cohort of patients on home nocturnal HD had similar survival with a US cohort of cadaveric-donor transplanted patients (84.5% vs 86.2% over 5 years) [219]. In another study a similar Canadian patient cohort on nocturnal HD had inferior survival to a Canadian transplanted patient cohort [224]. A more recent study in a single center found similar patient survival of 116 patients on intensive HD to 3,073 patients after cadaveric kidney transplantation done in the same geographical area [225].

Short daily HD is associated with higher patient survival in observational studies [143, 226] and data from the USRDS database show that patients on this regimen experience survival rates similar to deceased-donor kidney transplanted patients [227, 228]. In addition, a comparative study showed that home daily HD was associated with fewer hospital admissions and hospital days, as well as a significantly lower risk for modality switch when compared to conventional HD and home PD [229]. Patients on the short daily schedule using the NxStage machine, compared to thrice weekly HD controls, exhibited fewer CVD-related hospital admissions, higher infection-related admissions, and slightly better patient survival rates [230, 231]. Analysis of patients on the daily arm of the FHN trial revealed a survival benefit for frequent compared to conventional HD, suggesting that daily HD should be considered for selected patients [232]. In contrast to the daily arm, a follow-up study of the FHN trial showed a higher mortality rate in the nocturnal arm compared to the conventional home HD [220]. The results contradict data from observational studies and were largely unexpected. Yet, the study presents several limitations. The sample size was small. Additionally, the observation period included one year after the completion of the FHN trial, during which several patients changed modality and finally the control group had an unexpectedly low mortality rate compared to historical controls [220].

Patients on intensive home HD regimens compared retrospectively with patients on conventional in-center thrice-weekly HD also exhibited lower mortality rates (13% *vs* 21%) [233, 234]. Australia /New Zealand data along with DOPPS data suggest an association between length of dialysis and patient survival, a phenomenon not merely associated with increased dialysis dose [235, 236].

In a retrospective study of 10,710 patients on PD and 706 patients on home HD from the Australia/New Zealand dialysis and transplantation registry, patients on home HD had a better 5-year survival rate (85%) than PD (44%) p<0.001) [237]. Selection biases may have affected the results.

In a review of the literature by Miller et al., in 10 out of the 13 studies that met their selection criteria (out of total 146), there was a 13-52% reduction in mortality rates on home HD compared to in-center HD [238].

In a retrospective study, 1,993 and 16,514 patients who transferred from in-center HD to home HD and PD, respectively, within the first year of HD had the same survival rates. Patients who transferred after the first year of in-center HD to home HD had higher survival rates than patients who transferred to PD, possibly reflecting the early beneficial effect of residual renal function on PD outcomes [239].

A study found that patients on in-center daily HD had a lower survival rate compared to patients on the thrice-weekly regimen [78]. Yet, the authors admit to limitations of the study including an indication bias as patients were converted to the daily regimen probably due to associated comorbidities, which was likely the reason for the increased mortality rates.

In a cohort study of 1,310 Canadian home HD patients, 600 on conventional home HD, 508 on nocturnal HD, and 202 on short daily HD, after multivariate adjustments the survival advantage of intensive HD was lost [240]. Technique failure was lower in the nocturnal HD group, as was the patient survival in the 'as treated' analysis.

Technique failure of patients on intensive home HD is variable. In a Canadian study, the unadjusted 1- and 2-year technique survival and overall survival were 90% and 83%, and 94% and 87%, respectively. Treating center was a strong predictor of technique failure and mortality [241]. Higher attrition rate was reported on daily HD using mainly the NxStage machine, although more recently lower attrition rates were reported [90, 242].

In summary, all of the evidence suggests decreased hospitalization rates and improved patient survival rates on intensive HD regimens. The exception is the patients who were converted to in-center short daily HD because of comorbidities. All the studies addressing mortality rates represent retrospective cohort studies and are possibly subjected to selection biases. The RCTs did not have mortality as an end point and the nocturnal trials were underpowered [243]. It is unlikely that an RCT will address patient mortality rates in the future.

Conclusion

In-center HD thrice weekly, the most prevalent dialysis modality, is associated with poor outcomes and high cost. The prevalent rates of home HD have declined over the years and despite some exceptions and a recent resurgence in the US, it is used only by about 2% of the dialysis population. Intensive hemodialysis, a collective term including increased length and or more frequent hemodialysis, is associated with better outcomes based on a large number of cohort studies and a small number of RCTs. These studies point to improvement in cardiovascular end points, BP control, mineral metabolism, sleep apnea, reproductive physiology and in some of them with improvement in quality of life and possibly increased patient survival. There are also potentially significant socioeconomic benefits associated with intensive HD.

Lack of adequate education and experience with home HD and financial disincentives represent significant barriers to the adoption of home HD. The recent establishment of the Kidney Health Initiative and the Advancing American Kidney Health Initiative in the US, mandating the adoption of home dialysis and transplantation by 80% of the incident patient population by the year 2025 is encouraging. Investing in new technology, creating financial incentives, providing patient support at home and education of patients and the members of the dialysis team, promise to increase the utilization of home dialysis.

REFERENCES

[1] Han Y, Saran R. Global Dialysis Perspective: United States. *Kidney 360*. 2020: 10.34067/KID.00.

[2] USRDS. *USRDS annual data report.* 2020 Date accessed Nov 14, 2020. Available from: https: //adr.usrds.org/2020/end-stage-renal-disease.

[3] Abra G, Schiller B. Public policy and programs - Missing links in growing home dialysis in the United States. *Semin Dial.* 2020; 33(1): 75-82.

[4] NKF-DOQI clinical practice guidelines for hemodialysis adequacy. National Kidney Foundation [published erratum appears in *Am J Kidney Dis* 1997 Oct; 30(4 Suppl 3): preceding table of contents]. *Am J Kidney Dis.* 1997; 30(3 Suppl 2): S15-S66.

[5] Gotch FA, Sargent JA. A mechanistic analysis of the National Cooperative Dialysis Study (NCDS). *Kidney Int.* 1985; 28(3): 526-34.

[6] Eknoyan G, Beck GJ, Cheung AK, Daugirdas JT, Greene T, Kusek JW, et al. Effect of dialysis dose and membrane flux in maintenance hemodialysis. *N Engl J Med.* 2002; 347(25): 2010-9.

[7] Charra B, Calemard M, Laurent G. Importance of treatment time and blood pressure control in achieving long-term survival on dialysis. *Am J Nephrol.* 1996; 16(1): 35-44.

[8] Buoncristiani U. Fifteen years of clinical experience with daily haemodialysis. *Nephrol Dial Transplant.* 1998; 13 Suppl 6: 148-51.

[9] Pierratos A, Ouwendyk M, Francoeur R, Vas S, Raj DS, Ecclestone AM, et al. Nocturnal hemodialysis: three-year experience. *J Am Soc Nephrol.* 1998; 9(5): 859-68.

[10] Pierratos A. Daily hemodialysis: why the renewed interest? *Am J Kidney Dis.* 1998; 32(6 Suppl 4): S76-S82.

[11] Culleton BF, Walsh M, Klarenbach SW, Mortis G, Scott-Douglas N, Quinn RR, et al. Effect of frequent nocturnal hemodialysis vs conventional hemodialysis on left ventricular mass and quality of life: a randomized controlled trial. *JAMA.* 2007; 298(11): 1291-9.

[12] Rocco MV, Lockridge RS, Jr., Beck GJ, Eggers PW, Gassman JJ, Greene T, et al. The effects of frequent nocturnal home hemodialysis: the Frequent Hemodialysis Network Nocturnal Trial. *Kidney Int.* 2011; 80(10): 1080-91.

[13] Group FHNT, Chertow GM, Levin NW, Beck GJ, Depner TA, Eggers PW, et al. In-center hemodialysis six times per week versus three times per week. *N Engl J Med.* 2010; 363(24): 2287-300.

[14] Haroon S, Davenport A. Haemodialysis at home: review of current dialysis machines. *Expert Rev Med Devices.* 2018; 15(5): 337-47.

[15] Mehrotra R. Advancing American Kidney Health: An Introduction. *Clin J Am Soc Nephrol*. 2019; 14(12): 1788.
[16] Hager D, Ferguson TW, Komenda P. Cost Controversies of a "Home Dialysis First" Policy. *Can J Kidney Health Dis*. 2019; 6: 2054358119871541.
[17] Ghaffari A, Kalantar-Zadeh K, Lee J, Maddux F, Moran J, Nissenson A. PD First: peritoneal dialysis as the default transition to dialysis therapy. *Semin Dial*. 2013; 26(6): 706-13.
[18] Pierratos A, Tremblay M, Kandasamy G, Woodward G, Blake P, Graham J, et al. Personal Support Worker (PSW)-supported home hemodialysis: A paradigm shift. *Hemodial Int*. 2017; 21(2): 173-9.
[19] Morton RL, Lioufas N, Dansie K, Palmer SC, Jose MD, Raj R, et al. Use of patient-reported outcome measures and patient-reported experience measures in renal units in Australia and New Zealand: A cross-sectional survey study. *Nephrology (Carlton)*. 2020; 25(1): 14-21.
[20] Flythe JE, Hilliard TS, Ikeler K, Keller S, Gipson DS, Grandinetti AC, et al. Toward Patient-Centered Innovation: A Conceptual Framework for Patient-Reported Outcome Measures for Transformative Kidney Replacement Devices. *Clin J Am Soc Nephrol*. 2020; 15(10): 1522-30.
[21] Centers for M, Medicaid Services HHS. Medicare program; end-stage renal disease prospective payment system. Final rule. *Federal register*. 2010; 75(155): 49029-214.
[22] Golper TA. The possible impact of the US prospective payment system ("bundle") on the growth of peritoneal dialysis. *Perit Dial Int*. 2013; 33(6): 596-9.
[23] Plumb TJ, Alvarez L, Ross DL, Lee JJ, Mulhern JG, Bell JL, et al. Safety and efficacy of the Tablo hemodialysis system for in-center and home hemodialysis. *Hemodial Int*. 2020; 24(1): 22-8.
[24] Weinhandl ED, Collins AJ. Relative risk of home hemodialysis attrition in patients using a telehealth platform. *Hemodial Int*. 2018; 22(3): 318-27.
[25] Lew SQ, Sikka N. Operationalizing Telehealth for Home Dialysis Patients in the United States. *Am J Kidney Dis*. 2019; 74(1): 95-100.
[26] Hayashi A, Yamaguchi S, Waki K, Fujiu K, Hanafusa N, Nishi T, et al. Testing the Feasibility and Usability of a Novel Smartphone-Based Self-Management Support System for Dialysis Patients: A Pilot Study. *JMIR research protocols*. 2017; 6(4): e63.
[27] Rosner MH, Lew SQ, Conway P, Ehrlich J, Jarrin R, Patel UD, et al. Perspectives from the Kidney Health Initiative on Advancing Technologies to Facilitate Remote Monitoring of Patient Self-Care in RRT. *Clin J Am Soc Nephrol*. 2017; 12(11): 1900-9.
[28] Ong SW, Jassal SV, Miller JA, Porter EC, Cafazzo JA, Seto E, et al. Integrating a Smartphone-Based Self-Management System into Usual Care of Advanced CKD. *Clin J Am Soc Nephrol*. 2016; 11(6): 1054-62.
[29] Krishna VN, Managadi K, Smith M, Wallace E. Telehealth in the Delivery of Home Dialysis Care: Catching up With Technology. *Adv Chronic Kidney Dis*. 2017; 24(1): 12-6.
[30] Nayak KS, Ronco C, Karopadi AN, Rosner MH. Telemedicine and Remote Monitoring: Supporting the Patient on Peritoneal Dialysis. *Perit Dial Int*. 2016; 36(4): 362-6.
[31] Sharma MK, Wieringa FP, Frijns AJ, Kooman JP. On-line monitoring of electrolytes in hemodialysis: on the road towards individualizing treatment. *Expert Rev Med Devices*. 2016; 13(10): 933-43.

[32] Pierratos A. Nocturnal home haemodialysis: an update on a 5-year experience. *Nephrol Dial Transplant*. 1999; 14(12): 2835-40.

[33] Hoy CD. Remote Monitoring of Daily Nocturnal Hemodialysis. *Hemodial Int*. 2001; 5(1): 8-12.

[34] Kennedy C, McGrath-Chong M, Arustei D, d'Gama C, Faratro R, Fung S, et al. A prototype line clamp for venous access bleeding in hemodialysis: A prospective cohort study. *Hemodial Int*. 2019; 23(2): 151-7.

[35] Diaz-Buxo JA, Schlaeper C, Vanvalkenburgh D. Evolution of home hemodialysis monitoring systems. *Hemodial Int*. 2003; 7(4): 353-5.

[36] Pierratos A, Francoeur R, Ouwendyk M. Delayed Dialyzer Reprocessing for Home Hemodialysis. *Hemodial Int*. 2000; 4(1): 51-4.

[37] Ayus JC, Achinger SG, Mizani MR, Chertow GM, Furmaga W, Lee S, et al. Phosphorus balance and mineral metabolism with 3 h daily hemodialysis. *Kidney Int*. 2007; 71(4): 336-42.

[38] Clark WR, Turk JE, Jr. The NxStage System One. *Semin Dial*. 2004; 17(2): 167-70.

[39] Kohn OF, Coe FL, Ing TS. Solute kinetics with short-daily home hemodialysis using slow dialysate flow rate. *Hemodialysis int*. 2010; 14(1): 39-46.

[40] Diaz-Buxo JA, White SA, Himmele R. Frequent hemodialysis: a critical review. *Semin Dial*. 2013; 26(5): 578-89.

[41] Pierratos A. Daily nocturnal home hemodialysis. *Kidney Int*. 2004; 65(5): 1975-86.

[42] Mahadevan K, Pellicano R, Reid A, Kerr P, Polkinghorne K, Agar J. Comparison of biochemical, haematological and volume parameters in two treatment schedules of nocturnal home haemodialysis. *Nephrology (Carlton)*. 2006; 11(5): 413-8.

[43] Su WS, Lekas P, Carlisle EJ, Cowin R, Bellamy J, Margetts PJ, et al. Management of hypophosphatemia in nocturnal hemodialysis with phosphate-containing enema: a technical study. *Hemodial Int*. 2011; 15(2): 219-25.

[44] Lockridge R, Cornelis T, van EC. Prescriptions for home hemodialysis. *Hemodial Int*. 2015; 19 Suppl 1: S112-S27.

[45] Huang SS, Qi K, Louzada M, Lindsay RM, Rehman F, Ke H, et al. Using dalteparin in quotidian and nocturnal hemodialysis patients: A prospective study. *Hemodial Int*. 2020; 24(2): 195-201.

[46] Bugeja A, Harris S, McCormick B, Brown PA, Liberty C, Krepelka T, et al. Safety and Efficacy of Tinzaparin Anticoagulation during Nocturnal Hemodialysis. *Am J Nephrol*. 2019; 50(4): 255-61.

[47] Suri RS, Larive B, Sherer S, Eggers P, Gassman J, James SH, et al. Risk of vascular access complications with frequent hemodialysis. *J Am Soc Nephrol*. 2013; 24(3): 498-505.

[48] Mustafa RA, Zimmerman D, Rioux JP, Suri RS, Gangji A, Steele A, et al. Vascular access for intensive maintenance hemodialysis: a systematic review for a Canadian Society of Nephrology clinical practice guideline. *Am J Kidney Dis*. 2013; 62(1): 112-31.

[49] Brunelli SM, Njord L, Hunt AE, Sibbel SP. Use of the Tego needlefree connector is associated with reduced incidence of catheter-related bloodstream infections in hemodialysis patients. *Int J Nephrol Renovasc Dis*. 2014; 7: 131-9.

[50] Twardowski ZJ. Update on cannulation techniques. *J Vasc Access*. 2015; 16 Suppl 9: S54-60.

[51] MacRae JM, Ahmed SB, Atkar R, Hemmelgarn BR. A randomized trial comparing buttonhole with rope ladder needling in conventional hemodialysis patients. *Clin J Am Soc Nephrol*. 2012; 7(10): 1632-8.

[52] Nesrallah GE, Cuerden M, Wong JH, Pierratos A. Staphylococcus aureus bacteremia and buttonhole cannulation: long-term safety and efficacy of mupirocin prophylaxis. *Clin J Am Soc Nephrol*. 2010; 5(6): 1047-53.

[53] Lok CE, Sontrop JM, Faratro R, Chan CT, Zimmerman DL. Frequent hemodialysis fistula infectious complications. *Nephron Extra*. 2014; 4(3): 159-67.

[54] Nesrallah GE. Pro: Buttonhole cannulation of arteriovenous fistulae. *Nephrol Dial Transplant*. 2016; 31(4): 520-3.

[55] Di Nicolo P, Cornacchiari M, Mereghetti M, Mudoni A. Buttonhole Cannulation of the AV Fistula: A Critical Analysis of the Technique. *Semin Dial*. 2017; 30(1): 32-8.

[56] Nadeau-Fredette AC, Johnson DW. Con: Buttonhole cannulation of arteriovenous fistulae. *Nephrol Dial Transplant*. 2016; 31(4): 525-8.

[57] Pauly RP, Eastwood DO, Marshall MR. Patient safety in home hemodialysis: quality assurance and serious adverse events in the home setting. *Hemodial Int*. 2015; 19 Suppl 1: S59-S70.

[58] Ibrahim A, Chan CT. Managing Kidney Failure with Home Hemodialysis. *Clin J Am Soc Nephrol*. 2019; 14(8): 1268-73.

[59] National Kidney F. KDOQI Clinical Practice Guideline for Hemodialysis Adequacy: 2015 update. *Am J Kidney Dis*. 2015; 66(5): 884-930.

[60] Suri R, Depner TA, Blake PG, Heidenheim AP, Lindsay RM. Adequacy of quotidian hemodialysis. *Am J Kidney Dis*. 2003; 42(1 Suppl): 42-8.

[61] Leypoldt JK, Cheung AK, Carroll CE, Stannard DC, Pereira BJ, Agodoa LY, et al. Effect of dialysis membranes and middle molecule removal on chronic hemodialysis patient survival. *Am J Kidney Dis*. 1999; 33(2): 349-55.

[62] Cheung AK, Rocco MV, Yan G, Leypoldt JK, Levin NW, Greene T, et al. Serum beta-2 Microglobulin Levels Predict Mortality in Dialysis Patients: Results of the HEMO Study. *J Am Soc Nephrol*. 2006; 17(2): 546-55.

[63] Cheung AK, Sarnak MJ, Yan G, Berkoben M, Heyka R, Kaufman A, et al. Cardiac diseases in maintenance hemodialysis patients: results of the HEMO Study. *Kidney Int*. 2004; 65(6): 2380-9.

[64] Raj DS, Ouwendyk M, Francoeur R, Pierratos A. beta(2)-microglobulin kinetics in nocturnal haemodialysis. *Nephrol Dial Transplant*. 2000; 15(1): 58-64.

[65] Fagugli RM, Vanholder R, De Smet R, Selvi A, Antolini F, Lameire N, et al. Advanced glycation end products: specific fluorescence changes of pentosidine-like compounds during short daily hemodialysis. *Int J Artif Organs*. 2001; 24(5): 256-62.

[66] Fagugli RM, De Smet R, Buoncristiani U, Lameire N, Vanholder R. Behavior of non-protein-bound and protein-bound uremic solutes during daily hemodialysis. *Am J Kidney Dis*. 2002; 40(2): 339-47.

[67] Sirich TL, Fong K, Larive B, Beck GJ, Chertow GM, Levin NW, et al. Limited reduction in uremic solute concentrations with increased dialysis frequency and time in the Frequent Hemodialysis Network Daily Trial. *Kidney Int*. 2017; 91(5): 1186-92.

[68] Brunati CCM, Gervasi F, Cabibbe M, Ravera F, Menegotto A, Querques M, et al. Single Session and Weekly Beta 2-Microglobulin Removal with Different Dialytic Procedures: Comparison between High-Flux Standard Bicarbonate Hemodialysis, Post-Dilution

Hemodiafiltration, Short Frequent Hemodialysis with NxStage Technology and Automated Peritoneal Dialysis. *Blood Purif.* 2019; 48(1): 86-96.
[69] Brunati CCM, Gervasi F, Casati C, Querques ML, Montoli A, Colussi G. Phosphate and Calcium Control in Short Frequent Hemodialysis with the NxStage System One Cycler: Mass Balance Studies and Comparison with Standard Thrice-Weekly Bicarbonate Dialysis. *Blood Purif.* 2018; 45(4): 334-42.
[70] Block GA, Klassen PS, Lazarus JM, Ofsthun N, Lowrie EG, Chertow GM. Mineral metabolism, mortality, and morbidity in maintenance hemodialysis. *J Am Soc Nephrol.* 2004; 15(8): 2208-18.
[71] DeSoi CA, Umans JG. Phosphate kinetics during high-flux hemodialysis. *J Am Soc Nephrol.* 1993; 4(5): 1214-8.
[72] Mucsi I, Hercz G, Uldall R, Ouwendyk M, Francoeur R, Pierratos A. Control of serum phosphate without any phosphate binders in patients treated with nocturnal hemodialysis. *Kidney Int.* 1998; 53(5): 1399-404.
[73] Daugirdas JT, Chertow GM, Larive B, Pierratos A, Greene T, Ayus JC, et al. Effects of frequent hemodialysis on measures of CKD mineral and bone disorder. *J Am Soc Nephrol.* 2012; 23(4): 727-38.
[74] VAN Eps CL, Jeffries JK, Anderson JA, Bergin PT, Johnson DW, Campbell SB, et al. Mineral metabolism, bone histomorphometry and vascular calcification in alternate night nocturnal haemodialysis. *Nephrology (Carlton).* 2007; 12(3): 224-33.
[75] Chan CT, Blankestijn PJ, Dember LM, Gallieni M, Harris DCH, Lok CE, et al. Dialysis initiation, modality choice, access, and prescription: conclusions from a Kidney Disease: Improving Global Outcomes (KDIGO) Controversies Conference. *Kidney Int.* 2019; 96(1): 37-47.
[76] Ting GO, Kjellstrand C, Freitas T, Carrie BJ, Zarghamee S. Long-term study of high-comorbidity ESRD patients converted from conventional to short daily hemodialysis. *Am J Kidney Dis.* 2003; 42(5): 1020-35.
[77] Chan C, Floras JS, Miller JA, Pierratos A. Improvement in ejection fraction by nocturnal haemodialysis in end-stage renal failure patients with coexisting heart failure. *Nephrol Dial Transplant.* 2002; 17(8): 1518-21.
[78] Suri RS, Lindsay RM, Bieber BA, Pisoni RL, Garg AX, Austin PC, et al. A multinational cohort study of in-center daily hemodialysis and patient survival. *Kidney Int.* 2013; 83(2): 300-7.
[79] Li JW, Wong JHS, Chak WL, Chau KF. Effect of incident nocturnal home hemodialysis versus incident continuous ambulatory peritoneal dialysis on employment rate, clinical, and laboratory outcomes: A 1-year retrospective observation study. *Hemodial Int.* 2018; 22(3): 308-17.
[80] Halpern SD, Berns JS, Israni AK. Willingness of patients to switch from conventional to daily hemodialysis: looking before we leap. *Am J Med.* 2004; 116(9): 606-12.
[81] Weinhandl ED, Gilbertson DT, Collins AJ. Mortality, Hospitalization, and Technique Failure in Daily Home Hemodialysis and Matched Peritoneal Dialysis Patients: A Matched Cohort Study. *Am J Kidney Dis.* 2016; 67(1): 98-110.
[82] Bonenkamp AA, van Gelder MK, Abrahams AC, Boereboom FTJ, Cornelis T, Luik AJ, et al. Home haemodialysis in the Netherlands: State of the art. *Neth J Med.* 2018; 76(4): 144-57.

[83] Auguste BL, Girsberger M, Kennedy C, Srithongkul T, McGrath-Chong M, Bargman J, et al. Are adverse events in newly trained home dialysis patients related to learning styles? A single centre retrospective study from Toronto, Canada. *BMJ open*. 2020; 10(1): e033315.

[84] Hercz G. The Trauma of Dialysis Initiation. *J Am Soc Nephrol*. 2017; 28(10): 2835-7.

[85] Bowman BT. Transitional Care Units: Greater Than the Sum of Their Parts. *Clin J Am Soc Nephrol*. 2019; 14(5): 765-7.

[86] Lockridge R, Weinhandl E, Kraus M, Schreiber M, Spry L, Tailor P, et al. A Systematic Approach To Promoting Home Hemodialysis during End Stage Kidney Disease. *Kidney360*. 2020; 1(9): 993-1001.

[87] Bowman B, Zheng S, Yang A, Schiller B, Morfin JA, Seek M, et al. Improving Incident ESRD Care Via a Transitional Care Unit. *Am J Kidney Dis*. 2018; 72(2): 278-83.

[88] Cherukuri S, Bajo M, Colussi G, Corciulo R, Fessi H, Ficheux M, et al. Home hemodialysis treatment and outcomes: retrospective analysis of the Knowledge to Improve Home Dialysis Network in Europe (KIHDNEy) cohort. *BMC Nephrol*. 2018; 19(1): 262.

[89] Auguste BL, Al-Muhaiteeb A, Chan CT. The Effect of Learning Styles on Adverse Events in Home Hemodialysis Patients. *Clin J Am Soc Nephrol*. 2018; 13(5): 782-3.

[90] Weinhandl ED, Collins AJ. Relative risk of home hemodialysis attrition in patients using a telehealth platform. *Hemodial Int*. 2018; 22(3): 318-27.

[91] Nadeau-Fredette AC, Chan CT, Bargman JM, Copland MA, Finkle SN, Oliver MJ, et al. Predictors of Care Gaps in Home Dialysis: The Home Dialysis Virtual Ward Study. *Am J Nephrol*. 2019; 50(5): 392-400.

[92] Saran R, Robinson B, Abbott KC, Agodoa LYC, Bhave N, Bragg-Gresham J, et al. US Renal Data System 2017 Annual Data Report: Epidemiology of Kidney Disease in the United States. *Am J Kidney Dis*. 2018; 71(3 Suppl 1): A7.

[93] Chan CT, Collins K, Ditschman EP, Koester-Wiedemann L, Saffer TL, Wallace E, et al. Overcoming Barriers for Uptake and Continued Use of Home Dialysis: An NKF-KDOQI Conference Report. *Am J Kidney Dis*. 2020; 75(6): 926-34.

[94] Walker RC, Howard K, Morton RL. Home hemodialysis: a comprehensive review of patient-centered and economic considerations. *Clinicoecon Outcomes Res*. 2017; 9: 149-61.

[95] Cafazzo JA, Leonard K, Easty AC, Rossos PG, Chan CT. Patient-perceived barriers to the adoption of nocturnal home hemodialysis. *Clin J Am Soc Nephrol*. 2009; 4(4): 784-9.

[96] Nickel M, Rideout W, Shah N, Reintjes F, Chen JZ, Burrell R, et al. Estimating patient-borne water and electricity costs in home hemodialysis: a simulation. *CMAJ Open*. 2017; 5(1): E61-E5.

[97] Chan CT, Wallace E, Golper TA, Rosner MH, Seshasai RK, Glickman JD, et al. Exploring Barriers and Potential Solutions in Home Dialysis: An NKF-KDOQI Conference Outcomes Report. *Am J Kidney Dis*. 2019; 73(3): 363-71.

[98] Golper TA. A View of the Bundle from a Home Dialysis Perspective: Present at the Creation. *Clin J Am Soc Nephrol*. 2018; 13(3): 471-3.

[99] Wilk AS, Hirth RA, Zhang W, Wheeler JRC, Turenne MN, Nahra TA, et al. Persistent Variation in Medicare Payment Authorization for Home Hemodialysis Treatments. *Health Serv Res*. 2018; 53(2): 649-70.

[100] Lin E, Cheng XS, Chin KK, Zubair T, Chertow GM, Bendavid E, et al. Home Dialysis in the Prospective Payment System Era. *J Am Soc Nephrol.* 2017; 28(10): 2993-3004.

[101] Gee PO. Kidney Health Initiative Roadmap for Kidney Replacement Therapy: A Patient's Perspective. *Clin J Am Soc Nephrol.* 2020; 15(5): 585-6.

[102] Patel S, Boehler A, Uehlecke N. A Vision for Advancing American Kidney Health: View from the US Department of Health and Human Services. *Clin J Am Soc Nephrol.* 2019; 14(12): 1789-91.

[103] Hippen BE, Reed AI, Ketchersid T, Maddux FW. Implications of the Advancing American Kidney Health Initiative for kidney transplant centers. *Am J Transplant.* 2020; 20(5): 1244-50.

[104] Evans RW, Manninen DL, Garrison LP, Jr., Hart LG, Blagg CR, Gutman RA, et al. The quality of life of patients with end-stage renal disease. *N Engl J Med.* 1985; 312(9): 553-9.

[105] McFarlane PA, Bayoumi AM, Pierratos A, Redelmeier DA. The impact of home nocturnal hemodialysis on end-stage renal disease therapies: A decision analysis. *Kidney Int.* 2006.

[106] Van Eps CL, Jeffries JK, Johnson DW, Campbell SB, Isbel NM, Mudge DW, et al. Quality of life and alternate nightly nocturnal home hemodialysis. *Hemodial Int.* 2010; 14(1): 29-38.

[107] Mohr PE, Neumann PJ, Franco SJ, Marainen J, Lockridge R, Ting G. The case for daily dialysis: its impact on costs and quality of life. *AmJ Kidney Dis.* 2001; 37(4): 777-89.

[108] Buoncristiani U, Cairo G, Giombini L, Quintaliani G, Bonforte G. Dramatic improvement of clinical-metabilic parameters and quality of life with daily dialysis. *Int J Artif Organs.* 1989; 12: 133-6.

[109] Kooistra MP, Vos J, Koomans HA, Vos PF. Daily home haemodialysis in The Netherlands: effects on metabolic control, haemodynamics, and quality of life. *Nephrol Dial Transplant.* 1998; 13(11): 2853-60.

[110] McPhatter LL, Lockridge RS, Jr., Albert J, Anderson H, Craft V, Jennings FM, et al. Nightly home hemodialysis: improvement in nutrition and quality of life. *Adv Ren Replace Ther.* 1999; 6(4): 358-65.

[111] Levenspiel B. My experience with daily dialysis. *ASAIO J.* 2001; 47(5): 469.

[112] Lindsay RM. Patient testimonials—'back in the land of the living'. As told by quotidian hemodialysis patients. *Contrib Nephrol.* 2004; 145: 117-21.

[113] Lindsay RM, Heidenheim PA, Nesrallah G, Garg AX, Suri R, Daily Hemodialysis Study Group London Health Sciences C. Minutes to recovery after a hemodialysis session: a simple health-related quality of life question that is reliable, valid, and sensitive to change. *Clin J Am Soc Nephrol.* 2006; 1(5): 952-9.

[114] McFarlane PA, Bayoumi AM, Pierratos A, Redelmeier DA. The quality of life and cost utility of home nocturnal and conventional in-center hemodialysis. *Kidney Int.* 2003; 64(3): 1004-11.

[115] Heidenheim AP, Muirhead N, Moist L, Lindsay RM. Patient quality of life on quotidian hemodialysis. *Am J Kidney Dis.* 2003; 42(1 Suppl): 36-41.

[116] Troidle L, Hotchkiss M, Finkelstein F. A thrice weekly in-center nocturnal hemodialysis program. *Adv Chronic Kidney Dis.* 2007; 14(3): 244-8.

[117] Manns BJ, Walsh MW, Culleton BF, Hemmelgarn B, Tonelli M, Schorr M, et al. Nocturnal hemodialysis does not improve overall measures of quality of life compared to conventional hemodialysis. *Kidney Int*. 2009; 75(5): 542-9.
[118] Unruh ML, Larive B, Chertow GM, Eggers PW, Garg AX, Gassman J, et al. Effects of 6-times-weekly versus 3-times-weekly hemodialysis on depressive symptoms and self-reported mental health: Frequent Hemodialysis Network (FHN) Trials. *Am J Kidney Dis*. 2013; 61(5): 748-58.
[119] Garg AX, Suri RS, Eggers P, Finkelstein FO, Greene T, Kimmel PL, et al. Patients receiving frequent hemodialysis have better health-related quality of life compared to patients receiving conventional hemodialysis. *Kidney Int*. 2017; 91(3): 746-54.
[120] Jardine MJ, Zuo L, Gray NA, de Zoysa JR, Chan CT, Gallagher MP, et al. A Trial of Extending Hemodialysis Hours and Quality of Life. *J Am Soc Nephrol*. 2017; 28(6): 1898-911.
[121] Smyth B, van den Broek-Best O, Hong D, Howard K, Rogers K, Zuo L, et al. Varying Association of Extended Hours Dialysis with Quality of Life. *Clin J Am Soc Nephrol*. 2019; 14(12): 1751-62.
[122] Trinh E, Chan CT. Intensive Home Hemodialysis Results in Regression of Left Ventricular Hypertrophy and Better Clinical Outcomes. *Am J Nephrol*. 2016; 44(4): 300-7.
[123] Chan CT, Floras JS, Miller JA, Richardson RM, Pierratos A. Regression of left ventricular hypertrophy after conversion to nocturnal hemodialysis. *Kidney Int*. 2002; 61(6): 2235-9.
[124] Fagugli RM, Reboldi G, Quintaliani G, Pasini P, Ciao G, Cicconi B, et al. Short daily hemodialysis: blood pressure control and left ventricular mass reduction in hypertensive hemodialysis patients. *Am J Kidney Dis*. 2001; 38(2): 371-6.
[125] Wald R, Goldstein MB, Wald RM, Harel Z, Kirpalani A, Perl J, et al. Correlates of left ventricular mass in chronic hemodialysis recipients. *Int J Cardiovasc Imaging*. 2014; 30(2): 349-56.
[126] Culleton BF, Walsh M, Klarenbach SW, Mortis G, Scott-Douglas N, Quinn RR, et al. Effect of frequent nocturnal hemodialysis vs conventional hemodialysis on left ventricular mass and quality of life: a randomized controlled trial. *JAMA*. 2007; 298(11): 1291-9.
[127] Wald R, Yan AT, Perl J, Jiang D, Donnelly MS, Leong-Poi H, et al. Regression of left ventricular mass following conversion from conventional hemodialysis to thrice weekly in-centre nocturnal hemodialysis. *BMC nephrology*. 2012; 13: 3.
[128] Ong JP, Wald R, Goldstein MB, Leipsic J, Kiaii M, Deva DP, et al. Left ventricular strain analysis using cardiac magnetic resonance imaging in patients undergoing in-centre nocturnal haemodialysis. *Nephrology (Carlton)*. 2019; 24(5): 557-63.
[129] Chan CT, Greene T, Chertow GM, Kliger AS, Stokes JB, Beck GJ, et al. Determinants of left ventricular mass in patients on hemodialysis: Frequent Hemodialysis Network (FHN) Trials. *Circ Cardiovasc Imaging*. 2012; 5(2): 251-61.
[130] Covic A, Goldsmith DJ, Georgescu G, Venning MC, Ackrill P. Echocardiographic findings in long-term, long-hour hemodialysis patients. *Clin Nephrol*. 1996; 45(2): 104-10.

[131] Karur GR, Wald R, Goldstein MB, Wald R, Jimenez-Juan L, Kiaii M, et al. Association between conversion to in-center nocturnal hemodialysis and right ventricular remodeling. *Nephrol Dial Transplant*. 2018; 33(6): 1010-6.

[132] Weinreich T, De los RT, Gauly A, Passlick-Deetjen J. Effects of an increase in time vs. frequency on cardiovascular parameters in chronic hemodialysis patients. *Clin Nephrol*. 2006; 66(6): 433-9.

[133] Fagugli RM, Pasini P, Pasticci F, Ciao G, Cicconi B, Buoncristiani U. Effects of short daily hemodialysis and extended standard hemodialysis on blood pressure and cardiac hypertrophy: a comparative study. *J Nephrol*. 2006; 19(1): 77-83.

[134] Liu F, Sun Y, Xu T, Sun L, Liu L, Sun W, et al. Effect of Nocturnal Hemodialysis versus Conventional Hemodialysis on End-Stage Renal Disease: A Meta-Analysis and Systematic Review. *PLoS One*. 2017; 12(1): e0169203.

[135] Susantitaphong P, Koulouridis I, Balk EM, Madias NE, Jaber BL. Effect of frequent or extended hemodialysis on cardiovascular parameters: a meta-analysis. *Am J Kidney Dis*. 2012; 59(5): 689-99.

[136] Dell'Italia LJ. The right ventricle: anatomy, physiology, and clinical importance. *Curr Probl Cardiol*. 1991; 16(10): 653-720.

[137] Chan CT, Kaysen GA, Beck GJ, Li M, Lo J, Rocco MV, et al. Changes in Biomarker Profile and Left Ventricular Hypertrophy Regression: Results from the Frequent Hemodialysis Network Trials. *Am J Nephrol*. 2018; 47(3): 208-17.

[138] Chan CT, Li GH, Valaperti A, Liu P. Intensive Hemodialysis Preserved Cardiac injury. *ASAIO J*. 2015; 61(5): 613-9.

[139] Roumeliotis A, Roumeliotis S, Chan C, Pierratos A. Cardiovascular Benefits of Extended-Time Nocturnal Hemodialysis. *Curr Vasc Pharmacol*. 2020.

[140] Inrig JK, Patel UD, Gillespie BS, Hasselblad V, Himmelfarb J, Reddan D, et al. Relationship between interdialytic weight gain and blood pressure among prevalent hemodialysis patients. *Am J Kidney Dis*. 2007; 50(1): 108-18, 18 e1-4.

[141] Merchant A, Wald R, Goldstein MB, Yuen D, Kirpalani A, Dacouris N, et al. Relationship between different blood pressure measurements and left ventricular mass by cardiac magnetic resonance imaging in end-stage renal disease. *J Am Soc Hypertens*. 2015; 9(4): 275-84.

[142] Charra B. Is there a magic in long nocturnal dialysis? *Contrib Nephrol*. 2005; 149: 100-6.

[143] Woods JD, Port FK, Orzol S, Buoncristiani U, Young E, Wolfe RA, et al. Clinical and biochemical correlates of starting "daily" hemodialysis. *Kidney Int*. 1999; 55(6): 2467-76.

[144] Buoncristiani U, Quintaliani G, Cozzari M, Giombini L, Ragaiolo M. Daily dialysis: long-term clinical metabolic results. *Kidney Int*. 1988; 24: S137-S40.

[145] Laurent G, Charra B. The results of an 8 h thrice weekly haemodialysis schedule. *Nephrol Dial Transplant*. 1998; 13 Suppl 6: 125-31.

[146] Nesrallah G, Suri R, Moist L, Kortas C, Lindsay RM. Volume control and blood pressure management in patients undergoing quotidian hemodialysis. *Am J Kidney Dis*. 2003; 42(1 Suppl): 13-7.

[147] Graham-Brown MP, Churchward DR, Smith AC, Baines RJ, Burton JO. A 4-month programme of in-centre nocturnal haemodialysis was associated with improvements in patient outcomes. *Clin Kidney J*. 2015; 8(6): 789-95.

[148] Thumfart J, Pommer W, Querfeld U, Muller D. Intensified hemodialysis in adults, and in children and adolescents. *Deutsches Arzteblatt international*. 2014; 111(14): 237-43.
[149] Walsh M, Culleton B, Tonelli M, Manns B. A systematic review of the effect of nocturnal hemodialysis on blood pressure, left ventricular hypertrophy, anemia, mineral metabolism, and health-related quality of life. *Kidney Int*. 2005; 67(4): 1500-8.
[150] Kotanko P, Garg AX, Depner T, Pierratos A, Chan CT, Levin NW, et al. Effects of frequent hemodialysis on blood pressure: Results from the randomized frequent hemodialysis network trials. *Hemodial Int*. 2015; 19(3): 386-401.
[151] Bugeja A, Dacouris N, Thomas A, Marticorena R, McFarlane P, Donnelly S, et al. In-center nocturnal hemodialysis: another option in the management of chronic kidney disease. *Clin J Am Soc Nephrol*. 2009; 4(4): 778-83.
[152] Chan CT, Harvey PJ, Picton P, Pierratos A, Miller JA, Floras JS. Short-term blood pressure, noradrenergic, and vascular effects of nocturnal home hemodialysis. *Hypertension*. 2003; 42(5): 925-31.
[153] Wald R, Goldstein MB, Perl J, Kiaii M, Yuen D, Wald RM, et al. The Association Between Conversion to In-centre Nocturnal Hemodialysis and Left Ventricular Mass Regression in Patients With End-Stage Renal Disease. *Can J Cardiol*. 2016; 32(3): 369-77.
[154] Demirci MS, Celik G, Ozkahya M, Tumuklu M, Toz H, Asci G, et al. Effects of thrice weekly nocturnal hemodialysis on arterial stiffness. *Atherosclerosis*. 2012; 220(2): 477-85.
[155] Charra B, Chazot C. The neglect of sodium restriction in dialysis patients: a short review. *Hemodial Int*. 2003; 7(4): 342-7.
[156] Ganesh SK, Stack AG, Levin NW, Hulbert-Shearon T, Port FK. Association of elevated serum PO(4), Ca x PO(4) product, and parathyroid hormone with cardiac mortality risk in chronic hemodialysis patients. *J Am Soc Nephrol*. 2001; 12(10): 2131-8.
[157] Yuen D, Pierratos A, Richardson RM, Chan CT. The natural history of coronary calcification progression in a cohort of nocturnal haemodialysis patients. *Nephrol Dial Transplant*. 2006; 21(5): 1407-12.
[158] Moe SM, O'Neill KD, Reslerova M, Fineberg N, Persohn S, Meyer CA. Natural history of vascular calcification in dialysis and transplant patients. *Nephrol Dial Transplant*. 2004; 19(9): 2387-93.
[159] Schnabel R, Blankenberg S, Lubos E, Lackner KJ, Rupprecht HJ, Espinola-Klein C, et al. Asymmetric dimethylarginine and the risk of cardiovascular events and death in patients with coronary artery disease: results from the AtheroGene Study. *Circ Res*. 2005; 97(5): e53-9.
[160] Chan CT, Harvey PJ, Boger R, Pierratos A, Floras JS. Dissociation between the short-term effects of nocturnal hemodialysis on endothelium dependent vasodilation and plasma ADMA. *Arterioscler Thromb Vasc Biol*. 2005; 25(12): 2685-6.
[161] Chan CT, Jain V, Picton P, Pierratos A, Floras JS. Nocturnal hemodialysis increases arterial baroreflex sensitivity and compliance and normalizes blood pressure of hypertensive patients with end-stage renal disease. *Kidney Int*. 2005; 68(1): 338-44.

[162] Szmitko PE, Fedak PW, Weisel RD, Stewart DJ, Kutryk MJ, Verma S. Endothelial progenitor cells: new hope for a broken heart. *Circulation*. 2003; 107(24): 3093-100.

[163] Sen S, McDonald SP, Coates PT, Bonder CS. Endothelial progenitor cells: novel biomarker and promising cell therapy for cardiovascular disease. *Clin Sci (Lond)*. 2011; 120(7): 263-83.

[164] Pauly RP, Chan CT. Reversing the risk factor paradox: is daily nocturnal hemodialysis the solution? *Semin Dial*. 2007; 20(6): 539-43.

[165] Verma S, Kuliszewski MA, Li SH, Szmitko PE, Zucco L, Wang CH, et al. C-reactive protein attenuates endothelial progenitor cell survival, differentiation, and function: further evidence of a mechanistic link between C-reactive protein and cardiovascular disease. *Circulation*. 2004; 109(17): 2058-67.

[166] Chan CT, Li SH, Verma S. Nocturnal hemodialysis is associated with restoration of impaired endothelial progenitor cell biology in end-stage renal disease. *Am J Physiol Renal Physiol*. 2005; 289(4): F679-84.

[167] Ranpuria R, Hall M, Chan CT, Unruh M. Heart rate variability (HRV) in kidney failure: measurement and consequences of reduced HRV. *Nephrol Dial Transplant*. 2008; 23(2): 444-9.

[168] Drawz PE, Babineau DC, Brecklin C, He J, Kallem RR, Soliman EZ, et al. Heart rate variability is a predictor of mortality in chronic kidney disease: a report from the CRIC Study. *Am J Nephrol*. 2013; 38(6): 517-28.

[169] Nishimura M, Hashimoto T, Kobayashi H, Fukuda T, Okino K, Yamamoto N, et al. Association between cardiovascular autonomic neuropathy and left ventricular hypertrophy in diabetic haemodialysis patients. *Nephrol Dial Transplant*. 2004; 19(10): 2532-8.

[170] Zoccali C, Mallamaci F, Parlongo S, Cutrupi S, Benedetto FA, Tripepi G, et al. Plasma norepinephrine predicts survival and incident cardiovascular events in patients with end-stage renal disease. *Circulation*. 2002; 105(11): 1354-9.

[171] Ferrario M, Raimann JG, Larive B, Pierratos A, Thijssen S, Rajagopalan S, et al. Non-Linear Heart Rate Variability Indices in the Frequent Hemodialysis Network Trials of Chronic Hemodialysis Patients. *Blood Purif*. 2015; 40(1): 99-108.

[172] Burton JO, Jefferies HJ, Selby NM, McIntyre CW. Hemodialysis-induced repetitive myocardial injury results in global and segmental reduction in systolic cardiac function. *Clin J Am Soc Nephrol*. 2009; 4(12): 1925-31.

[173] Jefferies HJ, Virk B, Schiller B, Moran J, McIntyre CW. Frequent hemodialysis schedules are associated with reduced levels of dialysis-induced cardiac injury (myocardial stunning). *Clin J Am Soc Nephrol*. 2011; 6(6): 1326-32.

[174] Chan CT, Chertow GM, Daugirdas JT, Greene TH, Kotanko P, Larive B, et al. Effects of daily hemodialysis on heart rate variability: results from the Frequent Hemodialysis Network (FHN) Daily Trial. *Nephrol Dial Transplant*. 2014; 29(1): 168-78.

[175] Zilch O, Vos PF, Oey PL, Cramer MJ, Ligtenberg G, Koomans HA, et al. Sympathetic hyperactivity in haemodialysis patients is reduced by short daily haemodialysis. *J Hypertens*. 2007; 25(6): 1285-9.

[176] Chan CT, Hanly P, Gabor J, Picton P, Pierratos A, Floras JS. Impact of nocturnal hemodialysis on the variability of heart rate and duration of hypoxemia during sleep. *Kidney Int*. 2004; 65(2): 661-5.

[177] Roumeliotis S, Dounousi E, Eleftheriadis T, Liakopoulos V. Association of the Inactive Circulating Matrix Gla Protein with Vitamin K Intake, Calcification, Mortality, and Cardiovascular Disease. A Review. *Int J Mol Sci*. 2019; 20(3).
[178] Al Hejaili F, Kortas C, Leitch R, Heidenheim AP, Clement L, Nesrallah G, et al. Nocturnal but not short hours quotidian hemodialysis requires an elevated dialysate calcium concentration. *J Am Soc Nephrol*. 2003; 14(9): 2322-8.
[179] Gangji AS, Windrim R, Gandhi S, Silverman JA, Chan CT. Successful pregnancy with nocturnal hemodialysis. *Am J Kidney Dis*. 2004; 44(5): 912-6.
[180] Block GA, Hulbert-Shearon TE, Levin NW, Port FK. Association of serum phosphorus and calcium x phosphate product with mortality risk in chronic hemodialysis patients: a national study. *Am J Kidney Dis*. 1998; 31(4): 607-17.
[181] Lockridge RS, Albert J, Anderson H, Barger T, Coffey L, Craft V, et al. Nightly Home Hemodialysis: Fifteen Months of Experience in Lynchburg, Virginia. *Home Hemodial Int*. 1999; 3(1): 23-8.
[182] Van Eps CL, Jeffries JK, Anderson JA, Bergin PT, Johnson DW, Campbell SB, et al. Mineral metabolism, bone histomorphometry and vascular calcification in alternate night nocturnal haemodialysis. *Nephrology (Carlton)*. 2007; 12(3): 224-33.
[183] Mucsi I, Hercz G, Uldall R, Ouwendyk M, Francoeur R, Pierratos A. Control of serum phosphate without any phosphate binders in patients treated with nocturnal hemodialysis. *Kidney Int*. 1998; 53(5): 1399-404.
[184] Lindsay RM, Alhejaili F, Nesrallah G, Leitch R, Clement L, Heidenheim AP, et al. Calcium and phosphate balance with quotidian hemodialysis. *Am J Kidney Dis*. 2003; 42(1 Suppl): 24-9.
[185] Walsh M, Manns BJ, Klarenbach S, Tonelli M, Hemmelgarn B, Culleton B. The effects of nocturnal compared with conventional hemodialysis on mineral metabolism: A randomized-controlled trial. *Hemodial Int*. 2010; 14(2): 174-81.
[186] Kim SJ, Goldstein M, Szabo T, Pierratos A. Resolution of massive uremic tumoral calcinosis with daily nocturnal home hemodialysis. *Am J Kidney Dis*. 2003; 41(3): E12.
[187] Toussaint N, Boddington J, Simmonds R, Waldron C, Somerville C, Agar J. Calcium phosphate metabolism and bone mineral density with nocturnal hemodialysis. *Hemodial Int*. 2006; 10(3): 280-6.
[188] Hanly PJ, Pierratos A. Improvement of sleep apnea in patients with chronic renal failure who undergo nocturnal hemodialysis. *N England J Med*. 2001; 344(2): 102-7.
[189] Kimmel PL, Miller G, Mendelson WB. Sleep apnea syndrome in chronic renal disease. *Am J Med*. 1989; 86(3): 308-14.
[190] Lyons OD, Inami T, Perger E, Yadollahi A, Chan CT, Bradley TD. The effect of fluid overload on sleep apnoea severity in haemodialysis patients. *Eur Respir J*. 2017; 49(4).
[191] Unruh ML. Sleep apnea and dialysis therapies: things that go bump in the night? *Hemodial Int*. 2007; 11(4): 369-78.
[192] Zoccali C, Mallamaci F, Tripepi G. Nocturnal hypoxemia: a neglected cardiovascular risk factor in end-stage renal disease? *Blood Purif*. 2002; 20(1): 120-3.
[193] Hanly P. Sleep disorders and home dialysis. *Adv Chronic Kid Dis*. 2009; 16(3): 179-88.
[194] Beecroft JM, Hoffstein V, Pierratos A, Chan CT, McFarlane P, Hanly PJ. Nocturnal haemodialysis increases pharyngeal size in patients with sleep apnoea and end-stage renal disease. *Nephrol Dial Transplant*. 2008; 23(2): 673-9.

[195] Elias RM, Chan CT, Paul N, Motwani SS, Kasai T, Gabriel JM, et al. Relationship of pharyngeal water content and jugular volume with severity of obstructive sleep apnea in renal failure. *Nephrol Dial Transplant.* 2013; 28(4): 937-44.
[196] Tang SC, Lam B, Ku PP, Leung WS, Chu CM, Ho YW, et al. Alleviation of Sleep Apnea in Patients with Chronic Renal Failure by Nocturnal Cycler-Assisted Peritoneal Dialysis Compared with Conventional Continuous Ambulatory Peritoneal Dialysis. *J Am Soc Nephrol.* 2006.
[197] Orr JE, Malhotra A, Sands SA. Pathogenesis of central and complex sleep apnoea. *Respirology.* 2017; 22(1): 43-52.
[198] Beecroft JM, Duffin J, Pierratos A, Chan CT, McFarlane P, Hanly PJ. Decreased chemosensitivity and improvement of sleep apnea by nocturnal hemodialysis. *Sleep medicine.* 2009; 10(1): 47-54.
[199] Schwartz DI, Pierratos A, Richardson RM, Fenton SS, Chan CT. Impact of nocturnal home hemodialysis on anemia management in patients with end-stage renal disease. *Clin Nephrol.* 2005; 63(3): 202-8.
[200] Ornt DB, Larive B, Rastogi A, Rashid M, Daugirdas JT, Hernandez A, et al. Impact of frequent hemodialysis on anemia management: results from the Frequent Hemodialysis Network (FHN) Trials. *Nephrol Dial Transplant.* 2013; 28(7): 1888-98.
[201] Ikizler TA, Flakoll PJ, Parker RA, Hakim RM. Amino acid and albumin losses during hemodialysis. *Kidney Int.* 1994; 46(3): 830-7.
[202] Galland R, Traeger J, Arkouche W, Cleaud C, Delawari E, Fouque D. Short daily hemodialysis rapidly improves nutritional status in hemodialysis patients. *Kidney Int.* 2001; 60(4): 1555-60.
[203] Chazot C, Vo VC, Blanc C, Hurot JM, Jean G, Vanel T, et al. Stability of nutritional parameters during a 5-year follow-up in patients treated with sequential long-hour hemodialysis. *Hemodial Int.* 2006; 10(4): 389-93.
[204] Spanner E, Suri R, Heidenheim AP, Lindsay RM. The impact of quotidian hemodialysis on nutrition. *Am J Kidney Dis.* 2003; 42(1 Suppl): 30-5.
[205] Raj DSC, Ouwendyk M, Francoeur R, Pierratos A. Plasma amino acid profile on nocturnal hemodialysis. *Blood Purif.* 2000; 18(2): 97-102.
[206] Rocco MV, Dwyer JT, Larive B, Greene T, Cockram DB, Chumlea WC, et al. The effect of dialysis dose and membrane flux on nutritional parameters in hemodialysis patients: Results of the HEMO Study. *Kidney Int.* 2004; 65(6): 2321-34.
[207] Agar JW, Pierratos A. Changes in hemoglobin and albumin concentration during nocturnal home hemodialysis. *Hemodial Int.* 2007; 11(3): 303-8.
[208] Kaysen GA, Greene T, Larive B, Mehta RL, Lindsay RM, Depner TA, et al. The effect of frequent hemodialysis on nutrition and body composition: frequent Hemodialysis Network Trial. *Kidney Int.* 2012; 82(1): 90-9.
[209] Gotch F, Kotanko P, Handelman G, Levin N. A kinetic model of calcium mass balance during dialysis therapy. *Blood Purif.* 2007; 25(1): 139-49.
[210] Holley JL, Schmidt RJ, Bender FH, Dumler F, Schiff M. Gynecologic and reproductive issues in women on dialysis. *Am J Kidney Dis.* 1997; 29(5): 685-90.
[211] Pinciaroli AR. Hormonal changes in daily hemodialysis. *Semin Dial.* 1999; 12(6): 455-61.
[212] Hou SH. Pregnancy in women on haemodialysis and peritoneal dialysis. *Baillieres Clin Obstet Gynaecol.* 1994; 8(2): 481-500.

[213] Barua M, Hladunewich M, Keunen J, Pierratos A, McFarlane P, Sood M, et al. Successful pregnancies on nocturnal home hemodialysis. *Clin J Am Soc Nephrol*. 2008; 3(2): 392-6.

[214] Hladunewich MA, Hou S, Odutayo A, Cornelis T, Pierratos A, Goldstein M, et al. Intensive hemodialysis associates with improved pregnancy outcomes: a Canadian and United States cohort comparison. *J Am Soc Nephrol*. 2014; 25(5): 1103-9.

[215] Moist LM, Port FK, Orzol SM, Young EW, Ostbye T, Wolfe RA, et al. Predictors of loss of residual renal function among new dialysis patients. *J Am Soc Nephrol*. 2000; 11(3): 556-64.

[216] Daugirdas JT, Greene T, Rocco MV, Kaysen GA, Depner TA, Levin NW, et al. Effect of frequent hemodialysis on residual kidney function. *Kidney Int*. 2013; 83(5): 949-58.

[217] Skeat L, Masterson R, Tjipto AC, Karschimkus C, Toussaint ND. Residual kidney function in nocturnal vs conventional haemodialysis patients: a prospective observational study. *Int Urol Nephrol*. 2020.

[218] Johansen KL, Zhang R, Huang Y, Chen SC, Blagg CR, Goldfarb-Rumyantzev AS, et al. Survival and hospitalization among patients using nocturnal and short daily compared to conventional hemodialysis: a USRDS study. *Kidney Int*. 2009; 76(9): 984-90.

[219] Pauly RP, Gill JS, Rose CL, Asad RA, Chery A, Pierratos A, et al. Survival among nocturnal home haemodialysis patients compared to kidney transplant recipients. *Nephrol Dial Transplant*. 2009; 24(9): 2915-9.

[220] Rocco MV, Daugirdas JT, Greene T, Lockridge RS, Chan C, Pierratos A, et al. Long-term Effects of Frequent Nocturnal Hemodialysis on Mortality: The Frequent Hemodialysis Network (FHN) Nocturnal Trial. *Am J Kidney Dis*. 2015; 66(3): 459-68.

[221] Choo SZ, See EJ, Simmonds RE, Somerville CA, Agar JWM. Nocturnal home haemodialysis: The 17 years experience of a single Australian dialysis service. *Nephrology (Carlton)*. 2019; 24(10): 1050-5.

[222] Lacson E, Jr., Xu J, Suri RS, Nesrallah G, Lindsay R, Garg AX, et al. Survival with three-times weekly in-center nocturnal versus conventional hemodialysis. *J Am Soc Nephrol*. 2012; 23(4): 687-95.

[223] Lacson E, Jr., Wang W, Lester K, Ofsthun N, Lazarus JM, Hakim RM. Outcomes associated with in-center nocturnal hemodialysis from a large multicenter program. *Clin J Am Soc Nephrol*. 2010; 5(2): 220-6.

[224] Tennankore KK, Kim SJ, Baer HJ, Chan CT. Survival and hospitalization for intensive home hemodialysis compared with kidney transplantation. *J Am Soc Nephrol*. 2014; 25(9): 2113-20.

[225] Nishio-Lucar AG, Bose S, Lyons G, Awuah KT, Ma JZ, Lockridge RS, Jr. Intensive Home Hemodialysis Survival Comparable to Deceased Donor Kidney Transplantation. *Kidney Int Rep*. 2020; 5(3): 296-306.

[226] Blagg CR, Kjellstrand CM, Ting GO, Young BA. Comparison of survival between short-daily hemodialysis and conventional hemodialysis using the standardized mortality ratio. *Hemodial Int*. 2006; 10(4): 371-4.

[227] Kjellstrand CM, Buoncristiani U, Ting G, Traeger J, Piccoli GB, Sibai-Galland R, et al. Short daily haemodialysis: survival in 415 patients treated for 1006 patient-years. *Nephrol Dial Transplant*. 2008; 23(10): 3283-9.

[228] Kjellstrand C, Buoncristiani U, Ting G, Traeger J, Piccoli GB, Sibai-Galland R, et al. Survival with short-daily hemodialysis: association of time, site, and dose of dialysis. *Hemodial Int*. 2010; 14(4): 464-70.

[229] Suri RS, Li L, Nesrallah GE. The risk of hospitalization and modality failure with home dialysis. *Kidney Int*. 2015; 88(2): 360-8.

[230] Weinhandl ED, Nieman KM, Gilbertson DT, Collins AJ. Hospitalization in daily home hemodialysis and matched thrice-weekly in-center hemodialysis patients. *Am J Kidney Dis*. 2015; 65(1): 98-108.

[231] Weinhandl ED, Liu J, Gilbertson DT, Arneson TJ, Collins AJ. Survival in daily home hemodialysis and matched thrice-weekly in-center hemodialysis patients. *J Am Soc Nephrol*. 2012; 23(5): 895-904.

[232] Chertow GM, Levin NW, Beck GJ, Daugirdas JT, Eggers PW, Kliger AS, et al. Long-Term Effects of Frequent In-Center Hemodialysis. *J Am Soc Nephrol*. 2016; 27(6): 1830-6.

[233] Nesrallah GE, Lindsay RM, Cuerden MS, Garg AX, Port F, Austin PC, et al. Intensive hemodialysis associates with improved survival compared with conventional hemodialysis. *J Am Soc Nephrol*. 2012; 23(4): 696-705.

[234] Jun M, Jardine MJ, Gray N, Masterson R, Kerr PG, Agar JW, et al. Outcomes of extended-hours hemodialysis performed predominantly at home. *Am J Kidney Dis*. 2013; 61(2): 247-53.

[235] Marshall MR, Byrne BG, Kerr PG, McDonald SP. Associations of hemodialysis dose and session length with mortality risk in Australian and New Zealand patients. *Kidney Int*. 2006; 69(7): 1229-36.

[236] Saran R, Bragg-Gresham JL, Levin NW, Twardowski ZJ, Wizemann V, Saito A, et al. Longer treatment time and slower ultrafiltration in hemodialysis: associations with reduced mortality in the DOPPS. *Kidney Int*. 2006; 69(7): 1222-8.

[237] Nadeau-Fredette AC, Hawley CM, Pascoe EM, Chan CT, Clayton PA, Polkinghorne KR, et al. An Incident Cohort Study Comparing Survival on Home Hemodialysis and Peritoneal Dialysis (Australia and New Zealand Dialysis and Transplantation Registry). *Clin J Am Soc Nephrol*. 2015; 10(8): 1397-407.

[238] Miller BW, Himmele R, Sawin DA, Kim J, Kossmann RJ. Choosing Home Hemodialysis: A Critical Review of Patient Outcomes. *Blood Purif*. 2018; 45(1-3): 224-9.

[239] Choi SJ, Obi Y, Ko GJ, You AS, Eriguchi R, Wang M, et al. Comparing Patient Survival of Home Hemodialysis and Peritoneal Dialysis Patients. *Am J Nephrol*. 2020; 51(3): 192-200.

[240] Tennankore KK, Na Y, Wald R, Chan CT, Perl J. Short daily-, nocturnal- and conventional-home hemodialysis have similar patient and treatment survival. *Kidney Int*. 2018; 93(1): 188-94.

[241] Pauly RP, Rosychuk RJ, Usman I, Reintjes F, Muneer M, Chan CT, et al. Technique Failure in a Multicenter Canadian Home Hemodialysis Cohort. *Am J Kidney Dis*. 2019; 73(2): 230-9.

[242] Seshasai RK, Mitra N, Chaknos CM, Li J, Wirtalla C, Negoianu D, et al. Factors Associated With Discontinuation of Home Hemodialysis. *Am J Kidney Dis*. 2016; 67(4): 629-37.

[243] Vinson AJ, Perl J, Tennankore KK. Survival Comparisons of Home Dialysis Versus In-Center Hemodialysis: A Narrative Review. *Can J Kidney Health Dis*. 2019; 6: 2054358119861941.

In: Issues in Kidney Disease – Dialysis
Editors: Stephen Z. Fadem and José A. Moura-Neto
ISBN: 978-1-68507-000-7

Chapter 12

HOME HEMODIALYSIS

Ankur Shah[1], MD, Devin McKelvey[2], DO and Rebecca Kurnik Seshasai[2,*], MD

[1]Warren Alpert Medical School of Brown University, Providence, RI, USA
[2]Perelman School of Medicine at the University of Pennsylvania, Philadelphia, PA, USA

ABSTRACT

The original outpatient hemodialysis modality, home hemodialysis, has seen a revitalization in the last decade in the United States. Evidence is limited but points to improved patient quality of life, better blood pressure control, better phosphorus control, LV mass reduction, opportunity for employment, and greater cost effectiveness compared to traditional in-center hemodialysis. Treatment schedules include short daily hemodialysis, nocturnal hemodialysis, hybrid therapies, and home adapted thrice weekly conventional hemodialysis. There are a number of FDA approved devices on the market as well as multiple devices currently seeking approval. Each device has a different approach in regards to the prescription to achieve adequate dialysis, including small solutes, middle molecules, fluid removal, and consideration to burden of treatment. In addition to individual patient considerations, program development and retention efforts are necessary to grow and maintain a home hemodialysis program and these efforts are detailed in the following chapter.

Keywords: dialysis, home hemodialysis, chronic kidney disease

INTRODUCTION

First utilized in 1963, home hemodialysis was the predominant dialysis modality in the United States (US) until 1972 when an amendment to the Medicare Social Security Act resulted in fiscal benefits supporting in-center hemodialysis [1]. In the early days of dialysis,

* Corresponding Author's E-mail: rebecca.seshasai@pennmedicine.upenn.edu.

approximately 40 percent of dialysis patients dialyzed at home via hemodialysis [1], although its prevalence fell significantly from that level. Home hemodialysis can be performed on several different schedules, including thrice weekly conventional, short daily, nocturnal, and hybrid. Short daily hemodialysis was initially described in 1969 but had a revival in 1990s as it became more fiscally viable, owing to cost savings in supplies and labor [2]. Daily nocturnal hemodialysis was reintroduced in Toronto in 1994 [3]. In the past decade, there has been a resurgence of home HD with more patient friendly equipment available as well as improved financial incentives in the US under the expanded prospective payment system [4, 5].

There has been a recent renewal in interest in home modalities in the United States with the 2019 executive order on Advancing American Kidney Health which set forth a goal of improving access to and quality of person centered treatments for kidney failure, with a specific target of having 80 percent of new ESKD patients in 2025 dialyzing at home or receiving a preemptive kidney transplant. In order to achieve this goal, reimbursement models that support dialysis at home are being developed.

In this chapter, we provide an overview of the most frequently used home hemodialysis regimens, available technology, epidemiology, patient outcomes, program factors including recruitment, training, discontinuation, and safety.

Epidemiology and Demographics

Despite its early success, there has been low usage of home hemodialysis (HHD) in the United States. According to the US Renal Data System [6], there were approximately 124,500 incident and 726,331 prevalent cases of ESKD in the US in 2017. More than half (62.7%) of all prevalent ESKD patients in the US were treated by HD (98 percent of whom dialyze in-center, and 2 percent dialyze at home). In the last decade, there has been significant growth in the use of home hemodialysis with a 120.8% increase in prevalence in 2017 compared to 2007. Four percent of incident ESKD patients in 2017 used home hemodialysis as a modality. Factors positively associated with increased home hemodialysis at the facility level include prevalence of peritoneal dialysis, unit size, patient employment, younger patient population, and vintage of unit [7]. Significant international variations exist in home hemodialysis uptake with New Zealand, Australia, Finland, Denmark, and Canada having the highest utilization [8].

Definition and Equipment

Home hemodialysis is a modality of kidney replacement in which hemodialysis is performed in the home setting. This can be done with the assistance of a care partner or solo. Several different schedules are commonly used, including conventional thrice weekly dialysis, short daily hemodialysis, and nocturnal hemodialysis. Short-daily hemodialysis (SDHD) typically consists of two-to-three hour sessions, 5-6 days per week and nocturnal hemodialysis (NHD) is performed overnight while sleeping and consists of six-to-ten hour sessions, generally four to six nights per week. These modalities are both performed at home and generally considered together when discussing home hemodialysis. Frequent hemodialysis is defined as hemodialysis performed more than thrice weekly and is often discussed in tandem with home hemodialysis as it is most often performed in the home setting. In the United States, home hemodialysis is most frequently performed using the low dialysate volume approach, in contrast to the conventional hemodialysis approach using much larger dialysate volumes per treatment [9]. The low dialysate volume approach uses flow rates that are much slower than the blood flow rate, resulting in an increased extraction rate of solutes and higher saturation of dialysate. This approach results in less dialysate used, at the expense of time. Conventional hemodialysis uses higher dialysate flow rates, sacrificing efficiency for time. As with in-center hemodialysis, vascular access with an arteriovenous fistula, arteriovenous graft, or tunneled central venous catheter is necessary. Arteriovenous fistula is the preferred access due to infection risk and longevity concerns.

While any conventional hemodialysis machine can be used in the home setting, this is not ideal for most patients as the conventional machines are large, heavy, and complex. Kjellstrand described the ideal HHD machine as one that allows a flexible regimen, is simple to set up and take down, allows patient controlled infusions, does not require systemic anticoagulation, is interactive, and has safety features including requiring minimal or no disinfection [10]. A number of dialysis machines are available for home use. These include machines that are optimized for the low dialysate volume approach and machines that are optimized for conventional blood and dialysate flows.

Low Dialysate Volume Approach

The low dialysate volume approach (LDVA) is broadly used in two different manners. The first, short daily hemodialysis, is an approach in which shorter more frequent treatments are performed. With this approach, flexibility is allowed in the choice of treatment days and times. Nocturnal hemodialysis is an alternate approach in which dialysis treatments are completed overnight. The following devices are typically used with the low dialysate volume approach.

NxStage – The NxStage System One consists of a cycler with a user-friendly interface that administers the therapy and disposable cartridges. The device is compact and does not require modifications to home plumbing systems. Blood flow rates can range from 100ml/min to 300ml/min. Dialysate flow rate is up to 300ml/min. Dialysate is available either in sterile prepared bags or can be generated using the PureFlow SL system which can generate batches of up to 60L of dialysate at a time, which can be used up to 96 hours after generation. The PureFlow SL can generate pure dialysate from regular tap water. Using the Nx2me connected health system treatment data is easily reviewed via an iPad device and remotely transferred to the dialysis unit staff. For patients choosing nocturnal therapies, a venous needle dislodgement device and fluid detection system are required; an infusion pump, cartridge with heparin line, and dual lumen needle are available. A unique aspect is the availability of single needle dialysis. This device is FDA approved in the USA.

Outset Tablo – The outset tablo is a cartridge-based device that was developed with the user interface and simplicity in mind. Touchscreen guidance is available to the end user and the system is wholly contained requiring only an electrical outlet and tap water. The machine produces ultrapure dialysate in real time from tap water. Blood flow rate ranges 50-400 ml/min and dialysate flow rate is up to 300ml/min. The device is FDA approved in the US for home use. Features include an integrated blood pressure cuff, automated saline bolus and tracking, one-touch rinseback, and automated self-cleaning. Similar to the NxStage System One, it can be used for both home dialysis and continuous renal replacement therapy in critical care settings.

Physidia S3 – The Physidia S3 is a device that is developed particularly for use in SDHD or every other day dialysis with the LDVA. The device is the lightest HHD machine, weighing only 23 kg. It includes a cartridge system with automated priming. On-line dialysate generation is not available, with only pre-bagged sterile dialysate available, however this dialysate meets ultrapure standards. Blood flow rate ranges 200-350 ml/min and dialysate flow rate is up to 200ml/min. This is the only HHD machine that can perform hemodiafiltration in addition of hemodialysis. It is approved for use in Europe, but FDA approval is still pending in the US.

Quanta SC+ – The Quanta SC+ is a compact, lightweight touchscreen-based device that uses a single-use cartridge-based design. The device is 20.4 x 14.5 x 21.6 inches and weighs 32 kg. Blood flow rates up to 450ml/min, dialysate flow rates up to 500ml/min, and treatments up to 8 hours in duration are supported. The device is notable for its simplicity with only 11 steps required for the full treatment. The device requires a standalone reverse osmosis device for water preparation or can be connected to a clinic central water feed. This device is available in the UK and Europe but not FDA approved in the USA.

Conventional Approach in Home

Fresenius 2008K@home – The Fresenius 2008K@home is a modified in-center hemodialysis machine that has been simplified for home use. Similar to standard in-center hemodialysis equipment, a stand-alone water purification system is needed. The machine has been modified with a simpler interface and has an automated prime, rinse back, blood pressure pump, and heparin pump integrated into the device. Dialysate concentration can be adjusted similar to in-center equipment. Portability is limited and often renovation in the home is needed.

The LDVA can be used with the 2008K@home or dialysis can be performed in a manner that mimics conventional in-center hemodialysis.

Clinical Outcomes

SDHD and NHD are generally studied independently of each other and have demonstrated different outcomes in observational studies. For the purpose of this chapter we will evaluate both of these home modalities.

Frequent Hemodialysis Network

In 2010 and 2011, the Frequent Hemodialysis Network (FHN), two randomized controlled trials, evaluated the effects of short daily hemodialysis and nocturnal hemodialysis versus conventional thrice weekly HD. In the FHN daily trial, a group of patients was randomized into an in-center SDHD arm with 125 patients receiving HD 6 days per week (average 5.2 sessions per week) and a CHD arm with 120 patients received standard thrice-weekly dialysis. The nocturnal trial had a total of 87 patients that were randomized into NHD 5-6 nights per week (n = 45) vs standard thrice weekly CHD (n = 42). The primary outcomes evaluated in both studies were: 1) All-cause mortality at 12 months or one-year change in left ventricular mass; and 2) All-cause mortality or one-year change in physical health based on RAND health survey data [11].

Compared to the CHD, there were significant improvements in the primary composite outcomes for the SDHD arm in the daily trial, while the NHD arm in the nocturnal study showed no significant improvements. Secondary outcomes evaluated included cognitive performance, depression, nutrition, mineral biomarkers, anemia control, blood pressure, hospitalization rates, and vascular access interventions which are discussed in detail in the following sections. There are several important limitations to the FHN nocturnal trial. One, there were likely type II error from low enrollment. Two, more than 50% of participants were new to dialysis and may have more residual kidney function, which could have blunted the improvement seen. Finally, although the control CHD group was intended to be in-center, in the nocturnal arm, many performed these treatments at home, which may have led to less of a difference seen between the two groups.

Left Ventricular Mass

Cardiac remodeling, particularly left ventricular hypertrophy, is highly prevalent in ESKD and associated with increased cardiac mortality [12]. Several studies have sought to evaluate the role of home hemodialysis on left ventricular mass. In 2007, Culleton et al. reported the results of a two-group, parallel, randomized controlled trial at two Canadian university centers [13]. A total of 52 patients were enrolled between August 2004 and December 2006, receiving either frequent NHD or CHD with the primary goal in evaluating change in left ventricular mass as assessed by cardiac MRI. The study showed the frequent NHD was associated with significant improvements in systolic blood pressure ($p = 0.01$), reduction in prescribed antihypertensives in 16 of the 26 in the NHD group compared to 3 of the 25 CHD group ($p = < 0.001$), and a significant improvement in left ventricular mass with a mean left ventricular mass (LVM) difference of 15.3 g ($p = 0.04$) between the groups. These findings are congruent with a previous observational study showing improvements in blood pressure ($p = 0.004$) and LVM ($p = 0.001$) after conversion from CHD to NHD [14].

The effects of SDHD on LVM has been evaluated in prospective observational studies as well. In 2005, Ayus et al. assessed the effects of SDHD, 6 sessions/week of 3 hours duration, and CHD, 3 sessions/week of 4 hours duration on LVM [15]. A total of 26 SDHD patients and 54 matched CHD patients were enrolled and the primary outcomes of LVM index and C-reactive protein levels were assessed at 12 months. The study noted significant decrease in LVM of 30% in the SDHD compared to the matched cohort of CHD patients. This was congruous with an earlier small study of 12 CHD patients that were randomly assigned in a cross over fashion to receive six months of CHD followed by six months of SDHD showing significant improvement in LVM index ($p = 0.01$) after the SDHD period [16].

Survival

Several large retrospective cohorts have been evaluated for difference in mortality amongst dialysis modality. Notably, these studies are severely limited by residual confounding. Marshall et al. reported the outcomes of 26,016 patients with 856,007 patient-months of follow-up. Compared to CHD, home hemodialysis patients had significant improvement in adjusted mortality (HR 0.51 95% CI, 0.44-0.59) [17]. A longitudinal study of NHD patients on a regimen of 6-10 hours per night, 6 nights per week over a 5.5-year period showed statistically significant improvement in the need for antihypertensive medications and phosphate binders, SF36 scores, calcium/phosphorus product, blood pressure, number of hospital admissions, and number of days of stay in the hospital. These improvements were associated with an improved mortality rate of 2.4% deaths per patient-year (95% CI 0.9% - 9.4%) [9]. In another study of 415 patients, over 1,006 patient-years, survival of patients on SDHD (n = 265) was 2-3 times better when compared to CHD (n = 150) [18].

Blood Pressure

Poorly controlled blood pressure is a major cause of morbidity and mortality in ESKD patients [19]. The prevalence of hypertension in the ESKD population from 2010-2012 was 86% as assessed by the ESRD medical evidence report [20]. In the DOPPS (Dialysis Outcomes and Practice Patterns Study) the prevalence of hypertension in ESKD patients was at least 60% as of 2015 [21]. Furthermore, it has been shown that active management of hypertension in ESKD patients on HD leads to significant reduction in mortality and cardiac events. In 2009, a meta-analysis looking at 1,679 dialysis patients showed an improvement in cardiovascular events ($p = 0.009$), all-cause mortality ($p = 0.014$), and cardiovascular mortality ($p = 0.044$) in patients actively treated for hypertension compared to control regimens [22].

It is clear that practices designed to better control blood pressure in ESKD patients will lead to improved outcomes for these patients. In a 2015 follow up to FHN, Kotanko et al. assessed the effects of frequent HD on blood pressure [23]. The more frequent HD patients, including both the SDHD and NHD patients, were noted to require significantly fewer antihypertensive medications; and in the first two months of FHN, the home dialysis patients were noted to have reduced pre-dialysis systolic blood pressures (SDHD 7.7 mmHg and NHD 7.3 mmHg) compared to the CHD group. In further analysis of the FREEDOM study, patients were noted to have a reduction in antihypertensive medications with daily home dialysis compared to CHD, with the number of patients on no antihypertensive medications rising from 21% to 47% [24].

Phosphate Control

Improvement in phosphorus control has been shown in many studies with home hemodialysis, though there is variation based on modality, likely owing to the mechanism of phosphorus removal on dialysis. Dialytic phosphate clearance is achieved in two phases with initial removal from the extracellular fluid, followed by a delayed secondary phase as the intracellular equilibrates and phosphate shifts extracellularly. It is thought that this second, slower phase is best addressed with longer treatments and may benefit more from NHD, with its generally longer treatment times, compared to shorter treatments on SDHD.

SDHD does show modest improvement in phosphorus control and possibly some reduction in phosphate binder use [15, 25]. However, the response is not as robust as in NHD. Culleton et al. showed that there was significant improvement in phosphorous levels and decreased/discontinued phosphate binders in 19 of the 26 patients in the NHD arm compared to 3 of the 25 patients in the CHD arm ($p = 0.001$) [13]. In addition, 73% of the 87 patients in the FHN trial had improvement in their phosphorus levels to the point of not requiring phosphorus binders at all, and 42% even required supplemental phosphorus to maintain normal levels [25]. Patients using NHD often require fewer, if any, phosphorus binders and are able to follow a much more liberal diet [15]. Patients receiving NHD can even require the addition of phosphate to dialysate to avoid overt hypophosphatemia.

Obstructive Sleep Apnea/Restless Leg Syndrome

Sleep disturbances, including sleep apnea and restless leg syndrome (RLS), are common, underdiagnosed problems in ESKD patients, and can lead to significant morbidity and mortality if left untreated. In a survey of 883 Italian patients on either HD or hemodiafiltration therapy, the prevalence of sleep apnea was 24%, according to the Berlin questionnaire [26]. However, this may be an underestimation based on self-reporting bias. A 2015 study of 104 Swiss patients on CHD showed the prevalence of sleep apnea to be 56% when tested using nocturnal polygraphy [27]. Only 19% of the patients tested had been aware of their diagnosis.

In a 2001 study of 14 patients who converted from CHD to NHD for 8-10 hours per night, episodes of sleep apnea and hypopnea per hour, as well as hypoxia, were improved with NHD. With CHD, there was a mean of 25 ± 25 (SD) episodes of apnea and hypopnea per hour, whereas with nocturnal HD there was a mean of 8 ± 8 episodes per hour. Oxygen saturation during sleep was higher with NHD compared to CHD (95.9% vs 93.8%) [28].

Restless leg syndrome is also common in ESKD patients. A recent study shows the prevalence of RLS to be 18.7% in ESKD patients [29]. However, it was much higher, 40%, in the FREEDOM trial [30]. This condition can impact level of fatigue, mood, and overall quality of life [29]. In a follow up to the FREEDOM trial analysis, Jaber et al. noted significant improvements in the prevalence and severity of RLS and other sleep disturbances [30].

Quality of Life

Overall quality of life is a wide-ranging topic that is difficult to assess and frequently under-addressed. Patients on conventional HD are frequently unable to work given the time requirements for in-center HD. Patients on home hemodialysis on the other hand have much greater flexibility in terms of when they complete their sessions. This allows for more time with family and friends, as well as maintaining the ability to work and earn a living, bringing with them all the psycho-social benefits that these entail. In the FREEDOM study group looking at the effect of daily hemodialysis on quality of life and depression symptoms, patients noted a significant improvement in quality of life as measured by the SF-36 survey at the initiation of SDHD. There was a robust response measured out at 4 months and 12 months after initiation

[24]. In a follow-up analysis assessing depressive symptoms in these patients, there was noted improvements in depressive symptoms using the Beck Depression Inventory (BDI) survey [24].

Fertility

In both males and females, ESKD is associated with decreased fertility through a multitude of factors. In a registry of 6,230 women in the United States between the ages of 14 and 44 years receiving either hemodialysis or peritoneal dialysis between 1992 and 1996, pregnancy was observed in only 2% [31]. That same year, a Belgian study showed an incidence of pregnancy in just 0.3 per 100 patients years in 1,472 women between the ages of 18 and 44 from 1975 through 1999 [32]. There is limited data on improvements in fertility rates among home hemodialysis patients. A small 2008 study by Barua et al. of 45 women receiving NHD showed a conception rate of 15.6% [33].

Maternal/Fetal Outcomes

In addition to poor fertility rates among CHD patients, pregnancy in ESKD is associated with an exceedingly high infant mortality rate compared to the non-dialysis population. In a 1994 survey of 1,281 women of childbearing age on CHD, only 1.5% became pregnant and of these only 37% resulted in surviving infants [31]. Jesudason et al. noted that women who conceived before starting dialysis had a significantly higher live birth rate of 91% compared to 63% in women who conceived after initiating dialysis [34]. This increase in infant mortality was largely due to significantly higher rates of early pregnancy loss before 20 weeks.

Home hemodialysis, both SDHD and NHD, has been shown to have a positive effect on maternal-fetal outcomes with increased likelihood of surviving pregnancies, perhaps owing to better volume and blood pressure control, normalized BUN, improved endothelial function, and possibly reduced inflammation, though the exact mechanism is unclear [9]. A study published in 2014 comparing more intensive hemodialysis regimens in Canada to more conventional hemodialysis regimens in America showed significant improvement in live birth rates (86.4% compared to 61.4%, $p = 0.03$) [35]. Interestingly, a dose response curve was noted showing dialysis intensity directly correlated to pregnancy outcomes, with live birth rates of 48% in women dialyzed ≤ 20 hours per week and 85% in women dialyzed > 36 hours per week ($p = 0.02$). In line with these findings, Barua et al. noted in a study consisting of five pregnant patients on NHD that there were six live births out of seven pregnancies with few maternal-fetal complications [33].

Dosing and Adequacy

A dialysis prescription can be considered adequate if it provides adequate solute removal and fluid removal while allowing the patient to achieve their goals, particularly considering quality of life. A prescription that is adequate for one patient may not be for another and a prescription that is adequate in one aspect, e.g., kt/v urea, may not be in another, e.g., fluid removal or burden.

Small Solute

Small solute clearance in practice has become synonymous with kt/v urea; however, it should be noted that urea is not the only small uremic solute. In fact, high degrees of azotemia can be tolerated [36]. In-center hemodialysis treatments are evaluated with a single pool kt/v (spkt/v), but these cannot merely be added together to compare more frequent treatments. Patients dialyzing more frequently need to be equilibrated to the same amount of time, thus the use of a weekly kt/v urea or standard kt/v (std kt/v). The std kt/v is the same for all modalities that produces the same mid-week pre-dialysis BUN. While this model has not been clinically validated, KDOQI guidelines recommend a std kt/v of 2.0 as this is the equivalent of three treatments a week achieving a spkt/v of 1.2, the KDOQI guideline for in-center hemodialysis [37]. A number of Kt/v pitfalls should be noted, including the limited evidence of toxicity of urea, the kinetics of urea not representative of all uremic solutes, the effects of edema, frailty, and obesity on the relation between the Watson equation derived V and the volume of distribution of urea, and the assumption that a single treatment approximates all treatments [38-40].

Middle Molecule

Middle molecules are defined as molecules between 500 Daltons and 60 kilodaltons in size. Two classically described examples are B2-Microglobulin and Vitamin B12. Small molecules with significant protein binding or large volume of distribution can have similar clearance characteristics to middle molecules, an example of which is phosphate. Increasing treatment time significantly increases middle molecule clearance, a possible advantage of nocturnal hemodialysis [41].

Volume

Perhaps the greatest benefit of home dialysis is in control of hypervolemia. Sodium can be considered to be the most overlooked uremic toxin, and patients receiving shorter, more frequent therapies are less reliant on plasma refill during the treatment. Evidence from in-center hemodialysis has demonstrated that increasing ultrafiltration rates are associated with worsening mortality, and maintenance of ultrafiltration rate below 10-13 ml/kg/min should be maintained [42]. Patients receiving nocturnal hemodialysis rarely encounter this issue as their weekly time on dialysis but are typically 2-3 times longer than that of patients receiving SDHD or conventional hemodialysis. If intradialytic weight gain regularly exceeds this rate, then dialysis can be extended, additional treatments added, or diet can be addressed.

As discussed earlier in this chapter, patients dialyzing via SDHD or nocturnal hemodialysis require significantly fewer hypertension medications [13, 14, 16]. When transitioning a patient to either of these modalities, antihypertensives should be decreased by 50%. Most patients will see an early reduction in dry weight followed by a later gain in tissue mass and increase in dry weight without accompanying edema or hypertension. Patients dialyzed with nocturnal home hemodialysis can often significantly reduce the number of blood pressure medications they require.

Conventional Prescription

When using the Fresenius 2008K@home or conventional hemodialysis equipment, a conventional in-center hemodialysis prescription is used. Typically, treatments are 3-4 hours with blood flow rates of approximately 400-450 ml/min and dialysate flow rates of 600-800 ml/min. If adequacy is not met, blood flow rate, dialysate flow rate, or time can be increased. Dialysate composition is varied to maintain normokalemia and prevent acidemia or alkalemia. Dialysate sodium, potassium, bicarbonate, and calcium can all be individualized.

LDVA Prescription

In contrast with the traditional approach, the low dialysate volume approach decreases the dialysate flow increasing the contact time of blood and dialysate and therefore increases the saturation of dialysate. In this approach, water is conserved, and saturation is greater than in hemodialysis, at the cost of time. The dialysis prescription when using the low dialysate volume approach should achieve normalization of potassium, acid base status, uremic symptoms, and euvolemia. In the US, a weekly standard kt/v urea of 2.1 is most commonly used as a surrogate of adequacy. In order to obtain a weekly standard kt/v urea of 2.1, single pool kt/v needs to be 1.2 if dialyzing thrice weekly, approximately 0.75 if dialyzing 4 times weekly, approximately 0.6 if dialyzing 5 times weekly, and approximately 0.5 if dialyzing 6 times weekly. Single pool kt/v urea cannot simply be added from multiple treatments to equal a weekly kt/v urea as this does not account for time that has passed while not on dialysis.

The variables utilized in the prescription vary with the equipment being used for the home hemodialysis treatments. NxStage inputs include blood flow rate, total dialysate volume, and flow fraction while other machines use blood flow rate, dialysate flow rate, and time. Flow fraction is defined as the ratio of dialysate flow rate to blood flow rate and can be used to estimate urea saturation of dialysate. Conceptually a fixed flow fraction guarantees that clearance will not be sacrificed if blood flow rate is limited as time will be extended. One can convert amongst these inputs using the following equations.

Flow Fraction x Blood Flow Rate = Dialysate Flow Rate
Time x Dialysate Flow Rate = Total Volume

In the low dialysate volume approach, flow fractions of 0.3-0.5 are typically used while in the standard approach flow fraction is typically 1.5 to 2. A flow fraction of 0.3-0.5 results in a dialysate urea saturation of 85-93%. A flow fraction of 1.5 to 2 results in a dialysate urea saturation far lower.

Patient Recruitment

All patients should be offered home dialysis modalities and provided education in the advanced stages of chronic kidney disease. We specifically entitled this section "patient recruitment" and not "patient selection" because we feel patients should not be selected as appropriate for the modality. Instead, patients should be educated so that they can make an informed choice. Patients with CKD 4 and 5 should attend at least one CKD education session, but several can be very helpful. Family members and potential care partners should be included in education sessions. Data suggests that when exposed to a good CKD education program, about 8% of patients will choose HHD, far more than the national average [43]. In addition to recruiting patients from the CKD population, patients who are already on in-center hemodialysis should be offered ongoing HHD education. Patients with failing kidney transplants or CKD as a result of another organ transplant are often highly motivated to perform dialysis at home and should be educated about HHD as an option. Patients using peritoneal dialysis may need or desire to switch modalities and should be offered HHD early to avoid temporary dialysis catheters. Oftentimes a fistula can be placed and mature while the patient is still on PD and then can easily transition within the home program without ever going in-center. Even when patients need to have dialysis acutely started, modality education can be successful at recruiting patients to home modalities. In one study approximately 10% of acute start dialysis patients eventually performed HHD after exposure to an in-hospital CKD education program [44].

Patient Screening

Although our aim in education and recruiting is to cast a broad net, it is important to appropriately screen patients before beginning HHD training [45]. The dialysis staff and providers should help to make sure the decision to start training is the right decision by fully informing the patient and any involved family or care partner (s) about the training process, and program expectations. There are some contraindications to HHD including lack of stable housing, significant psychiatric or neurologic impairment, certain physical ailments, which cannot be overcome with a care partner or technology, or drug and alcohol addiction which may impair a patient's ability to make sound decisions or make it dangerous to self-cannulate a vascular access.

HHD program staff typically have the patient visit the unit for ongoing modality education and discussion prior to beginning training and they may also arrange for a home visit to make sure the home environment can be arranged in a suitable way to accommodate HHD. Broadly, program staff should discuss with patients the reasons they are interested in HHD as a modality, their home environment, supplies and equipment, patient cognitive and psychosocial status, patient and care partner expectations and a medical history.

Patient Training

The initial HHD training period can take 4-6 weeks depending on how quickly the patient learns the material and whether they are concurrently learning how to cannulate their access.

Patients who are transitioning from in-center hemodialysis (ICHD) can be taught self-cannulation while still receiving ICHD. It is important to have a standard curriculum for HHD training so that each topic can be taught, reviewed and evaluated [45]. If a care partner will be training with the patient, respective duties of the patient and care partner should be discussed ahead of time. As discussed elsewhere in this chapter, the patient – care partner relationship is important to understand and support, in order to increase the overall success of HHD for the patient. Patients are adult learners and will have different educational backgrounds and preferred learning methods. If possible, the HHD nurse should consider the most effective way to review material with the patient, and ask their learning preferences ahead of time. At the end of training, there should be an assessment that all parties are comfortable with the patient transitioning home and the nurse should ideally help the patient with the first treatment in the home to ease anxiety and give the patient confidence that they can succeed at home. It is important that training not stop once the patient goes home. Patients should be re-trained on an ongoing basis. Once patients grow comfortable with dialyzing at home, they may grow complacent and so reinforcing proper technique on a continual basis is vital to avoid complications.

BARRIERS TO GROWTH, TECHNIQUE SURVIVAL, AND DISCONTINUATION

There are many reasons for low utilization of HHD in the United States. Barriers include psychosocial concerns of the patient or care partner, insufficient patient education, infrastructure limitations, misconceptions and inadequate training for physicians, economic disincentives and importantly, high rates of discontinuation [46].

Commonly cited psychosocial barriers include denial of chronic kidney disease diagnosis, fear of self-cannulation, medicalization of the home, fear of catastrophic event in the home, and concern about social isolation and burden on family members [47]. There may be misconceptions of who is an appropriate candidate for HHD, or who can learn how to perform the necessary skills. Inadequate patient education about chronic kidney disease and dialysis modalities is a limitation to growth of HHD. Many patients receive limited CKD care prior to starting dialysis, and even those that do may receive little education about dialysis options. In order to grow and recruit home dialysis patients there must be adequate infrastructure, including a home dialysis training program, nurses who are skilled at caring for HHD patients and physicians who are motivated and skilled at prescribing the therapy. In some fellowship programs, young nephrologists receive limited training and exposure on caring for and prescribing HHD therapy. In an ASN survey of graduating nephrology fellows between 2004-2008, less than 20% felt well trained to care for HHD patients [48]. Additionally, there can be financial barriers including cost to patients or family members who need to take off work for a lengthy HHD training period or pay for modifications in the home.

Discontinuation, or technique failure, is another major limitation to the growth of HHD, and has been shown to be as high as 25% in the first year in the United States [49]. Although patients with more comorbid conditions and certain demographic characteristics have been associated with increased discontinuation, it appears that psychosocial reasons and burden of therapy drive the majority of discontinuations [50, 51].

Many strategies can be used to overcome barriers to HHD and reduce discontinuation. The patient and care partner relationship (if one exists) is an important dynamic in HHD. First, there may be a misconception that a partner is required, which indeed it is not. HHD without a care partner is common in other countries and is approved by the US FDA on one machine. When there is a care partner, it is important to include the partner early in the process. Ongoing support of the patient-care partner dyad is important and this relationship can evolve over time. Specifying early what the role of the partner will be and who will complete each task can help to avoid stress later. Patients as well as care partners need ongoing social and emotional support [52]. Peer support networks can help to normalize the process for patients and avoid social isolation. Using tools to assess patient's values and priorities as well as screen for underlying depression can be helpful.

Patient education early, and on an ongoing basis, is vital to the success of home modalities. Education is not only to offer HHD as an option, but also to dispel myths and reduce fear surrounding the process. Some programs offer CKD education programs – our program offers classes in CKD for our stage IV and V patients to introduce all modalities early. Patients are encouraged to subsequently visit our home dialysis center to learn more about those options and see the machines in person. Transitional care units can be utilized to provide intensive education and experience to new dialysis patients. The typical model is that all new dialysis patients spend 3-5 weeks receiving more frequent dialysis (4+ treatments/week with lower blood flow rates ("gentle dialysis") on a home dialysis machine and importantly, intensive and unbiased education about all renal replacement therapies [53].

Physicians need robust education on prescribing home modalities during fellowship. They should also be encouraged to seek out post fellowship training opportunities such as conferences or other educational programs, so that they are comfortable and confident prescribing home modalities. Nurses and technicians should also be educated on home dialysis. In-center staff are often a source of information for patients and they should have some baseline knowledge about home modalities.

Most HHD discontinuation is related to burn-out. Home dialysis programs should discuss stressors with the patient and care partner routinely. They can and should investigate ways in which technology may help to alleviate anxiety or reduce frequency of visits to the center with the use of telemedicine or monitoring platforms. They should have in place methods to offer respite care and offer this to patients when appropriate. Supporting patients' mental health and having open communication about frustrations is vital.

Safety

Patient safety is of paramount importance in ESKD patients on HD and home hemodialysis is not without complications. The two biggest safety concerns for home dialysis patients are infection and exsanguination. In a study by Weinhandl et al. looking at hospitalizations in 3,480 home hemodialysis patients and 17,400 CHD patients, all-cause hospitalizations were noted to be similar in both groups. However, hospitalizations for cardiac-related admissions was lower in the home hemodialysis group while hospitalizations for infections were higher [54]. These infections appeared to be access related as they were predominately bacteremia/sepsis, endocarditis, osteomyelitis, and vascular access infections. Interestingly when compared to matched CHD patients, home dialysis patients were at higher risk for infection as a cause for first admission, but not readmission. This is perhaps owed to reinforced training in sterile technique and hygiene following first admission, though the exact reason is unclear.

Despite the risk of infection however, home hemodialysis has been shown to be a safe option. In analysis of the data from two adult home HD programs in Canada from 2001 to 2012 with 190 patients, Wong et al. note a crude rate of 0.060 events per 1,000 dialysis treatments with six potentially fatal adverse events [55]. These events were noted to consist of 1 episode of exsanguination and five events related to human error. In another study of 29 patients that were converted from CHD to home hemodialysis and assessed for adverse events over a six month period, similar and/or potentially improved safety parameters were seen after conversion to home hemodialysis, with 12 patients having 69 adverse events (5.84/100 treatments) on CHD and 18 patients had 40 (3.34/100 treatments) on home HD [56].

VASCULAR ACCESS

There are two common means for patient self-cannulation: the rope ladder (standard needling) technique and the buttonhole technique. For the rope ladder technique, patients place the needles in different, rotating locations along the length of the fistula before returning to the original location. The purpose of this is to utilize a different location for each treatment. The buttonhole technique utilizes the same location, pierced sequentially with each treatment, allowing the formation of a scarred channel that the patient will continue to access. This channel is the "buttonhole", so named because of its appearance, and is accessed with a blunt needle once the tract is formed.

The buttonhole technique has become popular among home dialysis and CHD patients due to its perceived decrease in pain compared to the rope ladder technique. Studies have attempted to assess differences in pain between the two techniques before and shown no significant differences between the two techniques [57]. A 2012 study by MacRae et al. investigated this further [58]. Using pain scores as a primary outcome, the study looked at 140 CHD patients that were randomly assigned either buttonhole technique or rope ladder technique. At eight weeks the median pain scores for both techniques were similar and the differences insignificant ($p = 0.57$). At 12 months, there were three episodes of Staphylococcus aureus infections and nine needling site abscesses requiring intravenous antibiotics with the buttonhole technique compared to zero episodes of these complications with the rope ladder technique ($p = 0.003$).

This concern for infection and other access complications among patients using the buttonhole technique has been evaluated. A multicenter, prospective, open label, randomized controlled trial of 70 patients randomized into either buttonhole or rope ladder cannulation techniques showed increased rates of infection, hematoma, and site pain with the buttonhole technique when compared to the rope ladder technique [59]. Attempts have been studied to try and address the risk of serious infection such as using mupirocin prophylaxis. In a long-term, single-center, retrospective study of 56 NHD patients, patients were assessed for both pre and post mupirocin prophylaxis for a total of 93.4 and 193.5 patient years, respectively [60]. Complications noted in the pre-mupirocin group were significant with 10 episodes of Staphylococcus aureus infection including four patients with metastatic complications of Staphylococcus pneumonia, septic arthritis, and one fatal C3 epidural abscess. In comparison, there were no reported episodes of infection when the patients were adherent to mupirocin prophylaxis. There were two cases of Staphylococcus infection in the post-mupirocin however in patients that had been non-adherent to the mupirocin treatment for at least three weeks.

The method of cannulation chosen should be personalized based on the center experience and patient preference. In addition, while longer and straighter fistulas may be well suited for the rope ladder technique, patients may find it easier to cannulate shorter or deeper fistulas with buttonholes. Regardless of technique, patients should be taught and encouraged regularly to use appropriate sterile technique, antibiotic prophylaxis and to examine their fistula daily and communicate frequently with the dialysis staff about any problems.

Comparative evaluation for access complications between frequent home hemodialysis and CHD has been assessed. In a group of 87 NHD patients, the FHN trial group showed a trend towards increasing vascular access complications in the NHD group compared to the CHD group with 34 vascular access events in the NHD arm compared to 21 events in the CHD arm ($p = 0.10$) [61]. This trend appears to be more reflective of vascular interventions rather than access failures, as the access failure events were similar in both groups with 17 failures in the NHD group and 13 failures in the CHD group.

Whichever method is chosen it is important to periodically audit the patient's cannulation technique to assess for potential risks in both procedural technique, sterility, and use of prophylaxis. Auditing tools have been evaluated previously and have been shown to be of benefit [62].

REFERENCES

[1] Blagg CR. A brief history of home hemodialysis. *Adv Ren Replace Ther.* 1996; 3(2): 99-105.

[2] DePalma JR, Pecker EA, Maxwell MH. A new automatic coil dialyzer system for 'daily' dialysis. *Hemodial Int.* 2004; 8(1): 19-23.

[3] Pierratos A. Daily nocturnal home hemodialysis. *Kidney Int.* 2004; 65(5): 1975-86.

[4] Trinh E, Chan CT. The Rise, Fall, and Resurgence of Home Hemodialysis. *Semin Dial.* 2017; 30(2): 174-80.

[5] Rivara MB, Mehrotra R. The changing landscape of home dialysis in the United States. *Curr Opin Nephrol Hypertens.* 2014; 23(6): 586-91.

[6] *2019 USRDS annual data report: Epidemiology of kidney disease in the United States.* National Institutes of Health, National Institute of Diabetes and Digestive and Kidney Diseases. Bethesda, MD, 2019.

[7] Walker DR, Inglese GW, Sloand JA, Just PM. Dialysis facility and patient characteristics associated with utilization of home dialysis. *Clin J Am Soc Nephrol.* 2010; 5(9): 1649-54.

[8] Briggs V, Davies S, Wilkie M. International Variations in Peritoneal Dialysis Utilization and Implications for Practice. *Am J Kidney Dis.* 2019; 74(1): 101-10.

[9] Lockridge RS Jr, Pipkin M. Short and long nightly hemodialysis in the United States. *Hemodial Int.* 2008; 12 Suppl 1: S48-50.

[10] Kjellstrand CM, Kjellstrand P. The ideal home hemodialysis machine. *Hemodial Int.* 2008; 12 Suppl 1: S33-9.

[11] Group FHNT; Chertow GM, Levin NW, Beck GJ, Depner TA, Eggers PW, et al. In-center hemodialysis six times per week versus three times per week. *N Engl J Med.* 2010; 363(24): 2287-300.

[12] Silberberg JS, Barre PE, Prichard SS, Sniderman AD. Impact of left ventricular hypertrophy on survival in end-stage renal disease. *Kidney Int.* 1989; 36(2): 286-90.

[13] Culleton BF, Walsh M, Klarenbach SW, Mortis G, Scott-Douglas N, Quinn RR, et al. Effect of frequent nocturnal hemodialysis vs conventional hemodialysis on left ventricular mass and quality of life: a randomized controlled trial. *JAMA*. 2007; 298(11): 1291-9.

[14] Chan CT, Floras JS, Miller JA, Richardson RM, Pierratos A. Regression of left ventricular hypertrophy after conversion to nocturnal hemodialysis. *Kidney Int.* 2002; 61(6): 2235-9.

[15] Ayus JC, Mizani MR, Achinger SG, Thadhani R, Go AS, Lee S. Effects of short daily versus conventional hemodialysis on left ventricular hypertrophy and inflammatory markers: a prospective, controlled study. *J Am Soc Nephrol.* 2005; 16(9): 2778-88.

[16] Fagugli RM, Reboldi G, Quintaliani G, Pasini P, Ciao G, Cicconi B, et al. Short daily hemodialysis: blood pressure control and left ventricular mass reduction in hypertensive hemodialysis patients. *Am J Kidney Dis*. 2001; 38(2): 371-6.

[17] Marshall MR, Hawley CM, Kerr PG, Polkinghorne KR, Marshall RJ, Agar JW, et al. Home hemodialysis and mortality risk in Australian and New Zealand populations. *Am J Kidney Dis.* 2011; 58(5): 782-93.

[18] Kjellstrand CM, Buoncristiani U, Ting G, Traeger J, Piccoli GB, Sibai-Galland R, et al. Short daily haemodialysis: survival in 415 patients treated for 1006 patient-years. *Nephrol Dial Transplant.* 2008; 23(10): 3283-9.

[19] Alborzi P, Patel N, Agarwal R. Home blood pressures are of greater prognostic value than hemodialysis unit recordings. *Clin J Am Soc Nephrol*. 2007; 2(6): 1228-34.

[20] Saran R, Li Y, Robinson B, Ayanian J, Balkrishnan R, Bragg-Gresham J, et al. US Renal Data System 2014 Annual Data Report: Epidemiology of Kidney Disease in the United States. *Am J Kidney Dis*. 2015; 66(1 Suppl 1): Svii, S1-305.

[21] Health ARCf. *The DOPPS Practice monitor*. [cited 2020 10/19]. Available from: http://www.dopps.org/DPM/.

[22] Heerspink HJ, Ninomiya T, Zoungas S, de Zeeuw D, Grobbee DE, Jardine MJ, et al. Effect of lowering blood pressure on cardiovascular events and mortality in patients on dialysis: a systematic review and meta-analysis of randomised controlled trials. *Lancet*. 2009; 373(9668): 1009-15.

[23] Kotanko P, Garg AX, Depner T, Pierratos A, Chan CT, Levin NW, et al. Effects of frequent hemodialysis on blood pressure: Results from the randomized frequent hemodialysis network trials. *Hemodial Int*. 2015; 19(3): 386-401.

[24] Jaber BL, Lee Y, Collins AJ, Hull AR, Kraus MA, McCarthy J, et al. Effect of daily hemodialysis on depressive symptoms and postdialysis recovery time: interim report from the FREEDOM (Following Rehabilitation, Economics and Everyday-Dialysis Outcome Measurements) Study. *Am J Kidney Dis.* 2010; 56(3): 531-9.

[25] Daugirdas JT, Chertow GM, Larive B, Pierratos A, Greene T, Ayus JC, et al. Effects of frequent hemodialysis on measures of CKD mineral and bone disorder. *J Am Soc Nephrol*. 2012; 23(4): 727-38.

[26] Merlino G, Piani A, Dolso P, Adorati M, Cancelli I, Valente M, et al. Sleep disorders in patients with end-stage renal disease undergoing dialysis therapy. *Nephrol Dial Transplant*. 2006; 21(1): 184-90.

[27] Forni Ogna V, Ogna A, Pruijm M, Bassi I, Zuercher E, Halabi G, et al. Prevalence and Diagnostic Approach to Sleep Apnea in Hemodialysis Patients: A Population Study. *Biomed Res Int*. 2015; 2015: 103686.

[28] Hanly PJ, Pierratos A. Improvement of sleep apnea in patients with chronic renal failure who undergo nocturnal hemodialysis. *N Engl J Med*. 2001; 344(2): 102-7.

[29] Kutlu R, Selcuk NY, Sayin S, Kal O. Restless legs syndrome and quality of life in chronic hemodialysis patients. *Niger J Clin Pract*. 2018; 21(5): 573-7.

[30] Jaber BL, Schiller B, Burkart JM, Daoui R, Kraus MA, Lee Y, et al. Impact of short daily hemodialysis on restless legs symptoms and sleep disturbances. *Clin J Am Soc Nephrol*. 2011; 6(5): 1049-56.

[31] Okundaye I, Abrinko P, Hou S. Registry of pregnancy in dialysis patients. *Am J Kidney Dis*. 1998; 31(5): 766-73.

[32] Bagon JA, Vernaeve H, De Muylder X, Lafontaine JJ, Martens J, Van Roost G. Pregnancy and dialysis. *Am J Kidney Dis*. 1998; 31(5): 756-65.

[33] Barua M, Hladunewich M, Keunen J, Pierratos A, McFarlane P, Sood M, et al. Successful pregnancies on nocturnal home hemodialysis. *Clin J Am Soc Nephrol*. 2008; 3(2): 392-6.

[34] Jesudason S, Grace BS, McDonald SP. Pregnancy outcomes according to dialysis commencing before or after conception in women with ESRD. *Clin J Am Soc Nephrol*. 2014; 9(1): 143-9.

[35] Hladunewich MA, Hou S, Odutayo A, Cornelis T, Pierratos A, Goldstein M, et al. Intensive hemodialysis associates with improved pregnancy outcomes: a Canadian and United States cohort comparison. *J Am Soc Nephrol*. 2014; 25(5): 1103-9.

[36] Johnson WJ, Hagge WW, Wagoner RD, Dinapoli RP, Rosevear JW. Effects of urea loading in patients with far-advanced renal failure. *Mayo Clin Proc*. 1972; 47(1): 21-9.

[37] National Kidney Foundation. KDOQI Clinical Practice Guideline for Hemodialysis Adequacy: 2015 update. *Am J Kidney Dis*. 2015; 66(5): 884-930.

[38] Vanholder R, Glorieux G, Eloot S. Once upon a time in dialysis: the last days of Kt/V? *Kidney Int*. 2015; 88(3): 460-5.

[39] Chertow GM, Owen WF, Lazarus JM, Lew NL, Lowrie EG. Exploring the reverse J-shaped curve between urea reduction ratio and mortality. *Kidney Int*. 1999; 56(5): 1872-8.

[40] Lowrie EG, Li Z, Ofsthun N, Lazarus JM. Body size, dialysis dose and death risk relationships among hemodialysis patients. *Kidney Int*. 2002; 62(5): 1891-7.

[41] Masakane I, Sakurai K. Current approaches to middle molecule removal: room for innovation. *Nephrol Dial Transplant*. 2018; 33(suppl_3): iii12-iii21.

[42] Flythe JE, Kimmel SE, Brunelli SM. Rapid fluid removal during dialysis is associated with cardiovascular morbidity and mortality. *Kidney Int*. 2011; 79(2): 250-7.

[43] Goovaerts T, Jadoul M, Goffin E. Influence of a pre-dialysis education programme (PDEP) on the mode of renal replacement therapy. *Nephrol Dial Transplant*. 2005; 20(9): 1842-7.

[44] Rioux JP, Cheema H, Bargman JM, Watson D, Chan CT. Effect of an in-hospital chronic kidney disease education program among patients with unplanned urgent-start dialysis. *Clin J Am Soc Nephrol.* 2011; 6(4): 799-804.

[45] Joel D Glickman, RKS. *Patient Selection and Training*. Daphne Knicely EA-R, Keiko Greenberg editor: McGraw Hill.

[46] Chan CT, Wallace E, Golper TA, Rosner MH, Seshasai RK, Glickman JD, et al. Exploring Barriers and Potential Solutions in Home Dialysis: An NKF-KDOQI Conference Outcomes Report. *Am J Kidney Dis.* 2019; 73(3): 363-71.

[47] Cafazzo JA, Leonard K, Easty AC, Rossos PG, Chan CT. Patient-perceived barriers to the adoption of nocturnal home hemodialysis. *Clin J Am Soc Nephrol.* 2009; 4(4): 784-9.

[48] Berns JS. A survey-based evaluation of self-perceived competency after nephrology fellowship training. *Clin J Am Soc Nephrol.* 2010; 5(3): 490-6.

[49] Seshasai RK, Mitra N, Chaknos CM, Li J, Wirtalla C, Negoianu D, et al. Factors Associated With Discontinuation of Home Hemodialysis. *Am J Kidney Dis.* 2016; 67(4): 629-37.

[50] Seshasai RK, Wong T, Glickman JD, Shea JA, Dember LM. The home hemodialysis patient experience: A qualitative assessment of modality use and discontinuation. *Hemodial Int.* 2019; 23(2): 139-50.

[51] Jayanti A, Nikam M, Ebah L, Dutton G, Morris J, Mitra S. Technique survival in home haemodialysis: a composite success rate and its risk predictors in a prospective longitudinal cohort from a tertiary renal network programme. *Nephrol Dial Transplant.* 2013; 28(10): 2612-20.

[52] Suri RS, Larive B, Garg AX, Hall YN, Pierratos A, Chertow GM, et al. Burden on caregivers as perceived by hemodialysis patients in the Frequent Hemodialysis Network (FHN) trials. *Nephrol Dial Transplant.* 2011; 26(7): 2316-22.

[53] Lockridge R, Weinhandl E, Kraus M, Schreiber M, Spry L, Tailor P, et al. A Systematic Approach to Promoting Home Hemodialysis During End Stage Kidney Disease. *Kidney* 360. 2020; 1(9): 993-1001.

[54] Weinhandl ED, Nieman KM, Gilbertson DT, Collins AJ. Hospitalization in daily home hemodialysis and matched thrice-weekly in-center hemodialysis patients. *Am J Kidney Dis.* 2015; 65(1): 98-108.

[55] Wong B, Zimmerman D, Reintjes F, Courtney M, Klarenbach S, Dowling G, et al. Procedure-related serious adverse events among home hemodialysis patients: a quality assurance perspective. *Am J Kidney Dis.* 2014; 63(2): 251-8.

[56] Sands JJ, Lacson E, Jr., Ofsthun NJ, Kay JC, Diaz-Buxo JA. Home hemodialysis: a comparison of in-center and home hemodialysis therapy in a cohort of successful home hemodialysis patients. *ASAIO J.* 2009; 55(4): 361-8.

[57] Verhallen AM, Kooistra MP, van Jaarsveld BC. Cannulating in haemodialysis: rope-ladder or buttonhole technique? *Nephrol Dial Transplant.* 2007; 22(9): 2601-4.

[58] MacRae JM, Ahmed SB, Atkar R, Hemmelgarn BR. A randomized trial comparing buttonhole with rope ladder needling in conventional hemodialysis patients. *Clin J Am Soc Nephrol.* 2012; 7(10): 1632-8.

[59] Chow J, Rayment G, San Miguel S, Gilbert M. A randomised controlled trial of buttonhole cannulation for the prevention of fistula access complications. *J Ren Care.* 2011; 37(2): 85-93.

[60] Nesrallah GE, Cuerden M, Wong JH, Pierratos A. Staphylococcus aureus bacteremia and buttonhole cannulation: long-term safety and efficacy of mupirocin prophylaxis. *Clin J Am Soc Nephrol.* 2010; 5(6): 1047-53.

[61] Rocco MV, Daugirdas JT, Greene T, Lockridge RS, Chan C, Pierratos A, et al. Long-term Effects of Frequent Nocturnal Hemodialysis on Mortality: The Frequent Hemodialysis Network (FHN) Nocturnal Trial. *Am J Kidney Dis.* 2015; 66(3): 459-68.

[62] Rousseau-Gagnon M, Faratro R, D'Gama C, Fung S, Wong E, Chan CT. The use of vascular access audit and infections in home hemodialysis. *Hemodial Int.* 2016; 20(2): 298-305.

In: Issues in Kidney Disease – Dialysis
Editors: Stephen Z. Fadem and José A. Moura-Neto
ISBN: 978-1-68507-000-7

Chapter 13

ONLINE HEMODIAFILTRATION IN CHRONIC KIDNEY DISEASE - THROUGH CLINICAL PRACTICE TO EVIDENCE

José A. Moura-Neto[1], MD,
José Carolino Divino-Filho[2], MD, PhD,
Ikuto Masakane[3], MD, PhD and Bernard Canaud[4,*], MD, PhD

[1]Department of Internal Medicine, Bahiana School of Medicine and Public Health, Salvador, Bahia, Brazil
[2]Division of Renal Medicine, Department of Clinical Science, Intervention and Technology, CLINTEC, Karolinska Institutet, Campus Flemingsberg, Stockholm, Sweden;
Latin American Chapter (LAC-DD)-International Society for Peritoneal Dialysis
[3]Yabuki Hospital, Yamagata City, Japan
[4]Global Medical Office FMC, Bad Homburg, Germany and University of Montpellier, School of Medicine, Montpellier, France

ABSTRACT

Hemodiafiltration is an extracorporeal renal replacement "hybrid" therapy that combines diffusion and convection in the same hemodialyzer with an isovolumic online substitution of the ultrafiltered fluid. By combining diffusion and convection processes, hemodiafiltration maintains the high diffusive clearance of small molecules obtained in hemodialysis and enhances removal of larger molecules comparable to that obtained in hemofiltration. Short-term prospective studies have provided intermediary outcomes showing that hemodiafiltration enhanced solute removal of middle and large molecular size solutes, improved hemodynamic tolerance of sessions, reduced inflammatory profile and erythropoiesis-stimulating agent dose consumption, and improved patient nutritional status, are all associated with clinical benefits. In the last years, several prospective randomized trials have been conducted in Europe. Although far from rejecting the use of hemodiafiltration, there are still some gaps in evidence-based medicine that need to be

* Corresponding Author's E-mail: bernard.canaud@fmc-ag.com.

addressed before the superiority of this technique can be definitively proven. This chapter mainly discusses basic principles, prerequisites, substitution modalities, and the clinical evidence surrounding hemodiafiltration.

Keywords: chronic kidney disease, online hemodiafiltration, renal replacement therapy, convective therapies, evidence-based medicine

INTRODUCTION

Hemodiafiltration (HDF) was introduced in the 1970s to address performance limitations of standard low-flux hemodialysis (HD), namely the limited middle and large molecule clearances and the limited clearance of small molecules provided by high-flux hemofiltration (HF) [1-3]. In HD, solute removal occurs mostly by diffusive transport mechanisms, a process that decreases rapidly with increasing molecular size of uremic compounds [4]. In contrast, solute removal in HF relies mainly on membrane sieving convection and total ultrafiltered volume, a process that provides higher clearances for larger solutes than HD, but unfortunately was limited by total fluid volume exchanged during short treatment time [5, 6]. By combining diffusion and convection processes in the same high-flux hemodialyzer, HDF keeps the high diffusive clearance of small molecules obtained in hemodialysis and enhances removal of larger molecules comparable to that obtained in hemofiltration [1, 7]. The introduction of this combined therapy in the field of renal replacement therapy was intended to improve renal replacement therapy efficiency and patients' outcomes. However, mass removal of middle and large molecular weight compounds may remain a challenge in some oversized patients or higher metabolic demand patients with current short HDF treatment schedules that can be easily overcome by increasing treatment time and/or frequency of HDF sessions [8, 9].

Following initial pilot studies, it was soon identified that online production of substitution fluid was the only viable option to ensure development and broader clinical use of this therapeutic modality [10-12]. Online HDF relies on the production of substitution fluid from fresh dialysis fluid by a two-stage cold sterilization process (i.e., two sterilizing ultrafilters in series) made possible by a change of the hydraulic circuit of HD machine equipped with volumetric control system [13]. The adaptation consists in the adjunction of a pumping module that diverts an adjustable fraction of the fresh inlet dialysate produced and infuses it directly into patient's blood stream (pre or postfilter) via a venous port. Volumetric control system of the HD machine compensates then for the fluid diverted by ultrafiltering an equivalent fraction from patient's blood to compensate for missing fluid and keep patient's isovolemic condition. This technical option currently referring to external online hemodiafiltration has several advantages that are recognized worldwide [14, 15]: firstly, it is safe and reliable from a microbiological and toxicological perspective; secondly, it gives access to unlimited amount of sterile and non-pyrogenic substitution fluid at relatively low fare; thirdly, it is easily integrated in the hardware (i.e., additional substitution pump, sterilizing ultrafilters) and software (i.e., volume controller, pressure test) of hemodialysis machine; fourthly, it remains friendly to the user and is easily implemented in the regular workflow for patient care; fifthly, it permits to customize treatment (i.e., convective volume, treatment time, electrolyte prescription) to patient needs.

Online HDF relies on the combined use of a high-flux hemodialyzer fitted by a capillary synthetic membrane (i.e., ultrafiltration coefficient > 20 $mL/h/mmHg/m^2$ and a sieving coefficient for ß2-microglobulin of > 0.6) and an adequate surface (i.e., 1.5 to $2.2m^2$), with a certified online HDF machine capable of delivering adjustable convection volume (i.e., 20 to 40 liters per session in postdilution mode) while maintaining an appropriate fluid balance by infusing a sterile, non-pyrogenic fluid into the patient's blood [16]. As prerequisite, online HDF machines require to be fed with ultrapure treated water and to adhere to strict hygienic rules (i.e., monitoring, maintenance, disinfection) to prevent all microbial and toxicological hazards [17, 18]. In other words, a certified and validated water treatment system including a distribution loop able to deliver ultrapure water at point of care within the dialysis facility is requested before considering launching any online HDF treatment program [19]. Furthermore, education and training of caregivers, precise microbiological and chemical quality monitoring of water and dialysis fluid, including disinfection and precise hygienic protocols for maintenance, are required. We refer interested readers of this topic to textbooks and expert reviews on this matter [18-20].

From the early days, online HDF has been recognized for its clinical benefits (i.e., patient perception) and improved intermediary outcomes that include increased removal of small and middle molecular weight uremic retention solutes [7], reduced intradialytic hypotension [21, 22], improved dialysis tolerance [23], and reduced dialysis-related pathology, such as amyloidosis and accelerated atherosclerosis [24-26]. Over last few years, accumulating stronger evidences have been generated both from large observational and interventional studies, that tend to accreditate superior outcomes with HDF as compared to HD, in particular by reducing cardiovascular burden, provided the adequate convective dose is delivered [27-29].

Interestingly, HDF is gaining every year higher clinical acceptance worldwide. As indicated by a recent survey (2018), HDF was used to treat 286,000 patients worldwide of which 278,000 were treated by online HDF (97%) which represents the vast majority [30]. Focusing on two geographic areas where HDF is mainly used, online HDF is being used to routinely treat 120,000 patients in Europe and 144,000 patients in Japan. Interestingly, average growth rates over the period 2009-2017 are 8.5% and 24% in Europe and Asia-Pacific region. Furthermore, online HDF is growing much rapidly in Asia region and particularly in Japan and China, less rapidly in Latin America, whereas, for a variety of reasons online HDF was essentially not used in the United States [30].

In this chapter, we will address the following topics: 1) Basic principles of online HDF; 2) Prerequisites for developing HDF programs; 3) Substitution modalities and their advantages and disadvantages; 4) Prescription of HDF; 5) Review of clinical evidence supporting the use of HDF; and finally, 6) Evidence-based medicine "revisited" in light of HDF.

Basic Principles of Online HDF

Online HDF is an extracorporeal renal replacement "hybrid" therapy that combines diffusion and convection in the same hemodialyzer with online substitution of fluid ultrafiltered [31]. Medical practice currently applies various modalities of HDF worldwide. Despite this diversity, the common element of all these multipurpose modalities is the combination of convective and diffusive solute clearances with online production of substitution fluid to ensure isovolemic control [32]. At the end of the process, total solute removal is the result of the sum of diffusive and convective clearances.

Convection is the predominant mechanism of mass transport of middle molecular size solutes in hybrid convective-diffusive dialysis techniques. Convective solute removal results from the bulk movement of the solvent (plasma water) through a semipermeable membrane driven by the hydrostatic pressure gradient - a transmembrane pressure gradient (TMP) - between blood and dialysate compartments [33]. A TMP causing fluid movement is the key element of convection [32].

Although convection is constant over a vast spectrum of molecular weight solutes, it decreases as the molecular size increase nears the size of the semipermeable membrane pores and stops at the cutoff point of the membrane. Membrane characteristics of the dialyzer (pore radius and conformation, structure and electro-chemical properties) have a key role in this process [34-37]. The capacity of the dialyzer membrane to clear a solute by convection from plasma depends on its sieving properties, expressed as an index, the sieving coefficient[1] (S, dimensionless), which varies with each membrane and solute [38]. In addition to the solute sieving coefficient and membrane characteristics (i.e., hydraulic permeability [Kuf]; membrane charge and hydrophobicity), the clinical effectiveness of convection in total solute removal depends on a broader variety of factors, such as solute characteristics (i.e., hydrophilicity, charge, protein binding, intracorporeal kinetic), the solute concentration in plasma water and the ultrafiltration rate and clinical operating conditions (i.e.; blood flow, treatment time and frequency) [33, 39].

Diffusion is the major mechanism of transport of small molecules in hemodialysis as well as in hybrid convective-diffusive modalities. In this process, the solutes move in every possible direction. This random movement results in a passive passage of molecules from a region with higher concentration to one of lower concentration until the gradient is eliminated and equilibrium between solutions is reached. Besides the concentration gradient, in vivo solute diffusive clearance across the membrane varies according to the membrane characteristics (i.e., proportional to surface area, solute diffusion coefficient and inversely proportional to the thickness of the membrane), the solute considered (i.e., molecular weight, plasma free fraction, diffusivity coefficient), patient characteristics and operating conditions (i.e., blood and dialysate flow, treatment time) [32].

Diffusion loses its effectiveness as the solute's molecular weight increases – a 1,000 Dalton solute, for example, is removed at about half of the rate of a solute with 60 Dalton (Urea). While diffusive transport successfully removes small molecular size solutes, convection is preferred for clearing larger solutes [40]. Removing solutes over a broader molecular weight spectrum should be the therapy goal of not only HDF but of all renal replacement therapies.

Although both solute transport mechanisms take place simultaneously in HDF, convection and diffusion are applied to different extents in this hybrid therapy and vary with the respective molecular weight of the cleared solute. For a solute successfully removed by diffusive transport (urea, for example), little is left to be cleared by convective removal. Following the same logical assumption, solutes with larger molecular sizes not effectively removed by diffusive transport (ß2-microglobulin, for example) are available in higher concentrations for convective transport. The combination of both mechanisms of mass transport provides more total solute removal than when these transport principles are applied separately; convection (hemofiltration) or

---

[1] Sieving Coefficient (SCD) for a defined solute is defined as the ratio of its concentration in the filtrate (Cf) [SCD = Cf/Ci] and in plasma inlet (Ci). Mean Sieving Coefficient (SCA) is defined as the ratio of the solute concentration in filtrate (Cf) and mean concentration of inlet (Ci) and outlet (Co). SCA = 2Cf/(Ci-Co) [38].

diffusion (hemodialysis) [40]. Finally, it is noteworthy that the overall mass transport results from the interaction, not the simple sum, of the two separate components, which is marked at higher ultrafiltration rates of HDF. Despite previous attempts to quantify their combined effect in terms of solute clearance with mathematical equations, the individual effects of convective and diffusive transports cannot be distinguished precisely [33]. A mathematical modeling has established an empirical correlation for the overall clearance (K) valid for all solutes and blood flows between 200 and 500 mL/min is found to be K = KD + 0.43 QF + 8.3 x 10-3 Q2F when clearances and QF are in mL/ min [41].

Prerequisites for Developing HDF Programs

The main prerequisite for performing online HDF is the online production of sterile and non-pyrogenic substitution fluid through a cold sterilization process using fresh dialysis fluid. Failure in any stage of this process or suboptimal disinfection of the machine could ultimately result in endotoxins, peptidoglycans and other microbial-derived products entering the patient's bloodstream. Thus, the strict adherence to hygienic disinfection rules relating to water treatment system and online HDF machines, rigorous microbial monitoring and periodic replacement of sterilizing ultrafilters virtually eliminates the aforementioned risk. In addition, all online blood purification techniques require ultrapure water, which is fundamental for the online production of the sterile substitution fluid [42, 43].

At the conventional dialysate flow rate of 500 mL/min, for example, the patient on a 4-hour session thrice-weekly program is exposed to around 360 liters per week of dialysis fluid. Online HDF may require an additional 20-25 liters (i.e., 60-75 liters per week) of online-produced substitution fluid per session infused directly intravenously. The production of ultrapure dialysis and substitution fluids – from tap to patient – entails various stages, comprising water purification systems, special ultrafilters, in addition to dialyzers with endotoxin-retention capabilities, which guarantee microbiological and chemical purity of high volumes of fluid entering and contacting the blood system of patients [44].

Microbiological contamination of dialysis fluids is known to negatively affect dialysis patient outcomes due to the stimulation of inflammatory responses and pathways causing oxidative stress [44]. There is a risk of endotoxins and/or microbial-derived products (i.e., peptidoglycans, DNA fragments) entering the blood compartment of dialyzers during dialysis via back-transport mechanisms, especially back-filtration. Activation of leukocytes generates pro-inflammatory cytokines and reactive oxygen species, contributing to cardiovascular diseases. For this reason, several guidelines and recommendations propose maximum acceptable levels of microbiological contamination for water and dialysis fluid measured in terms of endotoxin units (EU/mL) and bacterial colony-forming units (CFU/mL) [44, 45]. Table 1 shows the maximum allowable levels of microbiological contaminants for water and dialysis fluids.

Table 1. Maximum permissible levels of microbiological contamination for dialysate [46]

	Standard dialysate	Ultrapure dialysate	Sterile, pyrogen-free infusion fluid
Bacterial limits, CFU/mL	< 100	< 0.1	< 0.000001
Endotoxin limits, EU/mL	< 0.5	< 0.03	< 0.03

Special sterilizing ultrafilters that have hollow-fiber membranes with a high adsorptive capacity for endotoxins help assure microbiological purity and safety of dialysis fluids. The hydrophobic part of the endotoxins (the fatty acid chain of the lipid A molecule) binds to hydrophobic domains of the polysulfone polymer of membrane, ultimately resulting in the retention of endotoxins in the dialyzer [47]. The integration of two such sterilizing ultrafilters placed in series onto the dialysis fluid pathway of dialysis machines is the final stage of the ultrapure dialysis fluid production offering furthermore a redundant microbiological protection. The sterilizing filters should be routinely disinfected, tested for preventing failure (air pressure bubble test) and used for a prespecified number of HDF sessions or during a certain period of time defined by the manufacturer. In order to improve the safety of the process, dialyzers containing hollow-fiber membranes made from synthetic polymers may add an additional line of microbiological protection. Regarding the microbiological and endotoxin retentive capacity of the membrane to ensure cold sterilization of dialysis fluid, some studies have shown differences among dialysis membranes [44, 48].

Online HDF marks an evolutionary milestone in extracorporeal renal replacement therapy. The entire process demands state-of-the-art renal replacement therapy machines that safely produce, infuse, monitor and adjust ultrapure sterile substitution fluid in the patient throughout the dialysis session. While physicians and evidence-based medicine (discussed later in this chapter) are still struggling to advocate a broader use of this technique, some already consider online HDF, including the HDF machines, the hemodiafilters, membranes, ultrafilters and all its equipment, a triumph in terms of engineering [49].

It is also imperative that online HDF use dialyzers with highly hydraulic permeability (KUF $\geq$ 50 mL/h/mmHg), high solute permeability (KoA urea > 600 and β2-microglobulin > 60 mL/min) and large surface area (1.50–2.10 m^2) [50].

Together with the use of proper equipment (water purification system, online HDF machines, ultrafilters, membranes, highly permeable dialyzers) and rigorous quality control of the online production systems of dialysis fluid, the application of best clinical practices ensure the safety of online HDF [51, 52]. As an example of good clinical practice, regularly evaluating clinical symptomatology and serial measurements of serum C-reactive protein of patients treated by online HDF on a monthly basis is recommended [43, 53].

Another requirement for HDF, this time patient-related, is adequate vascular access. In the postdilution mode of HDF (discussed in the following section of this chapter), an access capable of delivering blood flows of 350–400 mL/min is desirable in order to achieve high convective volumes on the conventional dialysis scheme of a 4-hour session thrice weekly. Relative high blood flows increase membrane shear stress, reduce protein cake formation, decrease transmembrane pressure and then facilitate ultrafiltration rates [50].

Finally, training and coaching healthcare personnel perform online HDF properly and safely is essential and therefore another prerequisite for implementing successfully HDF program within each dialysis unit. Table 2 summarizes all the prerequisites discussed in this section.

The safety of online HDF has been attested repeatedly by several publications in the past years; there are no studies so far reporting adverse outcomes of patients with this therapy. Recently, the CONTRAST study observed over 20,000 HDF sessions performed in ten renal replacement therapy facilities and its findings may be used to confirm the reliability of this modality [43, 54]. Online HDF is currently performed in 278,000 patients with chronic kidney disease G5 treated by dialysis (CKD G5D) patients in several different countries [30]. If all the aforementioned requirements are followed and checklisted (Table 2), it is definitely safe to perform online HDF.

Table 2. Prerequisites to perform online HDF safely

• Ultrapure water
• Online HDF machine
• Rigorous quality control: Hygienic disinfection rules relating to the online HDF machine, microbial monitoring and periodic substitution of sterilizing ultrafilters
• Adequate hemodiafilter: Highly permeable hemodiafilters (KUF ≥ 50 mL/h/mmHg, KoA urea >600, β2-microglobulin > 60 mL/min) with large surface area (1.50–2.10 m^2), low internal blood flow resistance and sieving coefficient for albumin (Sc alb < 0.001)
• Trained healthcare personnel to perform online HDF
• Adequate vascular access
• Good clinical practices: monitoring patients' signs and symptoms and dialysis adequacy, optimal anticoagulation

SUBSTITUTION MODALITIES

The site of infusion of the substitution fluid can affect the performance of the HDF [55]. The various online HDF modalities currently available are classified according to the substitution site [56]: predilution (infusion site before the hemodiafilter), mid-dilution (infusion between the ultrafiltration and diffusion compartment) [57, 58], mixed dilution (simultaneous infusion pre- and post-hemodiafilter) [59] and postdilution (infusion site after the hemodiafilter) [60]. Mid- and Mixed dilution have been recently proposed as alternative modalities for enhancing clearance performances while reducing fluid volume consumption [50, 61-63].

In the following paragraphs, we will focus on the two most common substitution modalities of HDF: postdilution and predilution. In addition, the Japanese experience with predilution modality is described in detail.

Postdilution HDF

Postdilution HDF is the most prevalent substitution modality in online HDF. In this modality, the HDF system produces sterile and apyrogenic substitution fluid online from the fresh dialysis fluid produced, which is infused after the hemodiafilter in order to replace the fluid lost by the patient during the ultrafiltration [43].

Postdilution HDF is widely regarded as the most efficient in removing middle molecular size solute [33, 39, 59, 64, 65]. However, hemoconcentration and excessive protein concentration polarization at the membrane interface along the length of the hollow fibers may occur depending on filtration fraction [55].

Hemoconcentration increases resistance to flow and blood viscosity within the hemodiafilter, particularly when high ultrafiltration rates are applied in postdilution HDF and when the patient has low capacity to recruit fluid from the extravascular space during dehydration [33]. The excessive protein concentration occurring along fibers of hemodialyzer tends to foul membrane and to decrease its nominal permeability leading to a high transmembrane pressure to maintain the prescribed ultrafiltration rates [55].

Several studies [66-69] suggest that CKD G5D patients receiving postdilution HDF may have a lower risk of death than HD, especially when high convective volume (23 liters) is reached per dialysis session [33]. To the conventional 4-hour thrice weekly session, high convective volumes in postdilution HDF are achieved through the application of high blood flows (Qb > 350 mL/min) which demands adequate vascular access as a prerequisite. This remains the main limitation to a broader application of this therapy among CKD G5D patients.

Predilution HDF

The predilution HDF may provide improved rheological and hydraulic conditions compared to the postdilution modality by conserving the membrane permeability, as the substitution fluid added to blood before the hemodiafilter reduces hemoconcentration and facilitates increased flow rate within the fibers with intensified shear-rate effect on the secondary protein layer [33]. To achieve a convective dose in predilution HDF equivalent to the targeted convective dose in postdilution HDF, the ultrafiltration volume should be multiplied by two [31].

The principal barriers to widespread use of predilution HDF result from: 1) the elevated cost, when compared to postdilution HDF, due to the increased amount of substitution fluid and electrolyte concentrates required; and 2) the reduced efficiency of small solute removal in the predilution modality, a consequence of the decrease in the diffusive component. Predilution HDF may benefit patients with high hematocrit to help in the anticoagulation of the extracorporeal circuit [33].

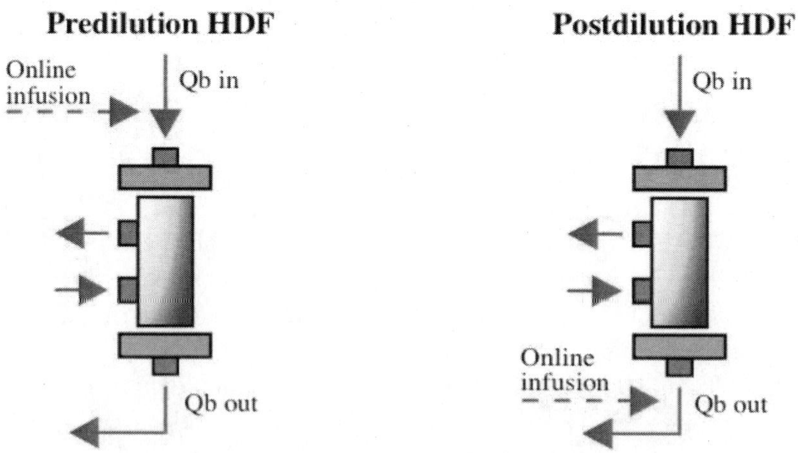

Figure 1. The main substitution modalities of HDF.

Figure 1 shows the two main substitution modalities of HDF discussed in this section; Table 3 presents the advantages and disadvantages of each of these modalities.

Table 3. Substitution modalities of HDF – advantages and disadvantages

Substitution Modalities	Advantages	Disadvantages
Predilution HDF	• Hemodilution • Lower hematocrit • Reduced protocrit • Lower viscosity • Reduced oncotic pressure • Increase shear rate and shear stress • Reduced fiber and membrane fouling • Permits HDF with lower blood flow or unfavorable hemorheological conditions • May enhance protein-bound solute clearance • Preserves hydraulic and solute membrane permeability (reduces membrane stress)	• Lower solute removal • Higher substitution volume needed (multiplied by two)
Postdilution HDF	• Higher efficiency in solute removal • Lower volume of substitution fluid than predilution, mid-dilution or mixed-dilution	• Necessity of a vascular access capable of delivering higher blood flow (350-400 mL/min) • Hemoconcentration Higher viscosity Higher oncotic pressure Increase in hematocrit and protocrit Potential membrane fouling • Reduced hydraulic and solute membrane permeability Reduced sieving coefficient Fiber clotting Potential alarms Increase in transmembrane pressure Increased membrane stress Potential albumin leakage

Adapted from Canaud et al, 2015 [31].

PREDILUTION HDF – THE JAPANESE EXPERIENCE

Predilution HDF Is the Mainstream of Online HDF in Japan

Online HDF with the use of ultrapure dialysis fluid has been utilized in Japan since the early 1990s. There have been three historical milestones in the development of online HDF in Japan: 1) the development of the Japanese Society for hemodiafiltration (JSHDF) in 1995; 2) the extra payment for ultrapure dialysis fluid in 2010; and 3) the extra payment for online HDF in 2012.

At the annual JSHDF meetings, many doctors and clinical engineers have met to discuss the clinical benefits, new technologies, and the water treatment of online HDF. Through these annual meetings, the trend of predilution online HDF in Japan has gradually been established. The first reimbursement for online HDF was introduced in 2010, but the extra payment for online HDF was established in 2012. It is an additional 500 JPY (equivalent to about 5 US dollars) for each conventional HD session. In the early days, offline HDF (bottle type) was the only reimbursed method, and it was provided only for dialysis related amyloidosis and intradialytic hypotension. However, these limited indications of HDF were totally withdrawn in 2012. Since then, the number of patients treated with HDF has been rapidly increasing; up to 38.3% (121,634/316,113) of all dialysis patients by the end of 2018 [70].

Dialysis fluid quality is an indispensable element for online HDF because bacteriological contamination of dialysis fluid deteriorates the safety of the therapy as well as the efficacy. The Japanese Society for Dialysis Therapy (JSDT) recommends that all dialysis modalities including online HDF should be provided with ultrapure dialysis fluid [71]. An extra payment for ultrapure dialysis fluid was also set in 2010 as additional 200 JPY (2 US dollars) for each session. It was reduced to 100 JPY (1 US dollar) in 2020. In the 2018 JSDT annual survey, ultrapure dialysis fluid had been achieved in 74.6% (3,168/4,244) of all facilities [70].

There are several kinds of HDF methods from the annual report from JSDT 2018: online HDF (70.9%), intermittent infusion HDF (IHDF) (26.0%) [72], acetate free biofiltration (AFBF) (0.1%), offline HDF (2.9%) and push-pull HDF (0.0%). As previously reported, the predilution mode is the mainstream of online HDF in Japan since the first JSDT survey for HDF in 2009. 95.6% of online HDF patients were treated by the predilution mode, whereas 86.6% of offline HDF patients were treated by the postdilution mode [73]. The average substitution volume was 39.9 liters in predilution and 10.2 liters in postdilution online HDF, whereas it was 12.0 liters in predilution and 8.0 liters in postdilution offline HDF [73]. The substitution volume was smaller in postdilution online HDF in Japan compared with previous reports, which emphasized the need for larger substitution volumes, greater than 20 liters per session, in order to achieve good clinical results [69, 74]. However, Japanese doctors use porous filters even for postdilution HDF as well as predilution HDF so we can achieve sufficient removal of low molecular weight proteins (LMWPs), even with small substitution volume in postdilution HDF [75].

Why Is the Predilution Mode the Mainstream in Japan?

Online HDF has been promoted in the world because with the intent to ameliorate QOL of dialysis patients and improve survival rate. Several studies have shown survival advantage or improvement of QOL for dialysis patients by online HDF [69, 76, 77]. Most of these trials were performed with postdilution HDF; however, predilution HDF has been the main stream of this modality uniquely in Japan. Why has predilution online HDF been the main stream in Japan?

In the early history of HDF therapy in Japan, several pioneer doctors found that aggressive removal of LMWPs with some albumin leakage occasionally ameliorated severe renal anemia [78, 79]. Since then, various small studies, which included clinical advantages of aggressive removal of LMWPs on dialysis related symptoms, have been reported. They evaluated bone/joint pain, skin itchiness, intradialytic hypotension restless leg syndrome (RLS) and general fatigue. In these trials, they used porous filters in the predilution mode of online HDF and accepted some albumin leakage, 3-5g or greater than 10g per session, depending on the patient's condition, in order to remove larger LMWPs [80, 81]. Unfortunately, most of these studies were reported in Japan. Interestingly, the Japanese experience did not spread outside the country, since protein leaking membrane and/or modality is being considered potentially harmful in this vulnerable population in Europe [82, 83].

The convective therapy developed to remove middle molecules effectively, and the efficacy of convective therapy mainly depends on the convection volume and the pore size distribution of the filter. Higher blood flow rate is indispensable in increasing the convection volume in the postdilution mode; on the other hand, it can be increased limitlessly in the predilution mode even though in a lower blood flow rate. However, caution should be implemented when observing small solutes under-dialysis in predilution HDF [84, 85]. In Japan, the average blood flow rate (around 200 mL/min) has been lower than the 300-400 mL/min commonly used in the rest of the world. Predilution HDF is able to increase the convection volume with lower blood flow rates [75]. However, sufficient Kt/V urea of around 1.5 has been reported in predilution HDF; no differences have been found among dialysis modalities [73].

When we try to remove larger LMWPs than ß2-microglobulin, we have to use more porous filters: high cut-off or medium cut-off filters. If we use these filters in the post dilution mode, we have a risk of unexpected amount of albumin leakage because of the protein concentrated layer on the membrane surface. In the predilution mode, we can control the albumin leakage by choosing a filter and titrating the substitution flow rate. In Japan, several dialysis companies have produced various types of filters with various solute removal properties composed by various membrane materials. Therefore, we can easily choose a proper filter for the patient condition and the target of solute removal.

Based on these key points, the predilution HDF with large substitution volume and porous filter has been the mainstream of HDF therapy in Japan. We usually use these types of filters for postdilution HDF with relatively lower substitution volume; however, we can get enough removal of LMWPs compared to postdilution HDF with large substitution volume, which is more commonly performed in the world [75]. These concepts of the convective therapy and the use of protein adsorptive membrane in HD in Japan could be said in short, "protein permeable dialysis" [80, 81].

As previously addressed, most of the trials about the clinical advantages of online HDF were performed in the postdilution mode, and there were few reports performed in the predilution mode, especially from Japan. Recently, Kikuchi et al. [86] reported the survival advantage of predilution online HDF compared with high flux HD from the JSDT data. Sakurai et al. reported that predilution HDF effectively ameliorated RLS according to increasing the intensity of larger LMWPs removal [87, 88]. Nagai et al. [89] reported the survival advantage of albumin leaky dialysis on patient survival.

Daily Practice Pattern of Online HDF in Japan

It is very important to set key and relevant parameters to assess quality and efficacy of HDF therapy; those parameters should be easy to use in clinical practices and also be connected to the patient's benefits. Convective therapy was developed to ameliorate uremic symptoms by intensively removing middle molecules, so we should have two types of parameters for adjusting and personalizing prescription to the patient's needs; one is the middle molecule removal, and the other is the patient's symptoms [81]. We should always consider the relationship between the solute removal and the symptoms.

The JSDT guideline recommends keeping the serum ß2-microglobulin concentration before dialysis below 30mg/L and 25mg/L, if possible [90]; this is the only guideline that addresses the removal of middle molecule in dialysis patients. However, there have been no guidelines or target values about the removal rate of ß2-microglobulin. Hoshino clearly showed the survival advantages in the dialysis patients treated with therapies with the removal rate of ß2-microglobulin as greater than 80% [91]. Recently, the targets of the middle molecule removal have become larger LMWPs, such as cytokines, free light chains and more [81, 85, 92]. There have been few studies that evaluated the relationship between the removal of LMWPs and improvement of dialysis related symptoms. Sakurai et al. [87] reported that removal rate of α1-microglobulin greater than 30% dramatically ameliorated RLS and the muscle rigidity caused by dialysis related amyloidosis. Through these experiences, the target level of the removal rate of α1-microglobulin has been set at greater than 35%. When we try to remove α1-microglobulin intensively, we have to accept some albumin leakage during dialysis session: 3-5 g, > 5 g or > 10 g per session, depending on the patient's condition. When we try these types of therapy, we have to be aware of the changes in serum albumin and should check the albumin concentration in the spent dialysate. The predilution mode is safer to effectively remove larger LMWPs avoiding the excessive albumin leakage than the postdilution mode, as previously addressed.

The first reason for prescribing HDF is to focus on the patient's symptoms. Is it skin itchiness, RLS, intradialytic hypotension, post-dialysis fatigue or something else? After we decide the targeted symptom of the therapy, we should evaluate it quantitatively or semi-quantitatively for the consequent evaluation of the intervention [81]. In Japan, the predilution mode is generally chosen for skin itchiness, RLS and hypotension, and the postdilution mode is chosen for bone/joint pain from dialysis related amyloidosis. We start predilution HDF with a mild protein permeable filter; the blood flow rate is generally 250-400 ml/min, the total dialysis fluid flow rate is 400-600 ml/min, and the substitution flow rate is around 12 liters/hour. When the targeted symptom improves, we keep the dialysis prescription until other symptoms possibly occur. If the symptomatology does not improve, we intensify the removal of larger LMWPs by monitoring the removal rate of ß2-microglobulin, α1-microglobulin as well as the albumin leakage during the dialysis session. If the symptomatology persists, we change the dialyzer (another membrane type) or the dilution mode to postdilution. Longer dialysis time and frequent dialysis are effective to ameliorate the symptoms, too. Protein leak therapies occasionally cause serum hypoalbuminemia and general fatigue. When we admit these signs, we have to downgrade the pore distribution of the filter or decrease the substitution flow rate.

PRESCRIPTION OF HDF

Although other treatment times and frequencies (short daily HDF, nocturnal HDF, etc.) are available, the conventional HDF scheme most commonly used worldwide is the same as conventional HD; a thrice-weekly 4-hour session. In this scheme, in order to obtain the best outcome, the goal of the therapy should be to achieve a convective volume per session of at least 23 liters in postdilution HDF and 46 liters in predilution HDF (twice the postdilution goal).

Not only the convective volume, but also the Kt/V should be evaluated periodically. If the goal is not achieved, changes in blood flow, dialysate flow, treatment time and/or frequency should be considered. The surface area of the hemodiafilter has to be sufficient to achieve the targeted Kt/V and a minimum KoA of 1000 should be prescribed. In case of higher filtration rates, it may be necessary to have a membrane with at least 30 ml/h/mmHg/m^2 of KuF. As mentioned before, a vascular access that provides adequate blood flow are important in order to avoid higher TMP, which may lead to fouling and clotting. A hemodiafilter with a larger surface area, KoA, KuF and different membrane should be considered if the therapy goals are not achieved after the initial maneuvers [74, 93].

The electrolyte prescription (e.g., Sodium, Potassium, Bicarbonate, Calcium, Magnesium) must be individualized according to the convective volume and metabolic needs of the patient [43]. Table 4 shows the usual electrolyte concentration in the dialysis fluid.

Table 4. Electrolyte concentration in the HDF dialysis fluid [31]

Electrolyte	Concentration
Sodium	135-138 mM
Potassium	2-4 mM
Bicarbonate	28–30 mM
Calcium	1.25–1.50 mM (2.5–3.0 mEq/L)
Magnesium	0.5 mM (1.0 mEq/L).

In comparison with conventional HD, HDF leads to increased blood pro-coagulatory activity due to forced ultrafiltration and potential loss of anticoagulant. Important to note that malfunction of the vascular access further increases the intradialytic coagulation risk, especially on postdilution HDF. Anti-thrombotic agent (ie, unfractionated heparin, LMWH) should not be logically administered as a bolus into the dialyzer inlet bloodline; up to 80% of low-molecular-weight, heparin and 50% of unfractionated heparin can be removed on first passage through a HDF setup. For this reason, the heparin bolus dose at the beginning of HDF should be administered preferably via the venous needle at least three minutes before initiating extracorporeal blood flow in order to mix the heparin with the patient's blood or alternatively for practical reason should be given via outlet venous bublle trap. Heparin dosage varies for each patient and a stepwise increase approach is required [31].

REVIEW OF CLINICAL EVIDENCE SUPPORTING THE USE OF HDF

It is of utmost importance to provide an historical, scientific and clinical perspective on where and how convective therapy began, as well as which clinical evidence along the way have been considered, as support for further development of its modalities and indications.

In the 1960s, Belding Scribner made an observation that patients maintained on intermittent peritoneal dialysis (IPD) did remarkably well clinically, even though peritoneal dialysis (PD) was much less efficient than HD at removing the commonly considered uremic toxins of small molecular weight, such as urea [94]. The longer IPD treatment time presumably permitted the slowly diffusing middle molecular weight solutes to be adequately removed. This "speculation" gave birth to the idea by Lee Henderson and Lewis W. Bluemle that convection would provide a superb tool to test the importance of the "middle molecule" hypothesis and possibly might offer a new treatment modality for uremia. The identification of convective solute transport in conjunction with water removal was achieved in an experiment with PD patients using the peritoneal membrane in 1966 [95].

Lee Henderson initially proposed hemofiltration to be called "diafiltration" to acknowledge the likely joint roles of convection and diffusion in the overall transport process [95]. The principal focus while using high-permeability synthetic membranes during the late 1960s to the mid-1970s was intermittent hemofiltration, which was wrongly called hemodiafiltration at the time. Subsequently, Benjamin Burton from the NIH, upon recognizing how little diffusion played a part, suggested in 1976 that they call it "hemofiltration" [96].

The *in vitro* and *in vivo* performance of this convective blood cleansing modality was rigorously described in two seminal papers in 1975 [5, 6]. So, it can be said that by the early 1970s, both hemofiltration and hemodiafiltration were already potential dialysis modalities for the treatment of CKD G5D patients.

As the volumes of fluids being infused further increased, an in-line ultrafilter was developed and demonstrated that a single pass through a fresh anisotropic, hydrophobic membrane with the appropriate molecular cutoff rendered ordinary dialysate sterile, pyrogen-free, and suitable for intravenous infusion during hemofiltration [97].

The recollections of the first clinical hemofiltration have been reported by Lee Henderson [98]; at that time, there were no human experimentation committees to relieve investigators' angst about these concerns. After long discussions, it was decided to employ a strategy of "creeping substitution," where a small hemofilter would run in parallel with the Travenol 100 liters tank twin coil dialyzer for maintenance dialysis. They gradually scaled up the area of the hemofiltration membrane (from 0.2 m^2 to 1.6 m^2, the blood flow rate from 100 to 300-400 ml/min), and the amount of ultrafiltrate exchanged (from 500 ml to 100 liters in a predilution mode). The latter estimates were guided by rough kinetics modeling of hemofilter performance. They were confident that the incremental approach would permit the identification of any deterioration in either the clinical or the laboratory status of the study subject [98]. Today this combined use of convection and diffusion is known as HDF [99].

The ease with which excess body water could be removed by the first patient to initiate the incremental protocol was remarkable; however, 10 to 15 liters of fluid exchange over the 5-hour treatment schedule produced a low-grade fever about half the time that resolved an hour or so following treatment. A second patient initiated the protocol and also presented frequent low-grade fevers that vanished promptly on conclusion of the session [100]. The cause for this fever subsequently turned out to be the use of pyrogen-containing water in the spinning process that adsorbed to the luminal surface of the fiber and was eluted by plasma, but not by saline. Their plan was to alternate two purely twin coil treatments with one predilution 15 liters HF treatment per week. The latter did not occur, as clinical hemofiltration was stopped, and they returned to animal work for the remainder of that year to track the cause of the fever.

The first patient to be fully maintained with 100 liters predilution hemofiltration as the only therapy was a woman with CKD-G5D due to severe hypertensive cardiovascular disease. After six months of therapy, there was no more hypertension or need of antihypertensive drugs, resolution of her cardiomegaly on chest x-ray, and the return to normal of her electrocardiogram (earlier compatible with left ventricular hypertrophy), whereas her biochemical profile showed no significant differences when compared with the one on routine HD [101].

Edward Quellhorst from Hannover was credited with the first in-depth clinical application of postdilution hemofiltration using the commercially available AN-69 membrane from Hospal and fluid cycling equipment of his own design. His group published their initial experience with hemofiltration (20 liters ultrafiltrate during one dialysis of five hours) in eight patients as a treatment for "dialysis-resistant" hypertension and hypotensive hyperhydration during a period of approximately one year (1/2 year to 1-1/2 years) [102]. His series of 100 patients followed for ten years is a landmark work [103] demonstrating that survival was comparable to, if not better than, that of hemodialysis patients who were treated three times per week for 5 hours, even though his hemofiltration patients were receiving a Kt/V for urea of only 1.65 per week.

Another group from Berlin reported on their clinical experience with more than 300 treatments obtained in seven uremic patients, treated three times weekly by chronic hemofiltration with each procedure lasting until 18 liters of filtrate [104]. The results suggested that hemofiltration would be superior to conventional hemodialysis. The main advantages of this treatment were characterized by its better control of hypertension, hyperhydration, improve hemodynamic response to ultrafiltration and possibly of uremic bone disease [105, 106]. Their next publication with experience compiled in more than 2400 HF and published in November 1978 confirmed that hemofiltration represented an alternative way of treating uremic patients [107].

The first published report of using the arteriovenous pressure gradient to drive transmembrane transport in patients for primarily fluid removal in patients with kidney failure was done by Silverstein et al. [108] with half square meter surface polysulfone membranes designed for experimental use in hemofiltration. Kramer et al. [109] applied this technically simple transport device for the treatment of acute kidney failure on a continuous basis, using only the arteriovenous pressure gradient to drive the system. Enclosed in their concept was the use of time to achieve quantitatively significant amounts of uremic toxin removal, i.e., mimicking the natural kidney. The next significant innovation in this pump-free technology came from Geronemus and Schneider [110]. They refocused attention on diffusive transport to increase small solutes clearance in patients with acute renal failure with a catabolic rate that exceeded the capacity of continuous arteriovenous hemofiltration to remove these toxins. They used low hydraulic permeability cellulosic membrane in hollow fiber format using the low blood flows of a pumpless system but with the addition of a slow flowing gravity-driven dialysate stream.

The next steps in the evolution of this technique involved complexity with re-introduction of tubing pumps to move blood from vein (or artery) to vein and the ultrafiltrate line to increase the gravity flow. Diffusion and convection were combined (hemodiafiltration) using high hydraulic permeability membranes plus a slow (10 to 15 ml/min) dialysate flow rate [111].

Two of the reasons why convective therapies did not develop as fast as they should, were the lack of technology to enable online production of sterile and pyrogen-free solutions for infusion as replacement fluid for convective therapy, and the cost of such fluids, then commercially prepared. In addition to the costs, these bags had three other disadvantages: the handling of heavy fully filled bags, volume limitation, and no possibility to individualize the composition of the replacement solution to each patient individual needs.

One last, but not least, reason was the regulatory mindset in approving online production of such solutions. Thirty to fifty liters of online solution was already available and administered to seven volunteer patients over 4-5 hours of hemofiltration with no side-effects in 1978 [97]. Even though this study demonstrated the clinical safety of the online technique, the possibility for wide application was delayed for many years due to the regulatory approving processes. The introduction of online HDF using ultrapure dialysis fluid as the source of the replacement fluid has allowed convective volume to be increased and reduced the cost of the procedure [112].

Randomized studies with limited sample sizes and non-randomized short studies have shown that online HDF improves hemodynamic stability and response to erythropoietin-stimulating agents (ESAs) and reduces the incidence of hemodialysis-associated amyloidosis and chronic inflammation [24, 113-117].

The effect of online HDF on patient survival was initially derived from non-controlled studies. Canaud et al. analyzed the data from Dialysis Outcomes and Practice Patterns Study (DOPPS) and reported that survival was associated with the amount of convection [66]. The European DOPPS Study was associated with a mortality risk reduction of 35% in patients treated with high-efficiency hemodiafiltration compared with those treated with conventional hemodialysis. These results were confirmed in other non-controlled studies conducted in several European countries, although two randomized studies (CONTRAST 2012, Turkish 2012/2013) recently failed to show differences in patient survival [67, 68].

Short-term prospective interventional studies have provided intermediary outcomes showing HDF enhanced solute removal of middle and large molecular size solutes [7, 114], improved phosphate control [118, 119], improved hemodynamic tolerance during sessions [120-122], reduced inflammatory profile reduction of AGEs levels [123], increased removal of Leptin [124], protein bound solutes [125, 126], plasma CRP and Il-6 levels [127], and pro-inflammatory potential reduction [117].

In a prospective study, 714 chronic hemodialysis Dutch patients were assigned to either online postdilution hemodiafiltration (n=358) or to continue low-flux hemodialysis (n=356) [67]. The primary outcome measure was all-cause mortality, and the main secondary endpoint was a composite of major cardiovascular events. After a mean three years of follow-up, it was not detected a significant difference between treatment groups with regard to all-cause mortality, whereas receiving high-volume hemodiafiltration was associated with lower all-cause mortality, a finding that persisted after adjusting for potential confounders and dialysis facility. The strengths of the study are its randomized design and the accurate and concise data collection. A potential limitation may be the inclusion of prevalent patients (as being survivors), as illustrated by a mean dialysis vintage of 2.9 years. Whether the inclusion of incident patients would have resulted in a different outcome could not be concluded from this study.

The aim of the Turkish online HDF study was to compare postdilution online HDF and high-flux HD in terms of morbidity and mortality [68]. This prospective, randomized, controlled trial enrolled 782 patients undergoing thrice-weekly HD and randomly assigned them in a 1:1 ratio. The mean follow-up period was 22.7 ± 10.9 months. The primary outcome was a composite of death from any cause and nonfatal cardiovascular events. The mean substitution volume in online HDF was 17.2 ± 1.3 liters. Primary outcome was not different between the groups, as well as cardiovascular and overall survival, hospitalization rate and number of hypotensive episodes. In a post hoc analysis, the subgroup of online HDF patients treated with a median substitution volume > 17.4 liters per session had significantly better cardiovascular and overall survival compared with the high-flux HD group. In adjusted Cox-regression analysis, treatment with high-efficiency online HDF was associated with a 46% risk reduction for overall mortality and a 71% risk reduction for cardiovascular mortality compared with high-flux HD. The study presented some constraints, such as the fact that a type II-error in the statistical analysis could not be excluded, enrolled patients were younger than the European dialysis patient population, patients had already been on dialysis for some years prior to enrollment, 87% of the patients had their blood pressure well controlled and 95% had an arteriovenous fistula when enrolled in the study.

Despite the aforementioned constraints of the study, the results nevertheless supported the possibility that higher substitution volumes in online HDF could provide a survival benefit in

HD patients. From this point of view, the study was in line with observational findings of the DOPPS database showing an association with better survival in patients with a higher convection volume [66] and with the results of the one year earlier published post hoc analysis of the CONTRAST study data [67].

Right after both studies were published, it was time for the ESHOL study (a Spanish multicenter, open-label, randomized controlled trial) to be reported [69, 128]. In this study, patients were assigned either to continue hemodialysis (n=450) or to switch to high-efficiency postdilution online HDF (n=456). The primary outcome was all-cause mortality, and secondary outcomes included cardiovascular mortality, all-cause hospitalization, treatment tolerability, and laboratory data. Compared with patients who continued on hemodialysis, those assigned to online HDF had a 30% lower risk of all-cause mortality, a 33% lower risk of cardiovascular mortality, and a 55% lower risk of infection-related mortality. The estimated number needed to treat suggested that switching eight patients from hemodialysis to online HDF could prevent one annual death. The incidence rates of dialysis sessions complicated by hypotension and of all-cause hospitalization were lower in patients assigned to online HDF.

This was the first prospective, randomized clinical trial showing that high-efficiency postdilution online HDF reduces all-cause mortality compared with conventional hemodialysis in the chronic prevalent population. The survival benefit observed in this study had sufficient statistical robustness to support the finding that online HDF was the major determinant of survival. Furthermore, the results were consistent in distinct subgroups of patients according to age, sex, diabetes mellitus, the Charlson comorbidity index, and vascular access. Although all patient groups benefitted from online HDF, the subgroups obtaining the greatest benefit were older, with no diabetes, arteriovenous fistula, and a higher Charlson comorbidity index.

The strengths of this study include the randomized design, the large sample size, and long follow-up, as well as the requirement of high convection volumes. Hemodialysis units participating in this clinical trial were trained to utilize high blood flow rates and long dialysis times in order to deliver a mean convective volume close to 24 liters/session. A limitation of the study was that a small proportion of patients (6.3%) were treated with low-flux membranes and, additionally, residual renal function was not monitored.

Based on the results of the CONTRAST and Turkish studies [67, 68], the convective volume seemed to be an important issue. In the *post hoc* analysis, both studies showed a 39% and 46% mortality risk reduction in patients receiving high convection volumes (22 and 20 liters/session, respectively). Similarly, the post hoc analysis in the ESHOL study [69] showed a 40% and 45% mortality risk reduction in patients receiving convection volumes between 23–25 liters/session and >25 L/session, respectively. These results provided randomized clinical trial evidence of the need to deliver high convection volumes to reduce all-cause mortality. In the ESHOL study, the mean blood flow rate was higher (387 mL/min) than in the CONTRAST and Turkish studies (300 and 310 mL/min, respectively) whereas the mean length of dialysis was longer (236 minutes) than in the CONTRAST study (226 minutes) and was similar to that of the Turkish study (236 minutes). These factors led to a higher mean delivered convection volume in the ESHOL study (23.7 liters/session) than in the CONTRAST (20.7 liters) and Turkish (20.7 liters) studies. These results indicate that the treatment modality could modify patient survival when a sufficient convective volume is reached. In view of these results, the authors suggested that online HDF may become the first-line option.

In the FRENCHIE study [77], a prospective, open-label randomized controlled trial, 381 elderly chronic hemodialysis patients (over age 65) were randomly assigned in a one-to-one ratio to either high-flux hemodialysis or online hemodiafiltration. The primary outcome was intradialytic tolerance (day 30-day 120). During the observational period for intradialytic tolerance, 85% and 84% of patients in high-flux hemodialysis and online hemodiafiltration arms, respectively, experienced at least one adverse event without significant difference between groups. As exploratory analysis, intradialytic tolerance was also studied, considering the sessions as a statistical unit according to treatment actually received. Over a total of 11,981 sessions, 2,935 were complicated by the occurrence of at least one adverse event, with a significantly lower occurrence in online hemodiafiltration with fewer episodes of intradialytic symptomatic hypotension and muscle cramps. By contrast, health-related quality of life, morbidity, and mortality were not different in both groups. An improvement in the control of metabolic bone disease biomarkers and β2-microglobulin level without change in serum albumin concentration was observed with online hemodiafiltration. Thus, overall outcomes favor online hemodiafiltration over high-flux hemodialysis in the elderly.

A wealth of convective therapy clinical experience has been gathered and a steady growing number of colleagues have been convinced of convection as an option in renal replacement therapy during the last decades. The quality and efficacy of convective therapies should not be evaluated only by convective volumes, solute removal patterns, survival rates, biocompatibility and hemodynamic stability during dialysis. Patients should also play an important part in this evaluation process, expressing their preferences in a shared-decision process in which their opinion on what is meaningful and important to them is part of the decision, even if the decision may not be aligned to guideline-based care. Patients usually have as main outcome goals their well-being, in addition to individual preferences and priorities; for example, time with the family, possibility to participate more actively in family/social life, work, and the absence of symptoms such as fatigue, itching and restless legs.

We should not only apply a disease-oriented approach, but also exercise what today is called a patient-centered approach. The Japanese experience with the dialysis prescription system based on the patient's feelings, named "Patient Oriented Dialysis" (POD) has been successful [129]. The ongoing CONVINCE study [130] shall generate important data on patient reported outcomes, which will give us new insights in the quest for the best individually tailored therapy and prescription for CKD G5D patients who strive to live as long as possible with the best possible Quality of Life.

EVIDENCE BASED MEDICINE REVISITED IN LIGHT OF HDF

What Is It and What Is It Not?

Evidence-based medicine (EBM) was introduced in the early nineties by UK physicians to rationalize clinical practices facing rapid development of medical knowledge to provide tangible evidence to promote better use of protocols to treat diseases, to support life with medical devices, or to indicate surgical interventions [131-133]. This approach was demanded by care practioners, public and health authority regulators. In 1996, Sackett et al. defined what EBM actually was and also clarified what it was not [134]. In this position statement, the authors clearly delineated that EBM was at the intersection of three domains that includes clinical expertise (i.e., doctor), patient centered values (i.e., patient) and relevant scientific evidences (i.e., science). Unfortunately, as is often the case in medicine, only some of the good things of the concept were incorporated in practice, while a limited understanding of the overall scenario led to a lot of misconception or misuse leading to disillusion and frustration [135-137].

What Is Its Role in Improving Clinical Practices?

Over the last few years, several authors have criticized the tyranny of EBM methods, arguing that they are an attempt to monopolize science for standardizing methods and research tools around a unique scientific truth, hiding other very important domains (i.e., clinical expertise, patient perception, ethical considerations) [138, 139]. A culminant point came in a provocative editorial of the British Medical Journal in 2014 claiming that evidence-based medicine was broken [140].

The EBM controversy arose from the fact that one would like to assimilate 'Medicine' to a pure "Science" when it is also an "Art." Debate over clinical utility of EBM will continue forever if one does not recognize that Medicine is an "art based on science" and not a "science based on medicine." To ensure a successful practice and preserve medicine's humanistic role, it is crucial to swing back the pendulum of medicine more towards the lost "art of medicine."

Where Do We Stand Now in Terms of Clinical Evidence with HDF?

Current debate and controversy on clinical benefits of HDF may serve to illustrate crisis of EBM in the nephrology field [141]. As preamble to HDF discussion, the use of EBM in CKD-G5D is already facing with a number of difficulties: Firstly, randomized controlled studies are scarce, weak or even inexistent, explaining why the present level of recommendations is relatively weak regarding best practice guidelines for dialysis and CKD-G5D. Secondly, most seminal interventional RCTs in dialysis have failed to reach their primary objective (e.g., the HEMO study [142], MPO study [143], Nocturnal FHN [144], IDEAL [145]). Thirdly, CKD-G5D and uremia are highly complex pathologies that combine several metabolic disorders interacting with one another with the consequence that specific interventions focusing on any one component are likely to fail to impact patient outcome [146-148]. Fourthly, dialysis patients are mostly elderly (~2/3 are over 65 years) having often multiple comorbid conditions giving them a high-vital risk profile [149]. Finally, practice patterns in the renal replacement field are highly diverse, as demonstrated by the DOPPS initiative, meaning that center or care provider effects are significant confounding factor towards the eventual clinical outcome of the dialysis patient [150].

Hemodiafiltration is obviously part of this debate with pros and cons arguing about its utility or futility [151-154]. HDF is widely recognized as the most innovative and most efficient dialysis modality for CKD-G5D patients [29, 155] and is also rightly the subject of scientific scrutiny, to assess the evidence-based facts that support its added value in the renal replacement field [156]. Considering HDF as the most advanced renal replacement modality available today in CKD- G5D patients, it was worthwhile to review facts in terms of clinical evidence in order to identify gaps and generate complementary research questions when needed [141, 157].

Short-term prospective interventional studies have provided intermediary outcomes showing that HDF enhanced solute removal of middle and large molecular size solutes (i.e., ß2-microglobulin, phosphate), improved hemodynamic tolerance of sessions, reduced inflammatory profile and ESA dose consumption, and improved patient nutritional status were associated with clinical benefits. Interestingly, all these clinical benefits are directly linked to the total convective dose delivered.

Several large cohort studies addressing hard clinical endpoints also identified that HDF improved patient survival. The prospective Dialysis Outcomes and Practice Patterns Study (DOPPS) suggested first that patients treated with relatively high volume HDF (15–25 liters/session) had a 35% lower mortality than those treated with low-flux HD [66], even if this landmark finding could not be confirmed in a recent analysis of DOPPS [158]. More recently, three large national cohort studies (French Registry, REIN [159]; Australia-New-Zealand Registry, ANZ [160]; Japan Registry, JSDT [86]) adjusted for main confounding factors have shown that patients receiving online HDF had significant improved survival expectancy (up to 30%) as compared to high flux hemodialysis paired groups. Interestingly, patient survival benefits relied on a reduced cardiac mortality [86].

Four main prospective randomized clinical trials (RCTs) were conducted in Europe (i.e., CONTRAST [67], TURKISH HDF [68], ESHOL [69], FRENCHIE [77]) over the last decade following initial DOPPS findings. As discussed earlier, only one out of the four-study - the ESHOL study - showed beneficial effects on all-cause or cardiovascular mortality. These findings sounded disappointing for the scientific medical community since they were not supportive of the superiority of HDF. However, it is interesting to note that far from rejecting the use of HDF, these findings stimulated research among medical community to scrutiny causes of failure and potential corrective actions. Apart from methodological concern of different studies, the main critical factor identified to be associated with patient's survival benefits was the total ultrafiltered volume per session, namely the convective dose. Interestingly, the convective dose delivered in postdilution HDF acted on survival in a dose-relationship manner with a minimum threshold volume (i.e., 22-23 liters per session in postdilution mode and 48 liters in predilution mode). Several causal factors reflecting mostly modifiable local policy and/or care practices patterns were identified (i.e., blood flow, vascular access, prescription, HDF machines, filters, substitution modality), thus offering potential ways of care improvement [74, 161, 162].

An individual-patient data meta-analysis (IPD-MA) being recognized as the gold standard for providing systematic review analysis [163, 164] was further developed based on pooled and completed dataset of the 2793 patients belonging to the four RCTs to overcome individual limitations of each one [76, 165]. In brief, HDF was associated with a reduction in relative risk of mortality (all-cause and cardiovascular) for patients in the highest tertile of convection volume, whatever anthropometric standardizing factor was used [165]. Again, the greatest benefit was for patients receiving the highest delivered convection volume (> 23 liters/session or 25.7 liters/1.73 m^2 body surface area).

What Is Missing to Bridge the Gap to Prove Superiority of HDF?

Renal replacement therapy is a continuous and steadily improving process that has led pioneers to develop innovation such as bicarbonate-buffered dialysate, high-flux membrane, ultrapure dialysate, ultrafiltration controller, and smart dialysis machines. Online hemodiafiltration is part of this evolutive process aiming to reduce burden of CKD-G5D patients. What remains to bridge the gap and prove superiority of HDF in a full EBM perspective? This question is currently being addressed by the CONVINCE study, a European Community-funded study, that started to enroll 1,800 prevalent CKD-G5D patients and planned to compare in two arms (of 900 patients each), high-flux HD and high-volume HDF (> 23 liters/session) over a three-year follow-up period [130]. To minimize concerns regarding dialysis dosing, targets were set on best practice guidelines both for the HD and the HDF. In addition, to further assess renal replacement treatment burden, the primary objective is focusing on mortality (all-cause and cardiovascular causes) while the secondary objective is focusing on patient perception (Patient Reported Outcome and Patient Reported Experience) using an innovative tool: PROMIS. In other words, within the same large scale multicenter international RCT study, we do hope that CONVINCE will provide definitive answers on patients' outcomes and patients' experiences.

REFERENCES

[1] Leber HW, Wizemann V, Goubeaud G, Rawer P, Schütterle G. Hemodiafiltration: a new alternative to hemofiltration and conventional hemodialysis. *Artif Organs.* 1978;2:150-3.

[2] Henderson LW, Silverstein ME, Ford CA, Lysaght MJ. Clinical response to maintenance hemodiafiltration. *Kidney Int Suppl.* 1975:58-63.

[3] Canaud B, Araujo A, Sany C, et al. A urea kinetic model for haemofiltration. *Life Support Syst.* 1985;3:15-25.

[4] Leypoldt JK. Solute fluxes in different treatment modalities. *Nephrol Dial Transplant.* 2000;15 Suppl 1:3-9.

[5] Henderson LW, Colton CK, Ford CA. Kinetics of hemodiafiltration. II. Clinical characterization of a new blood cleansing modality. *J Lab Clin Med.* 1975;85:372-91.

[6] Colton CK, Henderson LW, Ford CA, Lysaght MJ. Kinetics of hemodiafiltration. I. In vitro transport characteristics of a hollow-fiber blood ultrafilter. *J Lab Clin Med.* 1975;85:355-71.

[7] Maduell F, Navarro V, Cruz MC, et al. Osteocalcin and myoglobin removal in on-line hemodiafiltration versus low- and high-flux hemodialysis. *Am J Kidney Dis.* 2002;40:582-9.

[8] Maduell F, Navarro V, Torregrosa E, et al. Change from three times a week on-line hemodiafiltration to short daily on-line hemodiafiltration. *Kidney Int.* 2003;64:305-13.

[9] Maduell F, Arias M, Durán CE, et al. Nocturnal, every-other-day, online haemodiafiltration: an effective therapeutic alternative. *Nephrol Dial Transplant.* 2012;27:1619-31.

[10] Canaud B, N'Guyen QV, Lagarde C, Stec F, Polaschegg HD, Mion C. Clinical evaluation of a multipurpose dialysis system adequate for hemodialysis or for postdilution hemofiltration/hemodiafiltration with on-line preparation of substitution fluid from dialysate. *Contrib Nephrol.* 1985;46:184-6.

[11] Canaud B, Nguyen QV, Argiles A, Polito C, Polascheoo HD, Mion C. Hemodiafiltration using dialysate as substitution fluid. *Artif Organs.* 1987;11:188-90.

[12] Canaud B, Imbert E, Kaaki M, et al. Clinical and microbiological evaluation of a postdilutional hemofiltration system with in-line production of substitution fluid. *Blood Purif.* 1990;8:160-70.

[13] Canaud B, Bosc JY, Leray-Moragues H, et al. On-line haemodiafiltration. Safety and efficacy in long-term clinical practice. *Nephrol Dial Transplant.* 2000;15 Suppl 1:60-7.

[14] Canaud B, Vienken J, Ash S, Ward RA. Hemodiafiltration to Address Unmet Medical Needs ESKD Patients. *Clin J Am Soc Nephrol.* 2018;13:1435-43.

[15] Ward RA, Vienken J, Silverstein DM, Ash S, Canaud B. Regulatory Considerations for Hemodiafiltration in the United States. *Clin J Am Soc Nephrol.* 2018;13:1444-9.

[16] Tattersall JE, Ward RA. Online haemodiafiltration: definition, dose quantification and safety revisited. *Nephrol Dial Transplant.* 2013;28:542-50.

[17] Canaud B. 'On-site' preparation of sterile apyrogenic electrolyte solutions for hemofiltration and hemodiafiltration. In: Cambi V (eds.) *Short Dialysis Topics in Renal Medicine,* vol 3 Springer, Boston, MA 1987;3.

[18] Mion CM, Canaud B, Garred LJ, Stec F, Nguyen QV. Sterile and pyrogen-free bicarbonate dialysate: a necessity for hemodialysis today. *Adv Nephrol Necker Hosp.* 1990;19:275-314.

[19] Canaud BJM, Mion CM. Water Treatment for Contemporary Hemodialysis. In: Jacobs C, Kjellstrand CM, Koch KM, Winchester JF, eds. *Replacement of Renal Function by Dialysis*. Dordrecht: Springer Netherlands; 1996:231-55.

[20] Kessler M, Group EW. Dialysis fluid purity: Section IV. *Nephrol Dial Transplant.* 2002;17:45-62.

[21] Mion M, Kerr PG, Argiles A, Canaud B, Flavier JL, Mion CM. Haemodiafiltration in high-cardiovascular-risk patients. *Nephrol Dial Transplant.* 1992;7:453-4.

[22] Locatelli F, Altieri P, Andrulli S, et al. Hemofiltration and hemodiafiltration reduce intradialytic hypotension in ESRD. *J Am Soc Nephrol.* 2010;21:1798-807.

[23] Canaud B. Effect of online hemodiafiltration on morbidity and mortality of chronic kidney disease patients. *Contrib Nephrol.* 2007;158:216-24.

[24] Locatelli F, Marcelli D, Conte F, Limido A, Malberti F, Spotti D. Comparison of mortality in ESRD patients on convective and diffusive extracorporeal treatments. The Registro Lombardo Dialisi E Trapianto. *Kidney Int.* 1999;55:286-93.

[25] Floege J, Ketteler M. beta2-microglobulin-derived amyloidosis: an update. *Kidney Int Suppl.* 2001;78:S164-71.

[26] Takenaka T, Itaya Y, Tsuchiya Y, Kobayashi K, Suzuki H. Fitness of biocompatible high-flux hemodiafiltration for dialysis-related amyloidosis. *Blood Purif.* 2001;19:10-4.

[27] Canaud B, Bowry SK. Emerging clinical evidence on online hemodiafiltration: does volume of ultrafiltration matter? *Blood Purif.* 2013;35:55-62.

[28] Canaud B, Morena M, Leray-Moragues H, Chalabi L, Cristol JP. Overview of clinical studies in hemodiafiltration: what do we need now? *Hemodial Int.* 2006;10 Suppl 1:S5-s12.

[29] Canaud BJ. Changing paradigms of renal replacement therapy in chronic kidney disease patients: ultrapure dialysis fluid and high-efficiency hemodiafiltration for all? *Kidney Int.* 2009;76:591-3.

[30] Canaud B, Kohler K, Sichart JM, Moller S. Global prevalent use, trends and practices in haemodiafiltration. *Nephrol Dial Transplant.* 2020;35:398-407.

[31] Canaud B, Bowry S, Stuard S. Hemodiafiltration. In Daugirdas JT, Blake PG, Ing TS (eds.). *Handbook of Dialysis*. 5th ed. Philadelphia: Lippincott Williams & Wilkins; 2015.

[32] Ronco C, Cruz D. Hemodiafiltration history, technology, and clinical results. *Adv Chronic Kidney Dis.* 2007;14:231–243.

[33] Pedrini LA, Zerbi S. Convective Techniques. In Nubé MJ, Grooteman MPC, Blankestijn PJ (eds.). *Hemodiafiltration: Theory, Technology and Clinical Practice.* Springer International Publishing Switzerland, 2016.

[34] Floege J, Granolleras C, Deschodt G, et al. High-flux synthetic versus cellulosic membranes for beta 2-microglobulin removal during hemodialysis, hemodiafiltration and hemofiltration. *Nephrol Dial Transplant.* 1989;4:653–7.

[35] Kim ST. Characteristics of protein removal in hemodiafiltration. *Contrib Nephrol.* 1994;108:23–37.

[36] Morti SM, Zydney AL. Protein-membrane interactions during hemodialysis: effects on solute transport. *ASAIO J.* 1998;44:319–26.

[37] Ronco C, Heifetz A, Fox K, et al. Beta 2-microglobulin removal by synthetic dialysis membranes. Mechanisms and kinetics of the molecule. *Int J Artif Organs.* 1997;20:136–43.

[38] Weryński A, Malchesky PS, Lewandowski JJ, Waniewski J, Wójcicki J, Piatkiewicz W. Theoretical formulation of sieving coefficient evaluation for membrane plasma separation. *Artif Organs.* 1985;9(3):250-254.

[39] Lornoy W, Becaus I, Billiouw JM, Sierens L, Van Malderen P. Remarkable removal of beta-2-microglobulin by on-line hemodiafiltration. *Am J Nephrol.* 1998;18:105–8.

[40] Ledebo I. Principles and practice of hemofiltration and hemodiafiltration. *Artif Organs.* 1998;22(1):20–5.

[41] Jaffrin MY. Convective mass transfer in hemodialysis. *Artif Organs.* 1995;19(11):1162-1171.

[42] Cappelli G, Perrone S, Ciuffreda A. Water quality for on-line haemodiafiltration. *Nephrol Dial Transplant.* 1998;13 Suppl 5:12–6.

[43] Canaud B, Ledebo I. History and Current Status of Online Haemodiafiltration. In Nubé MJ, Grooteman MPC, Blankestijn PJ (eds.). *Hemodiafiltration: Theory, Technology and Clinical Practice.* Springer International Publishing Switzerland, 2016.

[44] Bowry SK. Membrane Requirements for High-Flux and Convective Therapies. *Contrib Nephrol.* 2011; 175: 57–68.

[45] Ward RA. Worldwide guidelines for the preparation and quality management of dialysis fluid and their implementation. *Blood Purif.* 2009;27:2–4.

[46] International Organization for Standardization. *Quality of dialysis fluid for haemodialysis and related therapies (ISO 23500-5:2019).* Geneva: International Organization for Standardization; 2019.

[47] Lonnemann G. Chronic inflammation in hemodialysis: the role of contaminated dialysate. *Blood Purif* 2000;18:214–223.

[48] Bowry SK, Gatti E, Vienken J. Contribution of polysulfone membranes to the success of convective dialysis therapies. *Contrib Nephrol.* 2011; 173: 110–118.

[49] Greenwood RN. The Machine and the Therapy Concept. *Contrib Nephrol.* 2011; 175: 27–34.

[50] Canaud BC, Chenine L, Renaud S, Leray H. Optimal therapeutic conditions for Online Hemodiafiltration. *Contrib Nephrol.* 2011; 168: 28–38.

[51] Vaslaki L, Karátson A, Vörös P, Major L, Pethö F, Ladányi E, Weber C, Mitteregger R, Falkenhagen D. Can sterile and pyrogen-free on-line substitution fluid be routinely delivered? A multicentric study on the microbiological safety of on-line haemodiafiltration. *Nephrol Dial Transplant.* 2000;15 Suppl 1:74–8.

[52] Di Felice A, Cappelli G, Facchini F, Tetta C, Cornia F, Aimo G, Lusvarghi E. Ultrafiltration and endotoxin removal from dialysis fluids. *Kidney Int Suppl.* 1993;41:S201–

[53] den Hoedt CH, Bots ML, Grooteman MP, van der Weerd NC, Mazairac AH, Penne EL, Levesque R, ter Wee PM, Nubé MJ, Blankestijn PJ, van den Dorpel MA, CONTRAST Investigators. Online hemodiafiltration reduces systemic inflammation compared to low-flux hemodialysis. *Kidney Int.* 2014;86(2):423–32.

[54] Penne EL, Visser L, van den Dorpel MA, van der Weerd NC, Mazairac AH, van Jaarsveld BC, Koopman MG, Vos P, Feith GW, Kremer Hovinga TK, van Hamersvelt HW, Wauters IM, Bots ML, Nubé MJ, Ter Wee PM, Blankestijn PJ, Grooteman MP. Microbiological quality and quality control of purified water and ultrapure dialysis fluids for online hemodiafiltration in routine clinical practice. *Kidney Int.* 2009;76(6):665–72.

[55] Ronco C. Hemodiafiltration: Technical and Clinical Issues. *Blood Purif.* 2015;40(1):2–11.

[56] Canaud B. Online hemodiafiltration. Technical options and best clinical practices. *Contrib Nephrol*. 2007; 158:110–122.

[57] Pedrini LA, Feliciani A, Zerbi S, Cozzi G, Ruggiero P. Optimization of middilution haemodiafiltration: technique and performance. *Nephrol Dial Transplant.* 2009;24:2816–2824.

[58] Feliciani A, Riva MA, Zerbi S, Ruggiero P, Plati AR, Cozzi G, Pedrini LA. New strategies in haemodiafiltration (HDF): prospective comparative analysis between on-line mixed HDF and mid-dilution HDF. *Nephrol Dial Transplant.* 2007;22:1672–1679.

[59] Pedrini LA, De Cristofaro V, Pagliari B et al. Mixed predilution and postdilution online hemodiafiltration compared with the traditional infusion modes. *Kidney Int.* 2000;58:2155-65.

[60] Canaud B, Lévesque R, Krieter D, Desmeules S, Chalabi L, Moragués H, Morena M, Cristol JP. On-line hemodiafiltration as routine treatment of end-stage renal failure: why pre- or mixed dilution mode is necessary in on-line hemodiafiltration today? *Blood Purif.* 2004;22(suppl 2):40–48.

[61] Pedrini LA, Zerbi S. Mixed dilution hemodiafiltration. *Contrib Nephrol.* 2007; 158: 123–130.

[62] Krieter DH, Falkenhain S, Chalabi L, Collins G, Lemke HD, Canaud B. Clinical cross-over comparison of mid-dilution hemodiafiltration using a novel dialyzer concept and post-dilution hemodiafiltration. *Kidney Int.* 2005;67:349–356.

[63] Santoro A, Ferramosca E, Mancini E, Monari C, Varasani M, Sereni L, Wratten M. Reverse mid-dilution: new way to remove small and middle molecules as well as phosphate with high intrafilter convective clearance. *Nephrol Dial Transplant.* 2007;22:2000–2005.

[64] Wizemann V, Kulz M, Techert F, Nederlof B. Efficacy of haemodiafiltration. *Nephrol Dial Transplant.* 2001;16 Suppl 4:27–30.

[65] Ahrenholz P, Winkler RE, Ramlow W, Tiess M, Muller W. On-line hemodiafiltration with pre and postdilution: a comparison of efficacy. *Int J Artif Organs.* 1997;20:81–90.

[66] Canaud B, Bragg-Gresham JL, Marshall MR, et al. Mortality risk for patients receiving hemodiafiltration versus hemodialysis: European results from the DOPPS. *Kidney Int.* 2006;69:2087–93.

[67] Grooteman MP, van den Dorpel MA, Bots ML, et al. Effect of online hemodiafiltration on all-cause mortality and cardiovascular outcomes. *J Am Soc Nephrol.* 2012;23:1087–96.

[68] Ok E, Asci G, Toz H, et al. Mortality and cardiovascular events in online haemodiafiltration (OL-HDF) compared with high-flux dialysis: results from the Turkish OL-HDF study. *Nephrol Dial Transplant.* 2013;28:192–202.

[69] Maduell F, Moreso F, Pons M, et al. High-efficiency postdilution online hemodiafiltration reduces all-cause mortality in hemodialysis patients. *J Am Soc Nephrol.* 2013;24:487–97.

[70] Nitta K, Masakane I, Hanafusa N, et al. 2018 Annual dialysis data report, JSDT renal Data Registry. *Japan J Dial* 2019; 52: 679-754.

[71] Kawanishi H, Akiba T, Masakane I, et al. Standard on microbiological management of fluids for hemodialysis and related therapies by the Japanese Society for Dialysis Therapy 2008. *Ther Apher Dial* 2009; 13: 161-166.

[72] Mineshima M, Takahashi S, Tomo T, et al. A Clinical Significance of Intermittent Infusion Hemodiafiltration Using Backfiltration of Ultrapure Dialysis Fluid Compared to Hemodialysis: A Multicenter Randomized Controlled Crossover Trial. *Blood Purif* 2019; 48: 368-381.

[73] Masakane I, Taniguchi M, Nakai S, et al. Annual Dialysis Data Report 2016, JSDT Renal Data Registry. *Renal Replacement Therapy* 2018; 4: 45.

[74] Chapdelaine I, de Roij van Zuijdewijn CL, Mostovaya IM, et al. Optimization of the convection volume in online post-dilution haemodiafiltration: practical and technical issues. *Clin Kidney J* 2015; 8: 191-198.

[75] Sakurai K, Hosoya H, Kurihara Y, et al. Evaluation of low-volume post-dilution online hemodiafiltration with Japanese high-performance hemodiafilters. *J Artif Organs* 2020:

[76] Peters SA, Bots ML, Canaud B, et al. Haemodiafiltration and mortality in end-stage kidney disease patients: a pooled individual participant data analysis from four randomized controlled trials. *Nephrol Dial Transplant* 2016; 31: 978-984.

[77] Morena M, Jaussent A, Chalabi L, et al. Treatment tolerance and patient-reported outcomes favor online hemodiafiltration compared to high-flux hemodialysis in the elderly. *Kidney Int* 2017; 91: 1495-1509.

[78] Saito A, Suzuki I, Chung TG, Okamoto T, Hotta T. Separation of an inhibitor of erythropoiesis in "middle molecules" from hemodialysate from patients with chronic renal failure. *Clin Chem* 1986; 32: 1938-1941.

[79] Yamada S, Kataoka H, Kobayashi H, Ono T, Minakuchi J, Kawano Y. Identification of an erythropoietic inhibitor from the dialysate collected in the hemodialysis with PMMA membrane (BK-F). *Contrib Nephrol* 1999; 125: 159-172.

[80] Tsuchida K, Minakuchi J. Albumin loss under the use of the high-performance membrane. *Contrib Nephrol* 2011; 173: 76-83.

[81] Masakane I, Sakurai K. Current approaches to middle molecule removal: room for innovation. *Nephrol Dial Transplant* 2018; 33: iii12-iii21.

[82] Krieter DH, Canaud B. High permeability of dialysis membranes: what is the limit of albumin loss?. *Nephrol Dial Transplant.* 2003;18(4):651-654.
[83] Ward RA. Protein-leaking membranes for hemodialysis: a new class of membranes in search of an application?. *J Am Soc Nephrol.* 2005;16(8):2421-2430.
[84] Masakane I, Kikuchi K, Kawanishi H. Evidence for the Clinical Advantages of Predilution On-Line Hemodiafiltration. *Contrib Nephrol* 2017; 189: 17-23.
[85] Maduell F, Broseta JJ, Rodas L, et al. Comparison of Solute Removal Properties Between High-Efficient Dialysis Modalities in Low Blood Flow Rate. *Ther Apher Dial* 2019.
[86] Kikuchi K, Hamano T, Wada A, Nakai S, Masakane I. Predilution online hemodiafiltration is associated with improved survival compared with hemodialysis. *Kidney Int* 2019; 95: 929-938.
[87] Sakurai K. Biomarkers for evaluation of clinical outcomes of hemodiafiltration. *Blood Purif* 2013; 35 Suppl 1: 64-68.
[88] Sakurai K, Saito T, Hosoya H, Kurihara Y, Yamauchi F. Therapeutic effect of high-efficiency online hemodiafiltration for recurrent restless legs syndrome in dialysis patients. *J Artif Organs* 2020.
[89] Nagai K, Tsuchida K, Ishihara N, et al. Implications of Albumin Leakage for Survival in Maintenance Hemodialysis Patients: A 7-year Observational Study. *Ther Apher Dial* 2017; 21: 378-386.
[90] Watanabe Y, Kawanishi H, Suzuki K, et al. Japanese society for dialysis therapy clinical guideline for "Maintenance hemodialysis: hemodialysis prescriptions." *Ther Apher Dial* 2015; 19 Suppl 1: 67-92.
[91] Hoshino J, Yamagata K, Nishi S, et al. Carpal tunnel surgery as proxy for dialysis-related amyloidosis: results from the Japanese society for dialysis therapy. *Am J Nephrol* 2014; 39: 449-458.
[92] Kirsch AH, Lyko R, Nilsson LG, et al. Performance of hemodialysis with novel medium cut-off dialyzers. *Nephrol Dial Transplant* 2017; 32: 165-172.
[93] Ronco C, Samoni S, De Rosa S. Dialyzers for Hemodiafiltration. In Nubé MJ, Grooteman MPC, Blankestijn PJ (eds.). *Hemodiafiltration: Theory, Technology and Clinical Practice*. Springer International Publishing Switzerland, 2016.
[94] Scribner BH: In Discussion. *Trans Am Soc Artif Intern Organs.* 1965; 81.
[95] Henderson LW. Peritoneal Ultrafiltration dialysis: enhanced urea transfer using hypertonic peritoneal dialysis fluid. *J Clin Invest.* 1966; 45: 950-5.
[96] Henderson LW. Hemofiltration. *Clin Nephrol.* 1978; 9: 43-4.
[97] Henderson LW, Beans E. Successful production of sterile pyrogen-free electrolyte solutions by ultrafiltration. *Kidney Int.* 1978;14: 522-25.
[98] Henderson LW. The Beginning of Clinical Hemofiltration: a Personal Account. *ASAIO J.* 2003; 513-7.
[99] Leber HW, Wizeman V, Goubaud G, Rawer P, Schutterle S. Simultaneous hemofiltration/hemodialysis: an effective alternative to hemofiltration and conventional hemodialysis in the treatment of uremic patients. *Clin Nephrol* 1978; 9: 115-21.
[100] Hamilton R, Ford C, Colton C, Cross R, Steinmuller S, Henderson L. Blood cleansing by diafiltration in uremic dog and man. *Trans Am Soc Artif Intern Organs.* 1971; 17: 259-65.

[101] Silverstein ME, Ford CA, Lysaght MJ, Henderson LW. Response to rapid removal of intermediate molecular weight solutes in uremic man. *Trans Am Soc Artif Int Organs.* 1974; 20B: 614-21.

[102] Schunemann B, Girndt J, Quellhorst E. Hemofiltration as a treatment for "dialysis-resistant" hypertension and hypotensive hyperhydration. *J Dial.* 1977; 1 (6): 575-83.

[103] Quellhorst E, Scheunnemann B, Hildebrand UH. Morbidity and mortality in long-term hemofiltration. *ASAIO J.* 1983; 6(4): 185-91.

[104] von Herrath D, Schaefer K, Hufler M, Asmus G, Hensel A. Clinical Aspects of Hemofiltration. *J Dial.* 1977; 1 (6): 545-58.

[105] Bergström J, Asaba H, Fürst P, Oulès R. Dialysis, ultrafiltration, and blood pressure. 1976. *Blood Purif.* 2006;24(2):222-231.

[106] Baldamus CA, Ernst W, Lysaght MJ, Shaldon S, Koch KM. Hemodynamics in hemofiltration. *Int J Artif Organs.* 1983;6(1):27-31

[107] Schaefer K, von Herrath D, Gullberg CA, Asmus G, Hufler M, Offermann G, Cremer H, Heuck CC, Ritz E. Chronic Hemofiltration: a critical evaluation of a new method for the treatment of blood. *Journal of Artificial Organs* 1978; 2 (4): 386-94.

[108] Silverstein ME, Ford CA, Lysagth MJ, Henderson LW. The treatment of severe fluid overload by ultrafiltration. *New Engl J Med.* 1974; 291: 747-51.

[109] Kramer P, Wigger W, Rieger J, Matthaei D, Scheler F. A new and simple method for treatment of overhydrated patients resistant to diuretics. *Klin Wschr.* 1977; 55: 1121-2.

[110] Geronemus R, Schneider W. Continuous arteriovenous hemodialysis: a new modality for treatment of acute renal failure. *Trans ASAIO.* 1984; 30: 610-3.

[111] Henderson LW. Hemofiltration: From the Origin to the New Wave. *Am J of Kidney Dis* 1996; 5 (S3): 105-7.

[112] Canaud B, Flavier JL, Argilés A, Stec F, Nguyen QV, Bouloux C, Garred LJ, Mion C: Hemodiafiltration with on-line production of substitution fluid: Long-term safety and quantitative assessment of efficacy. *Contrib Nephrol* 1994; 108: 12–22.

[113] Maduell F, del Pozo C, Garcia H, Sanchez L, Hdez-Jaras J, Albero MD, Calvo C, Torregrosa I, Navarro V: Change from conventional haemodiafiltration to on-line haemodiafiltration. *Nephrol Dial Transplant.* 1999; 14: 1202–07.

[114] Lornoy W, Becaus I, Billiouw JM, Sierens L, Van Malderen P, D'Haenens P. On-line haemodiafiltration. Remarkable removal of b2-microglobulin. Long-term clinical observations. *Nephrol Dial Transplant.* 2000; 15(1): 49–54.

[115] Ward RA, Schmidt B, Hullin J, Hillebrand GF, Samtleben W. A comparison of on-line hemodiafiltration and high-flux hemodialysis: A prospective clinical study. *J Am Soc Nephrol.* 2000 11: 2344–50.

[116] Wizemann V, Lotz C, Techert F, Uthoff S .On-line haemodiafiltration versus low-flux hemodialysis. A prospective randomized study. *Nephrol Dial Transplant.* 2000; 15(1): 43–8.

[117] Carracedo J, Merino A, Nogueras S, Carretero D, Berdud I, Ramírez R, Tetta C, Rodríguez M, Martín-Malo A, Aljama P. On-line hemodiafiltration reduces the proinflammatory CD14+CD16+ monocyte-derived dendritic cells: A prospective, crossover study. *J Am Soc Nephrol.* 2006; 17: 2315–21.

[118] Zehnder C, Gutzwiller JP, Renggli K. Hemodiafiltration: a new treatment option for hyperphosphatemia in hemodialysis patients. *Clin Nephrol* 1999; 52: 152-159.

[119] Penne EL, van der Weerd NC, van den Dorpel MA, Grooteman MPC, Lévesque R, Nubé MJ, Bots ML, Blankestijn PJ, ter Wee PM. Short-term effects of online hemodiafiltration on phosphate control: a result from the randomised controlled Convective Transport Study (CONTRAST). *Am J Kidney Dis.* 2010; 55: 77-87.

[120] Lin CL, Huang CC, Chang CT, Wu MS, Hung CC, Chien CC, Yang CW. Clinical improvement by increased frequency of on-line hemodialfiltration. *Ren Fail.* 2001; 23: 193–206.

[121] Donauer J, Schweiger C, Rumberger B, Krumme B, Böhler J. Reduction of hypotensive side effects during online-haemodiafiltration and low temperature haemodialysis. *Nephrol Dial Transplant.* 2003: 18, 8: 1616–1622.

[122] Vilar E, Fry AC, Wellsted D, Tattersall JE, Greenwood RN, Farrington K. Long-term outcomes in online hemodiafiltration and high flux hemodialysis: a comparative analysis. *Clin J Am Soc.* 2009; 4 (12) 1944-1953.

[123] Gerdemann A, Wagner Z, Solf A, Bahner U, Heidland A, Vienken J, Schinzel R. Plasma levels of advanced glycation end products during haemodialysis, haemodiafiltration and haemofiltration: potential importance of dialysate quality. *Nephrol Dial Transplant.* 2002; 17: 1045-1049.

[124] Lepenies J, Stahl C, Ludat K, et al. Elimination of leptin by different extracorporeal treatment modalities. *Nephrol Dial Transplant.* 2000;15:220.

[125] Bammens B, Evenepoel P, Verbeke K, Vanrenterghem Y. Removal of the protein-bound solute p-cresol by convective transport: a randomized crossover study. *Am J Kidney Dis.* 2004; 44:278-85.

[126] Bammens B, Evenepoel P, Keuleers H et al. Free serum concentrations of the protein-bound solute p-cresol predict mortality in hemodialysis patients. *Kidney Int.* 2006; 69: 1081-1087.

[127] Filipoulos V, Hadiyannakos D, Metaxaki P, Sideris V, Takouli L, Anogiati A, Vlassopoulos D. Inflammation and oxidative stress in patients on hemodiafiltration. *Am J Nephrol.* 2008; 28 (6): 949-57.

[128] Maduell F, Moreso F, Pons M, Ramos R, Mora-Macià J, Foraster A, Soler J, Galceran JM, Martinez-Castelao A, Online Hemodiafiltration Study Group from the Catalonian Society of Nephrology. Design and patient characteristics of ESHOL study, a Catalonian prospective randomized study. *J Nephrol.* 2011; 24: 196–202.

[129] Masakane I. High-Quality Dialysis: A Lesson from the Japanese Experience. *NDT Plus.* 2010; 3(1): i28-i35.

[130] Blankestijn PJ, Fischer KI, Barth C, et al. Benefits and harms of high-dose haemodiafiltration versus high-flux haemodialysis: the comparison of high-dose haemodiafiltration with high-flux haemodialysis (CONVINCE) trial protocol. *BMJ Open.* 2020;10:e033228.

[131] Richardson PE. David Sackett and the birth of Evidence Based Medicine: How to Practice and Teach EBM. *BMJ.* 2015;350:h3089.

[132] Sackett D. Evidence-based medicine. *Lancet* 1995;346:1171.

[133] Smith BH. Evidence based medicine. Rich sources of evidence are ignored. *BMJ* 1996;313:169; author reply 70-1.

[134] Sackett DL, Rosenberg WM, Gray JA, Haynes RB, Richardson WS. Evidence based medicine: what it is and what it isn't. *BMJ* 1996;312:71-2.

[135] Haynes B. Evidence-based medicine. *Lancet* 1995;346:1171.

[136] Maynard A. Evidence based medicine. Cost effectiveness and equity are ignored. *BMJ.* 1996;313:170-1.

[137] Miles A, Loughlin M, Polychronis A. Evidence-based healthcare, clinical knowledge and the rise of personalised medicine. *J Eval Clin Pract.* 2008;14:621-49.

[138] Goldenberg MJ. On evidence and evidence-based medicine: lessons from the philosophy of science. *Soc Sci Med.* 2006;62:2621-32.

[139] Greenhalgh T, Howick J, Maskrey N, Evidence Based Medicine Renaissance G. Evidence based medicine: a movement in crisis? *BMJ.* 2014;348:g3725.

[140] Spence D. Evidence based medicine is broken. *BMJ.* 2014;348:g22-g.

[141] Canaud B, Busink E, Apel C, Bowry SK. Is There Not Sufficient Evidence to Show That Haemodiafiltration Is Superior to Conventional Haemodialysis in Treating End-Stage Kidney Disease Patients? *Blood Purif.* 2018;46:7-11.

[142] Eknoyan G, Beck GJ, Cheung AK, et al. Effect of dialysis dose and membrane flux in maintenance hemodialysis. *N Engl J Med.* 2002;347:2010-9.

[143] Locatelli F, Martin-Malo A, Hannedouche T, et al. Effect of membrane permeability on survival of hemodialysis patients. *J Am Soc Nephrol.* 2009;20:645-54.

[144] Rocco MV, Daugirdas JT, Greene T, et al. Long-term Effects of Frequent Nocturnal Hemodialysis on Mortality: The Frequent Hemodialysis Network (FHN) Nocturnal Trial. *Am J Kidney Dis.* 2015;66:459-68.

[145] Cooper BA, Branley P, Bulfone L, et al. A randomized, controlled trial of early versus late initiation of dialysis. *N Engl J Med.* 2010;363:609-19.

[146] Twardowski ZJ, Misra M, Singh AK. Con: Randomized controlled trials (RCT) have failed in the study of dialysis methods. *Nephrol Dial Transplant* 2013;28:826-32; discussion 832.

[147] Singh AK, Kari JA, Twardowski ZJ, Misra M. Pro: The value of randomized controlled studies in dialysis methods. *Nephrol Dial Transplant.* 2013;28:834-5; discussion 5-6.

[148] Novak JE, Inrig JK, Patel UD, Califf RM, Szczech LA. Negative trials in nephrology: what can we learn? *Kidney Int.* 2008;74:1121-7.

[149] Gomez AT, Kiberd BA, Royston JP, et al. Comorbidity burden at dialysis initiation and mortality: A cohort study. *Can J Kidney Health Dis.* 2015;2:34.

[150] Robinson BM, Akizawa T, Jager KJ, Kerr PG, Saran R, Pisoni RL. Factors affecting outcomes in patients reaching end-stage kidney disease worldwide: differences in access to renal replacement therapy, modality use, and haemodialysis practices. *Lancet.* 2016;388:294-306.

[151] Mann JF. How does hemodiafiltration improve survival? *Kidney Int.* 2013;84:1287-8.

[152] Farrington K, Davenport A. The ESHOL study: hemodiafiltration improves survival-but how? *Kidney Int.* 2013;83:979-81.

[153] Kuhlmann MK. On-line hemodiafiltration: not a self-fulfilling prophecy. *J Am Soc Nephrol.* 2012;23:974-5.

[154] Golper TA. Is hemodiafiltration ready for broader use? *Kidney Int.* 2015;88:940-2.

[155] Maduell F, Moreso F. Should high-flux hemodialysis be replaced by online hemodiafiltration for treating end-stage renal disease patients? *J Comp Eff Res.* 2013;2:347-9.

[156] Mostovaya IM, Blankestijn PJ, Bots ML, et al. Clinical evidence on hemodiafiltration: a systematic review and a meta-analysis. *Semin Dial.* 2014;27:119-27.

[157] Schiffl H. Online hemodiafiltration and mortality risk in end-stage renal disease patients: A critical appraisal of current evidence. *Kidney Res Clin Pract.* 2019;38:159-68.

[158] Locatelli F, Karaboyas A, Pisoni RL, et al. Mortality risk in patients on hemodiafiltration versus hemodialysis: a 'real-world' comparison from the DOPPS. *Nephrol Dial Transplant.* 2018;33:683-9.

[159] Mercadal L, Franck JE, Metzger M, et al. Hemodiafiltration Versus Hemodialysis and Survival in Patients With ESRD: The French Renal Epidemiology and Information Network (REIN) Registry. *Am J Kidney Dis.* 2016;68:247-55.

[160] See EJ, Hedley J, Agar JWM, et al. Patient survival on haemodiafiltration and haemodialysis: a cohort study using the Australia and New Zealand Dialysis and Transplant Registry. *Nephrol Dial Transplant.* 2019;34:326-38.

[161] de Roij van Zuijdewijn CLM, Chapdelaine I, Nubé MJ, et al. Achieving high convection volumes in postdilution online hemodiafiltration: a prospective multicenter study. *Clin Kidney J.* 2017;10:804-12.

[162] Marcelli D, Scholz C, Ponce P, et al. High-volume postdilution hemodiafiltration is a feasible option in routine clinical practice. *Artif Organs.* 2015;39:142-9.

[163] Riley RD, Lambert PC, Abo-Zaid G. Meta-analysis of individual participant data: rationale, conduct, and reporting. *BMJ.* 2010;340:c221.

[164] Stewart LA, Tierney JF. To IPD or not to IPD? Advantages and disadvantages of systematic reviews using individual patient data. *Eval Health Prof.* 2002;25:76-97.

[165] Davenport A, Peters SA, Bots ML, et al. Higher convection volume exchange with online hemodiafiltration is associated with survival advantage for dialysis patients: the effect of adjustment for body size. *Kidney Int.* 2016;89:193-9.

In: Issues in Kidney Disease – Dialysis
Editors: Stephen Z. Fadem and José A. Moura-Neto
ISBN: 978-1-68507-000-7

Chapter 14

PALLIATIVE CARE IN DIALYSIS

Rebecca Schmidt*[*]*, DO and Anas Diab, MD
Department of Medicine, Section of Nephrology,
West Virginia University School of Medicine, Morgantown, WV, USA

ABSTRACT

Renal replacement therapy sustains life for patients with kidney failure, the benefits intended to outweigh the burdens and discomforts imposed by the procedure and its attendant complications. As a patient's clinical context changes and the hardships associated with dialysis become less acceptable, some patients come to desire a more conservative, less proactive approach to their overall care. Palliative care prioritizes comfort and patients' preferences for treatment in keeping with life goals and may be appropriate for patients contemplating withdrawal or wishing to de-escalate their care. The challenges of embedding palliative care into the continuum of care for patients on dialysis are multifactorial and juxtaposed against a culture of care evolving from the fundamental origins of dialysis and supported by longstanding regulatory and payment structures. This chapter addresses the challenges involved in embedding palliative practices and processes into the current culture of dialysis patient care, the rationale for a change in approach to dialysis care and the components needed to integrate a palliative focus into our care of patients dependent on dialysis for life.

Keywords: palliative care in ESRD, dialysis withdrawal, hospice, conservative management in ESRD, advance directives

INTRODUCTION

For patients with kidney failure, renal replacement therapy provides rescue from potentially fatal biochemical abnormalities and fluid accumulation, alleviating symptoms through partial correction of physiologic and volume balances. A semblance of normal life is restored by this process such that the benefits of dialysis for many patients outweigh the burdens

[*] Corresponding Author's E-mail: rschmidt@hsc.wvu.edu.

and discomforts imposed by the procedure and its attendant complications. Over time, as a patient's clinical context changes, the hardships associated with dialysis may enhance suffering and some patients choose to withdraw from dialysis. Other patients may wish to continue dialysis and pursue a more conservative, less proactive approach to their overall care.

Dialysis may be a decision of default for patients who present to physicians in dire clinical straits and those for whom the complexity of their medical status may supersede the immediacy of decision making about a life-sustaining therapy such as dialysis. Recognition of acute kidney injury also prompts dialysis to be initiated without consideration of future ramification because of the need for emergent action. Dialysis is sometimes provided as a time-limited trial to allow for contemplation while a patient's medical condition continues to evolve [1]. In many circumstances, once initiated, chronic maintenance dialysis is stopped only at death unless a conscious decision is made by the patient or surrogate decision maker to withdraw. Along with the growing literature and interest in conservative non-dialytic care for patients choosing to forego dialysis [2-5], there is increasing recognition and acceptance that conservative dialytic care is an appropriate palliative intervention for patients wishing to continue (or those not able to stop) dialysis [6-8].

As defined by the World Health Organization, palliative care is "an approach that improves the quality of life of patients and their families facing the problems associated with life-threatening illness, through the prevention and relief of suffering by means of early identification and impeccable assessment and treatment of pain and other problems, physical, psychosocial and spiritual [9]". Applied to dialysis patients, palliative care may be appropriate and implemented for patients contemplating withdrawal or when the desire to reduce one's active pursuit of new diagnoses or other active interventions constitute similar need for a defined palliative approach while continuing dialysis. Such an approach is one in which care prioritizes comfort and patients' preferences for treatment in keeping with life goals. The integration of palliative care into renal replacement therapy, thus includes the provision of supportive palliative care for patients who desire it, irrespective of whether withdrawal from dialysis is ultimately chosen. The challenges of embedding palliative care into the continuum of care for those dialysis patients who desire a less proactive approach are multifactorial and juxtaposed against a longstanding culture of care supported by regulatory and payment structures that may be at odds with psychosocial and emotional contextual considerations.

This chapter addresses the challenges inherent in embedding the practice of palliative care into the current culture of dialysis patient care, presents a rationale for changing our approach to dialysis care, and offers recommendations for integrating a palliative focus into care of those patients with dialysis-dependent kidney failure who desire a conservative approach.

Embedding the Option of Palliative Care into the Current Culture of Dialysis Care

Concept of Dialysis as a Life-Restorative Therapy vs. Life-Supportive or Life-Sustaining Care

With the passage of entitlement legislation in 1972, the opportunity to receive dialysis became a reality for most patients with end stage renal disease (ESRD), then a predominantly young population without chronic, progressive medical issues such as diabetes and heart disease [10]. Advances in medical care of cardiovascular and other diseases have contributed to longer life spans among patients with kidney failure and the indications for renal replacement therapy have since expanded to patients who historically would not have been offered dialysis by virtue of age or attendant medical problems [11, 12]. Subsequent advances in technology, improvements in effectiveness and the capacity for operationalizing the dialysis process have been accompanied by the unanticipated expansion of elderly patients initiating dialysis [13] and a prevalent ESRD population for which a standard approach to care may not meet the expectations and needs of individual patients whose reasons for both pursuing and continuing dialysis may be extremely disparate.

The introduction of palliation into the culture of dialysis care challenges the fundamental basis of renal replacement therapy as an essentially proactive treatment without which death may soon ensue. Resistance to the idea of palliative dialysis care may stem from the concept that dialysis was originally intended as a means to life restoration for those younger patients whose symptoms and complications of kidney failure precluded them from continuing employment or achieving activities of daily living [14, 15]. As a road to rehabilitation, the ESRD program was anticipated to foster and promote the return to work for its recipients, hence the evolution of structured processes and goals designed to maximize the benefits provided. The expectation that dialysis, if paid for, would make it possible for most recipients to return to work [16] did not come to pass and low employment rates among patients with advanced kidney disease continue to be reported [17-19]. As the population of patients starting renal replacement therapy has exploded to include older patients [13] with a multitude of medical issues, some progressive and some terminal, recognition that patients choose to pursue dialysis for different reasons has generated scrutiny of the generic nature of providing chronic dialysis. Rehabilitation is not a uniform goal among all patients with advanced kidney failure, some of whom initiate dialysis to avoid or forestall death or because they hope that dialysis can support them long enough to experience an upcoming event of life import [20]. Many older patients are significantly frail with what has been described as the "renal phenotype" [21] and the decision between dialysis or death was made under duress [22]. Commitment to continued care which might be intensive and require travel to hospitals or admission to nursing facilities for skilled care may be a less than desirable option for some older patients [23]. For those patients who do initiate dialysis, plans or even hopes that dialysis will allow rehabilitation or a return to previous levels of function may not be realized and wishes may change over time [24, 25]. As patients suffer clinical decline and the burdens of dialysis intensify, rehabilitation may no longer be a realistic goal (Figure 1). Changes in clinical status may be overt or subtle though not uncommonly the trajectory is one of continued decline [26, 27], and dialysis transforms from being life-restorative to life-sustaining with potential for prolonged suffering. The recognition that continuing dialysis is not the desire of every patient has accompanied efforts to instill palliative options into the dialysis culture of care [28, 29].

Disease-Focused, Facility-Focused and Population-Focused Culture

The provision of safe dialysis requires a complex infrastructure, staff with specialized knowledge and training and a comprehensive set of processes, systems and programs designed to assure that the process of dialysis is safely performed and patients are monitored for their response and/or benefit from dialysis as reflected by laboratory values and interdisciplinary assessments [30]. Although treatments are prescribed somewhat individually, dialysis care is generally focused on achieving clinical parameters that are associated with survival, fostering a culture of care that is designed to accommodate the needs of patients who desire aggressive rather than conservative care. The predominance of in-center dialysis commits a large majority of ESRD patients to group-focused, center-provided treatments rather than individual-focused, self-provided treatments at home. Whether dialyzing at home or in-center, patients may suffer a clinical decline that is acute, subacute or slow and progressive, any of which may warrant re-direction to a palliative approach to dialysis care.

Flexibility of scheduling and acceptance of less rigorous adherence to dialysis treatment times may align with a patient's individual goals but may result in suboptimal performance goals that count against the dialysis facility's quality metric scores [31]. The nephrologist is often interposed between population-based facility goals and those specific to an individual patient's preferences and as leader of the medical team must address and balance this disconnect. The provision of palliative care may command changes to the routine treatment paradigm of thrice-weekly dialysis or other flexibilities that will allow dialysis to better fit the needs of those patients who are suffering clinical decline and wish to individualize their treatments. The obligation to provide individual-directed care may collide with the opportunity to provide dialysis at all and speaks to the need for a shift in how we provide care to patients on dialysis.

Provider, System and Regulatory Barriers

A number of barriers pose challenges to integrating palliative care into a dialysis unit's practice (Table 1). A lack of training in palliative care or supportive options [32-35], lack of understanding, or lack of comfort with end of life conversations in general may underly some health care providers' reticence in offering care that is counter to aggressive, proactive management. Clinical practice guidelines are variably incorporated into practice but notably, do exist [36]. In addition, a conversation to explain and explore options takes time, a most precious commodity for most physicians, and an activity that takes away from day-to-day monitoring tasks and treatment urgencies. Poor communication, not surprisingly, adversely affects advance care planning [37]. Patients sometimes present with symptoms or signs warranting urgent or emergent dialysis, prompting its initiation at a time when more dire clinical circumstances preclude high level end of life care discussions between patients and the nephrologist who may be new to the patient's care team. A fragile elderly patient with severe co-morbid conditions might be most appropriate for conversation that includes the option of palliative care irrespective of whether dialysis is started, but discomforting symptoms or potentially fatal biochemical abnormalities command a delay of this type of conversation. Once on chronic dialysis, a multitude of specialists may be involved. This presents a challenge to coordination and can result in disjointed care that lacks a 'locus of responsibility' [38]. Decision making in dialysis may be emotionally burdensome [39], and morally distressing [40]. Previous patient experience may also impact a nephrologist's decision about when, how and for whom these conservations should be initiated.

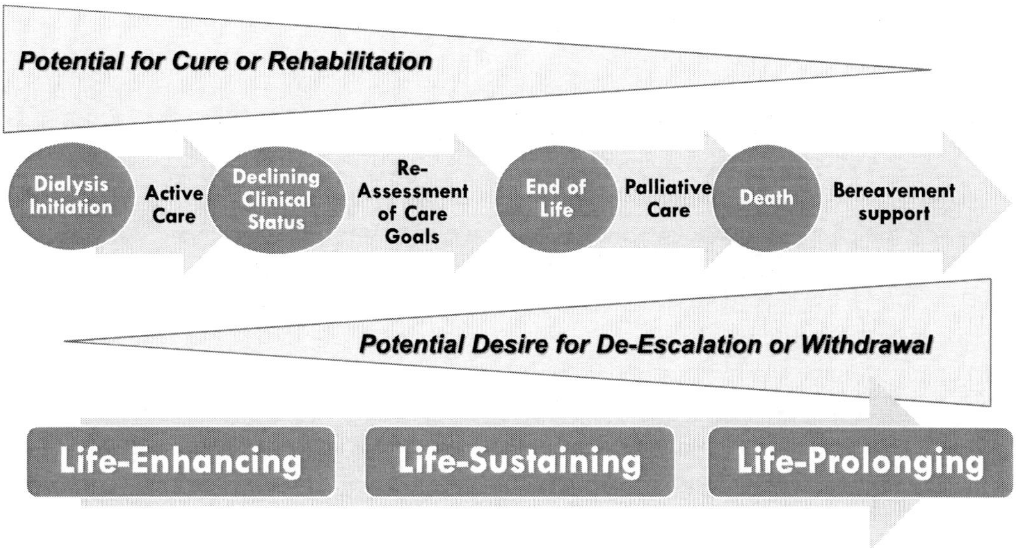

Figure 1. Continuum of care in dialysis from initiation through death.

Table 1. Barriers to integrating palliative care into dialysis patient and family

• Patient and Family:
• Lack of awareness of option
• Fear related to others' acceptance
• Unrealistic about condition and prognosis
• Lack of decision-making capacity
• Fear of outcome on remaining loved ones
• Fear that withdrawal signifies a lack of hope, which would influence the caregiver
• Health Care Provider
• Difficulty estimating prognosis
• Moral imperative to continue life-saving efforts
• Lack of understanding of patient's wishes
• Unrealistic expectations about prognosis
• Inability or unwillingness to offer this option
• Ethical opposition
• Emotional burden of recollection
• Health Care System
• Physician quality and performance metrics
• Facility quality and performance metrics
• Efficiency in dialysis unit operations
• One-size-fits all approach
• Historical origins of dialysis

Regulatory barriers in the form of targets also may serve as disincentives to the provision of less proactive care for the patient on renal replacement therapy. CMS-established requirements created to ensure that the level of care provided for patients receiving dialysis meets standards of acceptability are in keeping with the Triple Aim [41] as it relates to the large majority of ESRD patients entitled to Medicare for coverage [30]. Performance measure metrics making up the Quality Incentive Program of the ESRD prospective payment system (PPS) include a conglomerate of laboratory values, dialysis dose, and dialysis access, all based on the percentage of patients reaching population-based targets [31]. Incentives such as central venous catheter avoidance, while appropriate in general, may not be in the best interest of a patient who wishes short-term dialysis rather than a long-term therapy. While vascular access *per se* is often accomplished successfully in the elderly, the burden and risk of surgery may be anathema to many of these patients. Institutional-level barriers may be impactful in shaping a nephrologist's approach to this dialogue [40].

An additional barrier pertains to the provision of hospice for patients with advanced kidney disease. Regional payer differences may impact eligibility for the hospice benefit and this lack of uniformity among payers has created confusion. The frequency of hospice utilization among patients with ESRD, has increased somewhat over the last decade [42-45], but remains fairly low and even among those who have chosen to withdraw from dialysis, when utilized at all, is often engaged immediately prior to death [46]. A greater use of hospice has been associated with inpatient palliative care consultation, though even in this setting, hospice is infrequently engaged [47]. For patients who do withdraw from dialysis and no longer need the ESRD benefit to cover dialysis care, engaging hospice based on a terminal diagnosis of ESRD is a straightforward matter. For patients who wish to engage hospice but retain their ESRD Medicare benefit and continue dialysis, a terminal diagnosis other than ESRD is required to receive the hospice benefit (unless the hospice entity agrees to cover the dialysis procedure). Under these circumstances, patients without a terminal diagnosis distinct to ESRD may be unable to engage hospice without withdrawing [48].

Rationale for Change in Approach

Multiple Clinical Scenarios Cannot Be Addressed with a One-Size-Fits-All Approach

Although the clinical course of patients in general may follow a predictable trajectory [26, 27], patients have unique needs based on their individual experiences. The effects of hemodialysis on symptom burden may differ between ESRD patients suffering from different diseases with terminally ill ESRD patients having higher symptom severity scores [49]. For most patients, the clinical course will change over time which speaks to the multiplicity of potential patient scenarios that warrant observation. In contrast to the patient who is thriving, actively doing well and has no reason to change course and the patient who wishes all diagnostic and therapeutic efforts be continued no matter their potential for success, other patients may wish to pursue a palliative care approach [50]. Still others may show signs of decline despite being less than aware of their clinical circumstances or, despite an awareness, unable/unwilling to acknowledge their own decline. Signs of imminent or risk for decline may be marked by increasing frequency of hospitalization, admission to a nursing home [51, 52], diagnosis of a terminal non-renal illness, or acceleration of coexisting disease process. Decline may be subtle with gradual loss of functional capacity and independence leading to psychological and emotional distress and the loss of personal desire to continue dialysis. Key concerns will include the patient's understanding of their current clinical status and their potential for improvement. Providing a prognosis based on patient-specific estimates in real-time will be an important aspect of the patient-physician dialogue along with a low threshold for initiating or revising advance care planning [36, 53-55]. Patients already exhibiting symptoms suggesting that dialysis is no longer of benefit may need counsel about revising previously made decisions and active involvement of their surrogate and medical power of attorney should be sought. The offer of hospice and possibly withdrawal may be an appropriate next step and/or part of the conversation. Alternatively, a plan to continue dialysis but de-escalate other interventions without hospice engagement may be appropriate for patients who are satisfied with their life status or who are not ready to withdraw. Examples of patients likely to benefit from palliative approach to dialysis care are shown in Table 2. As dialysis transforms from a therapy that is life-enhancing to one that is life-prolonging, many patients and families may see less and less value or benefit to continuing the procedure [56].

Changes in Functional and Clinical Factors May Change Wishes and Goals for Care

Clinical factors and functional status evolve over time with the downhill trajectory of disease [27, 52] for ESRD often occurring abruptly and in parallel with high intensity care [57, 58] in the last weeks of life. That not all patients wish to undergo such treatment speaks to the need for early advance care planning and an approach that addresses the patient's unique clinical and psychosocial context [59]. Patients' preferences may follow changes in clinical circumstances and alternatives that fit with the evolving scenario warrant exploration [24, 25]. Patients with acute kidney injury may start dialysis abruptly when the time frame for needing renal replacement therapy is not known and projecting the likelihood of renal recovery is difficult to impossible. Dialogue about options for each potential outcome and monitoring of signs and symptoms that portend permanent need for dialysis will be important components of the conversation as well as the admonition that any decision can be changed. Reports of patients reporting decisional regret [60] about their decision to initiate dialysis speak to the importance of honest and clear communication.

Table 2. Scenarios likely to warrant palliative care approach in dialysis patients

• Patient who is declining subtly but wishes to continue dialysis
• Patient is declining abruptly
• Patients who started dialysis by default or for acute kidney injury which does not abate
• Patients on time-limited trial of dialysis
• Patients who do not wish to pursue active medical diagnostic searches or treatment
• Patients who are ready to withdraw or wish to de-escalate care

Patients on chronic maintenance dialysis may suffer clinical deterioration that is indolent and not life-threatening while comorbid illness accelerates often without overt clues and intercurrent problems attendant to ESRD (such as those associated with vascular access) take precedence by default. Ensuing loss of independence and declining functional status may be followed by failure to thrive; such patients may cease to benefit from dialysis, despite not being acutely ill (Figure 2). Frailty is common among ESRD patients [22, 61-63], particularly those on hemodialysis, the elderly and women. A greater incidence of falls and hospitalizations are important markers of decline and signal a poor prognosis. Reports that many elderly patients die within months of starting dialysis [52] speak to the high likelihood that clinical as well as functional changes will not only occur, but will be severe enough to warrant conversation about invoking a palliative approach. Further, elderly patients have multiple functional impairments, physical symptoms and a high rate of depression [64-66]. Sadly, many patients dying with advanced kidney disease receive little palliative care or bereavement support despite a high prevalence of pain [67], respiratory distress and anxiety [68].

Table 3. Potential triggers for considering a change in approach to care

• Accelerating co-morbid illness
• Increasing frequency of hospitalizations
• Admission to nursing home
• Dialysis of non-renal terminal illness
• Significant loss of functional abilities
• Loss of personal drive to continue dialysis
• Unrelenting, refractory depression
• Patient-specific prognosis that is poor
• Physician assessment that "no, I would not be surprised' at the patient's death

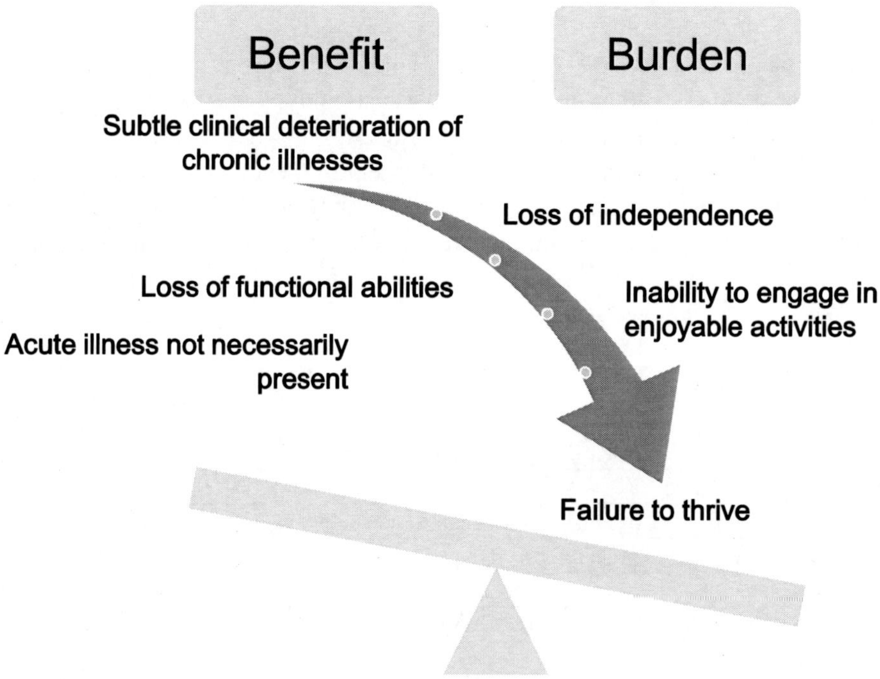

Figure 2. Changing benefit-burden balance for patients on dialysis.

Tools to aid in clinical decision making can help identify patients at risk for clinical decline [69, 70]. The Surprise Question ("Would you be surprised if this patient died within the next year?") is an intuitive, effective tool for predicting outcomes in patients on hemodialysis [71, 72]. Triggers for initiating or re-visiting conversations about future treatments include a negative response to the surprise question, increasingly frequent hospitalizations, admission to a nursing home, inability to care for oneself, depression refractory to treatment or an unrelenting desire to discontinue dialysis (Table 3). Clinical judgement, intuition and a solid relationship with the patient may trump surveys increasingly used in dialysis units to evaluate parameters presumed to reflect quality of life. The short-term health survey – 12 physical component score may not capture the wide range of patients who may be at risk for functional decline [73], and be less optimal for older patients (Hall) who have adapted to reductions in functional capacity and those who have succumbed to a new level of acceptance. Trajectory of illness models may be helpful in identifying the appropriate time to intensify dialogue about end of life wishes.

When Dialysis Becomes Life-Prolonging Rather than Life-Enhancing

Evidence that ESRD patients have received higher intensity treatment compared to patients with other chronic illnesses [58, 59], along with concerns that many patients may not actually desire such treatment, speaks to the need for careful, proactive and deliberate discussions about wishes for end of life care [28, 36, 74, 75]. Life expectancy after the initiation of long-term dialysis is often severely limited in the elderly, and it is becoming increasingly clear that many older patients who are receiving dialysis experience a significant burden of concomitant illness, functional limitation, and symptoms [27, 76]. Frail, older patients with ESRD are more likely to be hospitalized, have more than double the risk for death [77], and functionally, are more likely to decline than improve by virtue of dialysis [52, 53].

By contrast, palliative care needs are reported to be unmet in many ESRD patients [68], with physical and emotional burdens such as pain, depression and sexual dysfunction contributing to the fall in health-related quality of life seen in chronic maintenance hemodialysis patients over time [78]. Indeed, quality of end of life care has been reported to be significantly better for patients with cancer and dementia than for those with ESRD, cardiopulmonary failure and fragility [79], perhaps due to the higher penetrance palliative care interventions long embedded in the care of patients with diseases considered terminal. Sleep disturbances are highly prevalent in ESRD patients and were recently correlated to poorer physical and mental quality of life [80]. Better physical quality of life was noted in younger, more educated ESRD patients who had less pain and greater support. The perception of support was important in this group of patients – the more support perceived, the less likely were patients to have depressive symptoms [80].

Delays in recovering from intradialytic symptoms may add to an already reduced level of functionality between treatments that affects the quality of life, both physically and emotionally. The need for vascular access interventions and the logistics required of continuing hemodialysis in patients with a failed access or patients without available options for either additional vascular access or medical suitability for peritoneal dialysis may serve as the impetus for a patient's decision to deescalate care or withdraw from dialysis altogether [81-84].

In short, clinical decline and perhaps, other life-changing events may result in dialysis becoming life-prolonging rather life-enhancing. Priorities are relative and those of patients (free time away from dialysis, ability to travel) may differ from those their health care providers (dialysis adequacy, mechanics of dialysis) [85]. Quality of life may trump death in importance for patients, thus, addressing those symptoms and events specific to the dialysis process which may become less acceptable over time will be important to assuring that comprehensive care is provided [86].

ESSENTIAL COMPONENTS OF INTEGRATING PALLIATIVE CARE INTO DIALYSIS PATIENT CARE

Advance Care Planning across the Continuum

Integrating the tenets of palliative care into dialysis patient care involves preparedness planning and the use of shared decision making as the fulcrum from which care is directed [28, 33, 54]. Predicated on a heightened awareness and the mindset that advance care planning is crucial to patient-centered care, the provision of palliative care requires a milieu in which shared decision making is ingrained in the culture and process of care whereby patients are given the opportunity to learn about their disease and prognosis. Core components of palliative care in dialysis patients are presented in Table 4.

Establishing relationships and building trust will be key to the physicians' capacity to meaningfully assist a patient and their family in the decision making about whether continued dialysis is appropriate [87, 88]. Recognizing when patients and/or families lack awareness of their options or harbor fear that others may not accept a decision to change course may be difficult but a necessary part of a physician's responsibility to their patient. Patients may fear the outcome of their choices will negatively affect their loved ones or signify a loss of hope that will influence care decisions of their physician. Patients and families may harbor unrealistic expectations about prognosis and physicians may have difficulty estimating patient prognosis, both of which must be addressed in order to move forward.

Rapport established early on in the course of a patient's illness allows time for trust to build and values and preferences to be clarified. Patient and family focused discussions about goals of care are best initiated early on (preferably before or at the outset of dialysis) and often require serial conversations that occur over the continuum of the disease process and care. Setting the stage early on for patients with a poor prognosis may prove useful when additional changes in clinical status occur. Early, rather than late, conversations that clarify a patient's understanding of their prognosis and the potential for their health to further deteriorate despite continued dialysis may be useful starting points. Assuring that family members understand their loved one's wishes and will support any decision to deescalate or withdraw care should be actively acknowledged.

Preferences for continued treatment or decision to withdraw from dialysis may be dynamic and relative, requiring serial conversations and the acknowledgement that emotional, spiritual and social contextual factors may impact decision making [28, 33]. Fear or denial may drive a patient's ability to engage in a discussion of what is essentially a choice between life and self-imposed death [89]. Specific issues to address will include burdens and effect of dialysis on daily life, anticipated clinical course and prognosis, potential for functional decline and the option to withdraw [7, 36].

Advance care planning empowers patients and families faced with decisions about future treatments and can help guide physicians to identify and offer treatments that align with a patient's values and evolving clinical circumstances. A low threshold for reviewing advance directives and offering patients the opportunity to change their end of life directives is rarely inappropriate for dialysis patients and should be accompanied by the option to withdraw dialysis in the appropriate circumstances. Decisions should be proactive and deliberate and directed by the patient though perhaps guided by the physician when clinical circumstances become overwhelming.

Advance directives, informed consent, documentation, Physicians Orders for Life Sustaining Treatment (POLST) [90] are more than exercises in documentation done for legal protection but moreover, serve as guidance for patients, families and physicians alike. In some settings, use of palliative care specialists may be instrumental to discussions and documentation of care goals and code status [91]. Clarifying the differences between and need for documentation that is future-oriented, general and the responsibility of the patient and family (advance directives) and current-care focused, specific and the responsibility of the physician (POLST) will be key to assuring that patients and families are appropriately equipped to deal with whatever decisions are made about ongoing as well as end of life care. The complexities of providing informed consent are formidable [92] and confounded by preferences that change over time [24, 25]. Nephrologists are uniquely positioned to engage advance care planning and informed consent to facilitate decisions about dialysis and ensure that patients' wishes are respected.

Table 4. Core components of palliative care in dialysis

• Ongoing advance care planning throughout the continuum of the dialysis experience
• Shared decision making throughout the course the patient's illness
• Recognition of changing clinical and functional factors that impact goals of care
• Honest, direct dialogue with patient and family about goals of treatment, ramifications of decisions to continue or withdraw from dialysis and/or deescalate care
• Anticipatory, proactive symptom management
• Tailored goals for palliative care with and without withdrawal from dialysis

Recognizing Changes in Clinical, Functional and Psychosocial Factors that Impact Decision Making and Goals of Care

The initiation of dialysis is overwhelming to most patients and the magnitude and circumstances of life changes and the future may be difficult to comprehend and unimaginable to accept. The challenges posed by the process of dialysis itself, the symptoms and the illness trajectory of ESRD are interfaced by the reality of one's own mortality and the dependence on a machine to sustain one's life. Over time, changes in clinical as well as emotional status may cause patients to perceive dialysis differently and become both conflicted about its benefits and less accepting of its burdens. When the balance between benefit and burden or harm changes and the quality of life becomes less than acceptable, a change in the direction and/or type of care likely warrants discussion. High rates of withdrawal have been associated with frailty, acute medical complications [57], and increased frequency of hospitalizations [93], without the significant or universal use of palliative care (34 percent of withdrawals vs 17 percent among those who did not withdraw) [57].

Accelerating comorbid illness progression, worsening or inability to control pain, or other symptoms, may underlie emotional and psychosocial distress and constitute triggers for assessing whether providing continue dialysis is personally beneficial. Objective triggers which may be helpful in identifying patients for whom a change in the approach to care might be warranted are shown in Table 4. More difficult may be the patient with a deteriorating clinical status that is subtle but not immediately life-threatening whose decline in functional status has been slow though significant. Often labeled as 'failure to thrive,' patients for whom the engagement of enjoyable activities is no longer possible may not be benefiting from continued dialysis despite not being acutely ill. A low threshold for revisiting advance directives as well as a deliberate effort to address the change in clinical context with each new event is a crucial aspect of this process.

Ongoing assessment of the benefits being provided by dialysis and recognizing patients for whom withdrawal may be appropriate or patients whose wishes may conflict with those of their family wishes are key prerequisites to an individualized care approach. Consideration of withdrawal may also be appropriate for patients who no longer have decision making capacity and whose health care surrogate requests dialysis discontinuation, patients with irreversible and profound neurological impairment who lack awareness of self or purposeful behavior, patients who cannot longer cooperate with the dialysis procedure or patients with a terminal non-renal illness [7, 36].

Educating Patients and Families about their Choices

Advance care planning provides a structure by which physicians can help patients learn about, understand and implement the options available to them throughout the course of their illness [20, 33, 53, 54, 92]. Physicians and caregivers may have great influence [94] on patients faced with life or death decision about treatment options, hence the importance of providing thorough, comprehensive information on the ramifications of the options available to every individual patient. Patients may avoid discussion of end of life issues with their families [28, 29, 95], and look to their physicians to raise the issues [96], and provide advice [37, 54]. Adequate and complete information that meets the rigors of informed consent and gives the patient information with which to make an informed decision is even more critical in the case of dialysis where the treatment is life-sustaining and involved but may not address specific causes of patient suffering. Proactive discussions about options for end of life care can reinforce trust, promote hope [20], and impact patient choices [97, 98]. Informing patients of the contingencies of their consent is patient-centric and keeps patient wishes, preferences and values at the forefront of the conversation.

Most patients wish to receive detailed information on their condition to prepare for the future, including both negative and positive information about prognosis and life expectancy [55]. It may be appropriate to warn families about the potential for caregiver burden which is multifaceted and can become formidable, requiring substantial emotional, physical and psychosocial strength as well as the ability to navigate the health care system [99]. Personal choices will impact a patient's decision to pursue active, passive, conservative or palliative care that does not include dialysis; indeed some patients may choose to accept discomforting or even painful symptoms [100, 101], and the other burdens associated with dialysis based on the hope and expectation that it will extend life. Changes in clinical context command continued communication and assurance that patients understand the impact of such changes on their prognosis and quality of life. The high prevalence of cognitive impairment [102] and depression

[66] in patients with kidney disease underscores the importance of assuring that patients understand their options to withdraw from dialysis and/or deescalate care.

In contrast to patients for whom dialysis remains life-enhancing and the burdens of continued active care with dialysis acceptable, some patients may wish to continue dialysis to alleviate ESRD-related symptoms while pursuing a conservative approach to their other illnesses. Other patients may wish to discontinue dialysis altogether and pursue palliative/supportive care. For these patients it is important to assure them that cessation of dialysis does not mean cessation of care or herald abandonment and assure that maximal medical care with or without hospice is provided. Patients who wish to continue dialysis but wish to do so in a conservative manner may choose to de-escalate their care and continue dialysis for support of ESRD-related conditions such as respiratory distress induced by volume overload.

SUPPORTING PATIENTS THROUGH THE CONTINUUM OF THEIR CLINICAL AND PSYCHOSOCIAL JOURNEY

Contextual considerations are key to optimizing the chance for a smooth and comfortable course through the end of life with plans for care that align with the specific needs of each individual patient and prioritize a patient-centric rather than disease- or facility-centric approach (Figure 3). Preparing patients with a poor prognosis or declining clinical status with dialogue about the options of de-escalation or withdrawal of care may be helpful to patients who are struggling with physical/medical decline and the loss of independence or functional abilities. Recommendations for supporting patients who choose to de-escalate care or withdraw from dialysis are presented in Table 5.

	Patient-Centered	**Disease- or Facility-Centered**	**Strategies**
Concerns	• Dependent on family members • Functional, physiological or emotional decline • Too tired to engage in activities • "Tired" of traveling to and the logistics of dialysis • Lacking personal drive to continue dialysis	• Patient compliance with treatments • Patient compliance with medications	• Open, honest dialogue with shared decision making and advance care planning
Priorities	• Quality of remaining life • Ability to engage in activities • Being without symptoms • Optimize remaining functional capacity	• Attainment of quality and performance metrics • Minimal missed treatments • Avoidance of hospitalizations	• Low threshold for initiating or re-revisiting advance care planning conversation
Goals	• Physical and emotional comfort • Control of physical symptoms • No acute need for decisions	• Management of anemia, mineral metabolism, blood pressure, diabetes and dry weight	• Treatment the patient receives aligns with treatment patient desires
Discussion Issues	• Plans to deal with changing clinical needs • Establish triggers for withdrawal • Clarify medical power of attorney and health care surrogate • Work with dialysis staff to provide treatments that is aligned with and optimizes patient comfort	• Manage symptoms of fluid overload • Minimize phlebotomies • Inclination toward dialysis	• Consider withdrawal • Offer hospice

Figure 3. Patient-Centric Approach to End of Life Care in Dialysis.

Table 5. Recommendations for supporting patients who choose to de-escalate care or withdraw from dialysis

• Provide assurance that withdrawal or de-escalation of care does not mean termination of care or abandonment.
• Emphasize a plan for providing medical therapy that is patient-centric and individually focused.
• Address clinical, emotional and physical symptoms with a focus on pain and 'in the moment' suffering.
• Offer hospice to help provide clinical assistance and social support for both patient and family.
• Work with multidisciplinary team to keep care coordinated.
• Plan for managing non-acute but discomforting symptoms that could occur with reductions in or withdrawal of dialysis.
• Plan for acute symptom management to pre-empt the need for 'heat of the moment' decisions.
• Assure emotional, spiritual and patient and family support for psychological pain.

Discontinuation of dialysis occurs with significant frequency [103-110], and is an option for those patients who no longer wish to continue dialysis, accept the ramifications of stopping it and are ready to die. A barrier to withdrawal for some patients may be the fear of dying alone, the fear that all care will be withdrawn and that patients' families will be ill-equipped to provide at-home care moving through the dying process related to both physical and emotional needs. Patients who contemplate withdrawal from dialysis should be assured that withdrawal from dialysis does not mean that no care will be provided and assurances should be given to the contrary and arrangements made to assist the family in their care of the withdrawing family member. Estimates of the time from dialysis withdrawal to death may be helpful to family members and patients as they plan for imminent patient death. Patients who choose to withdraw from dialysis should be informed of common symptoms to anticipate and plans for managing acute and non-acute but discomforting symptoms which might occur. Medications should be reviewed and retained and continued for their impact on discomforting symptoms. Dietary restrictions should be lifted on an individual patient basis and blood draws eliminated.

Continuation of active care with plans to revisit the decision is appropriate for those patients who are unsure, those with conflicted family members or those whose clinical status has fluctuated and there may be potential for improvement in status over time. The possibility that health will further deteriorate should be clarified and rationale for the conversation provided to the patient and family along with open discussion of contextual and family issues that have changed over time. Frequent review of advance directives and POLST will help assure that the treatment provided is the treatment desired. Continuation of dialysis with palliative/supportive care for those patients who wish for support of ESRD-related symptoms such as volume overload may require alteration in the dialysis prescription and an acceptance on the part of the dialysis facility and nephrologist that metrics on the given patient are of lower priority.

A focus on symptom control, rather than achievement of target goals, is primary for patients who choose to withdraw from dialysis as well as those patients who wish to de-escalate care. Symptom management (Table 6) includes antiemetics, acidosis management to minimize anorexia, nausea and vomiting, metoclopramide, haloperidol for gastroparesis component, diuretics to minimize dyspnea and edema, topical agents, antihistamines or gabapentin for pruritus, treatment for restless leg syndrome, and analgesia for pain. The importance of emotional, spiritual and family support for psychological pain cannot be overemphasized.

Guidance for patients who choose to withdraw should secure documentation of and make available their advance directives, will and durable or medical power of attorney and inventory of financial information. Directions with regard to funeral preferences and a written, audio or video message to family and friends may be desired [7, 36].

Table 6. Symptom management for patients withdrawing from dialysis or de-escalating care

• Anticipate the development of symptoms and prescribe proactively
• Manage nausea and vomiting with prokinetics (metoclopramide, haloperidol) or if refractory, methotrimeprazine
• Minimize breathlessness and edema with diuretics or if refractory, fentanyl or hydromorphone
• Manage restlessness, agitation or delirium with haloperidol or if refractory, methotrimeprazine; lorazepam or midazolam for anxiety
• Offer topical agents, antihistamines, gabapentin may be needed for pruritis
• Offer specific treatment for symptoms of restless leg syndrome
• Consider erythropoietin-stimulating agents for anemia-associated fatigue
• Offer analgesia for serious physical pain

CONCLUSION

Clinical decline occurs often in patients with ESRD on dialysis but may be difficult for patients and families to acknowledge and accept. Many may be unaware of or not inclined to see options other than continued dialysis. Family members may harbor fears that their loved one will experience worsening of their suffering or feel guilt that a change in approach constitutes wrongdoing. Transitioning from a proactive to a palliative approach to care should be a conscious decision about one's clinical journey. Honest and open dialogue of contextual and family issues, acknowledgement and explanation of expectations for clinical status and/or recovery, and frequent review of advance directives and POLST will help assure that the treatment provided is the treatment desired.

Whether choosing continued or withdrawal care, patients deserve to understand the options available to them and the ramifications of the choices they make. A heightened awareness, communication and discussion, relationships and trust, along with shared decision making are prerequisite to creating a culture of care that speaks to the medical, clinical, emotional, physical, spiritual and psychosocial needs of patients on dialysis. Indeed, the distinction between opportunity to extend life and obligation to do so applies throughout the continuum of a patient's journey through ESRD and dialysis.

REFERENCES

[1] Scherer JS, Holley JL. The role of time–limited trials in dialysis decision making in critically ill patients. *Clin J Am Soc Nephrol.* 2016 Feb 5; 11(2): 344-53.

[2] Chandna SM, Da Silva-Gane M, Marshall C, Warwicker P, Greenwood RN, Farrington K.Survival of elderly patients with stage 5 CKD: comparison of conservative

management and renal replacement therapy. *Nephrol Dial Transplant.* 2011 May 1; 26(5): 1608-14.

[3] Carson RC, Juszczak M, Davenport A, Burns A. Is maximum conservative management an equivalent treatment option to dialysis for elderly patients with significant comorbid disease? *Clin J Am Soc Nephrol.* 2009 Oct 1; 4(10): 1611-9.

[4] Ellam T, El-Kossi M, Prasanth KC, El-Nahas M, Khwaja A. Conservatively managed patients with stage 5 chronic kidney disease—outcomes from a single center experience. *QJM.* 2009 Aug 1; 102(8): 547-54.

[5] Dalrymple LS, Katz R, Kestenbaum B, Shlipak MG, Sarnak MJ, Stehman-Breen C, Seliger S, Siscovick D, Newman AB, Fried L. Chronic kidney disease and the risk of end-stage renal disease versus death. *J Gen Intern Med.* 2011 Apr 1; 26(4): 379-85.

[6] Tamura MK, O'Hare AM, Lin E, Holdsworth LM, Malcolm E, Moss AH.Palliative care disincentives in CKD: changing policy to improve CKD care. *Am J Kidney Dis.* 2018 Jun 1; 71(6): 866-73.

[7] Davison SN, Levin A, Moss AH, Jha V, Brown EA, Brennan F, Murtagh FE, Naicker S, Germain MJ, O'donoghue DJ, Morton RL. Executive summary of the KDIGO Controversies Conference on Supportive Care in Chronic Kidney Disease: developing a roadmap to improving quality care. *Kidney Int.* 2015 Sep 1; 88(3): 447-59.

[8] Tamura MK, Meier DE. Five policies to promote palliative care for patients with ESRD. *Clin J Am Soc Nephrol.* 2013 Oct 7; 8(10): 1783-90.

[9] World Health Organization. *Definition of Palliative Care.* https: //www.who.int/cancer/ palliative/definition/en/ (Accessed June 4, 2020).

[10] Eggers PW. A quarter century of medicare expenditures for ESRD. *Semin Nephrol.* 2000 Nov; 20(6): 516-22.

[11] Committee on Chronic Kidney Disease, Gottschalk CW. *Report of the committee on chronic kidney disease.* 1967.

[12] Rosansky SJ, Eggers PW. Trends in the US end-stage renal disease population: 1973–1983. *Am J Kidney Dis.* 1987 Feb 1; 9(2): 91-7.

[13] United States Renal Data System. *2019 USRDS annual data report: Epidemiology of kidney disease in the United States.* National Institutes of Health, National Institute of Diabetes and Digestive and Kidney Diseases, Bethesda, MD, 2019.

[14] Levinsky NG. The Organization of Medical Care--Lessons from the Medicare End Stage Renal Disease Program. *N Engl J Med.* 1993 Nov 4; 329(19): 1395-9.

[15] Rettig RA. Special treatment—the story of Medicare's ESRD entitlement. *N Engl J Med.* 2011 Feb 17; 364(7): 596-8.

[16] Gutman RA, Stead WW, Robinson RR. Physical activity and employment status of patients on maintenance dialysis. *N Engl J Med.* 1981 Feb 5; 304(6): 309-13.

[17] Kutner NG, Brogan D, Fielding B. Employment status and ability to work among working-age chronic dialysis patients. *Am J Nephrol.* 1991; 11(4): 334-40.

[18] Rasgon S, James-Rogers A, Chemleski B, Ledezma M, Mercado L, Besario M, Trivedi J, Miller M, Dee L, Pryor L, Yeoh H. Maintenance of employment on dialysis. *Adv Ren Replace Ther.* 1997 Apr 1; 4(2): 152-9.

[19] Muehrer RJ, Schatell D, Witten B, Gangnon R, Becker BN, Hofmann RM. Factors affecting employment at initiation of dialysis. *Clin J Am Soc Nephrol.* 2011 Mar 1; 6(3): 489-96.

[20] Davison SN, Simpson C. Hope and advance care planning in patients with end stage renal disease: qualitative interview study. *BMJ*. 2006 Oct 26; 333(7574): 886.

[21] Swidler M. Considerations in starting a patient with advanced frailty on dialysis: Complex biology meets challenging ethics. *Clin J Am Soc Nephrol*. 2013 Aug 7; 8(8): 1421-8.

[22] Elliott BA, Gessert CE, Larson P, Russ TE. Religious beliefs and practices in end-stage renal disease: implications for clinicians. *J Pain Symptom Manag*. 2012 Sep 1; 44(3): 400-9.

[23] Jassal SV, Watson D. Dialysis in late life: benefit or burden. *Clin J Am Soc Nephrol*. 2009 Dec 1; 4(12): 2008-12.

[24] Moranne O, Fafin C, Roche S, Francois M, Allot V, Potier J, Babici D, Lobbedez T, Matignon M, Mariat C, Vigneau C. Treatment plans and outcomes in elderly patients reaching advanced chronic kidney disease. *Nephrol Dial Transplant*. 2018 Dec 1; 33(12): 2182-91.

[25] Elliott BA, Gessert CE, Larson P, Russ TE. Shifting responses in quality of life: People living with dialysis. *Qual Life Res*. 2014 Jun 1; 23(5): 1497-504.

[26] Holley JL. Palliative care in end-stage renal disease: illness trajectories, communication, and hospice use. *Adv Chronic Kidney Dis*. 2007 Oct 1; 14(4): 402-8.

[27] Murtagh FE, Sheerin NS, Addington-Hall J, Higginson IJ. Trajectories of illness in stage 5 chronic kidney disease: a longitudinal study of patient symptoms and concerns in the last year of life. *Clin J Am Soc Nephrol*. 2011 Jul 1; 6(7): 1580-90.

[28] Holley JL, Schmidt RJ. Conservative/palliative treatment and end-of-life care in chronic kidney disease. *In Management of Chronic Kidney Disease*, 2014 (pp. 451-461). Springer, Berlin, Heidelberg.

[29] Hines SC, Babrow AS, Badzek L, Moss AH. Communication and problematic integration in end-of-life decisions: Dialysis decisions among the elderly. *Health Commun*. 1997 Jul 1; 9(3): 199-217.

[30] US Department of Health and Human Services, Centers for Medicare and Medicaid Services. *Conditions for Coverage for ESRD Facilities*, final rule (42 CFR Part 494.80). Fed Regist. 2008, 20393.

[31] US Department of Health and Human Services, Centers for Medicare and Medicaid Services. *ESRD Quality Incentive Program*. https: //www.cms.gov/Medicare/Quality-Initiatives-Patient-Assessment-Instruments/ESRDQIP/index (accessed 6/4/2020).

[32] Davison SN, Jhangri GS, Holley JL, Moss AH.Nephrologists' reported preparedness for end-of-life decision-making. *Clin J Am Soc Nephrol*. 2006 Nov 1; 1(6): 1256-62.

[33] Holley JL, Carmody SS, Moss AH, Sullivan AM, Cohen LM, Block SD, Arnold RM. The need for end-of-life care training in nephrology: National survey results of nephrology fellows. *Am J Kidney Dis*. 2003 Oct 1; 42(4): 813-20.

[34] Combs SA, Culp S, Matlock DD, Kutner JS, Holley JL, Moss AH. Update on end-of-life care training during nephrology fellowship: a cross-sectional national survey of fellows. *Am J Kidney Dis*. 2015 Feb 1; 65(2): 233-9.

[35] Schell JO, Green JA, Tulsky JA, Arnold RM. Communication skills training for dialysis decision-making and end-of-life care in nephrology. *Clin J Am Soc Nephrol*. 2013 Apr 5; 8(4): 675-80.

[36] Renal Physicians Association. *Shared decision-making in the appropriate initiation of and withdrawal from dialysis.* Renal Physicians Association, 2000.

[37] Goff SL, Eneanya ND, Feinberg R, Germain MJ, Marr L, Berzoff J, Cohen LM, Unruh M. Advance care planning: a qualitative study of dialysis patients and families. *Clin J Am Soc Nephrol*. 2015 Mar 6; 10(3): 390-400.

[38] O'Hare AM, Szarka J, McFarland LV, Taylor JS, Sudore RL, Trivedi R, Reinke LF, Vig EK. Provider perspectives on advance care planning for patients with kidney disease: Whose job is it anyway?. *Clin J Am Soc Nephrol*. 2016 May 6; 11(5): 855-66.

[39] Wachterman MW, Leveille T, Keating NL, Simon SR, Waikar SS, Bokhour B. Nephrologists' emotional burden regarding decision-making about dialysis initiation in older adults: a qualitative study. *BMC Nephrol*. 2019 Dec 1; 20(1): 385.

[40] Ladin K, Pandya R, Kannam A, Loke R, Oskoui T, Perrone RD, Meyer KB, Weiner DE, Wong JB. Discussing conservative management with older patients with CKD, an interview study of nephrologists. *Am J Kidney Dis*. 2018 May 1; 71(5): 627-35.

[41] Berwick DM, Nolan TW, Whittington J. The triple aim: care, health, and cost. *Health affairs*. 2008 May; 27(3): 759-69.

[42] O'Hare AM, Hailpern SM, Wachterman M, Kreuter W, Katz R, Hall YN, Montez-Rath M, Tamura MK, Daratha KB. Hospice use and end-of-life spending trajectories in medicare beneficiaries on hemodialysis. *Health Affairs*. 2018 Jun 1; 37(6): 980-7.

[43] O'Hare AM, Rodriguez RA, Hailpern SM, Larson EB, Tamura MK. Regional variation in health care intensity and treatment practices for end-stage renal disease in older adults. *JAMA*. 2010 Jul 14; 304(2): 180-6.

[44] Murray AM, Arko C, Chen SC, Gilbertson DT, Moss AH. Use of hospice in the United States dialysis population. *Clin J Am Soc Nephrol*. 2006 Nov 1; 1(6): 1248-55.

[45] O'Connor NR. Hospice Among Hemodialysis Patients: Too Little, Too Late to Impact Care Delivery or Costs?. *Am J Kidney Dis*. 2018 Dec 1; 72(6): 903-5.

[46] Wachterman MW, Hailpern SM, Keating NL, Tamura MK, O'Hare AM. Association between hospice length of stay, health care utilization, and Medicare costs at the end of life among patients who received maintenance hemodialysis. *JAMA Intern Med*. 2018 Jun 1; 178(6): 792-9.

[47] Chettiar A, Montez-Rath M, Liu S, Hall YN, O'Hare AM, Tamura MK. Association of inpatient palliative care with health care utilization and postdischarge outcomes among Medicare beneficiaries with end stage kidney disease. *Clin J Am Soc Nephrol*. 2018 Aug 7; 13(8): 1180-7.

[48] Medicare Hospice Benefit. https: //www.medicare.gov/Pubs/pdf/02154-Medicare-Hospice-Benefits. Accessed June 4, 2020.

[49] Wu YL, Cheung DS, Takemura N, Lin CC. Effects of Hemodialysis on the Symptom Burden of Terminally Ill and Nonterminally Ill End-Stage Renal Disease Patients. *J Palliat Med*. 2019 Mar 1; 22(3): 282-9.

[50] Schell JO, Patel UD, Steinhauser KE, Ammarell N, Tulsky JA. Discussions of the kidney disease trajectory by elderly patients and nephrologists: a qualitative study. *Am J Kidney Dis*. 2012 Apr 1; 59(4): 495-503.

[51] Kurella Tamura M, Covinsky KE, Chertow GM, Yaffe K, Landefeld CS, McCulloch CE. Functional status of elderly adults before and after initiation of dialysis. *N Engl J Med*. 2009 Oct 15; 361(16): 1539-47.

[52] Jassal SV, Chiu E, Hladunewich M. Loss of independence in patients starting dialysis at 80 years of age or older. *N Engl J Med*. 2009 Oct 15; 361(16): 1612-3.

[53] Moss AH. Integrating supportive care principles into dialysis decision making: a primer for palliative medicine providers. *J Pain Symptom Manag*. 2017 Mar 1; 53(3): 656-62.
[54] Davison SN, Moss AH. Supportive care: meeting the needs of patients with advanced chronic kidney disease. *Clin J Am Soc Nephrol*. 2016 Oct 7; 11(10): 1879-80.
[55] Davison SN, Jhangri GS, Koffman J. Knowledge of and attitudes towards palliative care and hospice services among patients with advanced chronic kidney disease. *BMJ Support Palliat*. 2016 Mar 1; 6(1): 66-74.
[56] Chen JC, Thorsteinsdottir B, Vaughan LE, Feely MA, Albright RC, Onuigbo M, Norby SM, Gossett CL, D'Uscio MM, Williams AW, Dillon JJ. End of life, withdrawal, and palliative care utilization among patients receiving maintenance hemodialysis therapy. *Clin J Am Soc Nephrol*. 2018 Aug 7; 13(8): 1172-9.
[57] Eneanya ND, Hailpern SM, O'Hare AM, Tamura MK, Katz R, Kreuter W, Montez-Rath ME, Hebert PL, Hall YN. Trends in receipt of intensive procedures at the end of life among patients treated with maintenance dialysis. *Am J Kidney Dis*. 2017 Jan 1; 69(1): 60-8.
[58] Wong SP, Kreuter W, O'Hare AM. Treatment intensity at the end of life in older adults receiving long-term dialysis. *Arch Intern Med*. 2012 Apr 23; 172(8): 661-3.
[59] Davison SN. End-of-life care preferences and needs: perceptions of patients with chronic kidney disease. *Clin J Am Soc Nephrol*. 2010 Feb 1; 5(2): 195-204.
[60] Saeed F, Ladwig SA, Epstein RM, Monk RD, Duberstein, PR. Dialysis Regret Prevalence and Correlates. *Clin J Am Soc Nephrol*. 2020 Jul 1; 15(7): 957-963.
[61] McAdams-DeMarco MA, Tan J, Salter ML, Gross A, Meoni LA, Jaar BG, Kao WH, Parekh RS, Segev DL, Sozio SM. Frailty and cognitive function in incident hemodialysis patients. *Clin J Am Soc Nephrol*. 2015 Dec 7; 10(12): 2181-9.
[62] McAdams-DeMarco MA, Law A, Salter ML, Boyarsky B, Gimenez L, Jaar BG, Walston JD, Segev DL. Frailty as a novel predictor of mortality and hospitalization in individuals of all ages undergoing hemodialysis. *J Am Geriatr Soc*. 2013 Jun; 61(6): 896-901.
[63] Fried LP, Ferrucci L, Darer J, Williamson JD, Anderson G. Untangling the concepts of disability, frailty, and comorbidity: implications for improved targeting and care. *J Gerontol A Biol Sci Med Sci*. 2004 Mar 1; 59(3): M255-63.
[64] Blumenfield M, Levy NB, Spinowitz B, Charytan C, Beasley Jr CM, Dubey AK, Solomon RJ, Todd R, Goodman A, Bergstrom RF. Fluoxetine in depressed patients on dialysis. *Int J Psychiat Med*. 1997 Mar; 27(1): 71-80.
[65] Levy NB, Blumenfield M, Beasley Jr CM, Dubey AK, Solomon RJ, Todd R, Goodman A, Bergstrom RR. Fluoxetine in depressed patients with renal failure and in depressed patients with normal kidney function. *Gen Hosp Psychiatry*. 1996 Jan 1; 18(1): 8-13.
[66] Kimmel PL. Depression in patients with chronic renal disease: what we know and what we need to know. *J Psychosom Res*. 2002 Oct 1; 53(4): 951-6.
[67] Barakzoy AS, Moss AH. Efficacy of the world health organization analgesic ladder to treat pain in end-stage renal disease. *J Am Soc Nephrol*. 2006 Nov 1; 17(11): 3198-203.
[68] Axelsson L, Alvariza A, Lindberg J, Öhlén J, Håkanson C, Reimertz H, Fürst CJ, Årestedt K.. Unmet palliative care needs among patients with end-stage kidney disease: a national registry study about the last week of life. *J Pain Symptom Manage*. 2018 Feb 1; 55(2): 236-44.

[69] Bansal N, Katz R, De Boer IH, Peralta CA, Fried LF, Siscovick DS, Rifkin DE, Hirsch C, Cummings SR, Harris TB, Kritchevsky SB. Development and validation of a model to predict 5-year risk of death without ESRD among older adults with CKD. *Clin J Am Soc Nephrol*. 2015 Mar 6; 10(3): 363-71.

[70] Wick JP, Turin TC, Faris PD, MacRae JM, Weaver RG, Tonelli M, Manns BJ, Hemmelgarn BR. A clinical risk prediction tool for 6-month mortality after dialysis initiation among older adults. *Am J Kidney Dis*. 2017 May 1; 69(5): 568-75.

[71] Moss AH, Ganjoo J, Sharma S, Gansor J, Senft S, Weaner B, Dalton C, MacKay K, Pellegrino B, Anantharaman P, Schmidt R. Utility of the "surprise" question to identify dialysis patients with high mortality. *Clin J Am Soc Nephrol*. 2008 Sep 1; 3(5): 1379-84.

[72] Cohen LM, Ruthazer R, Moss AH, Germain MJ. Predicting six-month mortality for patients who are on maintenance hemodialysis. *Clin J Am Soc Nephrol*. 2010 Jan 1; 5(1): 72-9.

[73] Hall RK, Luciano A, Pieper C, Colón-Emeric CS. Association of Kidney Disease Quality of Life (KDQOL-36) with mortality and hospitalization in older adults receiving hemodialysis. *BMC Nephrol*. 2018 Dec 1; 19(1): 11.

[74] Davison SN. The ethics of end-of-life care for patients with ESRD. *Clin J Am Soc Nephrol*. 2012 Dec 1; 7(12): 2049-57.

[75] Moss AH. Ethical principles and processes guiding dialysis decision-making. *Clin J Am Soc Nephrol*. 2011 Sep 1; 6(9): 2313-7.

[76] Weisbord SD. Symptoms and their correlates in chronic kidney disease. *Adv Chronic Kidney Dis*. 2007 Oct 1; 14(4): 319-27.

[77] Johansen KL, Chertow GM, Jin C, Kutner NG. Significance of frailty among dialysis patients. *J Am Soc Nephrol*. 2007 Nov 1; 18(11): 2960-7.

[78] Murtagh FE, Addington-Hall JM, Higginson IJ. End-stage renal disease: a new trajectory of functional decline in the last year of life. *J Am Geriatr Soc*. 2011 Feb; 59(2): 304-8.

[79] Wachterman MW, O'Hare AM, Rahman OK, Lorenz KA, Marcantonio ER, Alicante GK, Kelley AS. One-year mortality after dialysis initiation among older adults. *JAMA Intern Med*. 2019 Jul 1; 179(7): 987-90.

[80] Shen Q, Huang X, Luo Z, Xu X, Zhao X, He Q. Sleep quality, daytime sleepiness and health-related quality-of-life in maintenance haemodialysis patients. *J Int Med Res*. 2016 Jun; 44(3): 698-709.

[81] O'Hare AM. Vascular Access for Hemodialysis in Older Adults: A "Patient First" Approach. *J Am Soc Nephrol*. 2013 Jul 31; 24(8): 1187.

[82] Vachharajani TJ, Moossavi S, Jordan JR, Vachharajani V, Freedman BI, Burkart JM. Re-evaluating the fistula first initiative in octogenarians on hemodialysis. *Clin J Am Soc Nephrol*. 2011 Jul 1; 6(7): 1663-7.

[83] Vachharajani TJ. Hemodialysis Access in the Elderly: Planning to Execution. In *Dialysis in Older Adults*, 2016 (pp. 45-55). Springer, New York, NY.

[84] Gomes A, Schmidt R, Wish J. Re-envisioning Fistula First in a patient-centered culture. *Clin J Am Soc Nephrol*. 2013 Oct 7; 8(10): 1791-7.

[85] Urquhart-Secord R, Craig JC, Hemmelgarn B, Tam-Tham H, Manns B, Howell M, Polkinghorne KR, Kerr PG, Harris DC, Thompson S, Schick-Makaroff K. Patient and

caregiver priorities for outcomes in hemodialysis: an international nominal group technique study. *Am J Kidney Dis*. 2016 Sep 1; 68(3): 444-54.

[86] Schmidt RJ, Moss AH. Dying on dialysis: the case for a dignified withdrawal. *Clin J Am Soc Nephrol*. 2014 Jan 7; 9(1): 174-80.

[87] Noble H, Chesser A, Kelly D. The cessation of dialysis in patients with end-stage renal disease: developing an appropriate evidence base for practice. *EDTNA-ERCA Journal*. 2005 Oct 12; 31(4): 208-11.

[88] Wilson FP, Yang W, Machado CA, Mariani LH, Borovskiy Y, Berns JS, Feldman HI. Dialysis versus nondialysis in patients with AKI: a propensity-matched cohort study. *Clin J Am Soc Nephrol*. 2014 Apr 7; 9(4): 673-81.

[89] Hussain JA, Flemming K, Murtagh FE, Johnson MJ. Patient and health care professional decision-making to commence and withdraw from renal dialysis: a systematic review of qualitative research. *Clin J Am Soc Nephrol*. 2015 Jul 7; 10(7): 1201-15.

[90] Citko J, Moss AH; Carley, M; Tolle, S. The national POLST paradigm initiative, 2nd edition # 178. *J Palliat Med*. 2011 Feb 1; 14(2): 241-2.

[91] Feely MA, Swetz KM, Zavaleta K, Thorsteinsdottir B, Albright RC, Williams AW. Reengineering dialysis: the role of palliative medicine. *J Palliat Med*. 2016 Jun 1; 19(6): 652-5.

[92] Schmidt RJ. Informing our elders about dialysis: Is an age-attuned approach warranted? *Clin J Am Soc Nephrol*. 2012 Jan 1; 7(1): 185-91.

[93] Wetmore JB, Molony JT, Liu J, Peng Y, Herzog CA, Collins AJ, Gilbertson DT. Readmissions following a hospitalization for cardiovascular events in Dialysis patients, a retrospective cohort study. *J Am Heart Assoc*. 2018 Feb 13; 7(4): e007231.

[94] Tonkin-Crine S, Okamoto I, Leydon GM, Murtagh FE, Farrington K, Caskey F, Rayner H, Roderick P. Understanding by older patients of dialysis and conservative management for chronic kidney failure. *Am J Kidney Dis*. 2015 Mar 1; 65(3): 443-50.

[95] Sellars M, Tong A, Silvester W, Pollock C, Luckett T, Morton RL, Detering KM, Spencer L, Clayton JM. P-52 Delivering advance care planning in chronic kidney disease (CKD): The perspectives of healthcare providers. *BMJ Support Palliat Care*. 2015;5:A59.

[96] Luckett T, Sellars M, Tieman J, Pollock CA, Silvester W, Butow PN, Detering KM, Brennan F, Clayton JM. Advance care planning for adults with CKD: a systematic integrative review. *Am J Kidney Dis*. 2014 May 1; 63(5): 761-70.

[97] Amro OW, Ramasamy M, Strom JA, Weiner DE, Jaber BL. Nephrologist-facilitated advance care planning for hemodialysis patients: a quality improvement project. *Am J Kidney Dis*. 2016 Jul 1; 68(1): 103-9.

[98] Schmidt RJ, Weaner BB, Long D. The power of advance care planning in promoting hospice and out-of-hospital death in a dialysis unit. *J Palliat Med*. 2015 Jan 1; 18(1): 62-6.

[99] Maddalena V, O'Shea F, Barrett B. An exploration of palliative care needs of people with end-stage renal disease on dialysis: family caregiver's perspectives. *J Palliat Care*. 2018 Jan; 33(1): 19-25.

[100] Abdel-Kader K, Unruh ML, Weisbord SD. Symptom burden, depression, and quality of life in chronic and end-stage kidney disease. *Clin J Am Soc Nephrol*. 2009 Jun 1; 4(6): 1057-64.

[101] Weisbord SD, Fried LF, Arnold RM, Fine MJ, Levenson DJ, Peterson RA, Switzer GE. Prevalence, severity, and importance of physical and emotional symptoms in chronic hemodialysis patients. *J Am Soc Nephrol.* 2005 Aug 1; 16(8): 2187 91.

[102] Murray AM, Tupper DE, Knopman DS, Gilbertson DT, Pederson SL, Li S, Smith GE, Hochhalter AK, Collins AJ, Kane RL. Cognitive impairment in hemodialysis patients is common. *Neurology.* 2006 Jul 25; 67(2): 216-23.

[103] Findlay MD, Donaldson K, Doyle A, Fox JG, Khan I, McDonald J, Metcalfe W, Peel RK, Shilliday I, Spalding E, Stewart GA. Factors influencing withdrawal from dialysis: a national registry study. *Nephrol Dial Transplant.* 2016 Dec 9; 31(12): 2041-8.

[104] Gessert CE, Haller IV, Johnson BP. Regional variation in care at the end of life: discontinuation of dialysis. *BMC Geriatr.* 2013 Dec 1; 13(1): 39.

[105] Chan HW, Clayton PA, McDonald SP, Agar JW, Jose MD. Risk factors for dialysis withdrawal: an analysis of the Australia and New Zealand Dialysis and Transplant (ANZDATA) Registry, 1999–2008. *Clin J Am Soc Nephrol.* 2012 May 1; 7(5): 775-81.

[106] Mizuno M, Ito Y, Tanaka A, Suzuki Y, Hiramatsu H, Watanabe M, Tsuruta Y, Matsuoka T, Ito I, Tamai H, Kasuga H. Peritonitis is still an important factor for withdrawal from peritoneal dialysis therapy in the Tokai area of Japan. *Clin Exp Nephrol.* 2011 Oct 1; 15(5): 727-37.

[107] Birmelé B, François M, Pengloan J, Français P, Testou D, Brillet G, Lechapois D, Baudin S, Grezard O, Jourdan JL, Fodil-Cherif M. Death after withdrawal from dialysis: the most common cause of death in a French dialysis population. *Nephrol Dial Transplant.* 2004 Mar 1; 19(3): 686-91.

[108] Seshasai RK, Mitra N, Chaknos CM, Li J, Wirtalla C, Negoianu D, Glickman JD, Dember LM. Factors associated with discontinuation of home hemodialysis. *Am J Kidney Dis.* 2016 Apr 1; 67(4): 629-37.

[109] Wetmore JB, Yan H, Gilbertson DT, Liu J. Factors Associated with Elective Withdrawal of Maintenance Hemodialysis: A Case-Control Analysis. *Am J Nephrol.* 2020; 51(3): 227-36.

[110] Qazi HA, Chen, H, Zhu M. Factors influencing dialysis withdrawal: a scoping review. *BMC Nephrol.* 2018 Dec 1; 19(1): 96.

In: Issues in Kidney Disease – Dialysis
Editors: Stephen Z. Fadem and José A. Moura-Neto
ISBN: 978-1-68507-000-7

Chapter 15

A 360° Global Peritoneal Dialysis Therapy Perspective: Health Economics, Programs and Policies

Natália Maria da Silva Fernandes[1], MD, PhD, Celso Souza de Moraes Junior[2], PhD, Nicola Wearne[3], MD, Bianca Davidson[3], MD, Talerngsak Kanjanabuch[4], MD and José Carolino Divino-Filho[5,*], MD, PhD

[1]Departments of Internal Medicine and Nephrology, Juiz de Fora Federal University, Juiz de Fora, Minas Gerais, Brazil

[2]Departments of Financial and Accounting and FADEPE (Foundation for Development, Teaching, Research and Extension), Juiz de Fora Federal University, Juiz de Fora, Minas Gerais, Brazil

[3]Division of Nephrology, Medicine, University of Cape Town, Cape Town, South Africa

[4]Division of Nephrology, Department of Medicine and Center of Excellence in Kidney Metabolic Disorders, Faculty of Medicine, Chulalongkorn University, Bangkok, Thailand and Peritoneal Dialysis Excellence Center, King Chulalongkorn Memorial Hospital, Bangkok, Thailand

[5]Division of Renal Medicine, Department of Clinical Science, Intervention and Technology, CLINTEC, Karolinska Institutet, Campus Flemingsberg, Stockholm, Sweden; Latin American Chapter (LAC-DD)-International Society for Peritoneal Dialysis

Abstract

The global cost of dialysis is high, being estimated at 87 billion USD (US dollars) in 2016, with an estimated value of 123 billion USD in 2023. The WHO 2019 global research report on the capacity of countries to act in the prevention and control of non-communicable diseases informed that 71% of Member States offer dialysis as a service,

* Corresponding Author's E-mail: jose.divino@ki.se.

usually made available through public funding, to at least 50% of people who depend on therapy. There are still many countries unable to develop a peritoneal dialysis (PD) program, mostly due to economic reasons. Furthermore, there is no consensus on a gold standard to measure cost, which may affect decision-making from the perspective of both the service payer and the service provider. In Africa, access to dialysis and PD is scarce. The median number of PD centers is 0.09 pmp (vs. 1.27 pmp globally). The scarcity of access and distribution of PD, the challenges of practicing PD in the context of dialysis rationing, poverty and the complications of high peritonitis, and communicable disease rates are elaborated in this chapter. However, successful PD program on the continent are also reported with comparable outcomes to the rest of the world and demonstrating how PD is saving lives in the setting of acute kidney injury. Thailand, an endemic area of tropical diseases, has slowly been overshadowed by non-communicable diseases. The introduction of the PD-First policy in 2008 is an important initiative in order to close the access to health services gap between the wealthy and the poor. Its success after ten years reinforces the role of the teamwork between healthcare members and policy makers toward concrete solutions for end-stage kidney disease patients. In this chapter, we concentrate on the PD global perspective covering three important topics: a global snapshot of PD and Health Economics, dialysis as a scarce resource and PD as an opportunity, and PD-first as a national policy.

Keywords: peritoneal dialysis, Health Economics, dialysis costs, policy, PD first, non-communicable diseases, scarce resource, rationing, PD access, poverty, outcomes, South Africa, Thailand

INTRODUCTION

In the 1950s, peritoneal dialysis (PD) was, even though taking its first steps as a renal replacement therapy (KRT), already saving and prolonging lives of patients with acute as well as chronic renal failure. Meanwhile, the initial clinical experience with hemodialysis (HD), by Professors Nils Alwall in Sweden and Wilhelm Kolff in the Netherlands, showed to be very promising, albeit its limited development. With the creation of a permanent natural vascular access for chronic patients by Cimino and Brescia, HD accelerated its development enabling dialysis for tens, hundreds, and today thousands of people around the world.

During the 60s and 70s, PD in the format of Intermittent PD (IPD), could not keep pace with HD. However, with the advent of a permanent peritoneal access (Tenckhoff catheter) and of the Continuous Ambulatory PD (CAPD), PD as a therapy finally took off on a long flight spreading the therapy, initially over the so called developed Western world and thereafter, slowly but continuously to the other continents and countries. There are still many countries unable to develop a PD program, mostly due to economic reasons and, in some countries where healthcare financial restrictions do not prevail, due to medical contra-indication based on biased preference (toward HD) by medical professionals.

Whereas the lack of financial funds impacts on the destiny of chronic kidney disease (CKD) patients in many countries in development, the patient survival rates in developed countries is satisfactory. KRT financial resources originate either from public healthcare or private sectors. For example, most of the prevalent HD patients in Portugal are treated in private-driven dialysis units; whereas in Cuba, all HD centers are operated and owned by the

State. Making the subject even more complex, there are globally many models of KRT reimbursement.

The reimbursement price per HD session in Greece is almost equivalent for the public and private sectors, and there is no increase in the state budget expenses and health budget with a rise in the number of private HD units; whereas, in Brazil, there is a huge difference in reimbursement for one HD session depending if the payment is made by the government or by a private health insurance (supplementary health).

There are countries, especially in the developing world, where PD is not indicated due to KRT financial constraints, whereas other countries have a PD-first program policy. México was, along with Hong Kong, the first country to operate successfully the PD-first policy in response to the 1985 earthquake that wiped out a great number of the public HD facilities in Mexico City. This presented an opportunity for an urgent need of dialysis therapy to be promptly covered by PD.

In this first, out of three PD chapters in this book, we focus on the PD global perspective covering three important topics: a global snapshot of PD and Health Economics, dialysis as a scarce resource and PD as an opportunity, and PD-first as a national policy.

HEALTH ECONOMICS AND PERITONEAL DIALYSIS: A GLOBAL SNAPSHOT

The average number of people receiving care for CKD globally is 759 per million population (pmp); this prevalence varies widely, from 4 pmp in Rwanda to 3392 pmp in Taiwan. Information on dialysis therapy (DT) (hemodialysis - HD or peritoneal dialysis - PD) is available in about 60% of countries and, similarly to CKD, the prevalence of patients with DT increases as the country's income increases (world average of 343 pmp, ranging from 0.5 pmp in Tanzania to 3251 pmp in Taiwan) [1].

The global cost of dialysis is high, being estimated at 87 billion USD in 2016, with an estimated value of 123 billion USD in 2023 [2]. Nonetheless, the World Health Organization (WHO) [3], in its 2019 global research report on the capacity of countries to act in the prevention and control of non-communicable diseases, addressed DT only superficially, showing that 71% of Member States offer dialysis as a service, usually made available through public funding, to at least 50% of people who depend on therapy (Figure 1).

Dialysis is offered to a greater extent in lower income countries when compared to kidney transplantation, which is offered in a much lesser extent. However, this chapter will focus specifically on dialysis therapy. In almost all the regions defined by the WHO, HD has been the most frequently offered therapy. Most impoverished countries, in particular, are burdened by the low number of nephrologists per million inhabitants (<5) and the inability of funding therapy through public means, which suggests that a mix of public and private resources is needed in these cases [4]. Studies have indicated that the high mortality rate in adults and children in sub-Saharan Africa is due to the inability of patients to finance part or all of the costs of dialysis therapy [5], demonstrating that despite dialysis being the most recurrent procedure in poor countries, it does not mean that therapy is offered to all and that it is possible to offer all modalities of therapy to people in need.

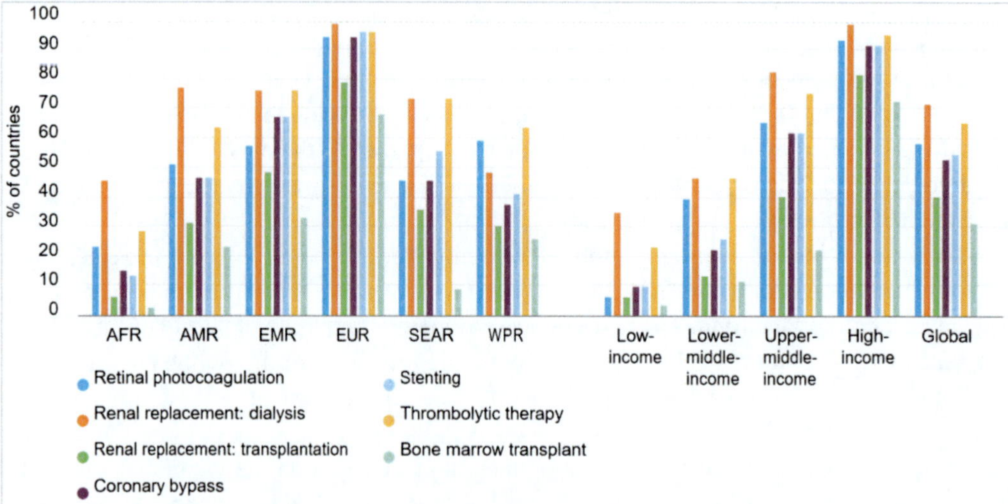

FR: WHO African Region; AMR: WHO Region of the Americas; EMR: WHO Eastern Mediterranean Region; EUR: WHO European Region; EAR: WHO South-East Asia Region; WPR: WHO Western Pacific Region.

Source: Assessing national CAPACITY for the prevention and control of non-communicable diseases (WHO, 2020).

Figure 1. Percentage of countries with procedures for the treatment of chronic non-communicable diseases reported as "usually available" in public funding for the health system, by WHO region and World Bank income group.

What determines the type of DT offered? Multiple variables are involved in this response. Although the country's income may be one of these determinants, it is worth noting that in Latin America, HD rates (67%) are similar to those of the USA (64%) but different from those of Europe (48%). PD rate, in turn, is around 7% in the USA and Europe and 10% in Latin America [6-8]. Asia shows heterogeneous rates of PD, reflecting the nature of the economy of Asian countries. To mention a few examples, in India, the proportions vary between 18% to 20%, in China 20%, in Hong Kong 79.6%, in Japan 3.1%, and in the Middle East 10.2% [9]. Therefore, we note that the greater offer of HD compared to the other therapy modalities suggests an economic contradiction regarding PD, which is a more viable cost option [10].

Another related variable is the country's public health policy. To mention an example in Latin America, Costa Rica has the highest rates of kidney transplantation, followed by PD and HD [8]. The health system of this country is based on three pillars: social security, public sector, and private sector. Other countries in Latin America share this type of health system; however, these countries have a large percentage variation between the types of DT. Data on European countries, in turn, with diverse types of health systems, also do not indicate the type of DT most prevalent in the country. However, the percentage of kidney transplantation in these countries is, on average, higher than in other parts of the world [1].

The impact of different dialysis reimbursement models was addressed by Piccoli et al. who differentiated the types of reimbursement by components, training, and package. There may be more than one type of reimbursement in the same country, as it occurs in France [11]. Government spending on reimbursement for DT services is allocated differently in a world separated by economic differences. Higher-income countries have greater availability of resources to cover the provision of health services related to KRT [12]. Therefore, knowing how much the DT modalities and transplantation cost may contribute to more efficient planning of public and private expenditures on DT worldwide.

Thus, we must consider that if no cost analysis demonstrating the cost of the therapy is performed, only estimates of expenses will be available, and the amount the country will spend on DT will be based on data that may differ from reality. This means that the amount of public funding directed to dialysis may not represent, in some countries, how much therapy costs. Understanding more deeply the composition of costs can help define variables to be investigated in future research on the differences between costs of the modalities of therapy and the cost constraints on quality coverage of procedures with the potential to reduce costs, such as PD in opposition to HD.

The main cost analyses used in economic assessments are the cost-minimization analysis[1]; cost-benefit analysis[2]; cost-effectiveness analysis[3]; and cost-utility analysis[4]. However, we agree that estimates of top-down costs may not be sufficient for a decision-maker [13]. This may be due to a country's wealth, which limits his budgetary capacity, or even due to a patient who has a limited capacity to afford the treatment. Thus, any policy proposals aimed at reducing the unequal access to DT will be conditioned to an answer for the question "how much it really cost or would cost" for a specific health system, service provider, or patient to cover that specific therapy.

Although efforts are made to reach a consensus on how clinical research methodologies should measure effectiveness, there is still no consensus on a gold standard to measure cost, which may affect decision-making. For this reason, we understand that cost information must be raised from the perspective of the service payer (top-down) and the service provider (bottom-up), which expands the power to detect possible cost constraints in a double and wider perspective. Furthermore, costing data (which considers the methods involved in micro-cost) can increase awareness of the DT cost components. This would increase the capacity of comparing regions and countries, in addition to allowing a more careful analysis of reimbursement payment methods by public and private health insurance systems.

We can mention the case of Brazil, where the non-determination of the DT cost prevented the country from having minimally adequate readjustments in the last ten years. The total expenditures paid by the Brazilian public health system ('Unified Health System' - SUS) represented a nominal growth[5] of expenditures of around 3.3% *per annum* from 2009 to 2018.

---

[1] Cost-minimisation analysis (CMS): is used to compare treatment costs between groups receiving clinically equivalent therapies (such as HD and PD). The result of the comparison is expressed in currency units such as dollars or euros [14].

[2] Cost-benefit analysis (CBA): is used to establish whether a therapy is considered beneficial or not. The benefits obtained (such as the years of life gained) from a program are first converted into currency units and then directly compared to the cost of providing the program. These costs and benefits are used to calculate a cost-benefit ratio (B:C), which is finally used to decide whether a program is economically beneficial or not. A program is considered economically beneficial if B: C > 1.0, and not economically beneficial if B: C <1.0.> Note that the term health benefits in currency units is not widely accepted [14].

[3] Cost-effectiveness analysis (CEA): in this type of study, a particular health benefit (or outcome), such as lowering blood pressure by X, and the total cost of therapy is converted into a cost-effectiveness ratio (CER). The lowest CER, or the lowest cost per outcome, is associated with the most economical therapy [14].

[4] Cost-utility analysis (CUA): is similar to a CER, but it also considers intangible quantities, such as patient preference and quality of life. Generally, an CUA describes each program in terms of Quality-Adjusted Life Year (QALY). A QALY refers to an entire year living a healthy life in a health person. For example, dialysis patients may consider 5 years of his life equal to 3 years of life in a healthy person or QALYs 3.0. A decision maker can choose the program that results in the maximum number of QALYs or the program that has the lowest cost per QALY achieved [14].

[5] Nominal: without considering inflation correction or a similar index.

However, the reality is that, over ten years, DT in Brazil has not even kept up with the variations of inflationary impacts, which has led to a negative discount rate in some services, such as PD. In general, DT obtained a real average rate of expenditure shrinkage in relation to inflation of -2.6% *per annum*. Figure 2 shows these accumulated percentage values. An average discount of -21.3% in 10 years is a severe indicator when it comes to the coverage of dialysis therapy by public health. When the values for PD and HD are assessed alone, one can see an increase in HD procedures and a reduction in the PD ones, as shown in Figure 2. Considering average values over ten years, analyzed per set of procedures, disregarding implants and training, HD maintained a nominal value (not adjusted for Brazilian inflation) of $6,995.20 and PD maintained a nominal value of $6,059.40 (exchange rate: US$ 1.00: R$ 3.87; 12/31/2018) [15].

Schreider et al. assessed the DT cost in Brazil from two perspectives, bottom-up and top-down, and found a constraint on the cost of DT both in the public sector and the supplementary health. In the case of PD, the difference between the bottom-up cost, assessed in percentage for three years, and the transfer of funds for PD by SUS (top-down) was - 29.8% [16].

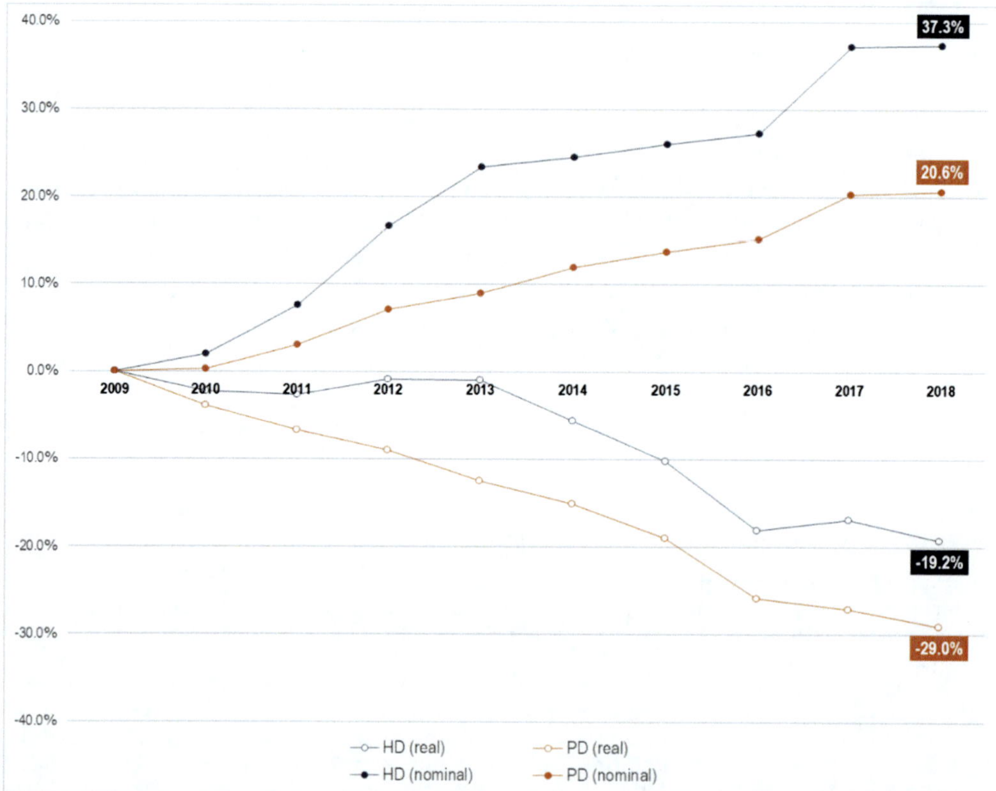

Source: Prepared by Moraes-Junior using data collected from the SUS DATASUS outpatient information system (SIA) database (2019) and the Brazilian Institute of Geography and Statistics (IBGE) (2019), HD- hemodialysis; PD- peritoneal dialysis.

Figure 2. Cumulative percentage evolution of total expenditures on Hemodialysis and Peritoneal Dialysis (nominal and real) from 2009 to 2018.

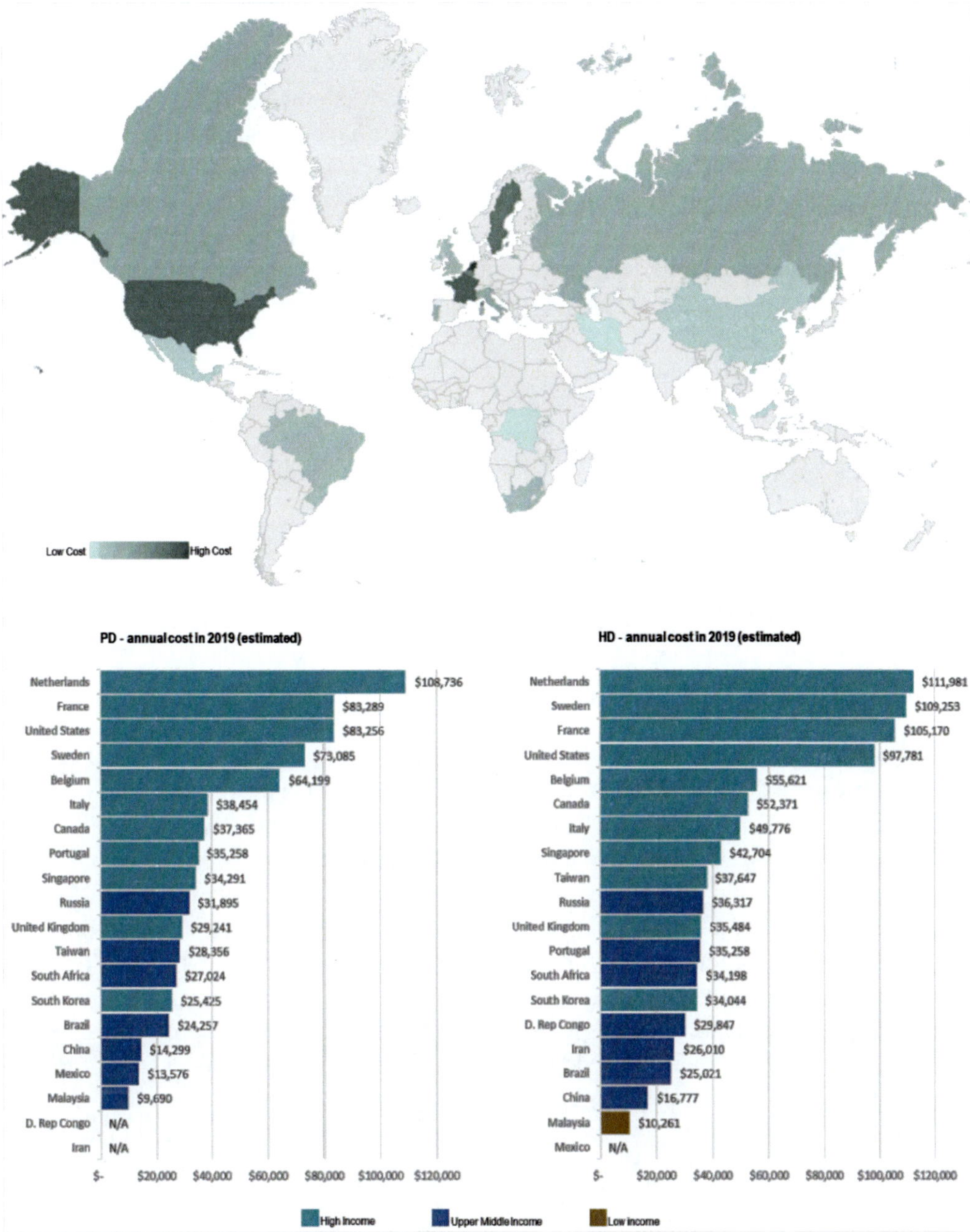

Figure 3. Map of the cost of PD and cost by type of dialysis therapy by country adjusted for inflation (values in US$) [17-36].

When analyzing studies assessing DT costs during the last ten years, identified through a search on Medline and EMBASE, we observed a relative heterogeneity of the methodologies used and a wide variation in the DT costs in the analysis of the composition of costs. A limitation of the data presented here refers to what can be compared, since the elements for the composition of costs were not clearly presented in some studies, even with DT following a highly similar clinical protocol worldwide.

We used the cost of the year mentioned in the study corrected by the country's inflation (data extracted from the Statista, Trading Economics, and Macrotrends Economic databases) and adjusted for the dollar exchange rate on 12/31/2019 for standardization and comparison purposes. Belgium, USA, France, Holland, and Sweden have a disproportionately high cost when compared to the other countries assessed (Figure 3). However, in all the countries analyzed (except for Belgium), PD still had a lower cost. This is always emphasized in comparative studies between HD and PD. The lowest PD costs were observed in Malaysia, Mexico, and China. It is important to note that these are estimates based on published data adjusted for inflation (up to 2019) and the dollar, which may result in data not consistent with reality.

The most up-to-date discussion about costs is based on value-based medicine. Above all, we understand that many issues on aspects of cost determination have yet to evolve in the field of economic health assessments. The study area of DT may be a forerunner in finding more robust ways to establish a gold standard on the definition of how much dialysis actually costs in the world.

Dialysis in Africa, a Scarce Resource: PD as an Opportunity

Background

The most recent Global Kidney Health Atlas (GKHA-Africa) reported that prevalence of CKD in Africa is 6.28%, which is lower than the global prevalence of 9.46%. However, the burden of end-stage kidney disease (ESKD) is pronounced in African countries, where access to treatment is often unaffordable and unavailable. Africa continues to be afflicted by poverty, poor infrastructure, and a massive burden of communicable diseases (HIV, malaria, tuberculosis and diarrheal illnesses). Given these significant challenges, addressing issues associated with non-communicable diseases, like ESKD, is a low priority for many governments [37].

In 2010, Liyanage and colleagues reported that Africa had the largest percentage difference between people needing and receiving KRT [38]. There is also paucity of information describing the extent and diversity of renal disease in Africa due to the lack of renal registry data. South Africa is the only country on the continent that has consistently reported country-wide data on KRT [39].

There are large disparities in work force for kidney care. In Africa, the number of nephrologists is 0.62 per million population (pmp), which is far lower than the global average of 9.95 pmp. Twenty- seven countries in Africa have less than 1 nephrologist pmp. In general, North Africa (except Libya) is better equipped with more than 10 nephrologists pmp [37]. There are significant shortages of all members of the kidney care team including: dialysis nurses, technicians, transplant coordinators, and surgeons. This is due to inadequate training and migration of specialists [40].

There are different models of funding kidney care in Africa. A combination of public and private systems fund KRT in 29% of African countries. Access creation and renal transplantation require payment out-of-pocket (OOP) in 26%, and 29% of countries, respectively [37]. The annual OOP costs of HD and PD are generally more than $10,000 higher in sub-Saharan Africa than in North Africa. Therefore, KRT is not affordable in most countries.

Why PD Makes Sense in Africa and PD-First in South Africa

CAPD should be an ideal form of KRT in Africa. It does not require advanced technologies, much infrastructure or need for dialysis staff support. It enables those living far from dialysis centers the convenience of home dialysis and allows flexibility with employment/schooling and for those caring for others. Furthermore, PD reduces the HD demand in urban areas. Evidence also supports PD-First prior to HD as there are known benefits for the preservation of residual renal function, protection of vascular access and an initial survival benefit [41]. Over the past two decades, the survival of patients treated with CAPD in developed countries, has steadily improved, both in absolute terms and in comparison, to those receiving HD [42-44].

Despite the advantages, HD remains the most common KRT in Africa with most centers located in big cities [37]. In South Africa, the demands for predominantly urban HD has led some provinces to practice "PD-First" unless there are compelling medical, physical, or psychosocial factors precluding PD. Patient survival, in a PD-First program in Cape Town, was not inferior to the survival in other PD-First programs or international registry data [45].

Distribution of PD in Africa

The recently updated GKHA-Africa has been published. Its mandate was to evaluate quality and availability of kidney care worldwide. In Africa, 42 of the 54 countries responded to the questionnaire. All countries reported the availability of HD services; however, access and quality varied geographically [37]. Several reports demonstrate a skewed distribution of KRT services in favor of a few large cities [46, 47]. The highest prevalence of chronic dialysis (both HD and PD) is found in North Africa with Tanzania having the lowest (0.5 pmp) [37].

PD is not the predominant form of dialysis in any country. Only 41% reported the availability of chronic PD. In Africa, the median number of PD centers is 0.09 pmp (vs. 1.27 pmp globally). Only 17% of countries reported the capacity to perform three to four PD exchanges daily. Efficient transport services prevent health care access in many rural areas, leaving millions of people with no access to KRT or long distances to travel [37].

South Africa and Tunisia perform the most PD in Africa with prevalence pmp of 23.3 and 36.8 respectively. The only countries to provide low or no cost dialysis are South Africa, Mauritius and Sudan [48]. A recent report from Egypt reported a decreasing prevalence of CAPD from 0.29 pmp to 0.1 pmp [37, 49]. Elzorkany expressed concerns that this was leading to decreased awareness of PD as the first option of KRT as well as lack of experienced physicians [49]. Sudan is the third largest country in Africa (population +/- 30 million); it has significant geographical odds yet has a functional PD program and currently supports 2.5 pmp on PD [37].

Challenges for PD Programs within an African Setting

Rationing Dialysis

In South Africa, with a population of 56.62 million, of the total number of patients accessing KRT, 7682 (71.5%) were on HD with 1199 (11.2%) on PD. The private sector currently has 7582 (855 pmp) on KRT, whereas the public sector, which serves 84% of the population, provides KRT for only 66 pmp [39]. Due to the severe resource constraints and the enormous disparity for access to KRT in the state sector, national guidelines have been developed. These guidelines mandate that only patients who can be transplanted are accepted onto public sector chronic dialysis programs. The South African Constitutional Court has ruled that rationing of dialysis is appropriate, given the resource scarcity [50]. In the Western Cape province, selection criteria guidelines were developed after extensive consultation with stakeholders, including patient representatives and ethics experts. The 'Accountability for Reasonableness' approach and the overarching ethical principle of utilitarianism were used in this process [51]. A review of the selection process over a 4-year period, reports that more than half (53.9%) of patients who were referred for KRT were not accepted [52]. Another center in the same province reported that 75% of all patients considered were declined [53].

Poverty – Exclusion for PD or an Obstacle?

The Human Development Index (HDI) is a statistical composite index of life expectancy, education, and per capita income indicators. In sub-Saharan Africa, HDI remains the lowest among all developing regions. There are also large discrepancies in the distribution of wealth within countries. Six of the 10 countries with the highest Gini index scores are in sub Saharan Africa [54, 55]. In addition, government spending on health is low. The WHO reported a 70-fold difference in healthcare spending between high- and lower-income countries, with the lowest spending in the countries of West, Central, and East Africa [56].

The role that socioeconomic status (SES) plays in PD continues to be debated in South Africa and abroad. Recent reports from South Africa have failed to demonstrate that SES was linked to poor survival or technique failure [57, 58]. In BRAZPD, economic status was not independently linked to outcomes [59]. Whether SES is an obstacle or poor predictive factor for outcome requires further investigation.

What remains clear is that poverty impacts patients practicing PD. In a recent unpublished review from Cape Town, South Africa (a public hospital in an urban setting), marked poverty was noted. In this cohort, only 29% were employed, 40% relied on disability grants or pensions, and the average income was low (R3 750 per month, equivalent to 199.79 US$). One fifth of patients reported hunger at some point over the past year. Amenities and sanitation were also challenging as thirty percent lived in an informal dwelling. Only 87.9% had access to running water and 19% did not have flushing toilets in their homes. Literature is limited on how PD is performed in more rural settings in Africa.

These challenges have been implicated in impacting on patient's QOL on PD. Within Africa most QOL studies have been performed in SA. An initial study reported no difference in QOL between HD and PD [60]. However subsequent studies have shown that PD patients have lower QOL scores with higher symptom burden [61-63]. Income within the cohort was one of the biggest determinants for QOL [62].

Lastly, environments alter PD practices. In Cape Town, South Africa, PD home visits are not allowed due to staff safety concerns [9]. Cape Town has one of the highest reported violent crime and murder rates (1,647/100,000 and 63/100,000 population, respectively) [64]. This is extremely high compared to the global average murder rate of 6.04/100,000 [65]. Home visits are shown to be essential for patient support, education, and decreasing peritonitis rates.

Cost of PD

Cost comparisons between CAPD and HD have been a subject of debate. Only South Africa and Kenya produce their own PD fluid locally [48]. Unfortunately, due to the lack of infrastructure, other African countries depend entirely on imported PD fluids, which make the cost excessively high. International transportation, import tariffs, and cost of storage, increase the cost [66, 67]. Therefore, the cost in many regions does not make PD economically sustainable.

When PD fluid is produced locally, the cost of PD decreases. In 2017, a public hospital in South Africa reported on micro costing differences between HD and PD. The study established that the costs of HD were higher than PD. This was mainly due to laboratory tests, HD solutions, as well as purchasing and maintaining the dialysis equipment [68]. This emphasizes the need to invest in fluid manufacturing (either nationally or regionally) in Africa to improve uptake of CAPD.

Peritonitis

Peritonitis is a major cause of morbidity (such as technique failure, transfer to HD, and catheter change) and is responsible for mortality in 2-6% of cases [69]. Predictors of peritonitis include baseline characteristics including age, gender, education level, reduced serum albumin, and presence of diabetes mellitus [70-72]. Weather and seasonal variation also influence the incidence of peritonitis with peaks in the months that are hot and humid [73]. However, the prevalence and causes of peritonitis vary depending on the region and the time period [69].

A systematic review of 1,512 PD patients in Africa reported on the prevalence and mortality of peritonitis. High rates of peritonitis were seen and ranged from 0.55–2.8 episodes/ patient-year. Recent studies demonstrated a decline in peritonitis rates compared to the earlier studies. All-cause mortality rates ranged 0-38.7% with peritonitis being the main contributor to death. Gram-positive organisms were the most common infection but, among the gram-negative infections, *Pseudomonas* predominated. Africa reported high rates of fungal infections in some regions (0.7-31%). Tuberculosis peritonitis ranged from 0.8-3%. High rates of culture negative peritonitis were reported in most studies (ranging from 12.5–62.5%) [74].

Table 1 reports recent published rates of peritonitis from large center within Africa, this ranged from 0.4–0.89 episodes/ patient-year. Many centers including Sudan and South Africa have described decreasing peritonitis rates over the last 15 years. This table confirms high rates of culture-negative peritonitis and a predominance of *Pseudomonas*.

Table 1. Peritonitis rates from large centres within Africa

	GDP $ Billion	Total health expenditure (% GDP)	N	Age years (mean)	DM	Peritonitis Events	Culture negative	Gram-Positive organisms	Gram-Negative organisms	Other	Deaths due to peritonitis
Morocco (2006-2011) [1]	298.6	5.5	36	49 +/-17	22%	18.59 (months X patients/ peritonitis)	26.3%	Gram-Positive (56.6%) *CNS (53.3%)* *Staph. aureas (36.6%)* *Non-groupable streptococcus (6.6%)*	Gram-negative (37.7%) *Pseudomonas (30%)* *Enterobacter 20%* *Klebsiella (15%)*	-	0
Senegal (2004 -2010) [2]	54.8	4.0	62	47 +/- 13	19%	1 episode/ 20 patient-months (0.60 episodes/ patient year)	51%	*Staph. aureas (18%)* *Streptococcus (2%)*	*Pseudomonas (16%)* *Klebsiella (2%)* *Serratia (2%)* *Acinetobacter (2%)*	Fungal (7%)	2/16
Egypt (1997-2010) [3]	1204.0	4.6	33	31.7	24%	1 episode/ 21.3 patient months (0.56 episodes/ patient year)	49%	*Staph. aureas (24%)*	*Pseudomonas (8%)*	Fungal (6%)	-
Tunisia (2006-2016) [4]	12.97	6.6	182	43.9+/-17	35%	1 episode/27.25 patient/months 0.44 episodes/patient-year	33.5%	-	-	-	-
Sudan (2005-2007) [5] (2010-2013)*[6]	177.4	6.3	111	56 (Mdn)		1 episode every 14 months (0.85 episodes/ patient year)	53% 46% (2010)* 5% (2012)*	*Staph. aureas (11.8%)** *Staph. epidermidis (5.9%)**	*E. coli (23.5%)** *Pseudomonas (21%)** *Klebsiella (5.9%)**	13.2%*	2/111
Nigeria (1995)[7]	1121.0	3.6	23	36.4	-	70% of cohort	88%	*Staph. aureas*	*Klebsiella*	-	-
SA: Limpopo (2007 – 2012) [8, 9]	767.2	8.2	152	36.8 +/- 11.4	9.9	0.82 episodes/ patient year	62.3%	Gram-positive (50.6%)	Gram negative (38%)	TB (7.6%) Fungal (3.8%)	-

	GDP $ Billion	Total health expenditure (% GDP)	N	Age years (mean)	DM	Peritonitis Events	Culture negative	Gram-Positive organisms	Gram-Negative organisms	Other	Deaths due to peritonitis
SA: Western Cape / GSH (2008 – 2015)[10]	767.2	8.2	199	39	9.8	0.87 episodes/ patient year	19.5%	*Staph. aureas 19.4%* *Staph. epidermidis (12.6%)* *CNS (15.12%)*	*Pseudomonas (3.7%)*	Fungal (4.2%)	-

GDP = gross domestic product, n = total in cohort, DM = diabetes, GSH = Groote Schuur hospital, Mdn = Median, *Staph. aureas* = Staphylococcus aureas, *Staph. epi* = Staphylococcus epidermidis, *CNS* = Coagulase-negative Staphylococci, *Pseudomonas* = Pseudomonas aeruginosa, *Klebsiella* = Klebsiella pneumonia, *E. Coli* = *Escherichia coli, Serratia* = Serratia plymunthica.

1. Bekaoui S, Haddiya I, Houti MS, Berkchi FZ, Ezaitouni F, Ouzeddoun N, et al. Infectious peritonitis profile in peritoneal dialysis at Ibn Sina University Hospital: a 6-year data report. Int *J Nephrol Renovasc Dis.* 2014;7:323-7. Epub 2014/09/05. doi: 10.2147/IJNRD.S42069..
2. Niang A, Cisse MM, Mahmoud SM, Lemrabott AT, Ka el HF, Diouf B. Pilot experience in senegal with peritoneal dialysis for end-stage renal disease. *Perit Dial Int*. 2014;34(5):539-43. Epub 2014/03/04. doi: 10.3747/pdi.2011.00327.
3. Mahmoud KM, Sheashaa HA, Gheith OA, Wafa EW, Agroudy AE, Sabry AA, et al. Continuous ambulatory peritoneal dialysis in Egypt: progression despite handicaps. *Perit Dial Int*. 2010;30(3):269-73. Epub 2010/04/29. doi: 10.3747/pdi.2009.00001.
4. Lasfar LB, Guedri Y, Zellama D, El Meknassi I, Azzebi A, Mrabet S, et al. Long-term clinical outcomes of peritoneal dialysis patients: 10-year experience of a single unit from Tunisia. *Saudi J Kidney Dis Transpl*. 2019;30(2):451-61. Epub 2019/04/30. doi: 10.4103/1319-2442.256852.
5. Elhassan EA, Kaballo B, Fedail H, Abdelraheem MB, Ali T, Medani S, et al. Peritoneal dialysis in the Sudan. *Perit Dial Int.* 2007;27(5):503-10. Epub 2007/08/21.
6. Kheir SM, Kafi SK, Ryden P, Elbir H, Soliman MA, Ali S, et al. Results of application of the ISPD guidelines to the management of peritoneal dialysis in a single center in Sudan. *J Infect Public Health*. 2017;10(3):348-52. Epub 2016/10/09. doi: 10.1016/j.jiph.2016.08.008.
7. Arije A, Akinlade KS, Kadiri S, Akinkugbe OO. The problems of peritoneal dialysis in the management of chronic uraemia in Nigeria. *Trop Geogr Med.* 1995;47(2):74-7. Epub 1995/01/01.
8. Isla RA, Mapiye D, Swanepoel CR, Rozumyk N, Hubahib JE, Okpechi IG. Continuous ambulatory peritoneal dialysis in Limpopo province, South Africa: predictors of patient and technique survival. *Perit Dial Int.* 2014;34(5):518-25. doi: 10.3747/pdi.2013.00334.
9. Tamayo-Isla RA, de la Cruz MC, Okpechi IG. Mycobacterial Peritonitis in CAPD Patients in Limpopo: A 6-Year Cumulative Report from a Single Center in South Africa. Perit Dial Int. 2016;36(2):218-22. Epub 2016/03/24. doi: 10.3747/pdi.2014.00322.
10. Davidson B, Crombie K, Manning K, Rayner B, Wearne N. Outcomes and Challenges of a PD-First Program, a South-African Perspective. *Perit Dial Int*. 2018;38(3):179-86. Epub 2018/06/01. doi: 10.3747/pdi.2017.00182

HIV and PD

In 2008, the first HIV positive donor to HIV positive recipient was pioneered at Groote Schuur Hospital, South Africa, thereby increasing the pool of donor kidneys. This was the turning point for HIV positive patients gaining access onto state funded KRT. The program has shown success with outcomes similar to non-HIV patients and better than those of extended criteria donor transplantation [76]. HIV-infected PD patients with a CD4 count < 200 cells/mm^3 have been shown to have an increased risk of peritonitis and relapsing peritonitis. HIV was not associated with technique failure [77].

Outcomes of PD on the African Continent

Table 2. Patient and technique survival in PD programmes in Africa

					Technique survival (%)				Patient survival (%)			
	Period	n	Age years (mean)	DM (%)	1 year	2 year	3 year	5 year	1 year	2 year	3 year	5 year
SA: Western Cape (GSH) [1]	2008 - 2015	199	39	9.8	85.0	75.2	-	45.0	91.3	79.6	-	50.2
SA: Western Cape (TBH) [2]	2008 - 2014	170	36	1.7	80.0	-	54.0	39.0	90.0	-	82.0	63.0
SA: Limpopo[3]	2007 - 2012	152	37	9.9	83.3	71.7	-	62.1	86.7	78.7	-	65.3
Egypt[4]	1997-2010	33	31.7	24	94.4	-	-	-	91.9	-	-	-
Senegal [5, 6]	2004-2010 2004 -2007*	62	Mdn 47 (+/- 13)	19.4	62*	45*	38*	-	63*	42*	-	-
Morocco[7]	2006-2011	36	Mdn 49 +/- 17	22	NA				NA			
Tunisia [8]	2006-2016	182	43.9+/-16.95	33.5	96.7	90	84.5	73.9	96.1	93.2	91.4	89.3

SA = South Africa, n= number in cohort, DM= diabetes, Mdn = median, GSH = Groote Schuur Hospital, TGB = Tygerberg Hospital, NA = not available.

1. Davidson B, Crombie K, Manning K, Rayner B, Wearne N. Outcomes and Challenges of a PD-First Program, a South-African Perspective. *Perit Dial Int*. 2018;38(3):179-86. Epub 2018/06/01. doi: 10.3747/pdi.2017.00182.
2. Kapembwa KB, N; Tannor, E; Davids, RM. Peritoneal dialysis technique survival at Tygerberg Hospital in Cape Town, South Africa. *Afr J Nephrol*. 2017;20(1):25-33.
3. Isla RA, Mapiye D, Swanepoel CR, Rozumyk N, Hubahib JE, Okpechi IG. Continuous ambulatory peritoneal dialysis in Limpopo province, South Africa: predictors of patient and technique survival. *Perit Dial Int*. 2014;34(5):518-25. doi: 10.3747/pdi.2013.00334.
4. Mahmoud KM, Sheashaa HA, Gheith OA, Wafa EW, Agroudy AE, Sabry AA, et al. Continuous ambulatory peritoneal dialysis in Egypt: progression despite handicaps. *Perit Dial Int*. 2010;30(3):269-73. Epub 2010/04/29. doi: 10.3747/pdi.2009.00001.
5. Niang A, Cisse MM, Mahmoud SM, Lemrabott AT, Ka el HF, Diouf B. Pilot experience in senegal with peritoneal dialysis for end-stage renal disease. *Perit Dial Int*. 2014;34(5):539-43. Epub 2014/03/04. doi: 10.3747/pdi.2011.00327.
6. Cisse MM, Hamat I, Gueye S, Seck SM, Ka el HF, Tall AO, et al. Peritonitis in patients on peritoneal dialysis: a single-center experience from Dakar. *Saudi J Kidney Dis Transpl*. 2012;23(5):1061-4. Epub 2012/09/18. doi: 10.4103/1319-2442.100953.
7. Bekaoui S, Haddiya I, Houti MS, Berkchi FZ, Ezaitouni F, Ouzeddoun N, et al. Infectious peritonitis profile in peritoneal dialysis at Ibn Sina University Hospital: a 6-year data report. *Int J Nephrol Renovasc Dis*. 2014;7:323-7. Epub 2014/09/05. doi: 10.2147/IJNRD.S42069.
8. Lasfar LB, Guedri Y, Zellama D, El Meknassi I, Azzebi A, Mrabet S, et al. Long-term clinical outcomes of peritoneal dialysis patients: 10-year experience of a single unit from Tunisia. *Saudi J Kidney Dis Transpl*. 2019;30(2):451-61. Epub 2019/04/30. doi: 10.4103/1319-2442.256852.

There is limited reported data on the outcomes of PD programs in Africa. Patient survival at 1 year ranged between 86.7–91.3%, and at five years is 50.2%–89% (Table 2). These results are comparable to those reported in international PD registries, middle-income countries, and in high-income countries. These results, however, need to be viewed in context. In certain countries in Africa (specifically SA), younger and healthier cohorts are selected for dialysis due to dialysis rationing. Even comparing cohorts within Africa, Northern African countries (Senegal and Egypt), have similar age and co-morbidity rates to international cohorts. However, sub-Saharan countries were dialysing younger cohorts (16–18 years younger than internal registries) with strikingly fewer diabetics (9.8% vs. 20–44%) (Table 2).

Reported mortality rates in countries where dialysis rationing is practiced needs to consider that a substantial proportion of PD patients (31%) who died with technique failure, could not be offered a modality switch to HD, due to non-transplantability. When a timely switch in this setting was performed, survival was excellent, with no deaths recorded at 5 years [45].

Factors associated with increased mortality included diabetes, low BMI, low serum albumin, low hemoglobin, and more than one episode of peritonitis [45, 58, 78]. The most common cause of technique failure was peritonitis throughout the African cohorts. Black African ethnicity and increased age were strong predictors of technique failure in both cohorts from Cape Town, South Africa [45, 78]. The reasons remain unclear but may include the impact of SES.

AKI and PD

Under-18s account for approximately 50% (+/- 600 million children) of the population in Africa, which has a major impact on healthcare resources [79]. Eleven percent of the admission in a Malawi paediatric emergency center were attributed to AKI with sepsis, malaria, and gastroenteritis identified as the cause in 85% [80]. Children typically have little comorbidity and, if able to survive the initial insult, frequently fully recover. Acute PD can therefore be highly cost-effective for young people who have the potential to complete schooling and become a significant contributor to the community [81]. Acute PD is potentially more cost-effective, requires minimal water and electricity, requires less training of staff, and alleviates the insertion of HD catheters, which can be challenging in the small child. In addition, two randomized controlled trials have shown earlier renal recovery with acute PD (34%) as compared to HD [82, 83].

The Saving Young Lives Program (SYL) was established in 2012 to develop sustainable acute PD programs to treat young patients with AKI in low-resource settings [84]. The program represents a partnership amongst 4 international nephrology organizations (ISN, IPNA, ISPD and Euro-PD) and the Sustainable Kidney Care Foundation. Within Africa, the program has reached out to 18 countries. A local champion is the most important factor, as the goal is for the SYL-supported units to become self-sufficient. A common problem has been difficulty obtaining commercial PD solutions, mixing PD solutions locally has been shown to be safe and an effective alternative, if fluids are not available [85].

Conclusion

There are still unacceptably high numbers of people unable to access KRT in Africa. Initiatives like SYL continue to strive to improve access to PD. However, despite many challenges, there are effective PD programs with outcomes that are comparable to large centers. Peritonitis rates in Africa remain a challenge. However, many centers have reported peritonitis rates meeting ISPD targets. Several countries including Sudan and South Africa have reported decreasing peritonitis rates over time. South Africa has demonstrated that a PD-First approach can be successful in a resource-limited setting. HIV and poverty remain pervasive problems throughout Africa but should be viewed as obstacles and not contraindications to receiving PD.

PD First Policy in Thailand

The number of patients with ESKD has been increasing worldwide. In Thailand, over 100,000 patients require dialysis [86], and >20,000 people start treatment with HD or PD every year [87]. Although the first HD and PD were performed in 1964 and 1982, respectively, the number of Thai patients treated with dialysis only gradually increased in the first three decades because of limited access arising from prohibitive costs, which precipitated catastrophic health expenditure for many families [88]. In 2008, the Thai government extended the scope of healthcare coverage to include KRT by launching the "PD First" policy. This provided Thai citizens with universal health coverage for dialysis, such that the numbers of dialyzed patients and dialysis centers increased exponentially. According to the United States Renal Data System annual report in 2018, Thailand was in the top five countries with the highest incidence rates of treated ESKD, 1,515 per million population/year in 2016 compared to 100 per million population/year in 2008 [89]. This short review elaborates on the principle and key success factors of the "PD First" policy, and how they have challenged and influenced dialysis treatment in Thailand.

Reimbursement System

Located in the middle of mainland Southeast Asia, Thailand is an agricultural country divided into 77 provinces and 13 healthcare regions with a current population of 66.6 million [90]. One-sixth of citizens live in the Bangkok metropolitan region. According to World Bank records, Thailand is classified as an upper-middle-income country, which has spent 6.5% of its gross domestic product on health [91]. Currently, there are three government health insurance schemes with different features and administrative management. Firstly, the Civil Servant Medical Beneficiary System (CSMBS), under the Ministry of Finance, covers 4.5 million civil servants and their immediate family members [92]. Secondly, the Social Security System (SSS), administered by the Social Security Office, Ministry of Labor, provides support for 12.6 million employees. The funding for this scheme originates from tripartite contributions, including employers, employees, and the government [93]. Lastly, the Universal Coverage Scheme (UCS), which is also known as the "30 Bahts (1 US Dollar) Scheme," managed by the National Health Security Office (NHSO), supports 51.6 million remaining citizens, who are self-employed and not employees of government, state enterprises, and private establishments [94].

The UCS was introduced in 2002; however, KRT compensation became established in 2008 [95]. Under the UCS, CAPD is provided as the first-line dialysis modality unless patients are not suitable for PD because of a PD contraindication or a history of PD technique failure. Such patients can access HD without additional payment. Patients who are medically suitable for PD can decline PD and choose HD as the first-line treatment, but they have to fully self-fund for dialysis-related costs [96, 97]. However, all the patients in the pre-dialysis program are introduced to both PD and HD. It is important to note that funding of kidney care medications, including PD bags, erythropoiesis-stimulating agents (ESA), iron supplements, and calcimimetic agents, are fully supported by the policy if the drugs are on the Thai National Medication List. Under the policy, PD bags are only provided as standard glucose-based, 2L-manual bags, capped at 5 bags daily, of international brands, but locally or regionally manufactured. Icodextrin, amino acid, and low-glucose degradation product (GDP)-based PD solutions can be prescribed but are not reimbursed by the policy. Only short-acting ESA is allowed for reimbursement and capped at 4,000 units twice weekly.

Making "PD First" Strategy Possible in Thailand

Table 3. Key success factors of implementing the PD First policy in Thailand

Nine key success factors
1. Fundamental changes in healthcare reimbursement systems by increasing incentives for clinicians and hospitals to initiate patients on CAPD
2. Cost containment, particularly for the procurement of PD solutions and ESA
3. Controlling the growing number of PD patients by expanding kidney transplantation programs and integrating "chronic care" and "palliative care" concepts into a CKD management model, as well as committing to educate the public and healthcare workers
4. Increasing the number of dedicated staff who have experience and expertise in PD, expanding the capacity of PD centers and strengthening the PD healthcare worker network
5. Setting up national support systems, including national courses to certify PD nurses and PD catheter insertion operators, service center model with multi-disciplinary care and home-visit practices, four regional training centers, standard textbook, web-based PD educational modules, and national PD patient network
6. Promoting research and innovation-oriented care. Holding an annually national meeting and offering rewards or recognition to frontline healthcare workers
7. Enhancing HD support as back-up to support PD patients who are at need of HD, either temporary or permanent
8. Integrating new technology into clinical care, such as telemedicine for home visiting
9. Developing national PD clinical practice guidelines, Thailand-specific key performance indicators (KPI)[98], and PD center accreditation (known as the supervisory visit)

In essence, the key success of implementing the "PD First" policy included nine elements [98], as demonstrated in Table 3. With these elements, a home delivery system for PD solutions has been introduced. The Government Pharmaceutical Organization (GPO) is responsible for the national procurement of the solution. The products are distributed mainly by the Thailand Post Co., Ltd, (THPD), whereas local logistics companies are subcontracted for the patients residing in rural areas [99]. All hospitals and PD clinics have to monthly key-in the prescription data for the amount of required PD consumables for each patient. THPD connects multi-partners using a web-based system and adopts the mobile Global Positioning System (GPS) to track the PD bags during the distribution and inform the patients ahead of the delivery [100]. The distribution system has been carried out effectively over the past decade, with more than 27 million bags being delivered to patients' homes each year; moreover, the system was capable of handling the major flood in the central region of Thailand during 2011 without a significant shortage of the supply [100]. The strength of this home delivery system over the traditional logistic system is reducing PD clinic/hospital burden and cost in the management of the stock. This is important, particularly in Thailand, where most of the public hospitals health workforces have tremendous workloads devoted to clinical, administrative and pharmaceuticals management as well as limited hospital space in order to store the PD bags in storage rooms.

Utility Rate of PD

Over the decade that the "PD First" policy has been in place, the number of PD patients and centers has grown exponentially. As of December 2016, the number of prevalent and incident PD patients was 26,450 (390 pmp) and 10,783 (159 pmp), respectively. PD penetration has now increased, respectively, 31% and 46% of all prevalent and incident dialysis patients when compared with < 10% before 2008 [87] (Figure 4). Almost 90% of PD patients are under the UCS [87]. Regional differences in the relative uptake of PD modality have also been noted, ranging from 17% in the Bangkok metropolitan region to 37% in rural regions [88].

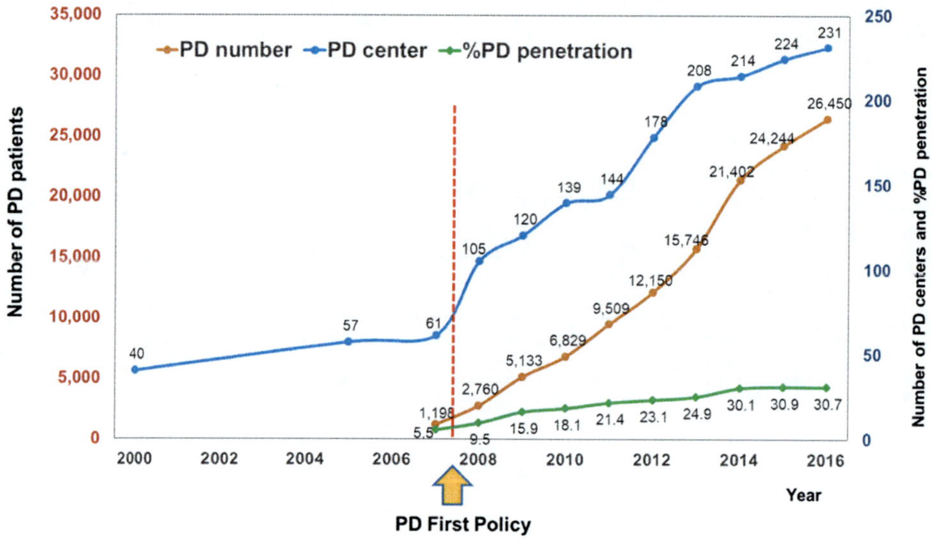

Figure 4. Peritoneal dialysis (PD) numbers, PD centers, and % PD penetration of prevalent dialysis patients (Pt) over time [87].

PD Centers and Patients Characteristics

Almost all PD facilities are affiliated with public/governmental hospitals, although an autonomous public organization owns one PD center and another center is a private clinic. Thai PD facilities are large, with an average of 102 (interquartile range: 48–208) PD patients per facility [101], and a low automated PD (APD) penetration (5%) [102]. The physician-to-patient ratio is 87:1, whereas the PD nurse-to-patient ratio is 70:1 [102]. Four facilities (out of 231 centers) have no nephrologists in charge, all of which belong to the community-based or standard hospitals. It is generally accepted that the optimal ratio of PD nurse-to-patient ratio should be below 20-25:1 [103, 104]. The workload of PD nurses is even harder if it counts on non-PD tasks and on-call, off-hour services. The burgeoning workload of medical staff in Thailand might be explained by the rapid implementation of the "PD First" policy. The number of active PD patients has risen ten times in a decade, while the growth of PD centers has increased only four times since the policy commenced.

Thai PD patients have an average age of 56 years, body weight of 58 kg, body mass index of 22.6 and body surface area (BSA) of 1.6 m^2. Furthermore, they have low education levels and household incomes; the majority at elementary school or lower level and household incomes lower than $5,000/year. These parameters are worse in patients located in provincial areas. CAPD is the dominant mode (95%); 82% of CAPD perform 2L x 4 exchanges a day. Less than 20% of the patients perform ≤3 or ≥5 exchanges a day. The average prescribed 24-hour exchange volume, normalized to BSA, is 8.7 L/1.73 m^2, whereas 81% of APD patients have no day dwell with an average total prescribed cycler volume per BSA of 11.0 L/1.73 m^2. Icodextrin is not used at all by CAPD patients and is limited to only 17% of APD patients. Neutral pH low GDP solutions is not prescribed in Thailand. Only 9% of PD patients use 3.86% PD solutions, and 73% do not use either of the high glucose PD solutions. The average weekly peritoneal Kt/V is 1.73 and 1.75 in CAPD and APD patients, respectively [102].

Hypokalemia and hypoalbuminemia are commonly observed in 37% and 67% of the patients, respectively. The average serum potassium and albumin are 3.7±0.6 mEq/L and 3.1±0.8 gm/dL. The mean hemoglobin level is 10.2 gm/dL, 42% has Hb levels below 10 gm/dL [105]. Most Thai PD patients are on a short-acting ESA, and 93% are using Epoetin-alpha [106]. According to the results of the Thailand Peritoneal Dialysis Outcomes and Practice Patterns Study (PDOPPS), over one-half of Thai PD patients require caregivers to assist with their PD exchanges (60%), which likely reflects the high prevalence of functional impairment in PD patients (47%) [107]. Patients who persistently or subsequently require caregivers to assist with PD exchange are associated with an increased risk of mortality, but not with peritonitis or HD transfer risk when compared to patients who never required caregivers to assist with PD [108].

PD Outcomes

PD-related infection is the leading cause of technique failure and death in Thai PD patients. In 2016, the crude peritonitis rate was 0.39 episodes/year, and the median facility peritonitis rate was 0.43 episodes/year [101]. The rates are comparable with those of low- and high-income countries, including Brazil (0.63 episodes/year) [109], Malaysia (0.27 episodes/year) [110], and at the upper end of the range reported in PDOPPS (0.28-0.40 episodes/year) (Figure 5) [101], indicating an improvement over a decade of the policy from 0.67 in 2008 [111] to 0.48 in 2011 [112] and 0.39 in 2017 [101]. Only 18% of the facilities failed to achieve the International Society for PD (ISPD) Guideline 2016 target of fewer than 0.5 episodes/year [101]. The Gram-negative rate has overtaken the Gram-positive bacterial peritonitis rate (0.12 versus 0.10 episodes/year) [101], and there is a notably high culture-negative peritonitis rate in Thailand (0.11 episodes/year) accounting for 28% of all peritonitis episodes [101]. Culture yields from PD effluent are greatly dependent on facility/laboratory practices. There is considerable variability in the capacity, capability, and practices of microbiology laboratories, with some lacking formal accreditation. Deviation from the ISPD guidelines is associated with culture-negative peritonitis rates [113].

However, the patient and technique survival rates have improved substantially. In 2016, the 1- and 5-year PD patient survival rates were 83% and 54%, respectively [114], compared with the 2012 rate with a one-year patient survival of 79%. These rates are comparable with those of Asia-Pacific countries, including Hong Kong (1-year, 91% and 5-year, 48%), China (1-year, 94% and 5-year, 64%), and Australia (1-year, 89% and 5-year, 39%) [115]. In addition, the technique survival rates (censored for death and kidney transplantation) are 95% and 81% in the first and fifth years of PD, respectively [114]. The technique survival rate is analogous with the previous reports, including China (1-year, 95% and 5-year, 86%), and Australia (1-year, 70% and 5-year, 10%) [115]. Moreover, Thai patients have slightly higher specific health-related quality of life (HRQoL) by the European Quality of Life-5 Dimensions (EQ-5D) questionnaire than the general PD populations [116] and have good spiritual well-being [117].

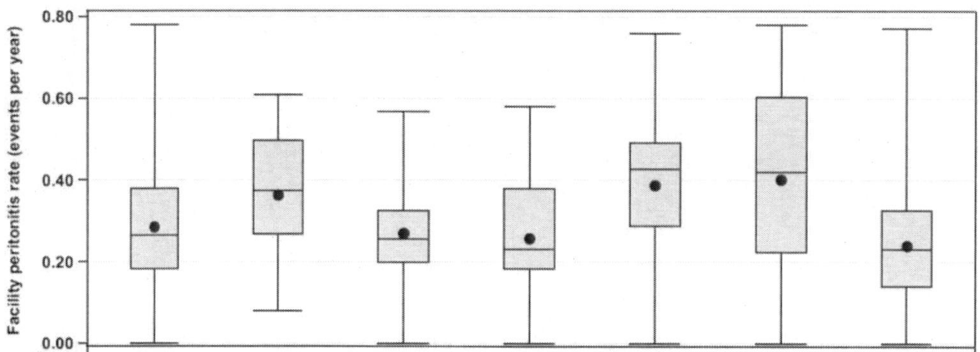

	Overall	Australia/NZ	Canada	Japan	Thailand	UK	US
Facility N	209	17	20	29	22	18	103
Mean	0.28	0.36	0.27	0.26	0.39	0.40	0.24
Min	0.00	0.08	0.00	0.00	0.00	0.00	0.00
10th	0.08	0.14	0.14	0.11	0.12	0.11	0.06
25th	0.18	0.27	0.20	0.18	0.29	0.22	0.14
50th	0.26	0.37	0.26	0.23	0.43	0.42	0.23
75th	0.38	0.50	0.32	0.38	0.49	0.60	0.33
90th	0.50	0.59	0.41	0.47	0.52	0.70	0.40
Max	0.78	0.61	0.57	0.58	0.76	0.78	0.77

Figure 5. Distribution of facility peritonitis rates by PDOPPS-participating country. Circle markers denote mean values. Boxes extend to 25th and 75th percentiles [16].

Challenges

The tremendous expansion of ESKD numbers in Thailand raises important national concerns regarding the sustainability of health financing and healthcare service delivery. Focused initiatives to mitigate CKD growth and expand kidney transplantation programs in regions outside of Bangkok should be further implemented as part of long-term cost-containment strategies. The centralization of resources and standardization of the financing mechanism of dialysis among three different health schemes could be considered, to promote more efficient use of national resources and create reimbursement equality. Several challenges require further research and improvement, including prevention of peritonitis-related death, avoidance of malnutrition and cardiovascular diseases, improvement of PD longevity, and reduction of caregiver dependency. In the short-term, improvements in PD-supporting systems in line with international standards, including culture techniques and nutritional support, are urgently needed for the sustainability of the "PD First" policy. Moreover, the growing amount of PD bag disposal is one recently environmentally concerned, generated greater than 5,000 tons yearly. Dispatched to the landfill or incarceration could pollute the environment. Recycling the PD bag county-wide is warranted.

The success of the policy, in terms of PD utilization rate, as well as patient and technique survivals, highlights the crucial role of the Thai healthcare teams in advocacy and collaboration with policymakers to work toward sustainable solutions for people living with kidney disease.

Conclusion

The global cost of dialysis is high, projected to be $123 billion by 2023 [2]. The WHO has reported that 71% of the Member-States offer dialysis as a service, generally available through public funding to, at least, 50% of people in need of dialysis [3]. As a global trend, the worldwide dialysis population is continuously increasing. However, there are tremendous gaps between chronic kidney disease (CKD) policies and KRT among countries and continents. Furthermore, there is no consensus on a gold standard to measure cost, which may affect decision-making from the perspective of both the service payer and the service provider.

Dialysis is a scarce resource in Africa, just like water in the desert. However, PD again is seen as an opportunity to bridge the gap in South Africa where a PD-first approach has been implemented with challenges such as dialysis rationing, poverty, cost of PD, peritonitis, and HIV. In spite of them, very good PD programs have been established and their outcome results do not lag behind the ones from large centers in other regions of the world.

Thailand, an endemic area of tropical diseases, has slowly been overshadowed by non-communicable diseases. The introduction of the PD-First policy in 2008 is an important initiative in order to close the access to health services gap between the wealthy and the poor. Its success after ten years reinforces the role of the teamwork between healthcare members and policy makers toward concrete solutions for ESKD patients.

The beauty of Peritoneal Dialysis is still its simplicity, flexibility, and availability. As PD evolved, new frontiers opened up, therapy options developed, and clinical indications proposed, tested, and established. Besides, Peritoneal Dialysis is also, cost-wise, a tantalizing KRT option for countries with constraint ESKD budgets.

References

[1] Bello AK, Levin A, Lunney M, Osman MA, Ye F, Ashuntantang G et al. *Global Kidney Health Atlas: A report by the International Society of Nephrology on the Global Burden of End-stage Kidney Disease and Capacity for Kidney Replacement Therapy and Conservative Care across World Countries and Regions*. International Society of Nephrology, Brussels, Belgium. 2019 in www.theisn.org/global-atlas.

[2] Brown, EN. Influence of Reimbursement Policies on Dialysis Modality Distribution Around the World. *Clin J of Am Soc Nephrol*. 2019:14(1):10-12. doi: 10.2215/CJN. 13741118.

[3] World Health Organization 2020. *Assessing national capacity for the prevention and control of noncommunicable diseases: report of the 2019 global survey*. Geneva: World Health Organization, 2020.

[4] Bilal Q, Mohamed A O , Levin A, Feehally J, Harris D, Jindal K et al. Kidney Care in Low- And Middle-Income Countries. *Clin Nephrol.* 2020:93(1): 21-30.

[5] Ashuntantang G, Osafo C, Olowu WA, Arogundade F, Niang A, Porter J et al. Outcomes in adults and children with end-stage kidney disease requiring dialysis in sub-Saharan Africa: a systematic review. *Lancet Global Health.* 2017: 5(4): e408-e417.

[6] *United States Renal Data System.* USRDS- https://www.usrds.org/2019/download/USRDS_2019_ES_final.pdf.

[7] *European Renal Association-European Dialysis and Transplant Association.* ERAEDTA- https://era-edta-reg.org/index.jsp?p=14.

[8] *Sociedade Latino-Americana de Nefrologia e Hipertensão.* SLANH- https://slanh.net/wp-content/uploads/2019/10/INFORME-2018.pdf.

[9] Navva PKR, Sreepada SV, Karopadi AN. Present Status of Renal Replacement Therapy in Asian Countries. *Blood Purif.* 2015:40:280-287. doi: 10.1159/000441574.

[10] Bello AK, Levin A, Lunney M, Osman MA, Ye F, Ashuntantang G et al. Status of care for end stage kidney disease in countries and regions worldwide: international cross sectional survey. *BMJ.* 2019: 367:l5873. doi.org/10.1136/bmj.l5873.

[11] Piccoli GB, Cabiddu G, Breuer C, Jadeau C, Testa A, Brunori G. Dialysis Reimbursement: What Impact do Different Models Have on Clinical Choices. *J Clin Med. 2*019: 8 (276): 1-17. doi:10.3390/jcm8020276.

[12] Van der Tol A, Lameire N, Morton RL, Van Biesen W, Vanholder R. An International Analysis of Dialysis Services Reimbursement. An International Analysis of Dialysis Services Reimbursement. *Clin J Am Soc Nephrol.* 2019:14(1): 84-93. doi:10.2215/CJN.08150718.

[13] Xu X, Nardini HKG and Ruger JP. Micro-costing studies in the health and medical literature: protocol for a systematic review. *Systematic Reviews.* 2014:47(3):1-7. doi:10.1186/2046-4053-3-47.

[14] Karopadi AN. Analysis of cost in Renal Replacement Therapy. *Perit Dial Int.* 2017:37(5):497-499. doi.org/10.3747/pdi.2017.00066.

[15] Souza de Moraes Jr C. [Custos com prestadores de serviços na atenção a Doença Renal Crônica em meio aos caminhos e descaminhos do SUS] / Celso Souza de Moraes Jr. -- 2019. 149 f.: il. PhD *Thesis - Universidade Federal de Juiz de Fora, Faculdade de Medicina.* Programa de Pós-Graduação em Saúde Brasileira, 2019.

[16] Schreider A, Moraes Junior CS, Fernandes NM. *Three years Evaluation of Peritoneal Dialysis and Hemodialysis absorption costing: the service provider's perspective compared to funds transfers from the public and private healthcare systems* (Submitted).

[17] Arefzadeh A, Lessanpezeshki M, Seifi S. The cost of hemodialysis in Iran. *Saudi J Kidney Dis Transpl* 2009; 20(2):307-311. Available from: http://www.sjkdt.org/temp/SaudiJKidneyDisTranspl202307-8132251_223522.pdf.

[18] Izeide PPM, Nlandu YM, Lepira FB, Makulo JRR, Engole YM, Mokoli VM, et al. Cost estimate of chronic hemodialysis in Kinshasa, the Democratic Republic of the Congo: A prospective study in two centers. *Hemodialysis International* 2019: doi:10.1111/hdi.12802.

[19] Surendra NK, Abdul Manaf MR, Hooi LS, Bavanandan S, Mohamad Nor FS, Firdaus Khan SS, et al. Cost utility analysis of end stage renal disease treatment in Ministry of Health dialysis centres, Malaysia: Hemodialysis versus continuous ambulatory

peritoneal dialysis. *PLoS ONE*. 2019: 14(10): e0218422. doi.org/10.1371/ journal. pone.0218422.

[20] Cortes-Sanabria L, Paredes-Cesena C, Herrera-Llamas RM, Cruz-Bueno Y, Soto-Molina H, Pazarın L et al. Comparison of Cost-Utility Between Automated Peritoneal Dialysis and Continuous Ambulatory Peritoneal Dialysis. *Archives of Medical Research*.2013: 44 655e661. doi.org/10.1016/j.arcmed.2013.10.017.

[21] Zhang H, Zhang C, Zhu S, Ye H an Zhang D. Direct medical costs of end-stage kidney disease and renal replacement therapy: a cohort study in Guangzhou City, southern China. *BMC Health Services Research*. 2020: 20:122. doi.org/10.1186/s12913-020-4960-x.

[22] Sbrissia D, Gouveia S, Bignelli AT, Hokazono SR, Danucalov I, Siemens TA et alm Analysis of economic impact among modalities of renal replacement therapy. *J Bras Nefrol*. 2017:39(2):162-171. doi: 10.5935/0101-2800.20170019.

[23] Kim SH, Jo MW, Go DS, Ryu DR., & Park J. Economic burden of chronic kidney disease in Korea using national sample cohort. *J Nephrol*. 2017: doi: 10.1007/s40620-017-0380-3.

[24] Makhele L, Matlala M, Sibanda M, Martin AP, Godman B. A Cost *Analysis of Haemodialysis and Peritoneal Dialysis for the Management of End Stage Renal Failure at an Academic Hospital in Pretoria, South Africa Pharmaco Economics*. 2019: Open https://doi.org/10.1007/s41669-019-0124-5.

[25] Tang CH, Chen HH, Wu MJ, Hsu BG, Tsai JC, Kuo CC et al. Out-of-pocket costs and productivity losses in haemodialysis and peritoneal dialysis from a patient interview survey in Taiwan. *BMJ Open*. 2019:9:e023062. doi: 10.1136/ bmjopen-2018-023062.

[26] Li B, Cairns JA, Fotheringham J, Tomson CR, Forsythe JL, Watson C et al. Understanding cost of care for patients on renal replacement therapy: looking beyond fixed tariffs. *Nephrol Dial Transplant*. 2015: 30: 1726–1734 doi: 10.1093/ndt/gfv224.

[27] Yagudina R, Kulikov A, Abdrashitova G, Serpik VG. Cost-Effectiveness Analysis of Medical Care for Chronic Renal Disease Patients in Need of Renal Replacement Therapy Via Peritoneal Dialysis and Hemodialysis in the Russian Health Care Environment. *Value in Health*. 2016: 19. A1-A318 (PUK12).

[28] Yang F, Lau T & Luo N. Cost-effectiveness of haemodialysis and peritoneal dialysis for patients with end-stage renal disease in Singapore. *Nephrology*. 2016: doi: 10.1111/ nep.12668.

[29] Rocha MJ, Ferreira S, Martins LS, Almeida M, Dias L, Pedroso S, Henriques AC, Almeida R, Cabrita A. Cost analysis of renal replacement therapy by transplant in a system of bundled payment of dialysis. *Clin Transplant*. 2011: doi: 10.1111/j.1399-0012.2011.01571.x.

[30] Beaudry A, Ferguson TW, Rigatto C, Tangri N, Dumanski S, Komenda. Cost of Dialysis Therapy by Modality in Manitoba. *Clin J Am Soc Nephrol*. 2018: 13. doi.org/ 10.2215/CJN.10180917.

[31] Roggeri A, Roggeri DP, Zocchetti C, Bersani M, Conte F AND ReNe (Renal Lombardy Network). Additional contributors from ReNe Network. Healthcare costs of the progression of chronic kidney disease and different dialysis techniques estimated through administrative database analysis. *J Nephrol*. 2016: doi: 10.1007/s40620-016-0291-8.

[32] Cleemput I, De Laet CA. Analysis of the costs of dialysis and the effects of an incentive mechanism for low-cost dialysis modalities. *Health Policy*. 2013:172–179. doi.org/10.1016/j.healthpol.2013.03.001.

[33] Eriksson JK, Neovius M, Jacobson SH, et al. Healthcare costs in chronic kidney disease and renal replacement therapy: a population-based cohort study in Sweden. *BMJ Open* 2016:6:e012062. doi:10.1136/bmjopen-2016- 012062.

[34] United States Renal Data System. *2019 USRDS annual data report: Epidemiology of kidney disease in the United States*. National Institutes of Health, National Institute of Diabetes and Digestive and Kidney Diseases, Bethesda, MD, 2019:in https://www.usrds.org/2019/viewDefault.aspx.

[35] Zambrowski J. Cou^t de la dialyse. *Ne´phrol ther*. 2016: doi.org/10.1016/j.nephro.2016.02.002.

[36] Mohnen SM, van Oosten MJM, Los J, Leegte MJH, Jager KJ, Hemmelder MH, et al. Healthcare costs of patients on different renal replacement modalities – Analysis of Dutch health insurance claims data. *PLoS ONE*. 2019: 14(8): e0220800. doi.org/10.1371/journal. pone.0220800.

[37] Bello AK, Johnson DW, Feehally J, Harris D, Jindal K, Lunney M, et al. Global Kidney Health Atlas (GKHA): design and methods. *Kidney Int Suppl*. 2017;7(2):145-53.

[38] Liyanage T, Ninomiya T, Jha V, Neal B, Patrice HM, Okpechi I, et al. Worldwide access to treatment for end-stage kidney disease: a systematic review. *Lancet*. 2015;385(9981):1975-82.

[39] Davids MR, Jardine T, Marais N, Zunza M, Jacobs JC, Sebastian S. South African Renal Registry Annual Report 2017. *Afr J Nephrol*. 2019;22(1):60-71.

[40] Swanepoel CR, Wearne N, Okpechi IG. Nephrology in Africa—not yet uhuru. *Nat Rev Nephrol*. 2013;9(10):610.

[41] Bargman JM, Thorpe KE, Churchill DN, Group CPDS. Relative contribution of residual renal function and peritoneal clearance to adequacy of dialysis: a reanalysis of the CANUSA study. *J Am Soc Nephrol*. 2001;12(10):2158-62.

[42] Heaf JG, Løkkegaard H, Madsen M. Initial survival advantage of peritoneal dialysis relative to haemodialysis. *Nephrol Dial Transplant*. 2002;17(1):112-7.

[43] Fenton SS, Schaubel DE, Desmeules M, Morrison HI, Mao Y, Copleston P, et al. Hemodialysis versus peritoneal dialysis: A comparison of adjusted mortality rates. *Am J Kid Dis*. 1997;30(3):334-42.

[44] Lukowsky LR, Mehrotra R, Kheifets L, Arah OA, Nissenson AR, Kalantar-Zadeh K. Comparing mortality of peritoneal and hemodialysis patients in the first 2 years of dialysis therapy: a marginal structural model analysis. *Clin J Am Soc Nephrol*. 2013;8(4):619-28.

[45] Davidson B, Crombie K, Manning K, Rayner B, Wearne N. Outcomes and Challenges of a PD-First Program, a South-African Perspective. *Perit Dial Int*. 2018;38(3):179-86.

[46] Wearne N, Okpechi IG, Swanepoel CR. Nephrology in South Africa: Not Yet ubuntu. *Kidney Dis*. 2019;5(3):189-96.

[47] Tannor EK, Awuku YA, Boima V, Antwi S. The geographical distribution of dialysis services in Ghana. *Ren Replace Ther*. 2018;4(1):3.

[48] Abu-Aisha H, Elamin S. Peritoneal dialysis in Africa. *Perit Dial Int*. 2010;30(1):23-8.

[49] Elzorkany KMA. Current state of continuous ambulatory peritoneal dialysis in Egypt. *Saudi J Kidney Dis Transpl*. 2017;28(6):1369.

[50] Moosa MR, Wearne N. Invited commentary should we be rationing dialysis in South Africa in the 21st century? *Perit Dial Int.* 2018;38(2):84-8.

[51] Moosa MR, Maree JD, Chirehwa MT, Benatar SR. Use of the 'accountability for reasonableness' approach to improve fairness in accessing dialysis in a middle-income country. *PloS one.* 2016;11(10):e0164201.

[52] Kilonzo KG, Jones ES, Okpechi IG, Wearne N, Barday Z, Swanepoel CR, et al. Disparities in dialysis allocation: An audit from the new South Africa. *PloS one.* 2017;12(4):e0176041.

[53] Moosa MR, Meyers AM, Gottlich E, Naicker S. An effective approach to chronic kidney disease in South Africa. *S Afr Med J.* 2016;106 (2):156-9.

[54] UN. United Nations Development Programme. *Human development data* (1990–2018). 2018. http://hdr.undp.org/en/data accessed 21 July 2020.

[55] CIA. Central Intelligence Agency. *Distribution of family income—GINI index.* https:// wwwciagov/library/publications/the-world-factbook/fields/223rankhtml accessed 21 July 2020.

[56] WHO. World Health Organization (WHO). *Global spending on health: a world in transition. 2019.* https://wwwwhoint/health_financing/documents/health-expenditure-report-2019/en/. accessed 21 July 2020.

[57] Katz IJ, Sofianou L, Hopley M. An African community-based chronic ambulatory peritoneal dialysis programme. *Nephrol Dial Transplant.* 2001;16(12):2395-400.

[58] Isla RAT, Mapiye D, Swanepoel CR, Rozumyk N, Hubahib JE, Okpechi IG. Continuous ambulatory peritoneal dialysis in Limpopo province, South Africa: predictors of patient and technique survival. *Perit Dial Int.* 2014;34(5):518-25.

[59] de Andrade Bastos K, Qureshi AR, Lopes AA, Fernandes N, Barbosa LM, Pecoits-Filho R, et al. Family income and survival in Brazilian Peritoneal Dialysis Multicenter Study Patients (BRAZPD): time to revisit a myth? *Clin J Am Soc Nephrol.* 2011;6(7):1676-83.

[60] Okpechi IG, Nthite T, Swanepoel CR. Health-related quality of life in patients on hemodialysis and peritoneal dialysis. *Saudi J Kidney Dis Transpl.* 2013;24(3):519.

[61] Okaka EI, Naidoo S, Ahmed MM, Davies M, Naicker S. Quality of life in patients on continuous ambulatory peritoneal dialysis in an African setting *Saudi J Kidney Dis Transpl.* 2015;26(3):631.

[62] Okaka E, Davies M, Ahmed M, Naidoo S, Naicker S. Impact of socio-economic factors on quality of life in patients on continuous ambulatory peritoneal dialysis in an African setting. *West Afr J Med.* 2014;33(2):125.

[63] Tannor EK, Archer E, Kapembwa K, Van Schalkwyk SC, Davids MR. Quality of life in patients on chronic dialysis in South Africa: a comparative mixed methods study. *BMC nephrology.* 2017;18(1):4.

[64] *Victims of crime survey* 2015/2016. https://www.statssa.gov.za/publications. (Accessed June 2017).

[65] *Global study on homicide executive summary*: https://www.unodc.org/documents/data-(Accessed February 2019).

[66] Wearne N, Kilonzo K, Effa E, Davidson B, Nourse P, Ekrikpo U, et al. Continuous ambulatory peritoneal dialysis: perspectives on patient selection in low-to middle-income countries. *Int J Nephrol Renovasc Dis.* 2017;10:1.

[67] Swanepoel CR, Wearne N, Okpechi IG. Nephrology in Africa--not yet uhuru. *Nat Rev Nephrol.* 2013;9(10):610-22.

[68] Makhele L, Matlala M, Sibanda M, Martin AP, Godman B. A cost analysis of haemodialysis and peritoneal dialysis for the management of end-stage renal failure at an Academic Hospital in Pretoria, South Africa. *PharmacoEconomics-open*. 2019;3(4):631-41.

[69] Mehrotra R, Devuyst O, Davies SJ, Johnson DW. The current state of peritoneal dialysis. *J Am Soc Nephrol*. 2016;27(11):3238-52.

[70] Chern Y-B, Ho P-S, Kuo L-C, Chen J-B. Lower education level is a major risk factor for peritonitis incidence in chronic peritoneal dialysis patients: a retrospective cohort study with 12-year follow-up. *Perit Dial Int*. 2013;33(5):552-8.

[71] Kotsanas D, Polkinghorne KR, Korman TM, Atkins RC, Brown F. Risk factors for peritoneal dialysis-related peritonitis: Can we reduce the incidence and improve patient selection? *Nephrology*. 2007;12(3):239-45.

[72] Chow KM, Szeto CC, Leung CB, Kwan B, Law MC, Li P. A risk analysis of continuous ambulatory peritoneal dialysis-related peritonitis. *Perit Dial Int.* 2005;25 (4):374-9.

[73] Szeto C-C, Chow K-M, Wong TY-H, Leung C-B, Li PK-T. Influence of climate on the incidence of peritoneal dialysis-related peritonitis. *Perit Dial Int*. 2003;23(6):580-6.

[74] Moloi M, Kajawo S, Noubiap J, Mbah I, Ekrikpo U, Kengne A, et al. Prevalence of peritonitis and mortality amongst patients on peritoneal dialysis in Africa: a systematic review. *BMJ Open*. 2018;8: e020464.

[75] Kapembwa KC, Bapoo NA, Tannor EK, Davids MR. Peritoneal dialysis technique survival at Tygerberg Hospital in Cape Town, South Africa. *Afr J Nephrol.* 2017;20(1):25-33.

[76] Muller E, Barday Z, Mendelson M, Kahn D. HIV-Positive–to–HIV-Positive Kidney Transplantation—Results at 3 to 5 Years. *N Engl J Med*. 2015;372(7):613-20.

[77] Ndlovu KC, Sibanda W, Assounga A. Peritonitis outcomes in patients with HIV and end-stage renal failure on peritoneal dialysis: a prospective cohort study. *BMC nephrology*. 2017;18(1):48.

[78] Kapembwa KC. Peritoneal dialysis technique survival at tygerberg Hospital in cape town, south Africa: Stellenbosch: Stellenbosch University; 2017.

[79] Desa U. United nations department of economic and social affairs, population division. world population prospects: The 2015 revision, key findings and advance tables. *Technical Report*: Working Paper No ESA/P/WP 2412015.

[80] Evans RD, Docherty M, Seeley A, Craik A, Mpugna M, Mann S, et al. Incidence, etiology, and outcomes of community-acquired acute kidney injury in pediatric admissions in Malawi. *Perit Dial Int*. 2018;38(6):405-12.

[81] Kilonzo KG, Akrabi HF, Yeates KE. Cost-effectiveness of acute peritoneal dialysis: Considerations from Africa. *Clin Nephrol*. 2019.

[82] Gabriel DP, Caramori J, Martim L, Barretti P, Balbi AL. High volume peritoneal dialysis vs daily hemodialysis: a randomized, controlled trial in patients with acute kidney injury. *Kidney Int*. 2008;73:S87-S93.

[83] Al-Hwiesh A, Abdul-Rahman I, Finkelstein F, Divino-Filho JC, Qutub H, Al-Audah N, et al. Acute kidney injury in critically ill patients: A prospective randomized study of tidal peritoneal dialysis versus continuous renal replacement therapy. *Ther Apher Dial*. 2018;22(4):371-9.

[84] Cullis B, Lalya F, Smoyer WE. Saving more young lives in Africa. *Perit Dial Int.* 2020:0896860820931662.

[85] McCulloch MI, Nourse P, Argent AC. Use of locally prepared peritoneal dialysis (PD) fluid for acute PD in children and infants in Africa. *Perit Dial Int.* 2020:0896860820920132.

[86] Krittayaphong R, Rangsin R, Thinkhamrop B, Hurst C, Rattanamongkolgul S, Sripaiboonkij N, Wangworatrakul W: Prevalence of chronic kidney disease associated with cardiac and vascular complications in hypertensive patients: A multicenter, nation-wide study in Thailand. *BMC Nephrol* 18: 115, 2017.

[87] Chuasuwan A, Praditpornsilpa K. *Thailand renal replacement therapy: Year 2015* [Internet]. Available at: http://www.nephrothai.org/images/Final_TRT_report_2015_%E0%B8%89%E0%B8%9A%E0%B8%9A%E0%B9%81%E0%B8%81%E0%B9%84%E0%B8%82.pdf. Accessed January 20, 2020.

[88] Kanjanabuch T, Takkavatakarn K. Global dialysis perspective: Thailand. *Kidney360.* April 2020 DOI: https://doi.org/10.34067/KID.0000762020.

[89] *United States Renal Data System: 2018 USRDS annual data report.* Chapter II: International comparisons. Available at: https://www.usrds.org/2018/download/v2_c11_IntComp_18_usrds.pdf. Accessed January 20, 2020.

[90] *Official Statistics Registration Systems Thailand*: 2019. Available at: http://stat.dopa.go.th/stat/st atnew/upstat_age.php. Accessed February 14, 2020.

[91] *Central Intelligence Agency: The world factbook: East Asia/Southeast Asia*: Thailand. Available at: https://www.cia.gov/library/publications/the-world-factbook/geos/th.html. Accessed January 20, 2020.

[92] Announcement of the Ministry of finance September 21, *1998: Determining the criteria and reimbursement rate of medical expenses for patients with kidney disease.* Available at: http://saraban-law.cgd.go.th/CGDWeb/simple_search.jsp. Accessed January 20, 2020.

[93] *Announcement of the medical committee under the social security act: Criteria and reimbursement rate of medical expenses for renal replacement therapy 2015.* Available at: https://www.sso.go.th/wpr/assets/upload/files_storage/_th/dfff6f731d973161024501fff69071d5.pdf. Accessed January 20, 2020.

[94] National Health Security Office. *NHSO Annual Report 2017.* Available at: http://stream.nhso.go.th/wp-content/uploads/ebooks/annual-2017. Accessed January 20, 2020.

[95] *The Secretariat of the Cabinet: The Cabinet resolution* 2007 [in Thai. Available at: https://cabinet.soc.go.th/soc/Program2-3.jsp?top_serl=214283. Accessed January 20, 2020.

[96] Chuengsaman P, Kasemsup V: PD First policy: Thailand's response to the challenge of meeting the needs of patients with end-stage renal disease. *Semin Nephrol.* 2017;37: 287–295.

[97] Tantivess S, Werayingyong P, Chuengsaman P, Teerawattananon Y. Universal coverage of renal dialysis in Thailand: promise, progress, and prospects. *BMJ.* 2013;346:f462. doi: 10.1136/bmj.f462.

[98] Pongpirul K, Kanjanabuch T, Puapatanakul P, Chuengsaman P, Dandecha P, Kingwatanakul P, et al. National feasibility survey of peritoneal dialysis key performance indicators in Thailand from provider perspective. *Nephrology* (Carlton). 2020;25(6):483-490.

[99] Takkavatakarn K, Puapatanakul P, Kanjanabuch T, Buanet T, Thongbor N, Pitakmongkol S, et al. An early experience of Check List to Improve Patient Self-care and Product Defect Report in Continuous Ambulatory Peritoneal Dialysis (CLIP SP) study. *Int J Artif Organs*. 2020;43(2):137-140.

[100] Thailand Post Distribution Co., Ltd [Internet]. 2020 [cited 2020, Feb 1]. Available from: https://www.thailandpost.co.th/un/article_detail/article/11/3951.

[101] Perl J, Fuller DS, Bieber BA, Boudville N, Kanjanabuch T, Ito Y, et al. Peritoneal dialysis-related infection rates and outcomes: Results from the peritoneal dialysis outcomes and Practice Patterns study (PDOPPS). *Am J Kidney Dis*. 2020;76(1):42-53.

[102] Wang AY, Zhao J, Bieber B, Kanjanabuch T, Wilkie M, Marshall MR, et al. International comparison of peritoneal dialysis prescriptions from the Peritoneal Dialysis Outcomes and Practice Patterns Study (PDOPPS). *Perit Dial Int.* 2020;40(3):310-319.

[103] Chaudhary K. Peritoneal Dialysis Drop-out: Causes and Prevention Strategies. *Int J Nephrol.* 2011;2011:434608.

[104] Moreiras-Plaza MM. Where we come from and where we are going in terms of peritoneal dialysis: identifying barriers and strategies for the future. *Nefrologia.* 2014;34(6):756-67.

[105] Kanjanabuch T, Puapatanakul P, Halue G, Lorvinidnun P, Tangjittrong K, Pongpirul K, et al. Implementation and Challenges of PDOPPS in a Middle Income Country: Thailand Experience. *Perit Dial Int.* 2020.

[106] Li PKT, Choy ASM, Bavanandan S, Chen W, Foo M, Kanjanabuch T, et al. Management of Anemia in Peritoneal Dialysis Patients –Asian Pacific Perspectives. *Manuscript in preparation.*

[107] Tennankore K, Zhao J, Karaboyas A, Bieber BA, Robinson BM, Morgenstern H, et al. The Association of Functional Status with Mortality and Dialysis Modality Change: Results from the Peritoneal Dialysis Outcomes and Practice Patterns Study (PDOPPS). *Perit Dial Int*. 2019;39:103-111.

[108] Puapatanakul P, Kanjanabuch T, Cheawchanwattana A, Tungsanga K, Tangjittrong K, Lowmseng N, et al. *Caregiver Requirement Status of Peritoneal Dialysis Patients in Thailand and Its Effects on Patient Outcomes: The Results of Thailand PDOPPS.* Manuscript in preparation.

[109] Figueiredo AE, Poli-de-Figueiredo CE, Meneghetti F, Lise GA, Detofoli CC, Silva LB. Peritonitis in patients on peritoneal dialysis: analysis of a single Brazilian center based on the International Society for Peritoneal Dialysis. *J Bras Nefrol*. 2013;35(3):214-9.

[110] Ong LM, Ch'ng CC, Wee HC, Supramaniam P, Zainal H, Goh BL, et al. Risk of Peritoneal Dialysis-Related Peritonitis in a Multi-Racial Asian Population. *Perit Dial Int.* 2017;37(1):35-43.

[111] Siriwong T. Why PD get in trend and why everyone love it? *Cardiovascular & Metabolic* (Thailand) 2011;24:43-4.

[112] Kanjanabuch T, Chancharoenthana W, Katavetin P, Sritippayawan S, Praditpornsilpa K, Ariyapitipan S, et al. The incidence of peritoneal dialysis-related infection in Thailand: a nationwide survey. *J Med Assoc Thai* 2011;94 Suppl 4:S7-12.

[113] Kanjanabuch T, Chatsuwan T, Udomsantisuk N, Nopsopon T, Puapatanakul P, Halue G. *Association of Local Peritoneal Dialysis (PD) Unit Sampling and Microbiology*

Laboratory Culture Practices with the Ability to Identify Causative Pathogens in PD-associated Peritonitis: Results of a National Survey. Manuscript in preparation.

[114] Changsirikulchai S, Sriprach S, Thokanit NS, Janma J, Chuengsaman P, Sirivongs D: Survival analysis and associated factors in Thai patients on peritoneal dialysis under the PD-first policy. *Perit Dial Int.* 2018;38:172–178.

[115] Li PK, Chow KM, Van de Luijtgaarden MW, Johnson DW, Jager KJ, Mehrotra R, et al. Changes in the worldwide epidemiology of peritoneal dialysis. *Nat Rev Nephrol.* 2017;13(2):90-103.

[116] Sakthong P, Kasemsup V. Health utility measured with EQ-5D in Thai patients undergoing peritoneal dialysis. *Value Health.* 2012; 15:S79-84.

[117] Cheawchanwattana A, Kanjanabuch T, Narenpitak S, Halue G, Tungsanga K, Tatiyanupanwong S, et al. *The Validity, Reliability, and Results of the WHOQOL-SRPB in Thai Peritoneal Dialysis Patients.* Manuscript in preparation.

In: Issues in Kidney Disease – Dialysis
Editors: Stephen Z. Fadem and José A. Moura-Neto
ISBN: 978-1-68507-000-7

Chapter 16

A 360° Global Peritoneal Dialysis Therapy Reality: Clinical Experience and Evidence

Ramón Paniagua[1], MD, Marcela Ávila Diaz[1], PhD, Abdullah Khalaf Al-Hwiesh[2], MD, Daniela Ponce[3], MD, PhD, Welder Zamoner[3], MD, André Luís Balbi[3], MD, PhD, Johan Rosman[4], MD, PhD and José Carolino Divino-Filho[5,*], MD, PhD

[1]Unidad de Investigación Médica en Enfermedades Nefrológicas.
UMAE Hospital de Especialidades Bernardo Sepúlveda Gutiérrez, Centro Médico Nacional Siglo XXI, Instituto Mexicano del Seguro Social, Mexico City, México
[2]King Fahd University Hospital, Imam Abdulrahman Bin Faisal University, Dammam, Saudi Arabia
[3]Department of Internal Medicine, University of São Paulo State - UNESP, Botucatu, Sao Paulo, Brazil
[4]Curtin University Medical School, Nephrologist Royal Perth Hospital, Perth, Western Australia, Australia
[5]Division of Renal Medicine, Department of Clinical Science, Intervention and Technology, CLINTEC, Karolinska Institutet, Campus Flemingsberg, Stockholm, Sweden;
Latin American Chapter (LAC-DD)-International Society for Peritoneal Dialysis

Abstract

Mexico needed to preserve peritoneal dialysis (PD) as a cheaper and accessible treatment without requiring large investments in hemodialysis (HD) facilities. The Mexican Social Security Institute (Spanish: Instituto Mexicano del Seguro Social) (IMSS) facilitated a randomized, multi-center clinical trial, the Adequacy of PD in Mexico (ADEMEX) study, which questioned the use of small molecule clearance to measure PD adequacy and thereby promoted a return to comprehensive clinical evaluation as the most

* Corresponding Author's E-mail: jose.divino@ki.se.

efficient dialysis measure. PD is underutilized in Saudi Arabia and in the Middle East; among the reasons, lack of pre-dialysis education programs and nephrologists expert in catheter insertion, later referral and expansion of outsourcing HD. The King Fahad University Hospital program must be considered one of the most prolific PD centers carrying out clinical studies on the subject. Interest in PD use to manage patients with AKI has been increasing recently. Today there is solid clinical evidence that hypervolemia, hyperpotassemia, acidosis, uremia and hypercatabolism can be well managed by PD in different scenarios. Many of these studies have been performed in a small Brazilian university city, Botucatu. The dilemmas of using PD in aboriginal patients in Australia is discussed here. The focus is on aboriginal people in very remote areas. Some personal views are presented as to the causes of the gap between outcomes for aboriginal and non-aboriginal patients and how the many failed attempts to close the gap could be addressed.

Keywords: peritoneal dialysis adequacy, randomized controlled trials, clinical evidence, acute kidney injury, indigenous, aboriginal, outcomes, deprivation, poverty

INTRODUCTION

Dr. Fred Boen wrote and defended his PhD thesis dissertation in Amsterdam in 1959 [1], containing a very thorough narrative of the peritoneal dialysis (PD) technique, including an initial literature review from 1877 until 1958. In the last part of his thesis, Dr. Boen presented complete case reports of twenty-two patients treated with 32 treatments, during the years 1951-1959, describing the results. The main indications were overhydration 16 times and hyperkalemia 16 times; most frequently a combination of these two factors was the reason to start PD. Nine patients recovered, seven of them with a clearance value above 60% the normal; these seven patients had reversible renal lesions: HgCl anuria, hemolysis (blood transfusion, prostatectomy, malaria), sulfa anuria, CCl_4 intoxication and post partum anuria. Two patients recovered with a low clearance value: one of them probably had bilateral cortical necrosis, the other sulfa anuria with pre-existing chronic glomerulonephritis. Furthermore, his thesis gave considerations to the management of acute kidney injury (AKI) and indications for PD.

Dr. Jon Gjessing, an anesthesiologist in Sweden, described in his 1967 thesis [2] new indications for PD such as severe hemorrhagic pancreatitis, new osmotic agents such as amino acids and dextran, pharmacokinetics of drugs administered intraperitoneally and as a diagnostic test in acute abdominal conditions, as well as the use of PD in the treatment of acute poisoning (more specifically, barbiturates, salicylates, and methyl-alcohol).

Mortality in AKI has unfortunately not changed in the last two decades, even though new kidney replacement therapies (KRT) have been developed and randomized controlled trials (RCT) with these new techniques published. These trials have shown that a dialysis dose threshold would exist below which there would be an impact on survival, but above which it would not appear to have increased benefit [3-5]. It is also unfortunate that, not rarely, physicians solely rely on one mathematical target, Kt/V, to make their decision on which KRT modality to prescribe. High-income countries may consider themselves privileged as they can tailor the decision of what modality to choose to each individual AKI patient, including PD; but middle and low-income countries should not feel underprivileged because, if all KRT modalities are sometimes not available, for sure PD as the most likely economical one, is always feasible to be used almost everywhere around the world.

ADEQUACY OF DIALYSIS ON MEXICO: ITS ORIGINS AND UNRESOLVED CONSEQUENCES

Chronic kidney disease (CKD) is a modern epidemic with a growing number of patients around the world; this continued growth is linked to the high incidence and prevalence rates of diabetes mellitus and hypertension. CKD is considered a challenge for health systems due to the large amount of resources that it demands human resources, infrastructure and financial funding [6-8].

Kidney transplantation is widely recognized as the most effective treatment for CKD, while the choice of dialysis modality, peritoneal dialysis (PD) or hemodialysis (HD), has been a subject of intense debate. Among the advantages of PD over HD are better quality of life, greater patient independence, and lower cost. Furthermore, when the patient's opinion intervenes in the selection of the treatment modality, PD is the most frequently chosen [9].

In spite of the above-mentioned advantages, for many years, HD was considered superior to PD because it had better technique survival rates. The PD technique failure is mainly due to peritonitis, which is the most frequent reason of patient transfer from PD to HD [10]. Currently, peritonitis rates have been significantly reduced thanks to the improvement in the disconnection systems and better patient training in therapy management and prevention of complications [11-13].

An important argument to support the preferential use of HD over PD has been the longer patient survival rates. In different earlier analyses, it was found that the HD advantage laid mainly on diabetic women over 65 years of age and in patients with significant comorbidities such as diabetes and heart failure [14]. The most recent cohort analyses have shown that survival rates are similar or even better in PD than in HD, at least in the first five years of treatment [15, 16].

Dialysis Environment before ADEMEX

Towards the middle of the 1990s, PD was intensely questioned, considering that the adequacy of dialysis was insufficient, if evaluated by the removal of small molecules such as urea and creatinine. In HD, urea removal measured by Kt/V could be substantially increased with the use of dialyzers with higher permeability, longer sessions, as well as with more frequent sessions per week. Fluid removal could also be increased according to the patient's requirements [17, 18].

An important argument was that PD had natural limits preventing a substantial increase in Kt/V. Continuous ambulatory peritoneal dialysis (CAPD) is time-limited to 24 hours, the volume of fluid infused is limited by the capacity of the peritoneal cavity and the patient size, whereas more than 5 exchanges per day limit the autonomy and quality of life of the patient [19]. Furthermore, the availability and use of PD solutions with high glucose concentrations to increase ultrafiltration made the metabolic management of the diabetic patient difficult, compromising the maintenance of fluid balance.

In 1996, the CANUSA (Canada-USA) study publication deepened doubts about the limits of the efficient removal of small molecules with CAPD by showing that the increase of 0.1 units of total Kt/V urea (peritoneal + renal) per week was associated with a 5% reduction in the risk of death, whereas an increase of 5 L/1.73m^2/week (peritoneal + renal) in creatinine clearance was associated with a 7% reduction in the risk of death. The study assumed equivalence between the Kt/V derived from the kidneys and that obtained by PD. These concepts justified that patients who did not reach a certain limit value of Kt/V, were transferred to HD with or without clinical evidence of insufficient dialysis. In clinical practice, this discouraged the use of PD and HD became the best option for dialysis modality [20].

The CANUSA conclusions were in contrast to non-interventional studies published only a few years later, in which renal Kt/V or residual renal function (RRF) were found to be associated with mortality, but not peritoneal Kt/V or peritoneal creatinine clearance [21- 23]. In a re-analysis of the CANUSA data published in 2001, urea and creatinine clearances were separated in their peritoneal and renal components; in this new approach, it was found that for every 5 L/wk/1.73 m^2 increase in glomerular filtration rate, the relative risk of death was reduced by 12%, but no association with peritoneal creatinine clearance was observed [24].

ADEMEX, the Study and Perception of the PD Community

ADEMEX enrolled 965 CAPD patients from 24 dialysis centers belonging to three different institutions in Mexico (Instituto Mexicano del Seguro Social, Instituto de Seguridad y Servicios Sociales pa los Trabajadores del Estado, y el Instituto de Ciencias Médicas y Nutrición Salvador Zubirán) between June 1998 and May 1999, and was terminated in 2001 when the last enrolled patient had completed two years follow-up and it was published in 2002 [25]. Four hundred eighty-four patients received CAPD in standard doses of 4x2 L daily and 481 patients received an optimized prescription to achieve a creatinine clearance ≥60L/wk/1.73 m^2 by increasing the volume of dialysis fluid from 2.0 to 3.0 L/Exchange, and/or the number of exchanges/day from 4 to 5; changes were made according to the dimensions and tolerance of the patients. The results showed that renal urea and creatinine clearance were associated with mortality, but peritoneal clearances in the ranges analyzed had no effect.

The study was first presented at the International Society for Peritoneal Dialysis Congress in Montreal in 2001; it has been extensively discussed and commented since then. At the time of its publication in 2002, in an editorial in the same issue, the excessive attention that was put on the study since its presentation, including the notes of the international press, were commented [26]. The editorial calls for taking the results objectively, without precipitating changes in the dialysis prescription, considered some reasonable doubts about the internal and external validity of the study, as **a**) incident and prevalent patients were included; **b**) the assessment of the type of peritoneal transport was performed with the dialysis adequacy and transport test (DATT) and not with traditional Peritoneal Equilibrium Test (PET); **c**) probably high transporters were underrepresented; and **d**) the causes of mortality were not exactly the same. Emphasis was placed on the smaller size and age of the Mexican patients compared to studies in other populations and on the exclusion of patients with manifestations of heart failure. Despite the doubts, the congruence with the results of the CANUSA re-analysis [24] and of previous non-interventional studies [21-23] was also pointed out. Other editorials highlighted the value of ADEMEX as an RCT and its strength as evidence [27].

In the same year, the first data from the Hemodialysis (HEMO) study [28], an RCT with 1846 patients where Kt/V urea values of 1.71 were compared with the standard Kt/V urea of 1.32, were published; no survival differences were observed. The two studies, ADEMEX and HEMO, were interpreted as evidence that urea and creatinine clearances are not reliable indexes for dialysis adequacy.

After these studies, the clearance of low molecular weight (MW) solutes (< 500 Da) became more seriously questioned as a parameter to evaluate dialysis prescription. In several publications, it has been suggested to evaluate the adequacy of dialysis by the removal of middle molecules (MW between 1000 and 50000 Da), and not small ones. However, when the concentration of some of these molecules was analyzed in patient samples in the HEMO study, no differences were found between the groups in all the analyzed molecules, suggesting that the Kt/V does not reflect the total concentration of these toxins (free fraction + protein-bound fraction) in patients treated with standard or high-flux HD. Moreover, it has not been shown that clearances of these molecules were related to survival [29].

Looking for New Adequacy Indexes

ADEMEX and HEMO are two large RCTs that have questioned how to prescribe the dialysis dose. However, their results do not promote overconfidence that the adequate dose of dialysis measured by Kt/V does not matter; they only indicate that there is no obvious advantage to obsessively increase the removal of low MW molecules. Indeed, the two studies have challenged the concept of adequacy and have prompted the search not for an isolated indicator, but for improving other aspects of patient care that are likely to improve clinical outcomes, particularly with regard to cardiovascular diseases [30-32].

Several opinion leaders have proposed a broad assessment of dialysis adequacy, based on the effect of some biochemical variables that are related to the survival of CKD patients [33]. Among these variables is the calcium and phosphorus metabolism. The association of hyperphosphatemia with comorbidity and cardiovascular mortality has been widely recognized, as well as improvement in survival with better control of phosphorus levels [34,35]. The prevention and treatment of secondary hyperparathyroidism also has considerable benefits in survival and cardiovascular risk [36].

Anemia is one of the earliest manifestations of CKD. Hemoglobin and hematocrit levels are non-linearly associated with mortality, hemoglobin levels between 12 and 13 g/dL appear to be optimal levels. Hemoglobin levels lower and higher than 12-13 g/dl ranges present higher mortality risks [37, 38]. In PD patients, as in HD, in addition to the use of erythropoietin, iron intake is an essential factor, without forgetting that chronic inflammation has a very important influence on the bioavailability of iron [39].

Malnutrition and especially the presence of malnutrition-inflammation-atherosclerosis (MIA) syndrome are associated with greater susceptibility to infections, cardiovascular damage, and death [40-42]. An important manifestation of uremic syndrome is loss of appetite. This factor, in addition to the increased intake of calories through glucose-containing dialysis solutions, may reduce the intake of important nutrients [43]. The losses of proteins, minerals, and water-soluble vitamins in the dialysis fluid are added to the factors that lead to the deterioration of the nutritional status [44]. Many of these negative aspects are susceptible to intervention via the integral prescription of PD.

Is Fluid Control a Good Index of PD Adequacy?

Almost twenty years have passed since the ADEMEX results were presented and a numerical indicator has not yet been found to measure the dose of PD. Control of extracellular volume is among the most useful indicators to assess adequacy. In the secondary analysis of CANUSA, the reduction in urinary volume was found to be a risk factor for mortality [24]. In the ADEMEX study, fluid removal and brain natriuretic factor were predictors for all-cause mortality, including cardiovascular [25, 45]. Other non-interventional studies have shown that fluid and sodium removal, but not Kt/V, are risk factors for mortality [46].

The growing utilization of electrical bio-impedance, as a non-invasive method to estimate fluid overload in both HD and PD patients, has allowed us to recognize that over-hydration is a frequent finding among PD patients. In some studies, up to 70% of patients may have some degree of over hydration [47].

Expansion of the extracellular fluid volume is associated with a higher ventricular mass index, abnormal remodeling of the left ventricle, reduction in the ejection fraction and the shortening fraction, diastolic dysfunction and intima/media thickening of the carotid artery. Fluid overload is related to mortality, particularly mortality of cardiovascular origin, as well as to the failure of the technique in patients with CAPD [46, 48, 49].

Patients with over-hydration generally have hypertension and loss of the circadian rhythm. Tight control of sodium intake and ultrafiltration lowers blood pressure. However, it is important to note that in some studies, hypertension is more related to peripheral resistance than to over-hydration. A significant number of patients with extracellular volume expansion have also been described as having normal blood pressure [46, 50, 51].

Fluid removal should be closely monitored as several of the pathophysiological mechanisms involved in the control of fluid overload are susceptible to modification with the prescription of dialysis. In some studies, the reduction of residual kidney function has been found to be related to volume overload, although the finding is inconsistent [46, 51]. Insufficient ultrafiltration is one of the most important factors, and may in turn be related to high peritoneal transport, thereby resulting in rapid loss of the osmotic gradient [52].

Fluid overload and the high peritoneal transport types are directly related to the increase in inflammation biomarkers [53-55]. Fluid overload and inflammation may have several links; one of them involves the passage of bacteria or bacterial products from the intestinal lumen into the circulation. The permeability of the intestinal epithelium in patients and animals with CKD is increased, and the toxicity of the uremic serum may intervene in this phenomenon [56]. Interestingly, in edematous states such as heart failure, edema of the intestinal wall also increases permeability and also the concentration of bacterial toxins in the blood [57]. This same mechanism has been invoked to explain the presence of endotoxemia in dialysis patients with fluid overload [58, 59]. In a study with HD and PD patients, splanchnic perfusion was measured and correlation was found between magnetic resonance images, endotoxemia, hydration markers, and cardiac morphology [60].

Overhydration can be controlled by prescribing dialysis adequately. The use of automated peritoneal dialysis (APD) with short dwell times in the cavity prevents loss of the osmotic gradient and increases ultrafiltration, more specifically for high transporters. Increasing osmolality with high glucose concentration has the same effect [47]; however, the use of icodextrin solutions, for the long dwell either in CAPD or APD, is more effective and also metabolically-friendly for diabetic patients [61].

Design, Planning, Validity, and Broad Collaboration

ADEMEX surprised many by its design, sample size, and results, which aroused disbelief in some, yet great expectation in others for the future of dialysis adequacy. There was also some concern about its internal and external validity because it was carried out in a Mexican population with smaller body dimensions and a high prevalence of diabetics and malnutrition. It was also surprising that it emerged from a country that, although it had PD as the dominant dialysis modality (applied to 90% of the end-stage kidney disease (ESKD) patients) [62, 63], also had less scientific development than many other Western countries.

Despite these limitations, Mexico also had characteristics that made it easier to carry out an important RCT in ESKD. As a developing country, the availability of resources for health was limited. Moreover, there was a concern that it would not be able to reach the adequacy goals and, therefore, PD would be replaced by HD, a more expensive and less accessible modality due to its technological requirements, specialized personnel and facilities [17-19]. It is important to underline that the existence of the Mexican Institute of Social Security (IMSS), an institution that provides health and social security services to more than 70 million Mexicans, was a determinant support to the success of the study. IMSS has a national network of 1,522 primary care clinics and 256 general hospitals, most of them with PD programs and 36 tertiary hospitals [64].

Important in the planning of the ADEMEX study was the experience of a previous successful multicenter RCT, in which the advantages of the twin bag disconnection system were demonstrated to reduce the rate of peritonitis and associated costs [65]. For this study, ADEMEX and other subsequent RCTs [66], besides the facilities of the Institution's hospital network, there was the advantage of having the support of its academic network, with a significant amount of training programs for specialist doctors and nurses as well as clinical research and training programs for researchers, programs in closely collaboration with internationally recognized universities.

Large RCTs demand great effort from many people and organizations. In an editorial comment to one of the former Mexican PD publications [67], the author advises a broad collaboration of nephrologists with government, pharmaceutical industry, and medical equipment manufacturers in order to face CKD growing problem [68]. The ADEMEX team had a decisive support from Mexican Medical Institutions, as well as from Baxter Management, Scientific/Medical Affairs, and clinical researchers, all together made the study possible.

ADEMEX changed the concept of PD adequacy stimulating a broader clinical evaluation instead of just a numerical target; however, searching for such targets remains active. Fluid balance may perhaps emerge as a good parameter of dialysis prescription.

A Middle East Unique PD Experience

The Middle East countries have altogether a population of about 280 million and a mean gross national income per capita of US $9500. The total number of patients with ESKD in the Middle East is about 120,000. PD was first started in Turkey in 1968 and subsequently introduced in the Kingdom of Saudi Arabia (KSA) and Iran 1980 [69]. KSA has a total population of 32 million inhabitants according to the 2016 Census. KRT started in KSA from a single center in 1970 and it substantially expanded to more than 243 centers by 2020. Diabetes mellitus is responsible for the majority of the patients (41%), followed by hypertension (35%).

By the end of 2019, the total number of ESKD dialysis patients in KSA was 19,659, according to The Saudi Center for Organ Transplantation (SCOT); 18,270 of them being treated by HD, whereas 1900 by PD in 35 PD centers with 77% of them being on APD [70]. It means that PD comprised 9.66% of the total dialysis patients in 2019, with a slight increase from 1372 patients in 2016.

Although most of the nephrologists encourage and support the idea of PD first, PD is still underutilized [71]. The reasons for PD underutilization in KSA have been elegantly illustrated by Dahlan et al. [72]; including lack of pre-dialysis education programs, patients not receiving proper counseling from their nephrologists, lack of nephrologists who are experts in PD catheter insertion, later referral and expansion of outsourcing HD programs [72]. The majority of dialysis centers are supervised by the Ministry of Health (MoH) followed by governmental non-MoH hospitals, private and charitable hospitals [73].

The population of the Saudi Eastern Province, where the King Fahad University Hospital (KFUH) is located, amounts to 4,780,619 and the total number of patients on dialysis 2257; 350 of them on PD, which constitutes the highest penetration in the Kingdom (15.5%). The KFUH PD program started with 15 patients in 2004, having treated 1300 patients throughout the next 16 years.

Over 100 manuscripts from the KFUH PD program have been published at reputable national and international journals; moreover, two new, percutaneous and laparoscopic, techniques for PD catheter insertion have been proposed [74, 75]. A triple-cuff low-entry (Saudi) PD catheter was also developed, which has improved catheter survival rate, totally eliminated catheter migration and significantly decreased peritonitis rate [74].

Peritonitis is a common and serious complication of PD and infection rates should be monitored and reported for every clinical dialysis program annually, as per the International Society of Peritoneal Dialysis (ISPD) recommendation [76]. There are no convincing data regarding the effect of PD catheter design and configuration on peritonitis risk. Eight randomized trials have compared straight and coiled Tenckhoff PD catheters and found no difference in peritonitis rates [77-88]. Several retrospective studies suggested that double-cuff Tenckhoff catheters are associated with a lower peritonitis rate than single-cuffed ones. However, the only randomized trial on this topic showed no difference in peritonitis risk between the two catheter types [87, 88]. The double-cuff Tenckhoff PD catheter was used from the start of the KFUH PD program until 2013. Thereafter, it was replaced with the previously described three-cuff low-entry Saudi catheter [74].

An observational prospective KFUH PD program study with 1123 PD patients was performed over twelve years, comparing the triple cuff Saudi catheter with the conventional double-cuff Tenckhoff catheter. The study aimed at determining the magnitude of the infection problem, identifying possible risk factors for PD-associated peritonitis and comparing the outcomes with these two PD catheter types as well as identifying the causative pathogens. Bacterial peritonitis were recorded in 70.8% of the patients with the double-cuff Tenckhoff catheter and in 29.2% of those with the triple-cuff Saudi catheter ($p = 0.0001$). The most frequent isolated pathogen was gram-positive and peritonitis episodes secondary to gram-positive organisms carried a better prognosis. In 24.8% of the episodes, the patients had to be transferred to HD because of unresolved peritonitis. Peritonitis rates varied significantly between the two types of PD catheter used; 0.11/patient-year in the three-cuff PD low-entry

Saudi catheter and 0.16/patient-year for episodes with the double-cuff conventional Tenckhoff catheter (p = 0.001). This positive result was attributed to the presence of three cuffs, which probably function as a triple barrier against infection. In addition, the relatively short portion of the three-cuff PD catheter inside the peritoneal cavity may play a role in minimizing the rate of peritonitis. This study demonstrated catheter survival rates that exceeded ISPD recommendations [89]. Infectious and non-infectious complications, before and after using triple-cuff Saudi catheter, are depicted in Figure 1 (Infectious complications) and Figure 2 (Catheter Malfunction complications).

A prospective randomized controlled clinical trial of 125 critically-ill patients with AKI comparing tidal peritoneal dialysis (TPD) (n = 63) versus continuous venousvenous hemodiafiltration (CVVHDF) (n = 63) was also conducted. The survival at 28 days was significantly better (69.8% vs. 46.8%, $p < 0.01$) and infectious complications were significantly less ($p < 0.01$) in the TPD group patients (9.5% vs. 17.7) when compared to the CVVHDF group. Moreover, recovery of kidney function (60.3% vs. 35.5%), median time to resolution of AKI [5 days (4-6) vs. 8 days (7-10)] and median duration of ICU stay [9 days (7-11) vs. 19 days (13-20)] ($p < 0.01$) were also significantly better for the TPD group patients. This important study was used as one of the references for the 2020 ISPD (International Society for Peritoneal Dialysis) guidelines for AKI. In addition, the KFUH PD program has been honored by participating in the 2020 AKI ISPD guidelines [90, 91].

A prospective observational study on instant-start life-saving PD, with 23 end-stage vascular access failure (ESVAF) patients who presented acutely to the hospital, was also carried out. The definition of ESVAF is the inability to create vascular access in both upper and lower limbs due to venous stenosis or thrombosis as documented by computer tomography or angiography. Urgent two-cuff curled Tenckhoff PD catheters were inserted percutaneously within a few hours, by the nephrology team, using the KFUH PD program catheter insertion method [75]. The conclusion was that instant-start PD as a life-saving modality is a feasible and safe alternative to HD in patients with ESVAF [92].

Peritonitis caused by S. aureus and gram-negative bacteria are usually severe and often require patient hospitalization and PD catheter removal. A prospective study was carried out with 203 patients, comparing mupirocin and gentamicin cream nasal application regimens in preventing exit-site infection (ESI) and peritonitis, in a warm climate country as Saudi Arabia. The rate of gram-positive ESI was 0.31/episode/patient-year vs. 0.22 episode/patient-year ($p < 0.05$) in favor of gentamicin, whereas the rate of gram-negative ESI was 0.28 episode/patient-year vs. 0.11 episode/patient-year ($p < 0.01$) in the mupirocin and gentamicin groups, respectively. Gram-positive ESI occurred in 17.1% vs 10.2% ($p < 0.05$), whereas 20% of and 5.1% of the patients ($p < 0.001$) had gram-negative ESI in the in the mupirocin group and gentamicin groups, respectively. Peritonitis rates were lower using gentamicin cream (0.17 episode/patient-year compared with mupirocin, 0.39 episode/patient-year, $p < 0.01$). The conclusion of the study was that prolonged use of mupirocin for ESI-prophylaxis is associated with the emergence of mupirocin-resistant S. aureus. Gentamicin cream is superior to mupirocin ointment in the prevention of PD catheter infections [93].

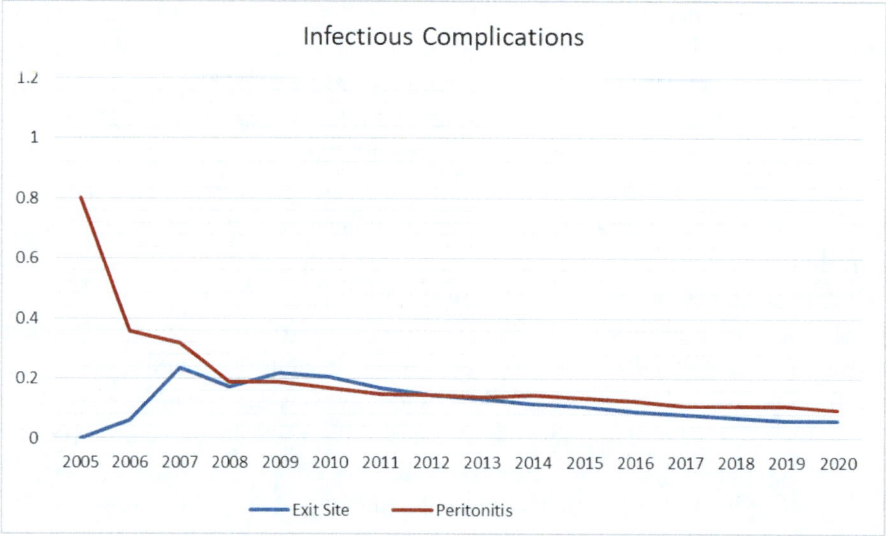

Figure 1. Infectious complications from year 2005 to 2020.

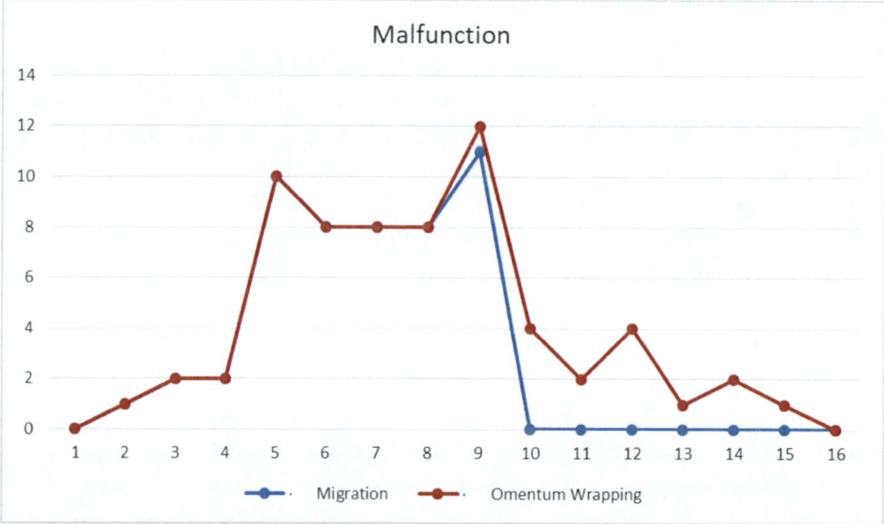

Figure 2. Catheter malfunction complications through 16 years.

Long-term peritoneal dialysis solution is considered the culprit for the pro-aggressive structural and functional alterations of the peritoneal membrane. The prominent findings in PD patients' peritoneal biopsies are mesothelial cell abnormalities, interstitial fibrosis, elastosis, and peritoneal membrane vasculopathy. The KFUH PD program published a randomized comparative trial in thirty-nine incident PD patients who were randomized into two groups: 19 patients with Dianeal® PD solution (Group A) and 20 patients with biocompatible Physioneal® PD solution (Group B). All patients used APD for a median period of 31 and 32 months, respectively.

The commonest change observed was peritoneal fibrosis, observed in 89.7% of the patients. The prevalence of vascular changes, moderate to severe fibrosis, as well as mesothelial cell abnormalities did not differ between the two solutions [94].

The 2016 ISPD Guidelines showed evidence favoring the use of prophylaxis antibiotics prior to colonoscopy. However, there has been little literature to support this recommendation. The KFUH PD program performed a prospective randomized study of 93 patients randomized into two age- and gender-matched groups; group A (46 patients) with intraperitoneal (IP) ceftazidime prior to colonoscopy and group B (47 patients) without prophylactic antibiotics. Post-colonoscopy peritonitis was documented in three (6.5%) and four (8.5%) patients of the groups A and B, respectively ($p > 0.05$). It was concluded that the relation between prophylactic antibiotic use prior to colonoscopy in APD patients and the risk of peritonitis does not stand. Only old age, diabetes mellitus, and low serum albumin appeared to be of significance [95].

Metformin use in ESRD patients has been prohibited for a long time. Little was known about the effect of PD on metformin clearance and the phantom of lactic acidosis, depriving ESRD patients from metformin therapeutic advantages. The KFUH PD program performed two studies with metformin in diabetic patients on APD. The first study involved 35 patients treated with Metformin at a daily oral dose in the range of 0.5 – 1.0 gram and followed up during one year [96]. This study demonstrated the feasibility of metformin use in APD, but it was not large enough to demonstrate safety. Therefore, a larger observational study with 83 type 2 diabetes mellitus APD patients [97] was executed. Metformin was administered in a daily dose of 500 mg. Patients were monitored for glycemic control, plasma lactate, and plasma metformin levels on a scheduled basis. The overall mean plasma lactate level across all blood samples was 1.44 + 0.6. Plasma lactate levels > 2 mmol/L and < 3 mmol/L were found in 11.8% and levels of 3.0-3.6 mmol/L in 2.4% of the samples. Hyperlactemia (level > 2 & < 5 mmol/L) was not associated with overt acidemia. None of the patients had lactic acidosis (levels > 5 mmol/L). Age > 60 was a predictor for hyperlactemia. No relationship between plasma metformin and lactate levels was found. We concluded that metformin may be used with caution in a particular group of ESRD patients who are on APD. Metformin allowed better diabetic control with significant reduction of BMI. PD appeared to be a safeguard against the development of lactic acidosis in this group of patients [97].

Another study involved APD patients with type-1 Cardiorenal syndrome (CRS). They were randomly assigned (n = 88) to a strategy of ultrafiltration (UF) therapy (n = 44) or tidal peritoneal dialysis (TPD) (n = 44). The primary end-point was the change from baseline serum creatinine level (Figure 3) and left ventricular function represented as ejection fraction (EF) (Figure 4), assessed 72 hours and 120 hours after random assignment. Patients were followed-up for 90 days after discharge from the hospital. We could demonstrate that TPD is a safe and effective means for removing toxins and large quantities of excess fluid from patients with intractable heart failure (HF). In patients with type 1 CRS, the use of TPD was superior to UF-therapy for the preservation of renal function, improvement of cardiac function and net fluid loss. UF-therapy was associated with a higher rate of adverse events [98].

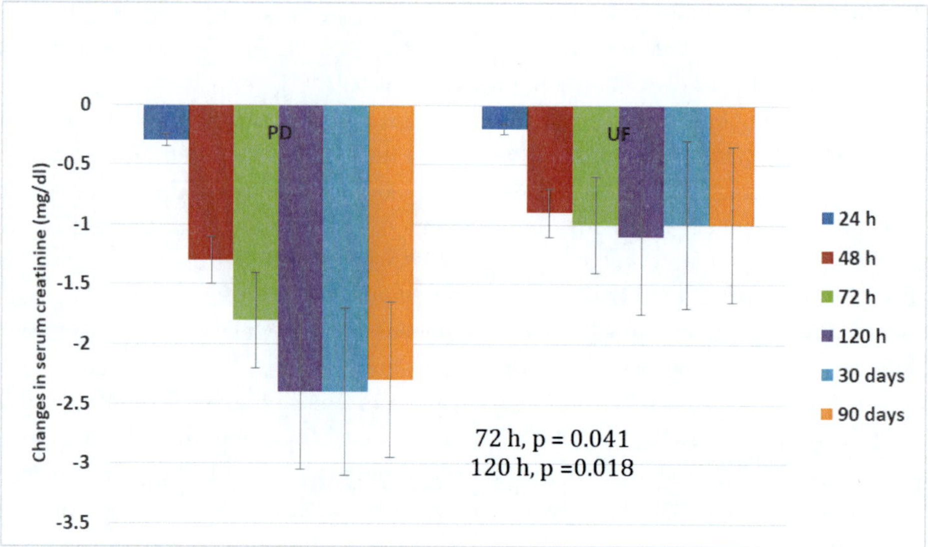

Figure 3. Mean changes in serum creatinine throughout the study period. PD = tidal peritoneal dialysis, UF = ultrafiltration, 30 days – 30 days after discharge, 90 days = 90 days after discharge. Error bars indicate 96% Cis.

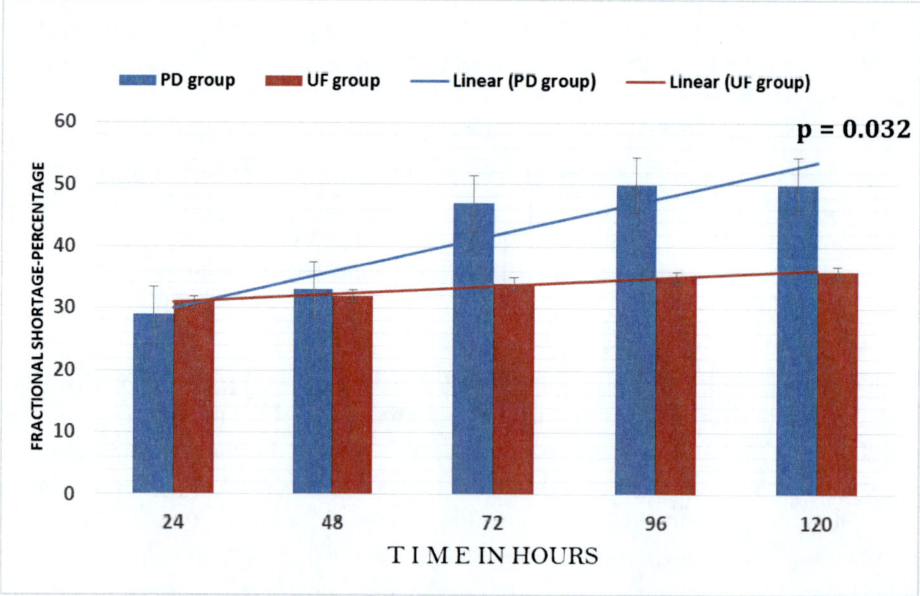

Figure 4. Left ventricular ejection fraction in relation to time in PD and UF groups. Error bars indicate 95% CIs. PD = tidal peritoneal dialysis, UF = ultrafiltration.

The Reborn of Peritoneal Dialysis in AKI

Decades ago, PD was widely accepted as treatment for AKI; however, its use declined in favor of HD. The interest in PD to treat AKI patients has been reignited and PD has been frequently used in developing countries due to its lower costs and minimal infrastructure requirements.

Technical Aspects and Controversies

The utilization of PD in AKI is facilitated by bedside placement of the Tenckhoff catheter, which can be safely performed by a nephrologist, radiologist, or surgeon. PD offers advantages over HD, such as lower risk of bleeding and technical simplicity.

The continuous and gradual characteristics of PD ensure prevention of disequilibrium syndrome, as well as significantly less cardiovascular stress, reducing the risk of kidney ischemia and fluid-electrolyte imbalance [99-106].

Besides the classical indication (uremic symptoms, fluid overload, acid-base disturbances or electrolyte disorders), PD can also be indicated to keep fluid balance in patients with congestive heart failure as well as to control hypo- and hyperthermia. In the setting of natural disasters and pandemia, when several victims might develop AKI and where damage to health care infrastructure makes access to power, clean water, and water treatment facilities unavailable, PD is an important and life-saving KRT modality [106-110].

It is also true that PD is not the most efficient therapy; for example, clearance per exchange may decrease if a shorter dwell time is applied; a lower efficiency may be observed in large-sized and severely hypercatabolic patients; fluid removal may be unpredictable; the risk of infection could also be a possibility; and possible issues with mechanical ventilation may also exist [103]. PD is relatively contra-indicated in patients with recent abdominal surgery, abdominal hernia, adynamic ileum, intra-abdominal adhesions, peritoneal fibrosis, or peritonitis. Table 1 shows PD advantages and disadvantages.

Since volume and solute removal are slow and unpredictable, PD may not be as efficient as HD techniques for the treatment of emergencies such as acute pulmonary edema or life-threatening hyperkalemia [108-114]. However, several studies have demonstrated PD as a life-saving therapy in many patients with hyperkalemia or acute pulmonary edema [115, 116]. Another possible limitation of PD in AKI is that associated protein losses may aggravate malnutrition. Protein losses as high as 48 g/day have been reported, but some reports document maintenance of serum albumin levels [116-120]. Protein supplementation, either enteral or parenteral (1.5 g/kg/day) is recommended for AKI patients treated by PD [121, 122].

The high glucose concentrations in peritoneal dialysate may cause hyperglycemia, even in non-diabetic patients. This is easily correctable through intravenous or intraperitoneal administration of insulin. Peritonitis occurring in patients with AKI using PD as a KRT modality can lead to poor outcomes, with older studies reporting a frequency as high as 40% [100,101,103]. With better catheter implantation techniques and automated methods, the incidence of peritonitis has been decreased and the risk of infection in PD is similar to extracorporeal blood purification for AKI [100, 101].

Table 1. Advantages and disadvantages of peritoneal dialysis (PD) in acute kidney injury (AKI)

Advantages	Disadvantages
Technically simple	It requires intact peritoneal cavity with adequate membrane function
No need for expensive equipment	It may not be adequate for severe edema or hyperkalemia
No vascular access needed	Peritonitis
Minimum blood loss	Ultrafiltration and clearance cannot be exactly predicted
Biocompatible	Protein losses
Useful in all types of AKI	It can cause hyperglycaemia and hypernatraemia
More rapid renal recovery	It may impair respiratory mechanics
It provides continuous renal replacement therapy and cardiovascular stability	Lactate buffer
Beneficial in selected patients population (children, heart failure, cirrhosis, bleeding diathesis)	

Previous studies have reported that PD can increase intra-abdominal pressure (IAP), leading to impaired diaphragm mobilization, as well as reduced pulmonary compliance and ventilation, which may cause or worsen respiratory failure [121, 122]. However, PD is seldom the cause of ventilation impairment in patients without pulmonary disease. Results from our group suggest increase in the pulmonary compliance without changes in IAP in AKI patients on PD [123].

Evidence and Guidelines

Interest in PD use to manage patients with AKI has recently been increasing. The first question that must be asked is whether PD can provide adequate metabolic control in AKI patients treated by PD. The Botucatu group has demonstrated that, with careful thought and planning, critically ill AKI patients can be successfully treated with PD [100, 107, 124-128]. To overcome some classic limitations of PD use in AKI (such as a low rate of ultrafiltration [UF], high risk of infectious and mechanical complications, and no metabolic control), the use of flexible catheters, cyclers, continuous therapy (24 hours), and high volumes (HV) of dialysis fluid has been proposed.

The efficacy of High Volume Peritoneal Dialysis (HVPD) was accessed in two prospective studies of 30 and 204 consecutive AKI patients, respectively [108,126]. PD was performed using a Tenckhoff catheter, 2 L exchanges, and 35–50 minutes dwell times. The prescribed Kt/V value was 0.6 per session, the duration of each session was 24 hours, and a total dialysate volume of 36–44 L/day was used. HVPD was effective in the correction of blood urea nitrogen (BUN), creatinine, bicarbonate, and fluid overload. Weekly Kt/V was around 3.5 and the mortality 57%. Older age and sepsis were identified as risk factors for death, while higher UF after three sessions were identified as favorable prognostic factors. It was concluded that HVPD is effective in selected patients. There were mechanical complications in 7.3% of AKI patients treated with HVPD and 12% of patients had infectious complications (peritonitis). Change of dialysis modality occurred in 13.3% of patients because of refractory peritonitis or mechanical complications (leakage or UF failure).

Dialysis dose adequacy in AKI is a controversial subject; there is very limited data on the effect of PD dose on AKI. Solute clearance in PD is limited by dialysate flow, membrane permeability, and surface area in contact with dialysate. Exchanges of 2 L lasting approximately one hour can achieve a saturation of the spent dialysate in the range of 50%. This means that, over 24 hours, a daily Kt/V of 0.5 can be achieved in a patient with a body weight between 60–65 kg [100, 106-108].

A trial with 61 septic AKI patients randomized to receive higher (n = 31) or lower (n = 30) intensity PD therapy (prescribed Kt/V of 0.8/session versus 0.5/session) was performed. The two groups had similar mortality after 30 days (55% versus 53%, p = 0.83). It was concluded that increasing the intensity of continuous HVPD therapy does not reduce mortality and does not improve control of urea, potassium, and bicarbonate levels [127].

According to the ISPD guidelines: PD for AKI recommendations, where resources permit, targeting a weekly Kt/V urea of 3.5 provides outcomes comparable to that of daily HD; targeting higher doses does not improve outcomes. This dose may not be necessary for many AKI patients and targeting a weekly Kt/V of 2.1 may be acceptable [128].

Following the previous guidelines on PD for AKI, Parapiboon et al. randomized 80 critically ill patients with AKI to two regimens recommended in the ISPD guidelines, aimed at achieving target weekly Kt/V of 3.5 and 2.1, respectively [129]. Patients were randomized to receive 1.5 L of PD fluid using manual PD and a single-bag open system delivered either hourly (36 L/24 hours) or every 2 hours (18 L/24 h) for the first 48 hours. Baseline characteristics were not significantly different between the 2 groups. However, it must be noted that the mean body weight was low (60.1kg ± 11.1) compared with that seen in other countries, and the dwell volumes were consequently low. The patients were similar to those in the study by Ponce-Gabriel et al. [130,131], with 88% on mechanical ventilation, 69% on inotropic support, and a mean APACHE II score of 26.1,2. Pre-dialysis BUN values were lower than those seen in the Brazilian studies (~75 mg/dl) and therefore may represent earlier initiation of dialysis.

The achieved Kt/V was 2.26 in the low intensity group and 3.3 in the high-intensity group. There was no significant difference in metabolic control although UF was higher in the high-intensity group. The mortality was 72% in the high-intensity and 63% in the low-intensity groups (p = 0.18), suggesting no advantage to the higher-intensity treatment. These results suggest there is unlikely to be any advantage in achieving a weekly Kt/V > 2.2.

The second question to consider is whether PD is comparable to other dialysis methods in AKI patients. Phu et al. [113] compared intermittent PD with continuous KRT, and demonstrated a worse outcome in patients treated with PD. Such reports should not be underestimated, although specific factors (such as the use of rigid catheters, acetate as buffer, manual exchanges, a too-short dwell time; i.e., 15 minutes, and no dialysis dose quantification) need to be seriously taken into consideration.

A randomized study performed by the Botucatu group with 120 AKI patients, compared HVPD versus daily intermittent HD [124]. Baseline characteristics were similar in both groups, which included older patients (mean age > 60 years), with high APACHE II scores, and patients using vasoactive drugs (> 60%). Both KRT modalities achieved metabolic and acid-base control. Mortality did not differ significantly between the two groups (58% versus 53%) either. Renal recovery was similar for both modalities, but HVPD was associated with a significantly shorter time to recovery (7.2 ± 2.6 versus 10.6 ± 4.7 days).

Table 2. Dialysis protocol technique, prescription, adequacy parameters, adverse events and outcome in different and recent studies on peritoneal dialysis (PD) in Acute Kidney Injury (AKI)

Study	Time period	Patients	PD prescription	Weeky Kt/V	UF (l/session)	Adverse events	Outcome
Ponce-Gabriel et al. [108] prospective study	2007	N = 30 59 ± 8 years 60% septic	Flexible cateter 36-44 l HVPD	3.8 ± 0.6	1.8 ± 0.6	17% Infectious: 17% Mechanical:7%	Mortality = 57% Not recovery of kidney function = 13%
Ponce-Gabriel et al. [125] randomized trial PD x dHD	2008	N = 120 64 ± 20 vs 62 ± 21 42 vs 47% septic	Flexible cateter 36-44 l HVPD	3.6 ± 0.6 vs. 5.8 ± 1.9 p < 0.01	2.1 ± 0.7 vs. 2.4 ± 0.7 p = 0.39	23 vs 24% p = 0.21 infectious:18vs13% mechanical:5vs13% p > 0.05	Mortality = 58 vs. 53% (p = 0.7[illegible]) Not recovery of kidney function = 17% vs. 23% (p = 0.61)
George et al. [132] randomized trial CVVHF vs. CPD	2011	N = 50 45 ± 17 vs 44 ± 16 48 vs 28% septic p > 0.05	Flexible cateter 24-48 l CPD	NR	2.9 ± 2.4 vs. 2.8 ± 4.1 p > 0.05	24 vs 12% p > 0.05 infectious: NR mechanical:24 vs.8% p > 0.05	Mortality = 84 vs. 72% (p = 0.71) Not recovery of kidney function = NR
Ponce et al. [126] Prospective study	2012	N = 150 64 ± 16 years 55% septic	Flexible cateter 36-44 l HVPD	3.6 ± 0.6	1.2 ± 0.7	18% infectious:12% mechanical:7.3%	Mortality = 57.3% Not recovery of kidney function = 6.6%
Ponce et al. [131] randomized trial PD x dHD	2013	N = 143 57 ± 21 vs 68 ± 24 p > 0.05 45 vs 51% septic p > 0.05	Flexible cateter 36-44 l HVPD	5.8 ± 1.6 vs. 3.6 ± 0.4 p < 0.01	2.5 ± 0.7 vs. 1.4 ± 0.7 p = 0.039	23 vs 24% p = 0.21 infectious:19vs16%echanical:15vs13% p > 0.05	Mortality = 63.3 vs. 63.9% (p = 0.91) Not recovery of kidney function = 9.6% vs.6.5% (p = 0.67)
Parapiboon et al. [129] randomized trial HVPD vs low volume PD	2017	N = 75 59 ± 21 vs 60 ± 24 p > 0.05 65 vs 61% septic p > 0.05	Flexible cateter 18-36 l HVPD	3.3 ± 0.6 vs. 2.2 ± 0.4 p < 0.05	2.5 ± 0.7 vs. 2.6 ± 0.4 p = 0.39	15 vs 8% p = 0.21 infectious:15vs 8% p > 0.05 mechanical: NR	Mortality = 72 vs. 63.9% (p = 0.81) Not recovery of kidney function = NR
Al-Hwiesh et al. [90] randomized trial CVVHDF vs TPD	2018	N = 120 44 ± 12 vs 45 ± 44 p > 0.05 60.3 vs 35.5% septic p > 0.05	Flexible cateter 25 l TPD	NR	1.9 ± 0.7 vs. 1.4 ± 0.4 p = 0.39	17 vs 9% p = 0.21 infectious:17vs 9% p < 0.05 mechanical: NR	Mortality = 69.8 vs. 46.8% (p = 0.04) Not recovery of kidney function = 60.3 vs 35.5% (p = 0.03)

NC: not calculated; NR: not reported; CPD: continuous peritoneal dialysis, HVPD: high volume PD, TPD: tidal PD; dHD: daily hemodialysis, CVVHDF: continuous venovenous hemodiafiltration; PHD: prol.

George et al. [132] performed a randomized study comparing continuous venovenous hemodialysis (CVVHD) and peritoneal dialysis (PD) in critically ill patients. No difference was observed in regard to correction of metabolic parameters and fluid overload. Urea and creatinine clearances were higher and fluid correction faster with CVVHDF. The mortality rates in both groups were similar. Unfortunately, the procedures were performed at different technological levels to the detriment of PD, in which rigid catheters, locally available PD fluids, and manual exchanges were used. The PD procedures utilized in George et al. study were very similar to the ones applied by Phu et al. [113].

In another prospective study, the effect of high volume peritoneal dialysis (HVPD) against extended daily hemodialysis (EHD) was compared on AKI patients' outcome [131]. The EHD and HVPD groups were similar in gender, severity, and etiology of AKI. There was a trend toward significant statistical difference regarding the presence of sepsis (62.3% in EHD group versus 44.9% in HVPD group, $p = 0.054$). Delivered Kt/V and UF were higher in the EHD group and there was no difference between the two groups in mortality and recovery of kidney function, or need for chronic dialysis.

In the most recent trial [90], Al-Hwiesh et al. compared 120 AKI patients randomized to treatment with TPD or CVVHDF. It is important to note that high volume TPD (25 liters per session) and a more biocompatible PD solution were used in this study. The survival at 28 days was significantly better in patients treated with TPD when compared to CVVHDF (69.8% vs. 46.8%, $p < 0.01$). Recovery of kidney function was also in favor of TPD (60.3% vs. 35.5%, $p < 0.01$). Table 2 shows the randomized controlled studies comparing PD vs. extracorporeal therapies and with high vs. low PD dose.

The largest cohort study providing patient characteristics, clinical practice, patterns, and their relationship to outcomes in a developing country has been published [133]. Its objective was to describe the main determinants of patient and technique survival, including trends over time of PD treatment in AKI patients. A total of 301 patients were included, 16.9% were transferred to HD during the study period. The main cause of technique failure (TF) was mechanical complication (47%) followed by peritonitis (41.2%). There was a change in TF during the study period; patients treated during 2009–2014 had a relative risk (RR) reduction of 0.86 (95% CI, 0.77–0.96) compared with patients treated between 2004 and 2008, and three independent mortality risk factors were identified: period of treatment (2009 and 2014), sepsis, and age > 65 years.

Very recently, all clinical experiences and studies on worldwide Nephrology practice, especially in countries in development, have supported the use of PD in COVID-19-related AKI, and APD is the preferred form to minimize the risk of exposure. Wherever APD is not available, CAPD could be used.

Peritoneal Dialysis in Indigenous Australians: A Personal View

Introduction

Australia has the landmass of the USA, but just 25 million inhabitants. Most live close to the coast, where resources and access to water are available. Demographically, Australia is very multi-cultural, predominantly Caucasian, and only 3.3% identify as Aboriginal (indigenous). Many of the Aboriginal Australians have integrated in coastal communities (300,000), but a significant number maintained their rural/remote live style in communities spread over the country; 350,000 in outer regional areas, 150,000 in often very difficult to access remote places, hundreds of kilometres from the next village. It is an indictment on post-colonization Australian history that indigenous people lived in this country for 50,000 years, before European violently settled, yet they were only recognized as Australian citizens and included in the census in 1967 [134]. Remote living aboriginals have the lowest socio-economic status and there is widespread poverty, childhood neglect and abuse, alcoholism, malnutrition and developmental disadvantage. Translated to renal disease, deprivation is correlated to glomerulomegaly, high incidence of diabetes and focal segmental glomerulosclerosis (FSGS) amongst others [135-138]. Statistically, this leads to an 8-32 fold incidence of renal replacement-dependent renal disease with excessive mortality rates at a young age [137]. The average life expectancy for remote aboriginals is 65.9 years for males and 69.6 years for females. This is on average 15-22 years less than for non-aboriginal people [134, 140]. These figures are even worse for renal patients.

This chapter will address the 'gap' between aboriginal and non -aboriginal health and the author will present personal experiences. Many past governments have tried to solve the problem by ever extending funding, which does not seem to have made a difference. Critical thinking about the future, from aboriginal as well as from non-aboriginal side is required.

Incidence and Prevalence of Renal Disease in Indigenous People

The median age of aboriginal people at diagnosis of ESKD is 30 years younger than a comparable group of non-aboriginal Australians [137], and the incidence of renal replacement therapy shows an 8-32 fold rate (400 patients per million in the city, with an extreme 1600 ppm in remote areas) compared to non-aboriginal Australians [138]. The real rate of dialysis dependency would be even higher as, for many reasons, indigenous patients do not reach dialysis treatment. These hurdles will be discussed below. Their transplant rates are also significantly lower than that of other Australians. Despite their extreme incidence and prevalence of dialysis, aboriginal patients contribute only 3% of total patients transplanted in 2016 [139].

Barriers to Peritoneal Dialysis in Indigenous Patients Globally

Indigenous patients in other countries have shown to have barriers regarding the use of PD [140[. This study had a prospective, observational cohort design in 3 remote areas in Canada. They found that indigenous patients started PD around 11 years earlier than non-indigenous patients. The two most significant barriers, as self-reported by indigenous patients, were lack of money and anxiety. The first barrier may seem unlikely in a country that, like Australia, has a universal health care program with no costs to any patient on any form of dialysis. However, inequality remains widespread in any western society. In a study by Mathew et al. [140], one of 67 participating non-indigenous patients died before initiation of dialysis against 5 of 32 indigenous patients. This could be an indication of a protracted decision process and resistance to start dialysis timely. Indeed, ANDATA statistics show that indigenous patients start KRT at a lower eGFR that non-Indigenous (7 ml/min vs. 11 ml/min), and many indigenous patients make a 'crash start,' being flown in by medivac and started on HD by Central Venous Catheters [139].

Prakash [142] reported in 2011 that when analyzing peritoneal dialysis in indigenous patients, mortality, technique failure, and peritonitis rates were significantly higher among indigenous patients and emphasized the importance of remoteness. These findings were later confirmed in an Australian study [138]. Also, dialysis treatment in remote areas is very expensive.

The Situation Specific to the Kimberley

Western Australia is the largest state of the country, slightly bigger than all of the European Union (EU). The capital is the 2 million inhabitant city of Perth with a well-developed infrastructure and 3 large tertiary hospitals. The author visits on a 6-8 weekly basis The Kimberley, a vast area in the North-west of Australia, with 50'000 inhabitants, 47% of them aboriginal. Only 3 towns have more than 2000 people. The Kimberley is partly coastal, partial desert, where aboriginal culture in small communities has been largely maintained with rituals and life style. Visits are made to 4 main towns that have haemodialysis centres and flights are taken in small planes to visit more remote communities to see patients. 4 months per year these communities are not accessible because of monsoon rain and disappearing sand-landing strips. Access by four-wheel drive is also not possible.

Aboriginals in The Kimberley accept western medicine, but only to a limited extent. Bush medicine (which comprises traditional medicines used by indigenous Australians) and healing play an eminent role. Presentation to renal clinics are usually very late, non-attendance rate in clinics over 45%, and urgent air evacuation to the closest tertiary hospital (Perth) is over 2000 km away. Haemodialysis units have been established in the towns of Broome, Derby, and Kununurra with each 10-14 dialysis chairs. Recently, Fitzroy Crossing (non-coastal) was added with 4 dialysis spots. The demand is much higher, causing aboriginal patients having to start in Perth, in an environment strange and perceived as hostile to them, with waiting times up to 18 months before they can return to 'country,' as they call their origin. There is a very strong connection in aboriginal culture to place of origin (land) and ancestors who lived there. This causes suffering, depression, non-compliance, alcohol abuse, and suicide in those forced to live away from home.

All forms of dialysis in Western Australia are outsourced to a private dialysis service provider, who is responsible for dialyzing all patients in Perth (5 large satellites, hospitals only having small units for inpatients and very sick dialysis patients), but also for the provision of home-based services in The Kimberley.

Since around a decade, there has been a strong push to use more home-based treatments, to make an early return to country possible, and also to allow for more autonomy. For countless reasons, the many projects that were launched have failed. These will be discussed under 'Barriers to Peritoneal Dialysis in The Kimberley.'

Increasing the numbers of indigenous people on home- based treatments, in particular peritoneal dialysis is a well-known challenge. Grace et al. [143] performed an Australian study, linking remoteness to the uptake of peritoneal dialysis, and found that rural and remote patients had a significantly lower uptake of peritoneal dialysis and postulated that they are more willing to relocate to places where haemodialysis is available. Their study, however, did not specifically address aboriginal patients as a subgroup. Marley et al. [144] analyzed the peritoneal dialysis outcomes of aboriginal Australians in The Kimberley (71 between 2003 and 2009) with other Australian aboriginals in the same time period (384) and non-aboriginals (5285). The median age at the start of PD was 10 years younger in aboriginals in general. They found a significantly shorter median time to first peritonitis, higher technique failure, and shorter median survival, despite the young age at which they started PD. They had double the number of peritonitis episodes, a real challenge in very remote areas. They concluded that the expansion of safer Kimberley HD options needed to continue. This conclusion may be the opposite of the international consensus amongst nephrologists and policy makers.

Barriers to Peritoneal Dialysis in the Kimberley

The author visits the main hubs and remote communities every 6-8 weeks for a full week to see dialysis patients and transplanted patients and review earlier CKD stages. There are many barriers to expand a PD program, but there has not been a comprehensive review apart from Marley et al. [144].

One of the authors (Johan Rosman) has his personal views and will introduce them below:

Accommodation

Aboriginal people often have no form of income, apart from social support. They often live in old, moldy and poor maintained social housing. The culture demands that the door is always open to anyone of the extended family. This may mean that at a given moment two people live in a two-bedroom house, and a few weeks later 15 in the same house. There is often no place for storage and PD bags can sometimes be found outside of the house in 40 degrees Celsius. Alcohol use and domestic violence are regretfully frequent and understandably, this is not the environment that is conducive for the hygiene dependent peritoneal dialysis. Infectious diseases, like sexually transmitted diseases (STD), Methicillin-resistant Staphylococcus infection (MRSA), and vancomycin-resistant enterococci (VRE) skin infections and leprosy are common. The complication rate and mortality, impacted by hesitations to see a doctor, and deliberate non-compliance, are high.

Culture

Aboriginal culture is one of mobility, largely by foot. Although the primary residence may be in a small community, many aboriginals adhere to the customs of 'going bush,' where they spend a significant time (weeks/months) away from home in the wilderness and exercise their important culture need for maintaining close contact to country. However, this is not compatible with PD, and also not to haemodialysis, leading to remote death, increased all-cause mortality, and urgent evacuations if help is available. There can also be a mistrust of western medicine, as patients in The Kimberley have seen relatives move to Perth to initiate dialysis and never saw them return. This is even stronger an argument against PD, as the high peritonitis rates with high mortality creates resistance against this method. As a person who offers help, such as a doctor, it can take years to be accepted in the aboriginal community and still be unable to achieve the compliance levels needed to provide adequate renal care. This is a challenge as few doctors are willing to live in The Kimberley, and hence the population is dependent on a constant flow of locums, often only staying for a few weeks.

Provider

In Western Australia, HD and PD are not provided by hospital, which have only very small HD units, meant for inpatients and very sick patients. The regular hemo-satellite and PD program is outsourced to a major global KRT player. This means that costs play an even more prominent role than in the public service and there is, for example, no PD nurse available anywhere in The Kimberley. The closest nurse is also in Perth, which is over 2000 km away. There is also no competition, as the State tendered the contract for HD as well as PD for thousands of patients to just the one provider.

In The Kimberley, the over-arching governance for aboriginal care lies with an aboriginal organization, the Kimberley Aboriginal Medical Services (KAMS) and all care provided is free, from primary to secondary care, medication and transport to and from clinics. Although KAMS as an extra bureaucratic layer adds to the complexity, it helps preserve the unique aboriginal attitude in our care.

Being Removed from Country

To receive a PD catheter, and later the PD training, patients will have to travel to Perth, as no hospital in The Kimberley implants PD catheters. The large city is intimidating for them, and has an average temperature about 10-15 degrees lower than that in The Kimberley, which is not acceptable for many aboriginal patients. They are deprived from their closest loved ones and away from country, as no family members are allowed to be in temporary housing in Perth with them. The situation is actually worse in HD, as the four units in The Kimberley cannot cope with demand and all patients need to start their dialysis in Perth. The waiting time to return home can be 12-18 months. This is a very bad scenario; alcohol problems, as well as depression and loneliness are very common in the city. Mothers do not see their young children for over a year. One would expect that this would be an incentive to choose PD, but interestingly, other factors prevail. Projects have failed to increase the number of patients on PD, mainly for reasons as outlined above. In 2011, the WA Government issued a 'Framework to improve home dialysis therapy in Western Australia.' After thorough analysis, it came to six key clinical recommendations. One of them was to have a nephrologist, who lives permanently in The Kimberley. Apart from lack of funding, it has not been possible to retain a nephrologist and the prospect of ever changing locum nephrologists is likely to make the situation worse. The other recommendations were in place already e.,g., 'adhere to evidence based guidelines'; and they could not contribute, as the decisive impediments to expansion, in particular overcrowded housing and cultural incompatibility with dialysis treatment, remain largely unsolved because of lack of compromise on aboriginal and non-aboriginal sides to change.

As of August 2020, The Kimberley has only 17 patients on PD, against 138 aboriginal patients on HD. This occurs despite 15 years of expensive quality improvement projects and the hard work of many who visit the country or travel to and from renal clinics in a professional capacity, which might include free healthcare, such as cost-free medication and transport.

The Future

It is not easy to foresee a rosy future for PD therapy in aboriginal communities. Since in The Kimberley, aboriginal people adhere strictly to their historic culture and belief systems. There is an ongoing 'clash of cultures,' leading to non -compliance with clinic visits, medication, and the will to start KRT. The incentive of being back in the country earlier in case of PD is failing because of extreme peritonitis rates with higher than usual mortality. The Australian government has, through the years, tried to solve the issue by investing more and more money, and by attracting more aboriginal people as liaison persons in the hospital workforce. But apart from first class dialysis satellite units being built in Australia's poorest environments, the outcome has not changed [145]. A summary of some ideas is listed below:

1. Adjustment of culture on both sides. An increasing number of especially younger aboriginal people, realize that to achieve success, a closer relation with western and aboriginal culture is required. There is an increased number of aboriginals in the workforce in hospitals, and elders have stepped up to warn youth about unhealthy eating, exercise, and many form of diabetes prevention. A leveling off of the incidence of renal disease in aboriginals has become apparent [139], although it is too early to cheer. From a governmental view, it is time to realize that housing/accommodation is the main issue. This is true for becoming sick, having a larger number of infections, and even AKI at a young age, related to CKD later in life, because of the housing situation. Investing money in housing will do more good than handing out cash payments that may be spent on alcohol. In one of the communities where we visit, a renal hotel is built, where aboriginal people can live, do their PD or HD and share their stories.
2. Reduce Anxiety amongst Aboriginal People. It is often underestimated that a large part of non-compliance, failure to attend clinic, and failed promises to comply with advice, are all actually driven by fear. For many aboriginal patients in The Kimberley, the doctors and nurses are highly regarded people in a place of authority, who intimidate. Breaking down this wall has been successfully attempted in the communites. Renal education, whether for CKD or dialysis, is always given with the appropriate tribal liaison person present and special tools are utliized, that are mainly of a visual nature, like drawings and pictures are used instead of text and DVDs.
3. Start with the children. A thorough school teaching program should be developed where health is a very important part of the curriculum. This may reduce the number of infections at a young age, rheumatic heart disease, and also diabetes. The children will bring these messages home, in the hope of achieving 'reverse teaching' of the parents.
4. Acknowledgement of the 'culture clash.' As long as neither side is willing to accept that aboriginal- and non-aboriginal cultures are inherently different, no progress will

be achieved. Non-aboriginal health care workers should realize that not every aboriginal patient will want to be 'saved' by certain KRT methods. The same is true for medication compliance. Aboriginal patients should understand that if they find value in living longer, then this can only be achieved by at least adopting the most basic principles of non-aboriginal care, being adherent, and following compliance. Also, the cherished long trips in the bush during the year will regretfully no longer be possible. For many of the non-aboriginal health care workers it is hard to understand that in the aboriginal people there are many who do not want to live 'at all costs.' Persisting in our western ways of thinking we see the very dramatic consequences of patients dying 2000 km away in Perth, whereas the patient's heart and soul is in country.

Unless we are ready for a massive change in cultural acceptance on both sides, nothing will change, as the gap has not closed since it first attempts in 2011 [147].

Final Remarks

ADEMEX has been the most importantly performed RCT for PD, challenging the concept of adequacy and prompting the search for improving other aspects of patient care that are likely to improve clinical outcomes. There may be a PD nephrologist or nurse who does not know the meaning of ADEMEX for the PD therapy, but most likely he or she is the exception.

The ADEMEX Study and Hemodialysis (HEMO) Study are two large RCTs that have questioned how to prescribe the dialysis dose. HDF, an alternative to standard HD, by adding the convective component to diffusion, removes middle molecules and larger low-molecular weight proteins more effectively. Greater convective volumes increase the clearance of the uremic toxins. It is interesting to point out that the identification of convective solute transport in connection with water removal was carried out in an experiment using the peritoneal membrane of ESKD patients maintained on chronic PD in 1966 [148].

This chapter provides information not only supporting PD as an alternative to extracorporeal therapy for both ESKD and AKI, but also clinical practice-based evidence addressing diverse topics in PD including adequacy, metabolism, infection, PD catheters, fluid balance, cardio-renal syndrome, antibiotic prophylaxis, metformin utilization, PD solution impact on the structure, and function of the peritoneal membrane. Important contributions have been continuously provided over the years from the Saudi Eastern Province by the KFUH PD Team, through clinical practice, publications of their own experience, and innovations such as their PD catheter insertion techniques.

The turning point in the utilization of PD for AKI was the publication by a group of nephrologists from a small university city in Brazil, Botucatu. They laid out a PD trailblazing expedition in 2007, which was exercised flawlessly, resulting in an attitude-changing AKI paper regarding PD indication and application of the "PD: state of the art" definition: Tenckhoff catheter, cycler, PD solution in plastic bags, closed system, and high volumes [108].

PD is a simple, safe, and efficient way to correct metabolic, electrolytic, acid-base, and volume disturbances generated by AKI; it can be used as a KRT modality to treat AKI in developing and developed countries, either in or out of the intensive care unit setting.

Furthermore, an improvement in patient and technique survival over the years, even after correction for several confounders, has been observed.

PD is a global therapy, being offered not only to educated but also to illiterate patients; not only in affluent areas but also in the less privileged suburbs of big cities; not only to people who can read and listen but also to the blind and deaf; not only to non-indigenous but also to indigenous people. Indigenous people in wealthy countries have outcomes of chronic disease that are comparable to those of patients in low socio-economic developing countries. Many are the barriers and cultural differences faced by patients in different corners, even the most remote, of the world. The personal view of a colleague, Johan Rosman, a nephrologist who has been working with the indigenous CKD population in Western Australia for many years is of extreme value and interest for all of us, regardless of where we live and work with CKD and KRT. It is a complex interplay, when deciding the dialysis modality, as many factors play a role, including socioeconomic, medical, cultural, and psychological. Besides, there is the need, as often as possible, of a shared decision-making together with the patient and family, weighing pros and cons as well as underscoring the values and preferences of the patient's culture. Dr. Rosman approaches from a personal perspective the causes of the gap between outcomes for aboriginal and non-aboriginal persons and how the many failed attempts to close the gap could be addressed.

From Mexico and Central America to the Kingdom of Saudi Arabia and from there to South America, continuing to Australia and then South Africa and landing at Thailand: a wealth of sound clinical evidence, unique experience, bold policy, targeted approach to create opportunities where they are scarce, cultural gaps being closed. There is still a lot more to learn about PD from everywhere as PD experience is a privilege of everyone and PD therapy a 360^0 global reality.

References

[1] Boen ST. *Peritoneal Dialysis: a clinical study of factors governing its effectiveness.* Dissertation thesis at University of Amsterdam. 1959; 1-166.

[2] Gjessing J. Studies of peritoneal dialysis. *Kidney Int.* 2008; 73: S18-S25.

[3] The RENAL Replacement Therapy Investigators. Bellomo R, Cass A, Cole L, Finfer S, Gallagher M, Lo S, et al. Intensity of renal-replacement therapy in critically ill patients. *New Engl J Med.* 2009; 361: 1627-38.

[4] The VA/NIH Acute Renal Failure Trial Network. Palevsky PM, Zhang JH, O'Connor TZ, Chertow GM, Crowley ST, Choudhury D. Intensity of renal support in critically ill patients with acute kidney injury. *New Engl J Med.* 2008; 359: 7-20.

[5] Ronco C, Bellomo R, Homel P, Brendolan A, Dan M, Picccinni P, La Greca G. Effects of different doses in continuous veno-venous hemofiltration on outcomes of acute renal failure: a prospective randomized trial. *Lancet.* 2000; 355: 26-30.

[6] GBD Chronic Kidney Disease Collaboration. Global, regional, and national burden of chronic kidney disease, 1990-2017: a systematic analysis for the Global Burden of Disease Study 2017. *Lancet.* 2020;395(10225):709-33.

[7] Jager KJ, Fraser SDS. The ascending rank of chronic kidney disease in the global burden of disease study. *Nephrol Dial Transplant.* 2017;32(suppl 2):ii121-ii128.

[8] Jha V, Garcia-Garcia G, Iseki K, Li Z, Naicker S, Plattner B, et al. Chronic kidney disease: global dimension and perspectives. *Lancet* 2013;382(9888):260-72.
[9] Struijk DG. Peritoneal Dialysis in Western Countries. *Kidney Dis* (Basel) 2015;1(3):157-64.
[10] Cho Y, Johnson DW. Peritoneal dialysis-related peritonitis: towards improving evidence, practices, and outcomes. *Am J Kidney Dis*. 2014;64(2):278-89.
[11] Monteón F, Correa-Rotter R, Paniagua R, Amato D, Hurtado ME, Medina JL, et al. Prevention of peritonitis with disconnect system in CAPD: A randomized control trial. *Kidney Int.* 1998;54(6):2123-128.
[12] Piraino B, Bernardini J, Brown E, Figueiredo A, Johnson D W, Lye W C, et al. ISPD position statement on reducing the risks of peritoneal dialysis-related infections. *Perit Dial Int.* 2011;31(6):614-30.
[13] Figueiredo AE, Moraes TP, Bernardini J, Poli-de-Figueiredo CE, Barretti P, Olandoski M, et al. Impact of patient training patterns on peritonitis rates in a large national cohort study. *Nephrol Dial Transplant.* 2015;30(1):137-42.
[14] Vonesh EF, Snyder JJ, Foley RN, Collins AJ. Mortality studies comparing peritoneal dialysis and hemodialysis: what do they tell us? *Kidney Int Suppl.* 2006;(103):S3-S11.
[15] Kumar VA, Sidell MA, Jones JP, Vonesh EF. Survival of propensity matched incident peritoneal and hemodialysis patients in a United States health care system. *Kidney Int* 2014;86:1016–22.
[16] Lukowsky LR, Mehrotra R, Kheifets L, Arah OA, Nissenson AR, Kalantar-Zadeh K. Comparing mortality of peritoneal and hemodialysis patients in the first 2 years of dialysis therapy: a marginal structural model analysis. *Clin J Am Soc Nephrol.* 2013;8(4):619-628.
[17] Keshaviah PR, Nolph KD, Van Stone JC. The peak concentration hypothesis: a urea kinetic approach to comparing the adequacy of continuous ambulatory peritoneal dialysis (CAPD) and hemodialysis. *Perit Dial Int.* 1989;9(4):257-60.
[18] Harty J, Boulton H, Venning M, Gokal R. Impact of increasing dialysis volume on adequacy targets: a prospective study. *J Am Soc Nephrol.* 1997;8(8):1304-10.
[19] Diaz-Buxo JA, Gotch FA, Folden TI, et al. Peritoneal dialysis adequacy: a model to assess feasibility with various modalities. *Kidney Int.* 1999;55(6):2493-2501.
[20] Churchill DN, Taylor DW, Keshaviah PR for the CANUSA Peritoneal Dialysis Study Group. Adequacy of dialysis and nutrition in continuous peritoneal dialysis: association with clinical outcomes. *J Am Soc Nephrol.* 1996;7(2):198-207.
[21] Diaz-Buxo JA, Lowrie EG, Lew NL, Zhang SM, Zhu X, Lazarus JM. Associates of mortality among peritoneal dialysis patients with special reference to peritoneal transport rates and solute clearance. *Am J Kidney Dis.* 1999;33(3):523-34.
[22] Szeto CC, Wong TY, Leung CB, Wang AY, Law MC, Lui SF, et al. Importance of dialysis adequacy in mortality and morbidity of chinese CAPD patients. *Kidney Int.* 2000;58(1):400-7.
[23] Rocco M, Soucie JM, Pastan S, McClellan WM. Peritoneal dialysis adequacy and risk of death. *Kidney Int* . 2000;58(1):446-57.
[24] Bargman JM, Thorpe KE, Churchill DN. CANUSA Peritoneal Dialysis Study Group. Relative contribution of residual renal function and peritoneal clearance to adequacy of dialysis: a reanalysis of the CANUSA study. *J Am Soc Nephrol.* 2001;12(10):2158-62.

[25] Paniagua R, Amato D, Vonesh E, Correa-Rotter R, Ramos A, Moran J, et al. Effects of increased peritoneal clearances on mortality rates in peritoneal dialysis: ADEMEX, a prospective, randomized, controlled trial. *J Am Soc Nephrol.* 2002;13(5):1307-20.

[26] Churchill DN. The ADEMEX Study: make haste slowly. *J Am Soc Nephrol.* 2002;13(5):1415-18.

[27] Blake P. ADEMEX: a landmark peritoneal dialysis study. Should we change our practice? *Perit Dial Int.* 2002;22(5):545.

[28] Eknoyan G, Beck GJ, Cheung AK, Daugirdas JT, Greene T, Kusek JW, et al. Hemodialysis (HEMO) Study Group. Effect of dialysis dose and membrane flux in maintenance hemodialysis. *N Engl J Med.* 200219;347(25):2010-9.

[29] Meyer TW, Sirich TL, Fong KD, Plummer NS, Shafi T, Hwang S, et al. Kt/Vurea and Nonurea Small Solute Levels in the Hemodialysis Study. *J Am Soc Nephrol.* 2016;27(11):3469-78.

[30] Prichard S. ADEMEX and HEMO trials: where are we going? *Blood Purif.* 2003;21(1):42-5.

[31] Tzamaloukas AH, Murata GH. Adequacy of peritoneal dialysis after the ADEMEX study. Back to the basics. *Int J Artif Organs.* 2002;25(9):827-31.

[32] Raymond T Krediet. The rise and fall of the K(t)/V concept in CAPD. *Nephrol Dial Transplant.* 2002;17(6):970-2.

[33] Perl J, Dember LM, Bargman JM, Browne T, Charytan DM, Flythe JE, et al. American Society of Nephrology Dialysis Advisory Group. The Use of a Multidimensional Measure of Dialysis Adequacy-Moving beyond Small Solute Kinetics. *Clin J Am Soc Nephrol.* 2017;12(5):839-847.

[34] Da J, Xie X, Wolf M, Disthabanchong S, Wang J, Zha Y, et al. Serum Phosphorus and Progression of CKD and Mortality: A Meta-analysis of Cohort Studies. *Am J Kidney Dis.* 2015;66(2):258-65.

[35] Galassi A, Cupisti A, Santoro A, Cozzolino M. Phosphate balance in ESRD: diet, dialysis and binders against the low evident masked pool. *J Nephrol.* 2015;28(4):415-29.

[36] Floege J, Kim J, Ireland E, Chazot C, Drueke T, de Francisco A, et al. Serum iPTH, calcium and phosphate, and the risk of mortality in a European haemodialysis population. *Nephrol Dial Transplant.* 2011;26(6):1948-55.

[37] Regidor DL, Kopple JD, Kovesdy CP, Kilpatrick RD, McAllister CJ, Aronovitz J, et al. Associations between changes in hemoglobin and administered erythropoiesis-stimulating agent and survival in hemodialysis patients. *J Am Soc Nephrol.* 2006;17(4):1181-91.

[38] Akizawa T, Okumura H, Alexandre AF, Fukushima A, Kiyabu G, Dorey J. Burden of Anemia in Chronic Kidney Disease Patients in Japan: A Literature Review. *Ther Apher Dial.* 2018;22(5):444-456.

[39] Zeidan A, Bhandari S. Anemia in Peritoneal Dialysis Patients; Iron Repletion, Current and Future Therapies. *Perit Dial Int.* 2017;37(1):6-13.

[40] Kiebalo T, Holotka J, Habura I, Pawlaczyk K. Nutritional Status in Peritoneal Dialysis: Nutritional Guidelines, Adequacy and the Management of Malnutrition. *Nutrients.* 2020;12(6):1715.

[41] Chung SH, Heimbürger O, Stenvinkel P, Qureshi AR, Lindholm B. Association between residual renal function, inflammation and patient survival in new peritoneal dialysis patients. *Nephrol Dial Transplant*. 2003;18(3):590-7.

[42] Qureshi AR, Alvestrand A, Divino-Filho JC, Gutierrez A, Heimbürger O, Lindholm B, et al. Inflammation, malnutrition, and cardiac disease as predictors of mortality in hemodialysis patients. *J Am Soc Nephrol*. 2002;13(Suppl 1):S28-36.

[43] Chung SH, Carrero JJ, Lindholm B. Causes of poor appetite in patients on peritoneal dialysis. *J Ren Nutr*. 2011;21(1):12-15.

[44] Jankowska M, Lichodziejewska-Niemierko M, Rutkowski B, Dębska-Ślizień A, Małgorzewicz S. Water soluble vitamins and peritoneal dialysis - State of the art. *Clin Nutr*. 2017;36(6):1483-1489.

[45] Paniagua R, Amato D, Mujais S, Vonesh E, Ramos A, Correa-Rotter R, et al. Predictive value of brain natriuretic peptides in patients on peritoneal dialysis: results from the ADEMEX trial. *Clin J Am Soc Nephrol*. 2008;3(2):407-15.

[46] Ateş K, Nergizoğlu G, Keven K, Sen A, Kutlay S, Ertürk S, et al. Effect of fluid and sodium removal on mortality in peritoneal dialysis patients. *Kidney Int*. 2001;60(2):767-76.

[47] Kim YL, Biesen WV. Fluid Overload in Peritoneal Dialysis Patients. Semin *Nephrol*. 2017;37(1):43-53.

[48] van der Sande FM, van de Wal-Visscher ER, Stuard S, Moissl U, Kooman JP. Using Bioimpedance Spectroscopy to Assess Volume Status in Dialysis Patients. *Blood Purif*. 2020;49(1-2):178-184.

[49] Demirci MS, Demirci C, Ozdogan O, Kircelli F, Akcicek F, Basci A, et al. Relations between malnutrition-inflammation-atherosclerosis and volume status. The usefulness of bioimpedance analysis in peritoneal dialysis patients. *Nephrol Dial Transplant*. 2011;26(5):1708-16.

[50] Cheng LT, Gao YL, Qin C, Tian JP, Gu Y, Bi SH, et al. Volume overhydration is related to endothelial dysfunction in continuous ambulatory peritoneal dialysis patients. *Perit Dial Int*. 2008;28(4):397-402.

[51] Tian JP, Du FH, Cheng LT, Tian XK, Axelsson J, Wang T. Peripheral resistance modulates the response to volume overload in peritoneal dialysis patients. *Perit Dial Int*. 2008;28(6):604-610.

[52] Davies SJ, Phillips L, Russell GI. Peritoneal solute transport predicts survival on CAPD independently of residual renal function. *Nephrol Dial Transplant*. 1998;13(4):962-8.

[53] Rumpsfeld M, McDonald SP, Johnson DW. Higher peritoneal transport status is associated with higher mortality and technique failure in the Australian and New Zealand peritoneal dialysis patient populations. *J Am Soc Nephrol*. 2006;17(1):271-8.

[54] Li PK, Ng JK, Mcintyre CW. Inflammation and Peritoneal Dialysis. *Semin Nephrol*. 2017;37(1):54-65.

[55] Davies SJ. Peritoneal solute transport and inflammation. *Am J Kidney Dis*. 2014 Dec;64(6):978-86.

[56] Vaziri ND, Zhao YY, Pahl MV. Altered intestinal microbial flora and impaired epithelial barrier structure and function in CKD: the nature, mechanisms, consequences and potential treatment. *Nephrol Dial Transplant*. 2016;31(5):737-746.

[57] Branchereau M, Burcelin R, Heymes C. The gut microbiome and heart failure: A better gut for a better heart. *Rev Endocr Metab Disord*. 2019;20(4):407-414.

[58] Anders HJ, Andersen K, Stecher B. The intestinal microbiota, a leaky gut, and abnormal immunity in kidney disease. *Kidney Int*. 2013;83(6):1010-1016.

[59] Simões-Silva L, Araujo R, Pestana M, Soares-Silva I, Sampaio-Maia B. The microbiome in chronic kidney disease patients undergoing hemodialysis and peritoneal dialysis. *Pharmacol Res*. 2018;130:143-151.

[60] Grant C, Harrison L, Hoad C, Marciani L, Cox E, Buchanan C, et al. Endotoxemia in Peritoneal Dialysis Patients: A Pilot Study to Examine the Role of Intestinal Perfusion and Congestion. *Perit Dial Int*. 2017;37(1):111-115.

[61] Goossen K, Becker M, Marshall MR, Bühn S, Breuing J, Firanek CA, et al. Icodextrin Versus Glucose Solutions for the Once-Daily Long Dwell in Peritoneal Dialysis: An Enriched Systematic Review and Meta-analysis of Randomized Controlled Trials. *Am J Kidney Dis*. 2020;75(6):830-846.

[62] Port FK. Worldwide demographics and future trends in end-stage renal disease. *Kidney Int Suppl*. 1993;41:S4-S7.

[63] Su-Hernández L, Abascal-Macías A, Méndez-Bueno FJ, Paniagua R, Amato D. Epidemiologic and demographic aspects of peritoneal dialysis in Mexico. *Perit Dial Int*. 1996;16(4):362-365. http://www.imss.gob.mx/sites/all/statics/pdf/informes/ 20192020/ 21-InformeCompleto.pdf.

[64] Monteón F, Correa-Rotter R, Paniagua R, Amato D, Hurtado ME, Medina JL, Salcedo RM, García E, Matos M, Kaji J, Vázquez R, Ramos A, Schettino MA, Moran J. Prevention of peritonitis with disconnect systems in CAPD: a randomized controlled trial. The Mexican Nephrology Collaborative Study Group. *Kidney Int*. 1998 Dec;54(6):2123-8.

[65] Paniagua R, Ventura MD, Avila-Díaz M, Cisneros A, Vicenté-Martínez M, Furlong MD, García-González Z, Villanueva D, Orihuela O, Prado-Uribe MD, Alcántara G, Amato D. Icodextrin improves metabolic and fluid management in high and high-average transport diabetic patients. *Perit Dial Int*. 2009 Jul-Aug;29(4):422-32.

[66] Su-Hernández L, Abascal-Macías A, Méndez-Bueno FJ, Paniagua R, Amato D. Epidemiologic and demographic aspects of peritoneal dialysis in Mexico. *Perit Dial Int*. 1996 Jul-Aug;16(4):362-5.

[67] Nissenson AR. Dialysis modality selection: harsh realities. *Perit Dial Int*. 1996 Jul-Aug;16(4):343-4.

[68] 69 - Najafi I. Peritoneal dialysis in Iran and the Middle East. *Perit Dial Int*. 2009; 29(S2): S217–S221.

[69] 70- Saudi Center for Organ Transplantation (SCOT). Dialysis in the Kingdom of Saudi Arabia, *Saudi J Kidney Dis Transpl* 2018; 29 (4):1012-1020.

[70] 71- Dahlan RA, Alsuwaida AO, Farrash MS, Qureshi MA, Hejaili F, Al Sayyari AA. Let Us Listen to Patients: Underutilization of Peritoneal Dialysis from Patients' Perspectives. *Perit Dial Int*. 2017; 37: 574–583.

[71] 72- Dahlan R, Qureshi M, Akeely F, Al Sayyari AA. Barriers to Peritoneal Dialysis in Saudi Arabia: Nephrologists' Perspectives. *Perit Dial Int.* 2016;36(5):564-566.

[72] 73- Shaheen F, B. Al-Attar, D. Santiago, P. Follero, H. Zakaria, and M. Kamal. Health Indicators for Renal Replacement Therapy in Saudi Arabia. *Transplant Proc*. 2019; 51 (2): 509-511.

[73] Al-Hwiesh AK. A modified peritoneal dialysis catheter with a new technique: Farewell to catheter migration. *Saudi J Kidney Dis Transpl*. 2016; 27(2):281-9.

[74] Al-Hwiesh AK. Peritoneal dialysis catheter insertion by a nephrologist: a new, simple and safe technique. *Perit Dial Int*. 2014; 34 (2): 204-11.

[75] Szeto CC, Wong TY, Chow KM, Leung CB, Li PK. Are peritoneal dialysis patients with and without residual renal function equivalent for survival study? Insight from a retrospective review of the cause of death. *Nephrol Dial Transplant*. 2003; 18:977–82.

[76] Akyol AM, Porteous C, Brown MW. A comparison of two types of catheters for continuous ambulatory peritoneal dialysis (CAPD). *Peritoneal Dialysis International* 1990; 10:63–6.

[77] Eklund BH, Honkanen EO, Kala AR, Kyllonen LE. Catheter configuration and outcome in patients on continuous ambulatory peritoneal dialysis: a prospective comparison of two catheters. *Perit Dial Int*. 1994; 14:70–4.

[78] Eklund BH, Honkanen EO, Kala AR, Kyllonen LE. Peritoneal dialysis access: prospective randomized comparison of the Swan neck and Tenckhoff catheters. *Perit Dial Int*. 1995; 15:353–6.

[79] Lye WC, Kour NW, van der Straaten JC, Leong SO, Lee EJ. A prospective randomized comparison of the swan neck, coiled, and straight Tenckhoff catheters in patients on CAPD. *Perit Dial Int*. 1996; 16 (Suppl 1): S333–5.

[80] Nielsen PK, Hemmingsen C, Friis SU, Ladefoged J, Olgaard K. Comparison of straight and curled Tenckhoff peritoneal dialysis catheters implanted by percutaneous technique: a prospective randomized study. *Perit Dial Int*. 1995; 15:18–21.

[81] Scott PD, Bakran A, Pearson R, Riad H, Parrott N, Johnson RW, Gokal R. Peritoneal dialysis access. Prospective randomized trial of 3 different peritoneal catheters – preliminary report. *Perit Dial Int*. 1994; 14:289–90.

[82] Johnson DW, Wong J, Wiggins KJ, Kirwan R, Griffin A, Preston J, et al. A randomized controlled trial of coiled versus straight swan-neck Tenckhoff catheters in peritoneal dialysis patients. *Am J Kidney Dis*. 2006; 48:812–21.

[83] USRDS. US Renal Data System Annual Data Report IV. Catheter-related fac¬tors and peritonitis risk in CAPD patients. *Am J Kidney Dis*. 1992; 20(Suppl 2):48–54.

[84] Honda M, Iitaka K, Kawaguchi H, Hoshii S, Akashi S, Kohsaka T, et al. The Japanese National Registry data on pediatric CAPD patients: a ten-year experience. A report of the Study Group of Pediatric PD Conference. *Perit Dial Int*. 1996; 16:269–75.

[85] Warady BA, Sullivan EK, Alexander SR. Lessons from the peritoneal dialysis patient database: a report of the North American Pediatric Renal Transplant Cooperative Study. *Kidney Int*. 1996; 53: S68–71.

[86] Nessim SJ, Bargman JM, Jassal SV. Relationship between double-cuff versus single-cuff peritoneal dialysis catheters and risk of peritonitis. *Nephrol Dial Transplant*. 2010; 25:2310–14.

[87] Eklund B, Honkanen E, Kyllonen L, Salmella K, Kala AR. Peritoneal dialysis access: prospective randomized comparison of single-cuff and double-cuff straight Tenckhoff catheters. *Nephrol Dial Transplant* 1997; 12:2664–6.

[88] Abdullah K. Al-Hwiesh, Ibrahiem Saeed Abdul-Rahman, Amani Al-Hwiesh, Abdulrahman Taha, Rawan Amir et al. Factors contributing to peritonitis in Peritoneal Dialysis: Comparing Triple Cuff Saudi Catheter to Double Cuff Tenckhoff Catheter. A 12-year observational study. *Accepted for publication at Saudi J Kidney Dis Transpl.*

[89] Al-Hwiesh A, Abdul-Rahman I, Finkelstein F, Divino-Filho JC et al. Acute Kidney Injury in Critically Ill Patients: A Prospective Randomized Study of Tidal Peritoneal

Dialysis versus Continuous Renal Replacement Therapy. *Ther Apher Dial.* 2018; 22(4):371–379.

[90] 91 Cullis B, Al-Hwiesh A, Kilonzo K, et al. ISPD guidelines for peritoneal dialysis in acute kidney injury: 2020 update (adults). *Perit Dial Int.* December 2020. doi:10.1177/0896860820970834.

[91] Al-Hwiesh AK, Abdul-Rahman IS, Al-Audah N, Al-Hwiesh A, Taha A, et al. (2019) Success of Instant-Start Life-Saving Peritoneal Dialysis in Patients with End-Stage Vascular Access Failure: Time to Rescue Patients. *Int J Nephrol Kidney Fail* 5(4): dx.doi.org/10.16966/2380- 5498.182.

[92] Al-Hwiesh AK, Abdul-Rahman IS, Al-Muhanna F, Al-Sulaiman MH, Al-Jondebi M, Divino-Filho JC. Prevention of peritoneal dialysis catheter infections in Saudi peritoneal dialysis patients: the emergence of high-level mupirocin resistance, *Int J Artif Organs* 2013; 36 (7): 473-483.

[93] Al-Hwiesh AK, Shawarby MA, Abdul-Rahman IS, Al-Oudah N, Al-Dhofairy B, Divino-Filho JC et al. Changes in peritoneal membrane with different peritoneal dialysis solutions: Is there a difference?. *Hong Kong Journal of Nephrology* 2016; 19: 7-18.

[94] Al-Hwiesh AK, Ibrahiem S Abdul-Rahman , Mohammad A Hussameldeen , Nadia Al-Audah , Abdalla Abdelrahman et al, Colonoscopy in Automated Peritoneal Dialysis Patients: Value of Prophylactic Antibiotics: A Prospective Study on a Single Antibiotic. *Int J Artif Organs*. 2017 Oct 13;40(10):550-557.

[95] Al-Hwiesh AK, Abdul-Rahman IS, El-Deen MA, Larbi E, Divino-Filho JC, Al-Muhanna FA, Gupta KL. Metformin in Peritoneal Dialysis: a Pilot Experience. *Perit Dial Int.* 2014 Jun; 34(4):368-75.

[96] Al-Hwiesh AK, Abdul-Rahman IS, Noor AS, Nasr-El-Deen MA, Abdelrahman A, El-Salamoni TS, Al-Muhanna FA, Al-Otaibi K, Al-Audah N. The Phantom of Metformin-Induced Lactic Acidosis in End-Stage Renal Disease Patients: Time to Reconsider with Peritoneal Dialysis Treatment. *Perit Dial Int.* 2017 1-2;37(1):56-62.

[97] Al-Hwiesh AK, Abdul-Rahman IS, Al-Audah N, et al.· Tidal peritoneal dialysis vs. ultrafiltration in type-1 cardiorenal syndrome: A prospective randomized study. *I J Artif Org* 2019; 42 (12): 684-94.

[98] Gabriel DP, Nascimento GV, Martim LC, Caramori JT, Barretti P, Balbi AL. Peritoneal dialysis in acute renal failure. *Ren Fail.* 2006; 28(6):451-6. doi: 10.1080/08860220600781245.

[99] Gabriel DP, Fernández-Cean J, Balbi AL. Utilization of peritoneal dialysis in the acute setting. *Perit Dial Int.* 2007 May/Jun; 27(3):328-31.

[100] Davenport A. Peritoneal dialysis in acute kidney injury. *Perit Dial Int.* 2008 Jul-Aug; 28(4): 423-4.

[101] Ponce D, Banin VB, Bueloni TVS, Caramori JT, Barretti P, Balbi AL. Different outcomes of peritoneal catheter percutaneous placement by nephrologists using a trocar versus the Seldinger technique: the experience of two Brazilian centers. *Int Urol Nephrol.* 2014 Oct; 46(10):2029-34. doi:10.1007/s11255-014-0738-6.

[102] Passadakis PS, Oreopoulos DG. Peritoneal dialysis in patients with acute renal failure. *Adv Perit Dial.* 2007; 23:7-16.

[103] Chionh CY, Ronco C, Finkelstein FO, Soni SS, Cruz DN. Acute peritoneal dialysis: what is the 'adequate' dose for acute kidney injury? *Nephrol Dial Transplant.* 2010 Oct; 25(10):3155-60.doi:10.1093/ndt/gfg178.

[104] Kronfol, N. Acute peritoneal dialysis prescription. In: Daugirdas JT, Ing TS, editors. *Handbook of Dialysis*. Ed (2). Boston: Little, Brown and Company, 1994. p. 301-9.

[105] Chionh CY, Soni S, Cruz DN, Ronco C. Peritoneal dialysis for acute kidney injury: techniques and dose. *Contrib Nephrol*. 2009 Jun; 163:278-84.

[106] Chitalia VC, Almeida AF, Rai H, Bapat M, Chitalia KV, Acharya VN, Khanna R. Is peritoneal dialysis adequate for hypercatabolic acute renal failure in developing countries? *Kidney Int*. 2002 Feb; 61(2):747-57.

[107] Gabriel DP, Nascimento GV, Martim LC, Caramori JT, Barretti P, Balbi AL. High volume peritoneal dialysis for acute renal failure. *Perit Dial Int*. 2007 May-Jun; 27(3):277-82.

[108] Amerling R, Glezerman I, Savransky E, Dubrow A, Ronco C. Continuous flow peritoneal dialysis: principles and applications. *Semin Dial*. 2003 Jul-Aug; 16(4): 335-40.

[109] Ronco C, Amerling R. Continuous flow peritoneal dialysis: current state-of-the-art and obstacles to further development. *Contrib Nephrol*. 2006;150: 310-20.

[110] Ronco C, Dell'aquila R, Rodighiero MP, Di Loreto P, Nalesso F, Spanò E, Parkhill R, Amerling R, Levin N. The ''Ronco'' catheter for continuous flow peritoneal dialysis. *Int J Artif Organs*. 2006 Jan; 29(1):101-12.

[111] Ronco C. Can peritoneal dialysis be considered an option for the treatment of acute kidney injury? *Perit Dial Int*. 2007 May-Jun; 27(3):251-3.

[112] Phu NH, Hien TT, Mai NT, Chau TT, Chuong LV, Loc PP, Winearls C, Farrar J, White N, Day N. Hemofiltration and peritoneal dialysis in infection-associated acute renal failure in Vietnam. *N Engl J Med*. 2002 Sep;347(12):895-902.

[113] Amerling R, DeSimone L, Inciong-Reyes R, Pangilinan A, Folden T, Ronco C, Gotch FA, Levin N. Clinical experience with continuous flow and flow-through peritoneal dialysis. *Semin Dial*. 2001 Sep-Oct; 14(5):388-90.

[114] Boen ST. Peritoneal dialysis: a clinical study of factors governing its effectiveness. *Kidney Int Suppl* 2008; 108: S5–S17).

[115] Ilabaca-Avendaño MB, Yarza-Solorzáno G, Rodriguez-Valenzuela J, Arcinas-Fausto G, Ramírez-Hernandez V, Hernández-Hernández DA, Jáuregui-Flores LA. Automated peritoneal dialysis as a lifesaving therapy in an emergency room: report of four cases. *Kidney Int Suppl*. 2008;(108):S173-6.

[116] Miller FN, Hammerschmidt DE, Anderson GL, Moore JN. Protein loss induced by complement activation during peritoneal dialysis. *Kidney Int*. 1984 Mar; 25(3):480-5.

[117] Blumenkrantz MJ, Gahl GM, Kopple JD, Kamdar AV, Jones MR, Kessel M, Coburn JW. Protein losses during peritoneal dialysis. *Kidney Int*. 1981 Apr; 19(4):593-602.

[118] Gordon S, Rubini ME. Protein losses during peritoneal dialysis. *Am J Med Sci*. 1967; 253(3):283-92.

[119] Góes CR, Berbel MN, Balbi AL, Ponce D. Metabolic implications of peritoneal dialysis in patients with acute kidney injury. *Perit Dial Int*. 2013;33(6):635-45.

[120] Bargman JM, Bick J, Cartier P, Dasgupta MK, Fine A, Lavoie SD, Spanner E, Taylor PA. Guidelines for adequacy and nutrition in peritoneal dialysis. Canadian Society of Nephrology. *J Am Soc Nephrol*. 1999;(10 Suppl 13):S311-21.

[121] Vieira JM, Jr Castro I, Curvello-Neto A, Demarzo S, Caruso P, Jr Pastore L, et al. Effect of acute kidney injury on weaning from mechanical ventilation in critically ill patients. *Crit Care Med*. 2013;35(1):184-91.

[122] Epstein SW. Effect of peritoneal dialysis fluid on ventilatory function. *Perit Dial* Bull. 1982; 2:120-2.

[123] Almeida CTP, Berbel MN, Balbi AL, Ponce D. Effect of Peritoneal Dialysis on Respiratory Mechanics in Acute Kidney Injury Patients. *Perit Dial Int.* 2014;34(5):1-6.

[124] Gabriel DP, Martin LC, Caramori JT, Barretti P, Balbi AL. High volume peritoneal dialysis vs daily hemodialysis: a randomized, controlled trial in patients with acute kidney injury. *Kidney Int.* 2008;108(Suppl 73):S87-S93.

[125] Ponce D, Berbel MN, Goes CR, Balbi AL. High Volume Peritoneal Dialysis in Acute Kidney Injury: Indications and Limitations. *Clin J Am Soc Nephrol.* 2012;7(6):887-94.

[126] Ponce D, Berbel MN, Abrão JMG, Goes CR, Balbi AL. Different Prescribed Doses of High-Volume Peritoneal Dialysis and Outcome of Patients with Acute Kidney Injury. *Advances in Peritoneal Dialysis*. 2011;118-24.

[127] Cullis B, Abdelraheem M, Abrahams G, Balbi A, Cruz DN, Frishberg Y, et al. ISPD guidelines/Recommendations Peritoneal Dialysis for Acute Kidney Injury. *Perit Dial Int.* 2014;34:494-517.

[128] Parapiboon W, Jamratpan T. Intensive Versus Minimal Standard Dosage for Peritoneal Dialysis in Acute Kidney Injury: A Randomized Pilot Study. Perit Dial *Int J Int Soc Perit Dial.* 2017;37(5):523–8.

[129] Ponce D, Caramori JT, Barretti P, Balbi AL. Peritoneal Dialysis in Acute Kidney Injury: Brazilian experience. *Perit Dial Int*. 2012;32(3):242-6.

[130] Ponce D, Berbel MN, Abrao JMG, Balbi AL. A randomized clinical trial of high volume peritoneal dialysis versus extended daily hemodialysis for acute kidney injury patients. *Int Urol Nephrol*. 2013;45(3):869-78.

[131] George J, Varma S, Kumar S, Thomas J, Gopi S, Pisharody R. Comparing continuous venovenous hemodiafiltration and peritoneal dialysis in critically ill patients with acute kidney injury: a pilot study. *Perit Dial Int*. 2011;31(4):422-9.

[132] Ponce D, Buffarah MNB, Goes CR, Balbi AL. Peritoneal Dialysis in Acute Kidney Injury: Trends in the outcome across time periods. *Plos One*. 2015;12;10(5):1-13.

[133] Australian Bureau of Statistics. Reflecting a Nation: Stories from the 2011 Census, July 2011, Cat No 2071.0.

[134] Mohan J, Atkinson DN, Rosman JB et al. Acute kidney injury in Indigenous Australians in the Kimberley: age distribution and associated diagnoses. *Med J Australia.* 2019; 211(1): 19-23.

[135] Hoy W. Kidney Disease in Aboriginal Australians: a perspective from the Northern Territory. *Clin Kidney J.* 2014; 7: 524-530.

[136] Hoy W, Mott SA, McDonald SP. An expanded view of chronic kidney disease in Aboriginal Australians. *Nephrology*. 2016; 21: 916-922.

[137] Lim W, Johnson DW, McDonald SP et al. Impending challenges of the burden of end-stage kidney disease in Australia. *Med J* Aust; 211(8): 374-381, 2019.

[138] Australian and New Zealand Dialysis and Transplant Registry, 41st report 2018. www.anzdata.org.au. Accessed on 21 August 2020.

[139] Mathew AT, Park J, Sachdeva M et al. Barriers to Peritoneal Dialysis in Aboriginal Patients. *Can J Kidney Health and Disease*; 5: 1-9, 2018.

[140] Gorham G, Howard K, Zhao Y et al. Cost of dialysis therapies in rural and remote Australia – a micro costing analysis. *BMC Nephrology*; 20: 231-242, 2019.

[141] Prakash S. An international perspective on peritoneal dialysis among indigenous patients. *J Int Soc Perit Dial.* 2011; 31: 390-398.

[142] Grace BS, Clayton PA, Gray NA et al. Socioeconomic Differences in the Uptake of Home Dialysis. *Clin J Am Soc Nephrol.* 2014; 9(5): 929-935.

[143] Marley JV, Moore S, Fitzclarence C et al. Peritoneal dialysis outcome of Indigenous Australian patients of remote Kimberley origin. *Aust J Rural Health.* 2014; 22(3): 101-108.

[144] Anderson K, Cunningham J, Devitt J et al. The IMPAKT study: using qualitative research to explore the impact of end-stage kidney disease and its treatments on aboriginal and Torres Strait Islander Australians. *Kidney Int;* Suppl; 3: 223-226, 2013.

[145] McDonald SP. End-stage kidney disease among indigenous peoples of Australia and New Zealand. *Kidney Int Suppl.* 2013;3(2): 170-173.

[146] Lim W, Johnson DW, McDonald SP et al. Impending challenges of the burden of end-stage kidney disease in Australia. *Med J Aust.* 2019; 211(8): 374-381.

[147] Henderson LW. Peritoneal ultrafiltration dialysis: enhanced urea transfer using hypertonic peritoneal dialysis fluid. *J Clin Invest.* 1966; 45: 950-5.

In: Issues in Kidney Disease – Dialysis
Editors: Stephen Z. Fadem and José A. Moura-Neto
ISBN: 978-1-68507-000-7

Chapter 17

PERITONEAL DIALYSIS EDUCATION: A GLOBAL PERSPECTIVE

Gustavo Moretta[1,7], MD, PhD, Susana Marcos[2,7], RN, Rosana Chaud[3,7], MD, Kleyton Bastos[4,7], MD, PhD, Carmen Arias Minaya[5,7], RN and José Carolino Divino-Filho[6,7,*], MD, PhD

[1]Escuela de Educación, San Andrés University, Buenos Aires, Argentina
[2]Argentina Society of Nephrological Nursing, Argentina
[3]FISSAL Comprehensive Health Insurance, Ministerio de Salud, Peru
[4]Department of Medicine, Federal University of Sergipe, Aracaju, Brazil
[5]National Coordinator of PD Hersil, Peru
[6]Division of Renal Medicine, Department of Clinical Science, Intervention and Technology, CLINTEC, Karolinska Institutet, Campus Flemingsberg, Stockholm, Sweden
[7]Latin-American Chapter (LAC-DD)-International Society for Peritoneal Dialysis

ABSTRACT

This chapter aims to bring the education sciences closer to the health workers. It will review the educational training contents that peritoneal dialysis patients must learn, with a focus on adult education and the development of skills or competencies. Moreover, it will present an assessment tool for the lessons learned, allowing communication among the health team members and, above all, for the patient to assess if she/he still needs to learn about chronic kidney diseases and peritoneal dialysis or if she/he is already an expert. If we consider therapeutic education a pillar of peritoneal dialysis, we must understand the need for evaluation of the educational program of the different institutions that train patients and propose the necessary steps required to initiate it. The focus will be on (I) Curriculum content and learning evaluation of peritoneal dialysis patients' educational programs; (II) The importance of the evaluation of PD educational programs; (III)

[*] Corresponding Author's E-mail: jose.divino@ki.se.

Therapeutic education and training of the health team for educational programs in peritoneal dialysis; and (IV) Review of some peritoneal dialysis learning experiences in Latin America

Keywords: learning evaluation, andragogy, use of rubrics, peritoneal dialysis, education, nephrolog, dialysis, health literacy

INTRODUCTION

Kidney replacement therapy (KRT) may present restrictions on a patient's lifestyle. The patient with chronic kidney disease (CKD) must overcome numerous barriers in order to survive; among them, the capacity to discern which KRT is the best choice, allowing a smoother adaptation to the new life situation. Home KRT such as peritoneal dialysis (PD) involve patients and/or their caregivers performing all required PD technique procedures at home, with a distant daily support of a multidisciplinary team or clinical staff. Moreover, they must also be aware of the possible complications and their management, adapting to the policies and procedures of the health system to which they belong.

The educational act becomes the central axis of this type of treatment, whereas the treatment should be tailored to each patient's individual needs and lifestyle. This independence may sometimes, unfortunately, lead to poor compliance and its possible consequences. Several authors have demonstrated the relationship of the relative risk of infectious complications by comparing patients who had a more detailed PD bag exchange protocol procedures with those who did not [1, 2]. The definition of education as the central axis of therapy is not a minor issue, because we are not talking about learning a succession of technical steps, but about developing skills that must be adapted to each person and to each health system.

This chapter aims to bring the education sciences closer to the health workers. In order to do so, we will review the educational content that PD patients must learn with a focus on skills development and the evaluation of lessons learned, training of facilitators (doctors and nurses) and their responsibilities in the way they train the patients, evaluation of educational programs and a proposal design for these programs, as well as the health authorities' responsibilities. We will finally review some PD learning experiences in Latin America and the world. Finally, one point to discuss is whether the formal educational levels (primary, secondary or higher) achieved by patients makes an impact on the results obtained either in PD training programs adapted for which learning is required or in therapy outcomes.

CURRICULUM CONTENT AND LEARNING EVALUATION OF PD PATIENTS' EDUCATIONAL PROGRAMS

The International Society for Peritoneal Dialysis (ISPD) has published recommendations related to PD patient training [3, 4]. They mention a number of factors that influence patient training outcomes, including facilitator-patient relationship, patient experience and knowledge, as well as educational methods such as protocols, time, training frequency, environment and training place [5]. While these guidelines together provide useful training recommendations, the training evaluation methods are not based on the acquisition of skills. There is no solid evidence that these interventions lead to increased adherence, reduced rates of peritonitis or other complications nor has a formal assessment been made of how well these guidelines have been implemented in clinical practice or, if performed, how much they have contributed to the clinical results obtained [6]. Regarding the curriculum, the ISPD guidelines recommend a well-developed PD training content program based on adult learning theory, a technique reported to produce a considerable increase in memory [7]. However, there have been very few studies evaluating the effect of the introduction of PD training programs based on adult learning theory.

The study representing the strongest evidence supporting the ISPD training guidelines recommendations is that of Hall et al. [8] who published an evaluation of a PD training curriculum based on adult, multicenter, non-randomized cluster training theory involving 620 PD patients. This curriculum was structured by learning levels, from lowest to highest, including memory, concept, principle, judgment/decision, problem solving, and demonstration. Patients trained by a curriculum based on adult learning (AL) theory (n=246) vs. conventional training (CT) programs (n=374) did not show any significant difference in neither peritonitis rates nor in interval between peritonitis episodes, over a 24-month follow-up period. As these results were not statistically significant, their statistical analysis has been questioned. However, there were statistically significant positive results for some clinical outcomes (less exit-site infections, less drop-out to HD due to infectious causes, better fluid balance as well as compliance scores) in the AL when compared to the CT group. Moreover, the conventional PD training curriculum and plan were not adequately described. Further clinical and research efforts are required in this area before firm recommendations can be made.

The teacher has an essential role in adult education as a "facilitator" in the apprentice's development of mental structures, so that the apprentice is able to build increasingly complex learning, so the action of the facilitator is that of a guide or tutor.

Gadola et al. [9] introduced, in Uruguay, a new PD educational program based on the adult learning theory emphasizing the training content focused on CKD and KRT modalities, basic PD mechanisms, cleanness and sterile concepts, hand washing, peritoneal solutions and supplies, bag exchanges, PD adequacy and timing, problem solving, nutrition, CKD complications and pharmacological treatment. In a retrospective design study with historical controls that led to the possibility of bias, the authors reported significantly lower peritonitis rates after 24 months of follow-up when compared with previous rates. Both studies refer to adult learning but do not describe the progress of structural learning or how to evaluate it or the characteristics of the educator.

Training, as Paulo Freire would say, is not the mechanical activation of human skills in order to achieve performance [10]. It is rather a critical exercise, which empowers, breaks free, and leads to autonomy. Each person has his own learning style; patients' learning capacity varies and, therefore, flexible methods are required. In Kolb's experiential learning theory (ELT) perspective, learners construct knowledge by experiencing, reflecting, thinking, and acting. The learning cycle shows that there are two ways in which we can grasp or take in experience – by Concrete Experience or Abstract Conceptualization. There are also two ways we can transform or deal with experience – by Reflective Observation or Active Experimentation [11].

There are patients with mental disabilities, low literacy levels, poor visual acuity, cultural diversity, different native language, advanced age, or pediatrics. This is the same situation faced by any teacher in daily life, with a unique aggravation that is the risk of life and the fear that it entails. Patients need to gain new knowledge that is really meaningful to their lives at that moment and also capable of internalizing them.

Taking Perkins' concepts [12], it is important to make visible the two deficiencies that can be applied to the PD teaching method: fragile knowledge and poor thinking. We refer to fragile knowledge when patients do not remember or actively use much of what they have supposedly learned. We encompass in this concept forgotten knowledge (if the patient will remember the taught facts and skills, the clinical results would improve), inert knowledge (for example, many PD training programs are initiated by explaining the function of the normal kidney to a person who no longer has any kidney function left, or delivering manuals with difficult medical terms that the patient will not require), naive knowledge (naive theories or stereotypes, for example, if one could not finish schooling, one will have difficulty in learning), and finally ritual knowledge (perhaps the common, for example, the so-called step by step, which only allows one to find mechanical solutions to the patients without generating a significant apprenticeship). The goal of education is to think about what is learned and the active use of what has been learned. Although repetition helps memorize, it is not as useful as other strategies that help you think. Many patients now spend one or two training days watching the nurse wash hands, or wash their own hands, without reflecting on the quality of the water they are going to use at home or the reason why they should dry their hands properly in order to avoid wet contamination. The workouts are not designed for the patient to think or be autonomous. Dong et al. [2] studying 130 incidents PD patients reported that after 6 months of follow-up, almost half of them neither washed their hands nor checked the expiration date of the PD bag or leaks, and 10% did not wear a cap or face mask when performing the PD exchange.

An Italian study by Russo et al. [1] demonstrated that after an average of 33 months, a PD re-training was needed for 47% of patients. Re-training every 6 months has been recommended by the ISPD [3]. Several teaching tools have been applied to improve PD training experiences, since Kennedy et al. [13] utilized dolls as a tool; among them, animations, visual images, audio tapes, and online courses. Everyone repeats the same educational experience based on what has been reported, without searching for an educational method where the patient or caregivers have to think.

Learning is a long-lasting change in conduct or ability to behave in a certain way and is the result of practice or other forms of experience. People learn when they acquire the ability to do something different. At the same time, we must remember that learning is inferential. We do not observe learning directly, but through its products or results. Learning is evaluated based on what people say, write, and do. This point is crucial for assessing PD patient skills.

However, we should add that learning involves a change in the ability to behave in a certain way, as people often learn skills, knowledge, beliefs, or behaviors without demonstrating it at the time of learning. Adults learn differently; a practical example may be the use of a new phone. How many people read the manual for use? One automatically starts using it. This allows one to distinguish, conceptualize, design and develop an andragogic fact or process in the field of education. Andragogy (from Greek ἀνήρ "man" and ἀγωγή "guide" or "driving") is the set of teaching techniques intended to educate adults [14]. Several theories explain how adult learning occurs, one of them is constructivism and the way to evaluate what can be learned is through the development of competencies. Constructivism states that apprentices develop their own comprehension of knowledge and skills. In the basic principles of the constructivism, it states that apprentices are more capable to remember information if the constructions contain a personal meaning to them.

The goal of adult education then involves the acquisition of knowledge, the development of skills, and the ability to apply these resources, in an appropriate manner, to each one of the situations arising in the daily life. An adult properly trained in the use of a PD device should have the appropriate competence to decide the physical space where to perform the dialysis procedure safely and to change whenever necessary.

Therefore, educational programs for patients admitted to PD require education focused on the development of competencies. Competencies are comprehensive actions taken, with suitability and commitment, against activities and problems in the context integrating know-how (attitudes and values), know-knowing (concepts and theories) and know-how (procedures) into a perspective of continuous improvement [15].

Learning is meaningful when the content is related in a non-arbitrary and substantial manner, not literally, to what the learner already knows. A non-arbitrary relationship should be understood as a concept, in which the ideas are related to some existing aspect, specifically relevant to the cognitive structure of the learner, such as an image, a significant symbol, a concept, or a proposition. An example of the daily practice of a patient being PD trained will be used to explain it. The diffusion process, that is usually in the curriculum, explain to the patient the removal of the toxins from the blood. For this purpose, graphs of two buckets are used separately where in one appears round figures, representing one toxin (for example, urea or creatinine) in greater amount (concentration) migrating to the other bucket containing a smaller amount (concentration) of the toxin, in order to equilibrate the concentrations across the buckets. The same knowledge can be applied with a "thinking" experiment. The patient is asked to place a tea infusion bag in a cup of hot water and describe what is going on. Why do you think it changes the color of the water in the cup? How much time does it take to change the color tone? Why does this phenomenon seem important? Educational activity has been transformed into an experience based on patient's prior knowledge, allowing him to infer new knowledge to be applied to his health situation. In order to remove toxins, it is necessary to fulfill the prescribed length of time that the PD solution will dwell in the peritoneal cavity.

An important task in a teaching sequence is to determine the problem to be addressed, what can be done in a general fashion and then, with the apprentices, to accomplish it in a specific environment. Here lies one of the main features of the competency model, that is, the training is carried out by addressing real problems with meaning and challenge, because that is precisely what a competency means: it is a comprehensive action to identify, interpret, argue and solve certain contextual problems [16]. Taking these concepts into account and with a self-criticism view of the PD educational programs, the patient-apprentice should be trained at home, in his context, where he will perform the dialysis procedure daily; however, the patient is usually trained at the dialysis center with its in-hospital structure, far away from the reality the patient will face at home.

Assessment is a fundamental element in the learning-teaching process, coordinating, regulating and guiding. Understood as a process, it is immersed in learning and teaching. Therefore, the evaluation process is part of any didactic approach and an integral element of the curriculum design, having an increasingly systematic and scientific approach of all elements involved in the learning and teaching processes: educator, apprentice, methodology, contexts, etc. Just as one has to think, plan and design the teaching activity, one should also think, plan and design the performance of the evaluation, with everything that involves time dedication, resource forecasting, time setting, decision on methodology and strategies, as well as selection of instruments [17]. The guidelines or parameters explaining the competency and allowing evaluation according to the context, present or future, are the performance criteria determining when the person's performance is adequate in certain areas of the learning/training. In order to evaluate these criteria, it is necessary to establish concrete and tangible evidence of what is being learnt of a competency. Evidence evaluation is based on established criteria, and it is necessary to evaluate them as a whole. For each criterion, indicators are established for each level of knowledge and thereby allowing its evaluation. The indicators are signs that show the level in which a competency has developed based on these criteria. Weighting consists in assigning a quantitative value to criteria and indicators in relation to their degree of contribution to the value of the competency. Competencies are usually evaluated within a quantitative range of 0% and 100%; any scale can be applied. In order to evaluate, a percentage is assigned to each one of the criteria taken into account when evaluating one competency, according with one or more evidences. It is necessary to compare the criteria among themselves and, then, for each individual criterion, to compare the indicators in order to determine its degree of relevance in the evaluation of the competency. Understanding the different items to be considered in the competency evaluation, it is important to create an instrument whose main purpose is to share the criteria to attain the learning tasks, and their evaluation among the apprentices (patients) and the educators.

This task roadmap, which will be called Rubric, describes the expectations, shared by the apprentice and educator, about one or several organized activities with different levels of accomplishment: from the least acceptable resolution to the unanimous one, from the most insufficient to the excellent. The Rubric is a powerful tool to evaluate any type of task, but its value should be especially emphasized in evaluating authentic tasks, real life tasks. It manifests itself as an ideal instrument for evaluating competencies, as it allows to analyze the complex tasks, generating a graduation starting from the simplest one to the most complex task. The Rubric is an instrument that, from the start and throughout the process, allows to share the criteria which will be applied to evaluate progress in a framework of formative and continuous evaluation. Furthermore, it reduces the subjectivity of the evaluation and facilitates different educators to coordinate and share the evaluation criteria, allows the apprentice to monitor his own activity, self-assess and promote responsibility for learning. The use of the Rubric facilitates almost immediate feedback, as it concedes substantial response time reduction by offering quantitative and qualitative results based on previously known standards for the development of the task.

Use of Rubrics in Peritoneal Dialysis

Table 1 shows an example of a Rubric for the evaluation of the learnings. The final results will enable one to classify PD learning levels as initial, basic, autonomous, or strategic according to the score achieved. Its design established two domains of knowledge, patient's dialysis safety and CKD management by the patient; each domain contains two competencies to be developed. The first domain requires the development of biosafety and connectology management whereas CKD requires management of complications associated with the technique or the chronic disease itself, as well as the correct use of the local health system.

Table 1. Weighted learning evaluation scale in patients on peritoneal dialysis

Domain	Criteria	Value	Weighted	Points
Biosecurity Management	1.1 Identifies healthiness while maintaining the hygiene of the place and staff. It is ordered during the dialysis procedure. Manages the importance of handwashing in terms of cleanness		2.5	6.25
	1.2. Recognizes and performs procedures recognized as biosecurity barriers. Manages correctly the catheter and cleaning of the exit-site.		5	12.5
	1.3 Identifies the various cleaning products used at home and disinfectants, knows their effects, latency times and inhibitors. Understands the basics of handwashing.	0.25	7.5	18.75
	1.4 It is responsible for the healthiness and cleanness of the home, associates the risk of contamination and evidence. Communicates if notice a difficulty and know how to manage it.		10	25
Managing Connectology and Solutions	2.1 The procedure meets the stages of healthiness and safe exchanges. Meets most pre-connection, connection and disconnection stages with all safety barriers.		3	10.5
	2.2 Meets all stages of pre-connection, connection and disconnection and all safety barriers. Understands the importance of the records.	0.35	6	21
	2.3. Know the concepts of diffusion, osmosis and ultrafiltration. It recognizes the effects of the PD solutions and the dwell time, relates them to weight, blood pressure and daily ultrafiltration.		8	28
	2.4 Understands the steps of the technique associated with the proper functioning of the peritoneum and acts accordingly. Knows how to communicate if he notices difficulties in the operation.		10	35
Managing Health control and using health networks	3.1. Organize your activities to attend monthly control with what you are asked for, effectively sample peritoneal fluid and know how to inject bag medication.		2.5	4.5
	3.2. Recognize long-term use medicines, dosage and importance. Manage the healthcare system Have a structured plan in case of an emergency.		5	9
	3.3. Learn about the use of prescribed medications. Understand the impact of carbohydrate consumption. Find out about the local healthcare system and verbalize about the local healthcare network.	0.18	7.5	13.5
	3.4. Demonstrate responsibility in self-care management.		10	18
Managing complications associated with the technique	4.1. Know the signs of peritoneum inflammation and, in case of evidence of cloudy fluid, act correctly and communicate with the dialysis unit by following the protocol action plan		2.5	5.5
	4.2. Manage water balance in relation to ingested fluids, water ultrafiltration (UF) and daily weight. Knowledge on how and when to use higher glucose concentration PD fluids to manage overhydration responsibly	0.22	5	11
	4.3. Learn the concept of glucose loading and the infection prevention steps. Verbalize these possibilities and actions.		7.5	16.5
	4.4 Demonstrate responsibility and act accordingly in decision-making in case of complications		10	22
Final Score	**Initial 0-27 p**	**Basic 28-53p**	**Autonomous 54-76p**	**Strategic 77-100p**

Table 2. Domain of competence: Safe peritoneal dialysis

Competence: Biosafety Management. 1. Handling of clean and sterile dirty concepts. 2. Recognize the effect of hand washing and the use of alcoholic gel. 3. Incorporate the concept of health at home. 4. Recognize the dialysis technique steps where exists the risk of bacterial contamination.	
Level: Startup program in PD. Days 1 and 2. Phase I	
Process Axis 1: Understand and relate biosafety with hygiene habits and the procedures that will be perform at home with the PD technique	
Criteria (or expected learnings / learning outcomes): 1.4 To demonstrate responsibility in managing self-care at home, to understand the steps of the technique associated with the risk of contamination, which is evidenced by: organized PD exchange room at home, organized technique learning steps according to comfort and maintaining biosecurity regardless of changes in habitat, to maintain self-care at home, to communicate any difficulty and agree with the PD team how to solve it (Expert Patient). 1.3 To identify the various cleaning products you use in your home (bleach, detergents) and disinfectants (alcoholic gel, iodine), know their mode of action, latency times and inhibitors, potential places where germs may exist and understand the basics of hand washing (know and understand). 1.2 To identify and act according to the concepts of dirty, clean and sterile. To recognize and perform procedures recognized as biosafety barriers: second hand washing, mask, prayer position, alcoholic gel, connection, prayer position, alcoholic gel, disconnection. To andles the catheter correctly and cleaning the exit hole. (know how to do) 1.1 To identify self-care at home, by maintaining the hygiene of the place, to be organized in relation to the dialysis procedure, to manage the importance of hand washing in terms of cleanliness and to verbalize when to wash hands. (know how to do).	**Evidence** 1.3/1.4 Organize the room where you will be dialysed according to your comfort, but based on what you have learned about health and hygiene. These behaviors are observed during the home visit. 1.1/1.2 To perform hand washing correctly, to be able to recognize where to place the dialysis products and to maintain order and cleanness at home.

For each competency, criteria have been established representing the tasks learned and the evidence of their learning. Each criterion is weighted on a scale in relation to its performance importance. For example, the domain of competence in the management of biosafety has as its axis of procedure that the patient understands and relates biosafety with hygiene procedures that will be carried out at home with the PD device.

The criteria for learning vary from the least to greatest (from 1 to 4). The Evaluation Rubric is shown in Table 1. Understanding that the criterion is evidenced by the health team, during the home visit, observing the correct actions of the apprentice. For example, perform hand washing correctly, select an adequate space where the PD exchanges will be performed and dialysis material stored, maintain a logical and comfortable order of actions to follow, and thereby not contaminating by touch. The Tables (2, 3, 4 and 5) show domains, criteria, and evidence to be evaluated in a PD patient training program.

Table 3. Domain of competence: Safe peritoneal dialysis

Competence: Management of Connectology and PD solutions. 1. Recognition and handling of PD dialysis bags, PD catheter, minicap, etc. as well as the steps to carry out the dialysis procedure at home. 2. To recognize the order in pre-connection, connection and disconnection steps of the PD exchange and to perform them safely. 3. To include the time required for the PD fluid to remain in the peritoneal cavity (the dialysis process). To incorporate the concepts of toxin diffusion and UF according to the sugar concentration in each PD bag. 4. Reflect properly the choice of the sugar concentration of the PD fluid and the amount of UF per day.

Level: Startup program in PD. Days 3 and 4. Phase ii	
Process Axis 2: Understand and relate the stages of the dialysis process in regard to the force of gravity (connection and disconnection) and the basic notions of the functioning of the peritoneal membrane during the dwell time. (diffusion and osmosis)	
Criteria (or expected learnings / learning outcomes) 1.4 To demonstrate responsibility in the handling of dialysis PD solutions, to understand the technical steps associated with the proper functioning of the peritoneum and to act accordingly: number of PD exchanges prescribed per day, infusion volume, dwell time, UF volume. These steps are evidenced by learning simulations; such as, water retention and use of the correct sugar concentration in the PD solution, decrease in UF in a single change. The patient shall communicate if observe difficulties in the functioning of the peritoneal dialysis (Expert Patient) 1.3 To know from examples of daily life the concepts of diffusion, osmosis and UF. One can recognize the effects of different solutions and the dwell time in daily UF. It relates to the control of bodyweight with the management of blood pressure (BP) and daily UF. (Know and understand). 1.2 To comply with all the stages of pre-connection, connection and disconnection of the PD system utilized and all the safety barriers. Understand the importance of the UF, body weight control and BP records requested. To monitor the UF volume by weighing the drained bag. To learn how and when to receive the monthly ordered PD supplies and to verify their delivered conditions. (Know how to do) 1.1 To act by being able to organize the space to carry out the procedure at home, fulfilling the concepts of health and safety. To fulfill the stages of pre-connection, connection and disconnection of PD system utilized and, also, all the barriers of security. (Know how to do)	**Evidence** 1.4 To combine the prescription of sugar concentrations in the PD solutions according to the diet, especially diabetic and hypertensive patients. Patient knows how to anticipate complications. 1.3 To monitor body weight, BP and UF logs daily in order to maintain body weight and BP under control. 1.1 /1.2 In the home visit, order is perceived and the change is made safely.

Table 4. Domain of competence: Management of chronic disease

Competence: Management of sanitary controls and use of networks. 1. Recognition and management of the various controls required when on dialysis, monthly laboratory control, echocardiogram, participation in educational workshops and home visits. 2. To recognize health goals, use of long-term medication and disease management in order to decide which of them is first priority to be approached. 3. To create a map of the neighborhood location of pharmacies, clinics or nearest hospitals as well as family doctor who can be contacted whenever needed. 4. To reflect on health-disease situation, to know the health system and network, to take appropriate action in case of risk using it and also when to call the dialysis unit.	
Level: Startup program in PD. Days 5 and 6. Phase III	
Process Axis 3: Understand and relate the concepts of chronic disease and its management using the health system correctly or setting it up if it is lacking. Understand the various controls to be received when in a chronic dialysis program and, through its compliance, incorporate the concepts of self-care and autonomy.	
Criteria (or expected learnings / learning outcomes) 1.4 To demonstrate responsibility in self-care management, based on own knowledge and acquired in the dialysis unit. To act accordingly in decision-making for the maintenance of own health and the dialysis technique (Expert Patient). 1.3 To manage the use of chronic medications; for example, which of them is associated with a higher risk of side-effect in case it should be discontinued (ex: cardiovascular). To understand the impact of carbohydrate (flour) consumption on weight control and dialysis. To find out more information about the health system and verbalize how his/her care network is like. (Know and Understand). 1.2 To recognize the list of long-term use medications, their prescribed dosage, and the importance of each one. To know where and how to request the long-term use medications. To know how to carry out the injection of a medication in a PD bag, if required. To structure what to do in case of an emergency, a contact list and a health center to attend. (know to do) 1.1 To organize your personal activities to attend the monthly control visit bringing what is requested (records, documentation, drained dialysis fluid sample or the whole drained PD bag, etc.). In case of need to bring to the monthly visit only a sample of drained PD fluid, the patient needs to know how to collect the peritoneal fluid sample. (know to do)	**Evidences:** 1.3/1.4 To participate in educational workshops. Discuss your experience and solutions to the problems to be faced. 1.1/1.2 To attend regularly the monthly visits to the Clinic and to bring all requested information by the Health care team.

Table 5. Domain of competence: Management of chronic disease

Competence: Management of complications associated with the technique. 1. Recognition and management of the most frequent complications related to the infusion and drainage of peritoneal fluid. 2. To recognize and properly care for the catheter exit site as well as to recognize the signs of infection, acting accordingly. 3. To recognize the normal characteristics of the drained fluid. To identify cloudy fluid as a sign of inflammation and act accordingly. To understand preventive modes of action to prevent peritonitis and exit-site infection. 4. To reflect adequately in search of the error that can lead to a technique complication and to verbalize with own words the most important points of prevention of complications.	
Level: Startup program in PD. Days 5 and 6. Phase III	
Process Axis 4: To understand and relate the concepts of health and personal hygiene to the appearance of infectious complications associated with the peritoneal dialysis technique. To understand the various controls that must be carried over your actions during the procedure and in case of complications, know how to act responsibly.	
Criteria (or expected learnings / learning outcomes)	**Evidence:**
1.4 To demonstrate responsibility in the management of self-care and of possible associated complications. Based on own knowledge acquired in the dialysis unit, the patient consequently acts in decision-making for the maintenance of own health and the dialysis technique. In case of complications, the patient acts in order to achieve the identification of the cause of the complication. (Expert Patient). 1.3 To know the concept of glucose load, its relationship with volume removal, its risks to the peritoneum and the calorie load involved. To know the steps to prevent infections related to intestinal symptoms (diarrhea-constipation), dental interventions, gynecological examinations and the care measures that may be required. (Know and understand).	1.3/1.4 Organize the different controls with other specialists. Manage body weight and diet. To have a critical view in relation to the treatment.
1.2 To manage adequately the water balance in relation to the liquids ingested by mouth, the daily UF and body weight. To know how to use the highest glucose concentration bags to handle overhydration responsibly. (know to do) 1.1 To carry out effectively hand washing and exit-site care. To recognize the signs of peritoneum inflammation and in case of the presence of cloudy fluid to know how to properly manage the peritonitis protocol utilized by the Clinic. (know to do)	1.1/1.2 Faced with a simulated "cloudy" bag, to evaluate how the patient reacts as if it were an infectious complication To recognize and correct biosecurity-related errors when exposed to a simulated situation.

EVALUATION OF EDUCATIONAL PROGRAMS ON PERITONEAL DIALYSIS

Education for patients with various chronic diseases is a challenge for health systems. Diseases such as hypertension, diabetes, obesity and CKD require educational programs provided by the health team so that people can develop skills or change behaviors. These non-formal adult education programs require training of their teachers in pedagogy knowledge and the evaluation of educational programs as well as their results. However, the biggest problem lies in the quality of educational programs and their correct evaluation.

Three core principles guide the planning, implementation, and evaluation activities of patient education programs. The first principle is that the program should be based on scientific evidence, including epidemiological and clinical studies. The second principle is that it should use effective communication strategies and appropriate teaching material to reach the selected recipients and finally, the evaluation should be an integral component of the planning and implementation of the program and used as part of an iterative process of re-planning and improvement of the program's activities [18].

Program evaluation is conceived as the process of measuring, comparing, and issuing a value judgment on the achievements achieved, through the application of methodological schemes that ensure the reliability of the processes and the objectivity of the information obtained. The evaluation of educational programs has existed for about forty years as a scientific discipline. A Program is a systematic plan designed by the educator in the service of educational goals. The educator plans his or her educational action for the apprentice or group, setting goals, selecting means, designing the right conditions, and establishing criteria and valuation guidelines [19]. The characteristics of an educational program can be seen in Table 6.

According to Stufflebeam and Shinkfield, evaluation should be considered a complex but unavoidable process [20]. One of the most conceptually powerful aspects is that the evaluation recognizes the action plan proposed by a program as a working hypothesis.

From this perspective, the evaluation reconstructs the expected causal relationships in key activities to products, from intermediate objectives (effects) to final objectives (impact). For example, the training of hand washing necessary in PD is an activity whose product is the prevention of touch-related infections, with intermediate objectives (lower gram + peritonitis rates) and final goals (better PD technique survival)

Thus, the design of the evaluation and the committed activities aim to put at the center of the analysis the focal problem to which the program seeks to solve and reconstruct the changes in those factors that have a more decisive impact on the resolution problem.

One of the focal problems to face is performing patient training based on safety and not on repetitive steps. In relation to the program, it is important to evaluate its components, objectives and goals, content, media, together with its implementation and development process. In reference to the methodology to be used, the technical quality of the program's own evaluation design is essential. Regardless of the evaluative model chosen, any minimal planning should establish the activities to be evaluated, set the evaluation criteria, choose strategies for obtaining and analyzing information, and then make decisions from it. Evaluation requires certain steps in terms of the program itself, its implementation and the analysis of its results [21].

Table 6. Educational program characteristics

1.	Educational goals and objectives adapted to the characteristics of the recipients in their context
2.	Clearly specify all the key elements to enable evaluability: recipients, agents activities, decisions, strategies and processes, staff roles and responsibilities, times , expected demonstrations
3.	Incorporate sufficient, adequate and effective resources for achieving goals and objectives.
4.	Have a system capable of assessing whether goals and objectives are achieved or not, and if not, where the dysfunctions and deficiencies occur and analyze their causes.

Source: Pérez Juste, R (2000)

Step 1: Evaluation of the Program as Such

It is the most important evaluation activity both because it is the first and basis of all others. It aims to establish the technical quality of the program, its practical feasibility and evaluability. Its function is basically formative, making in advance the improvement decisions that can raise the potential of the program.

The evaluation should collect data on the basic structure of the program, its formulation and the relationship to the needs, gaps, demands and expectations of the recipients (patients, physicians, nurses, nutritionists, social workers). The evaluation generally enables formative decision-making (pre-improvement, staff training e.g.,) and also, in extreme cases, summative decision-making (withdrawal of the program due to lack of resources). The required criteria are observed in Table 7.

The diversity of PD programs is large, but they have several problems in common. One is that the PD program rests entirely in the nurse, instead of having the participation of the entire health team. Moreover, the staff training in adult education methods (Andragogy) is scarce, basically empirical and absent in most of the curricular contents of nephrologists and nurses' training.

In general, institutions do not give sufficiency of the supports, means and resources, in particular on the training, involvement and commitment of the actors and others involved. A common view throughout Latin America is the variety in quantity and quality of allocated doctors and nurses' hours and the effective hours dedicated to patient education. There are countries where the nephrologist is not required for the management of the PD program, often related to lack of resources, but in the same countries their presence is required for hemodialysis sessions.

The feasibility of the program is largely related to the continuity in time of its participants; when a change is generated by high staff turnover, the program reveals a weakness by not having a training system for the new personnel, carrying risks for patients.

Step 2: Evaluation of the Program Implementation Process

This moment aims to facilitate the timely improvement in decision-making and accumulate information to be introduced into future editions of the program. Its function is basically formative. Information on intermediate results and unplanned effects is key to the methodology. It can be done through observation, dialogues, interviews with facilitators, analysis of tasks, intermediate training tests of the team, and subsequent analysis of the information. The criteria are compliance, institutional coherence, and satisfaction of those involved. For example, the number of average training hours received by patients is considered a compliance criterion.

A program is able to evaluate the number of patients who have their learning at initial, basic, autonomous or strategic levels and set up results indicators, for example 75% of their patients should be autonomous. The development of teaching material suitable for the target population is also crucial. The didactic triad in Andragogy and Constructivism places the facilitator, the apprentice and the content on an accessible level, a fact that distinguishes it from the behavioral model.

Learning is an active process where knowledge is built and modeled by experience. We have many times seen videos or manuals that aim to replace the teaching interaction of learning and avoid the creation of learning spaces based on experience, where the apprentice is the actor and not a single viewer.

Table 7. Criteria for the evaluation of educational programs as such

1. Quality, relevance and realism of goals and objectives.
2. Adequacy to recipients and context.
3. Adequacy of the support, means and resources to achieve the objectives, in particular on the training, involvement and commitment of the actors and others involved.
4. Technical quality of evaluation approaches.
5. Technical quality of the program: coherence with the theoretical basis and needs to which it seeks to respond; internal congruence among its components.
6. Program viability.
7. Evaluability: relevance, sufficiency, clarity and accessibility of the available program information necessary at the various times or stages of its implementation and evaluation. Analysis of the difficulties detected and foreseeable in assessing the program.

Step 3: Evaluation of the Results of the Implementation of the Program

The purpose of this stage is to check the effectiveness of the program. The function is fundamentally summative. The evaluation collects results information in relation to objectives. It takes as criteria the effectiveness, defined as a degree of achievement of the proposed objectives, as well as the efficiency of the results in relation to the available means and the circumstances in which the program is applied.

Take as references the starting situation: the program versus itself (progress) and pre-specified levels. The Rubric presented shows us domains that patients must achieve and the educator can teach. There are very clear indicators of the effectiveness of the programs, such as the peritonitis and exit-site infection (ESI) rates, indicating the degree of biosafety domain achieved by the patient. Another indicator associated with the PD technique, complications management, is evidenced by fluid overload, hypertension, or annual hospitalization rates. All these rates should be related to the hours of teaching activity, its quality, method used, facilitator qualification, and relevance of the developed content.

Step 4: Institutionalization of the Evaluation of the Program

Finally, and probably critical is the institutionalization of the educational PD programs evaluation. With the successive cycles of evaluation-improvement-evaluation- improvement, the full integration of the program and its evaluation is achieved, which results in the improvement of both the program and the methodology of the evaluation itself, as well as in the professional improvement of the facilitators. This point requires the integration of the entire nephrology team. For the program's evaluation, it is necessary to have a critical and continuous improvement oversight and to share with the whole nephrology team and patients the achievements, difficulties, and educational/clinical results of the year, as well as the goals for the next year. The PD program evaluation process will also be useful in educating funders regarding feasible, appropriate and accurate measures necessary for running a PD patient training program. Moreover, the evaluation process will enable the funders to correctly allocate economic and human resources by measuring the effectiveness of educational programs.

THERAPEUTIC EDUCATION AND TRAINING OF THE HEALTH TEAM FOR EDUCATIONAL PROGRAMS IN PD

Therapeutic education is administered by health care providers trained for patient education and designed to allow a patient (or family members) to manage the treatment and prevent complications while maintaining or improving the quality of life. Its main objective is to produce a therapeutic effect, in addition to that of all other interventions (pharmacological, physiotherapy, etc.) [22]. Patient therapeutic education has led to a significant decrease in the number of hospital admissions of patients with bronchial asthma or diabetic coma. Besides a decrease in lower limb amputations, it has also resulted in a better quality of life by delaying amputations in 75% of cases [23]. The WHO working with groups on patient therapeutic education report recommends two levels of therapeutic education training for chronic diseases: basic and post-basic. Basic training is designed to learn the educational, psychological and social methods required to educate chronically ill patients. It should also address the biomedical aspects of chronic diseases and the most significant and necessary teachings for patient treatment management. On the other hand, post-basic training is responsible for the ability to coordinate various training activities within an institution or a network of health services. It is designed to train health professionals to become coordinators of patient education programs including prevention, mainly secondary and tertiary [24].

Educational programs for the health team should include direct hands-on experience with patients (patient-based education) as an important part of learning programs. It should also be based on active learning and strengthening students' ability to plan and design their own continuing education (student-centered), based on patient health needs (problem-based). Unlike conventional education courses, facilitator training should be based on several additional disciplines such as communication, technology, psychology and sociology.

PD Patients Nurse Care Management with a Focus on Therapeutic Education

Today, the world faces a new social, economic, political, demographic and cultural reality, affected by unexpected contingencies such as Covid-19 Pandemic (2019 -2020), which demands a Health System capable of meeting the growing health needs of the population, especially in the approach of chronic processes.

There is a growing demand for nurses and their skills. Furthermore, the nephrological nursing competencies of the 21st century need to be evaluated in different environments in order to assess the strengths areas of improvement.

Identifying and applying nursing skills for the care of people treated with PD is a difficult task; this is a very vulnerable patient population, requiring complex care, consuming a lot of socio-health resources and demanding integrated and continuous care. The main focus of nurse care is on therapeutic education and PD nursing needs special training to fulfill its role. Approach strategies should be specific to the CKD patients on PD therapy, usually older adults with associated co-morbidity and poly-medication, who should learn how to perform self-care PD. They are models of clinical practice focused on the patient and his family; implementing instruments to ensure safety and continuity in long-term care. The nursing management we propose is in agreement with the Innovative Chronic Care Models (ICCM), in which "the care of people with chronic diseases requires moving from a reactive, disease-focused model to a proactive and planned model, focused on the person and its context, a model that ensures a good quality of care, promotes longitudinal follow-up and treatment adherence and persistence [25, 26].

The International Society for Peritoneal Dialysis (ISPD) in its recommendations 2020 proposes that, in order for the individual in PD to achieve high quality goals, the dialysis prescription should reflect a decision-making shared process between the patient and the health team in order to establish realistic objectives that maintain quality of life, as well as minimize symptoms and the burden of treatment [27]. To achieve this goal, the nursing education team must have strategies based on therapeutic education [28, 29]. More and more patients require assisted treatments with more emphasis on lower health costs and evidence-based practices; these needs concern patients, health organizations and their caregivers, payers and politicians [30].

The Nursing Care Plan (NCP) is the implementation tool of the Nursing Process and is shown in Figure 1. It assures hospitals of efficient nurse care, interdisciplinary collaboration (by putting everyone with the same care goal), and also meets the documentation requirements needed for insurers and governing bodies. It is a systematic and organized method for managing individualized care, according to the basic approach that each person or group responds differently to a real or potential health impairment. It is proposed to manage nurse care by applying standardized NCP for patients on PD who respond to predictive diagnoses with a focus on self-care and therapeutic education. When predictive diagnoses are identified, they should be ranked to identify nurse care priorities. NANDA International Diagnoses are used to identify appropriate care outcomes (Nursing Outcomes Classification "NOC") [31]; and to apply the best nursing interventions (Nursing Interventions Classification "NIC") [30]. Predictive Nurse Diagnoses, to be included in standardized NCP with a focus on PD patient and family education can be seen in Table 8 [32].

In the 21st century, chronic diseases are a challenge for health systems, due to the costs it generates, but it is also an opportunity for nursing to be present where advanced nursing care programs are needed, conducting case management and monitoring of complex chronic patients. A highly qualified ward is required to perform different functions such as sick case managers, liaison nurse and advanced practice nurse. Incorporating the role of the educator in nursing care practice requires specific training [33]. A minimal curriculum in therapeutic education (based on theories of Andragogy and Constructivism) is offered in the undergraduate and graduate programs for different health professionals working with CKD and dialysis. Furthermore, postgraduate training aimed at advanced PD nurses with a more exclusive dedication to the educational role are available in different countries [34]. Most nurse and physician training programs do not contain training content in therapeutic education in their curriculum. In its early years, PD care training was provided by nurses who had gained PD experience. Such training often focused on acquiring skills evaluated through repetitive actions and quality indicators oriented to the production process. Subsequently, nursing specialization programs were created in nephrological care with professionals who started teaching at the university without having training as teachers or educators. As they did not have the training, they ended up repeating the same traditional way of teaching that were presented to them, without preparation and updating in order to meet the new professional needs required by the labor market [35].

We now face a situation where it is not only enough to have experience to "teach – educate and train"; there is a need to transform this passive attitude into a reconstruction of the learning teaching process, where educational methodologies and techniques are incorporated strengthening the teaching role inherent in the nursing professional.

Table 8. Predictive nurse diagnosis to be included in standardized nursing care plans with a focus on PD patient and family education

NANDA –I Taxonomy	Domain	Diagnosis (Label)
Code 00078	Health Promotion	Ineffective Self-Health Management
Code 00079	Health Promotion	Non- compliance
Code 00126	Perception/Cognition	Deficient Knowledge
Code 00069	Coping/Stress Tolerance	Inefective Coping
Code 00004	Safety/Protection	Infection
Code 00061	Role Relationships	Caregiver Role Strain
Code 00064	Role Relationships	Parental Role Conflict

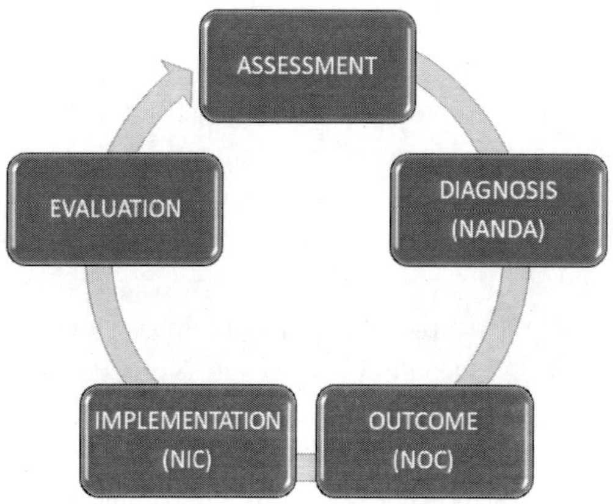

1. **Assessment**: Collecting and analyzing data to gain a hollstic understanding of patients´s needs and risk factors.
2. **Diagnosis**: Using data, patients feedback, and clinical judgement to form the nursing diagnoses.
3. **Outcome/Planning**: Setting short-term and long-term goals based on the nurse´s assessment and diagnosis, ideally with input from the patient. Determine interventions to meet those goals.
4. **Implementation**: Implementing nursing care according to the care plan based on patient´s health conditions and the nursing diagnosis.
5. **Evaluation**: Monitoring (and documenting) the patient's status and progress toward the goals and modifying the care plan as needed.

Figure 1. The Nursing process - five key steps.

If the curriculum of nursing schools manages to be unified, recognizing the importance of the therapeutic and educational activities, we would form nurses more committed to the profession [36]. Currently, WHO "has raised growing concern in health systems and in the educational and employment situation of nursing, identified as a group that will be increasingly important in the response of health systems to epidemiological conditions of populations" [37]. Therefore, the PD nurse training goes beyond knowledge of the disease and its treatment; the importance of its role lies in how to educate the chronic patient in improving health and quality of life." Unlike health education, which aims to promote health and prevent the onset of disease, patient education is a secondary or rather tertiary prevention, aimed exclusively at individuals affected by a chronic disease. Its purpose is to train patients in the treatment, monitoring, and prevention of complications arising from their own disease. In short, it is a question of the patient being able to manage his/her own disease [38]. Self-care patient education is characterized by an authentic planned and organized transfer of competencies (so far considered exclusive to health professionals) to the patient. In other words, the patient achieves as much autonomy as possible compared to dependence on care services. From this perspective, patient education is not simply about "informing the patient about aspects related to the illness. Information is not knowledge, but information can participate in building the knowledge if integrated into the experience".

Health Literacy, Educational Level and Health Outcomes

Health literacy and educational level formally achieved by the patients together with the quality of the educational PD programs compose a triangle, which needs to be analyzed for its impact on health outcomes. Health literacy reverberates in different spheres of patient behavior such as in the use of health services, self-management capacity, adherence to the treatment, search for information, decision-making, and commitment to preventive measures. Relationships between low levels of health literacy and an increased utilization of health services in the United States, as well as in Europe, have been reported. It seems that the possibility of complications occurrence increases as health literacy levels decrease [39, 40]. Patients with lower health literacy levels feel less able to manage their illnesses, get less involved in the decision-making in respect to their own clinical conditions and also present higher risk of hospitalization and mortality [41, 42]. Studies focused on the importance of educational achievements in the health outcomes of CKD patients are scarce [43].

Two small studies with patients treated with dialysis have indicated that a lower level of health literacy is associated with a 54% higher mortality risk (HR, 1.54; 95% CI, 1.01-2.35), whereas tertiary education is associated with ~~a~~ 46% lower mortality when compared to primary education (HR, 0.54; 95% CI, 0.32-0.91) [44]. Several authors have reported that formally achieved educational factors are associated to PD complications. In a large observational multicenter Brazilian PD study (BRAZPD), Martin et al. have demonstrated that the educational level of the patients is associated to the "peritonitis-free" survival risk (illiteracy versus university education level: HR=1.75, 95% CI=1.04-2.92; primary versus university education level: HR = 1.64; CI 95% = 1.06 – 2.54; and secondary versus university education level: HR = 1.57; CI 95% = 0.99 – 2.49) [45]. Chern et al. observed an association between a lower educational level and risk of peritonitis (HR=1.45; 95% CI = 1.01–2.06, p = 0.0454) [46]. Kim et al. reported similar results in a Korean population, where an intermediary or primary school level (< 9 years of schooling) was associated with a significant risk of peritonitis (HR 1,61; IC del 95%: 1,10–2,36) [47].

Zhi-Kai Yang et al., in a large-scale retrospective multicenter study, showed that a higher educational level for any member of the family was a predictive factor, independently of the PD outcome, except for death, cardiovascular event, or occurrence of a first episode of peritonitis, after adjusting for cofounding factors. This is the first study that provides information on the impact of the educational status of family members on the outcomes of PD patients [48]. Tong et al. confirmed the results of Yang et al. Besides presenting the close relationships among the family educational and income levels, rural residency and less medical attention, the multivariate analysis also validated that the predictive role of the family educational level is not confounded by these aforementioned factors [49]. Xu et al. reported that the educational level of patients and families do not have an impact on the occurrence of the first episode of peritonitis, probably due to the fact that the enrolled PD centers were well-developed with PD professionals as well as in relation to PD education programs for professionals and patients [50].

In a prospective cohort study of 1952 incident PD patients enrolled in BRAZPD from December 2004 to October 2007, cumulative patient survival was lower in the low educational level (EL) group (< 4 school years) when compared to high EL group (≥ 4 school years) - (Log Rank test $\chi^2 = 4.29$, $p = 0.03$); but technique survival did not vary significantly (Log Rank test $\chi^2 = 0.90$, $p = 0.34$) between the EL groups. However, in Cox-regression adjusted analyses comparing patients with < 4 years vs ≥ 4 years of education, similar hazard ratios of death (HR = 0.97; 95% CI = 0.73 - 1.29; p = 0.84) and technique survival (HR = 1.06; 95% CI = 0.81-1.38; p = 0.67) were observed (personal communication, by Bastos et al. - not published).

This conclusion refers to the importance of the PD Teams on the outcomes results. The best manner to achieve educational programs is not yet well-defined. Several authors have tried to identify training methods to prevent peritonitis and some protective factors have been identified. Methods utilized during the process of teaching-learning, such as the use of audio support along the practical and theoretical training, have suggested a lower risk of occurring new episodes of peritonitis after the first one [51]. In Uruguay, Gadola et al. have demonstrated that a PD educational program based on the principles of adult learning is associated with a lower peritonitis rate (0.29 episode per patient/year in comparison to 0.48 per patient/year with the former used educational program ($p < 0.05$)[9]. Following the same line, utilizing the principles of Andragogy, the CECODIAR study evaluated the impact of a randomized educational intervention on the residual renal function (RRF) and left ventricular mass (LVM) of incident PD and HD patients, followed-up for 36 months. The results showed improved cardiovascular (CV) outcomes in the group that received CV education [52].

The teaching method plays an important role in the outcomes results. BRAZPD demonstrated that a compounded training time longer than 15 hours was associated with a lower peritonitis rate (0.26 episode per patient/year) when compared to those patients with a training time shorter than 15 hours (0.32 episode per patient/year) ($p = 0.01$). Less than 60 minutes of training per day was associated with a higher peritonitis rate when compared to those patients with a training time between 60 and 120 minutes per day ($p = 0.03$). Being trained during the ten days immediately post PD catheter implantation was associated with a higher peritonitis rate when compared to training performed pre-catheter implantation. (0.32 vs 0.28 episode per patient/year)[53]. In an interesting study, Castro et al. investigated the importance of the training site and its impact on peritonitis rates. Their results showed an improvement in the peritonitis incidence, from one episode per 25 patient/months to one episode per 44 patient/months, after the implementation of home PD training (HR = 0.59; 95% CI = 0.43-0.81) [54]. Hsu et al. indicated that a multidisciplinary education program, previous to dialysis start, was associated to a longer peritonitis-free survival. PD theoretical learning and practical training may be a challenge for some patients and, therefore, the PD learning programs must be flexible and fit to each person individual needs [55].

One should pay special attention to patients with lower education levels, who may need adjusted learning methods/styles. When evaluating the knowledge and behavior of 191 Italian PD patients, Russo et al. [1] found that 47% of their patients needed retraining, at a certain point in time. We suggest that written PD education support is associated with a lower rate of peritonitis-free survival. It has been indicated that informative educational material directed to CKD patients are beyond the literacy level of the average patient. In consequence, many patients do not benefit from these offered written information as they lack the necessary skills to comprehend them [56].

The intention, sometimes, is to replace the role of the facilitator by a written or audiovisual support to the patients; thereby reducing the need for explanations and/or educational investment by part of the team during the learning process. The final product of this conduct is a worsening in the patient care and attention. The PD training programs should contain alternative forms, means and modes in order to offer the best education to each and every patient. As we write this chapter, a multicenter Peruvian study is ongoing, in order to evaluate the learning of utilizing one Rubric of PD competences evaluation similar to the one proposed in this chapter.

CONCLUSION

The educational activity, understood as a therapeutic act, requires the training of the professionals assigned to that task, with the necessary tools to evaluate the learning of patients and the quality of the programs. Today many patients around the world are being educated for PD, but the criteria and modes of training are changing rapidly.

It is time to create a common language for evaluation of educational activities, based on patient safety and to realize when the patient is ready to go home to perform his/her PD treatment. It is time to evaluate our educational programs from a 360-degree perspective. How are our nurses educated and to what extent do our physicians participate in the assessment of education? What awareness do we have of what the patient has learned when sent home? It is time to have a 360-degree view on what has been done in the PD educational field, but not return to the earlier times. Now, it is time to reflect and move forward to a full therapeutic education, based in Andragogy and Constructivism.

REFERENCES

[1] Russo R, Manili L, Tiraboschi G, Amar K, De Luca M, Alberghini E, et al. Patient re-training in peritoneal dialysis: Why and when it is needed. *Kidney Int*. 2006; 70 (Suppl103): S127–32.

[2] Dong J, Chen Y. Impact of the bag exchange procedure on risk of peritonitis. *Perit Dial Int*. 2010; 30(4): 440–7.

[3] Bernardini J, Price V, Figueiredo A. ISPD Guidelines/Recommendations Peritoneal Dialysis Training. *Perit Dial Int*. 2006; 26: 625–32.

[4] Piraino B. Innovations in Treatment Delivery, Risk of Peritonitis, and Patient Retention on Peritoneal Dialysis. *Semin Dial*. 2017; 30(2): 158-163.

[5] Prowant BF. Determining if characteristics of peritoneal dialysis home training programs affect clinical outcomes: Not an easy task. *Perit Dial Int*. 2006; 26: 643– 644,.

[6] Zhang L, Hawley CM, Johnson DW. Focus on peritoneal dialysis training: Working to decrease peritonitis rates. *Nephrol Dial Transplant*. 2016; 31(2): 214–22.

[7] Stonecypher K. Creating a patient education tool. *J Contin Educ Nurs*. 2009; 40(10): 462–7.

[8] Hall G, Bogan A, Dreis S, Duffy A, Greene S, Kelley K, et al. New directions in peritoneal dialysis patient training. *Nephrol Nurs J.* 2004; 31(2): 149-154,159-163.
[9] Gadola L, Poggi C, Dominguez P, Poggio MV, Lungo E, Cardozo C. Risk Factors and Prevention of Peritoneal Dialysis-Related Peritonitis. *Perit Dial Int.* 2018; (3): pdi.2017.00287.
[10] Dale J, Hyslop-Margison EJ. Paulo Freire: Teaching for Freedom and Transformation. Springer Science+Business Media B.V. 2010, editor. 2010.
[11] Kolb A. Elements of effective E-Learning. In: J. Armstrong and CVF, editor. *Handbook of Management Learning*, Education and Development. 2009. p. 4268.
[12] Perkins D. La escuela inteligente. *Anim Genet.* 2008; [Smart school]
[13] Kennedy J. One nurse's experience. The development of CAPD dialysable dolls. *J Nephrol Nurs.* 1985; 2(5): 231-235.
[14] Alonso Chacón P. La Andragogía como disciplina propulsora de conocimiento en la educación superior. *Rev Electrónica Educ.* 2012; 16(1): 15–26. [Andragogy as a knowledge-promoting discipline in higher education.]
[15] Tobón S, Pimienta J, García J. Secuencias Didácticas: Aprendizaje y Evaluación de Competencias. *Revista Mexicana de Educación a Distancia.* 2010; 12: 77–92. [Didactic Sequences: Learning and Evaluation of Competences. *Mexican Journal of Distance Education*]
[16] Villardon L. Evaluación del aprendizaje. *Educ siglo XXI.* 2006; 58(24): 57–76. [Learning Assessment]
[17] Brookhart SM. Educational Assessment Knowledge and Skills for Teachers. *Educ Meas Issues Pract.* 2011; 30(1): 3–12.
[18] Gallivan J, Greenberg R, Brown C. The national diabetes education program evaluation framework: How to design an evaluation of a multifaceted public health education program. *Prev Chronic Dis.* 2008; 5(4).
[19] Well C, Hernandez S, Alonso E. A brief history of program evaluation. University Editorial Group, editor. In *theory, models and methods of evaluation of programs.* Madrid; 2004. 9–30 p.
[20] Stufflebeam A, Shinkfield D. *Theoretical and practical guide Systematic evaluation.* Publication Center of the Ministry of Education and Science; editor. Madrid: Paidos; 1995.
[21] Pérez Juste R. Evaluación de programas educativos. *Bordón Rev Pedagog.* 1991; 43(4): 261–381. [Evaluation of educational programs]
[22] Assal JP et al. Patient education 2000. In: *New trends in patient education.* Amsterdam,: Elservier; 1995.
[23] Assal JP, Albeanu A, Peter-Riesch B, Vaucher J. [Cost of training a diabetes mellitus patient. Effects on the prevention of amputation]. *Diabete Metab.* 1993 Dec; 19(5 Suppl): 491—495.
[24] Martin PY, Droulez MG, Sexton-Dobby A, Marangon N, Hadaya K, Saudan P, et al. [The importance of education in the management of chronic kidney disease patient]. *Rev Med Suisse.* 2009 Feb; 5(192): 470-472,474.
[25] World Health Organization. Innovative Care for Chronic Conditions Framework [Internet]. *Innovative Care for Chronic Conditions: Building blocks for Action.* Washington, DC.; 2013. Available from: http://www.who.int/chronic_conditions/icccreport/en/.

[26] Wagner EH, Glasgow RE, Davis C, Bonomi AE, Provost L, McCulloch D, et al. Quality improvement in chronic illness care: a collaborative approach. *Jt Comm J Qual Improv*. 2001 Feb; 27(2): 63–80.

[27] Brown EA, Blake PG, Boudville N, Davies S, de Arteaga J, Dong J, et al. International Society for Peritoneal Dialysis practice recommendations: Prescribing high-quality goal-directed peritoneal dialysis. *Perit Dial Int*. 2020; 40(3): 244–53.

[28] Blake PG, Brown EA. Person-centered peritoneal dialysis prescription and the role of shared decision-making. *Perit Dial Int*. 2020 May; 40(3): 302–9.

[29] Gonzalez Mestre A. Autonomy of the patient with chronic diseases: From passive patient to active patient. *Rev Enfermería Clínica*. 2014; 24(1): 67–73.

[30] Moorhead S, Jhonson M, Maas M, Swanson E. Nursing Outcomes Classifications, NOC. 4ta. Ed. Universidad de Iowa., editor. Elservier; 2009. Pag. XIV.

[31] Herdman Header KS. NANDA *International Nursing Diagnoses Definitions & Classification*, 20. 2017. 500 p.

[32] Pisano González MM, González Pisano A. [Modifying habits and treatment adherence, essential for controlling the chronic disease]. *Enferm Clin*. 2014; 24(1): 59–66.

[33] OMS/FAO. Dieta, nutrición y prevención de enfermedades crónicas, Informe de una Consulta Mixta de Expertos. *Ser Inf técnicos* 916. 2003; 1: 1–152.

[34] Jansa M, Galindo M, Valverde M, Yoldi C, Vidal M, Isla P. The Spanish Diabetes Society (SED) statement on the curricular and professional profile of expert/specialized nurses caring for people with diabetes, their relatives or caregivers. *Av Diabetol*. 2014; 28(2): 35–7.

[35] Paim AS, Iappe NT, Rocha DLB. Métodos de enseñanza utilizados por docentes del curso de enfermería: Enfoque en la metodología de investigación. *Enferm Glob*. 2015; 14(1): 136–52. [Teaching Methods Used by Nursing Course Professors: Focus on Research Methodology]

[36] Ponti L. *La enfermería y su rol en la educación para la salud* بىبىب. Editorial Teseo, editor. ثب ب ث ب ث. Ciudad Autónoma de Buenos Aires; 2016. [*Nursing and its role in health education*]

[37] Malvarez Silvina, Famer Cristianne CM. Proyecto de Recursos Humanos para el Desarrollo de la Salud (DH) Área de Sistemas y Servicios de Salud (HSS). Proy Recur Humanos para el Desarro la Salud Área Sist y Serv Salud. 2008; 55. [*Human Resources Project for Health Development (DH) Health Systems and Services Area (HSS). Human Resources Project for Health Development Area Sist y Serv Salud. 2008; 55.*]

[38] Alfonso MT. Educación al Paciente Crónico. *Rev Of la Soc Española Enfermería Nefrológica*. 1996; 1(1992): 1–12. [Chronic Patient Education. Rev Of the Spanish Soc *Nursing Nephrology*.]

[39] Vandenbosch J, Van den Broucke S, Vancorenland S, Avalosse H, Verniest R, Callens M. Health literacy and the use of healthcare services in Belgium. *J Epidemiol Community Health*. 2016 Oct; 70(10): 1032–8.

[40] Bailey SC, Brega AG, Crutchfield TM, Elasy T, Herr H, Kaphingst K, et al. Update on health literacy and diabetes. *Diabetes Educ*. 2014; 40(5): 581–604.

[41] Palumbo R. Discussing the Effects of Poor Health Literacy on Patients Facing HIV: A Narrative Literature Review. *Int J Heal Policy Manag*. 2015 May; 4(7): 417–30.

[42] Mackey LM, Doody C, Werner EL, Fullen B. Self-Management Skills in Chronic Disease Management: What Role Does Health Literacy Have? *Med Decis Making*. 2016 Aug; 36(6): 741–59.

[43] Morton RL, Schlackow I, Mihaylova B, Staplin ND, Gray A, Cass A. The impact of social disadvantage in moderate-to-severe chronic kidney disease: an equity-focused systematic review. *Nephrol Dial Transplant*. 2016 Jan; 31(1): 46–56.

[44] Cavanaugh KL, Wingard RL, Hakim RM, Eden S, Shintani A, Wallston KA, et al. Low health literacy associates with increased mortality in ESRD. *J Am Soc Nephrol*. 2010 Nov; 21(11): 1979–85.

[45] Martin LC, Caramori JCT, Fernandes N, Divino-Filho JC, Pecoits-Filho R, Barretti P. Geographic and educational factors and risk of the first peritonitis episode in Brazilian Peritoneal Dialysis study (BRAZPD) patients. *Clin J Am Soc Nephrol*. 2011 Aug; 6(8): 1944–51.

[46] Chern YB, Ho PS, Kuo LC, Chen JB. Lower education level is a major risk factor for peritonitis incidence in chronic peritoneal dialysis patients: a retrospective cohort study with 12-year follow-up. *Perit Dial Int*. 2013; 33(5): 552–8.

[47] Kim HJ, Lee J, Park M, Kim Y, Lee H, Kim DK, Joo KW, Kim YS, Cho EJ, Ahn C, Oh KH. Lower Education Level Is a Risk Factor for Peritonitis and Technique Failure but Not a Risk for Overall Mortality in Peritoneal Dialysis under Comprehensive Training System. *PLoS One*. 2017 Jan 5; 12(1): e0169063.

[48] Yang ZK, Han QF, Zhu TY, Ren YP, Chen JH, Zhao HP, et al. The associations between the family education and mortality of patients on peritoneal dialysis. *PLoS One*. 2014; 9(5): 1–7.

[49] Tong A, Sainsbury P, Craig JC. Support interventions for caregivers of people with chronic kidney disease: a systematic review. *Nephrol Dial Transplant*. 2008 Dec; 23(12): 3960–5.

[50] Xu R, Zhuo M, Yang Z, Dong J. Experiences with assisted peritoneal dialysis in China. *Perit Dial Intl*. 2012; 32(1): 94–101.

[51] Lachenbruch PA. Comparisons of two-part models with competitors. *Stat Med*. 2001 Apr; 20(8): 1215–34.

[52] Moretta G, Viñuela A, Lara C, Duccase C et col. Impact of Randomized Educational Intervention on Residual Renal Function and Left Ventricular Mass Index in Incident PD and HD Patients. *J Am Soc Nephrol*. 2014; 25: 607.

[53] Figueiredo AE, Moraes TP de, Bernardini J, Poli-de-Figueiredo CE, Barretti P, Olandoski M, et al. Impact of patient training patterns on peritonitis rates in a large national cohort study. *Nephrol Dial Transplant*. 2015 Jan; 30(1): 137–42.

[54] Castro MJ, Celadilla O, Muñoz I, Martínez V, Mínguez M, Auxiliadora Bajo M, et al. Home training experience in peritoneal dialysis patients. *EDTNA ERCA J*. 2002; 28(1): 36–9.

[55] Hsu CK, Lee CC, Chen YT, Ting MK, Sun CY, Chen CY, et al. Multidisciplinary predialysis education reduces incidence of peritonitis and subsequent death in peritoneal dialysis patients: 5-year cohort study. *PLoS One*. 2018; 13(8): e0202781.

[56] Morony S, Flynn M, McCaffery KJ, Jansen J, Webster AC. Readability of Written Materials for CKD Patients: A Systematic Review. *Am J Kidney Dis*. 2015 Jun; 65(6): 842–50.

In: Issues in Kidney Disease – Dialysis
Editors: Stephen Z. Fadem and José A. Moura-Neto
ISBN: 978-1-68507-000-7

Chapter 18

DEVELOPMENTS IN IMPLANTABLE AND WEARABLE ARTIFICIAL KIDNEYS

Megha Salani*[*], *MD and Thomas Golper, MD
Vanderbilt University Medical Center, Nashville, TN, USA

ABSTRACT

Development of new devices for renal replacement therapy includes wearable and implantable models. Wearable artificial kidneys use sorbent columns to regenerate dialysate allowing for smaller, portable devices. The implantable artificial kidney mimics the kidney using cell culture and nanotechnology. These devices are currently in various stages of development. The mechanism of action and currently available data will be discussed in this chapter. Further studies are needed to show the safety and efficacy reasons and to prove non-inferiority to current dialysis modalities. Such studies can provide data regarding the clearance of small and middle molecules as well as the patient's experience and comfort of use. Over time, it will be important to ascertain how they affect performance status, nutritional status, quality of life, and mortality.

Keywords: implantable, wearable, portable

INTRODUCTION

Current home dialysis options allow for more patient autonomy and a potentially improved quality of life compared with in-center hemodialysis, but also impose a burden of care on the patient and their care partners. Thus, innovations in this field should be aimed at improving quality of life and reducing the burden of self-care. Wearable artificial kidneys (WAKs) and implantable artificial kidneys (IAKs) are promising new technologies that are currently undergoing testing. The need for large water and electric supplies and storage space for large/heavy dialysate may be prohibitive for home dialysis candidates. If mitigated with newer

[*] Corresponding Author's E-mail: megha.salani@vumc.org.

artificial kidney models, home dialysis may become more widely available. Ease of use and reduction in training time could also make these modalities more desirable for both physicians and patients. Portability can help with normalization of lifestyle for end-stage kidney disease patients. Although the patient and healthcare costs of such devices are not yet well-defined, widespread use of such devices may reduce the costs associated with in-center dialysis such as building, maintenance, and staffing costs. These devices can also reduce the impact of dialysis on the environment as in-center hemodialysis has a large carbon footprint and requires substantial amounts of water. This chapter will focus on how these technologies work, including potential advantages and disadvantages. Specifically, we will discuss the automated wearable artificial kidney (AWAK) and wearable artificial kidney (WAK), which have undergone small human trials, as well as the implantable artificial kidney (IAK), which is in preclinical testing.

PORTABLE DIALYSIS TECHNOLOGIES

To better understand the concept of portable dialysis, we will discuss the WAK and AWAK in more depth. Briefly, these devices run on batteries and use sorbent technology to regenerate dialysis so that they are not attached to large electric or water supplies. They are small enough to be worn on one's body, allowing the patient to move about while on dialysis [1, 2].

Sorbent-Based Dialysate Regeneration

Prior to discussing wearable artificial kidneys, it is worth discussing sorbent technology, which allows for regeneration of spent dialysate. This allows for less water/dialysate need, which allows the dialysis process to be more portable. The regeneration occurs when the dialysate runs through different sorbent columns that rid the dialysate of waste products (Table 1). The first column contains urease, resulting in the hydrolysis of urea into ammonia and carbon dioxide. Hydration with water molecules provides hydrogen and hydroxide ions - the hydrogen protonates ammonia molecules and the hydroxide ions combine with carbon dioxide to become bicarbonate. The next column contains zirconium phosphate, which has a negative charge to which hydrogen and sodium ions are initially bound at the time of manufacture. The hydrogen and sodium ions are exchanged for cations in spent dialysate, such as potassium, calcium, magnesium, and ammonium. The next layer of the sorbent column is composed of zirconium oxide and zirconium carbonate with bound bicarbonate and acetate, which exchange for negatively charged compounds including phosphate and sulfates. Organic toxins are then removed from the dialysate by a bed of activated charcoal. The dialysate is then recharged with calcium and magnesium to become fresh dialysate and returns to flow through the dialyzer again. Use of sorbent technology with dialysis in the past was sometimes complicated by ammonia breakthrough, leading to nausea and hypotension, and the generation of carbon dioxide bubbles due to the binding of released hydrogen with carbonate [3].

Table 1. Example of sorbent columns

Column	Binds	Releases
Urease Layer	-	Ammonium, bicarbonate
Zirconium Phosphate	Ammonium, calcium, magnesium, potassium, other cations	Sodium, hydrogen
Zirconium Oxide and Zirconium Carbonate	Phosphate, fluoride, heavy metals	Acetate, bicarbonate, sodium
Activated Carbon	Heavy metals, creatinine, uric acid, other organic molecules	-

Wearable Artificial Kidney

The WAK (Wearable Artificial Organs Inc.) is a wearable blood-based renal replacement device that can be worn like a belt or a vest (Figure 1). The device is less than 5 kg, is battery operated, and uses less than 400 mL of sterile water. The system is primed with 0.45% sodium chloride solution and connected to a dual-lumen HD catheter. Blood is anticoagulated with heparin using a syringe pump and proceeds to a 2-channel pump that alternately propels blood and dialysate to a small polysulfone hollow-fiber dialyzer. The blood pump compensates for low blood flows by alternating blood and dialysate pulses thus oscillating the dialyzer transmembrane pressure 60 to 70 times per minute. This is called a pulsating push-pull flow, where the blood compartment is at peak flow when dialysate flow is at its trough, and vice versa. When the blood exits the dialyzer, it goes through a bubble detector and the blood flow is halted if bubbles are present. Otherwise, the blood is returned to the patient. The spent dialysate is regenerated using sorbents as indicated above with the excess diverted via an ultrafiltration pump to a waste bag [4]. This system has been studied in preclinical trials and trials in humans [1, 5-7]. In one study in humans of 24-hour application of the WAK, average urea clearance was 22.7 mL/min. Electrolytes and pH were stable and ammonia was not detected. Complications included dialysate flow issues related to carbon dioxide bubbles, related to sorbents as discussed above, catheter clotting, and needle dislodgement from a fistula (which was detected by the safety mechanisms in place) [7]. Because of the risk for accidental disconnection, the WAK is likely to be used with a catheter rather than needles in a fistula. Proper aseptic technique combined with continuous use may help minimize infectious complications associated with catheter use, but the consequences of continuous catheter use are not well-defined. Because the dialysate used in the WAK is sterile (dialysate in conventional dialysis is not), there may be fewer stimuli for chronic inflammation, but this is yet to be seen. Dr. Victor Gura et al. are currently working on using lighter materials and combining pumps to make the device smaller and lighter during the day. Having a separate diurnal and nocturnal device can allow the patient to be even more mobile during the daytime, while still obtaining adequate clearance. Additional trials with these modifications to ensure safety and efficacy are needed before more widespread use of the WAK.

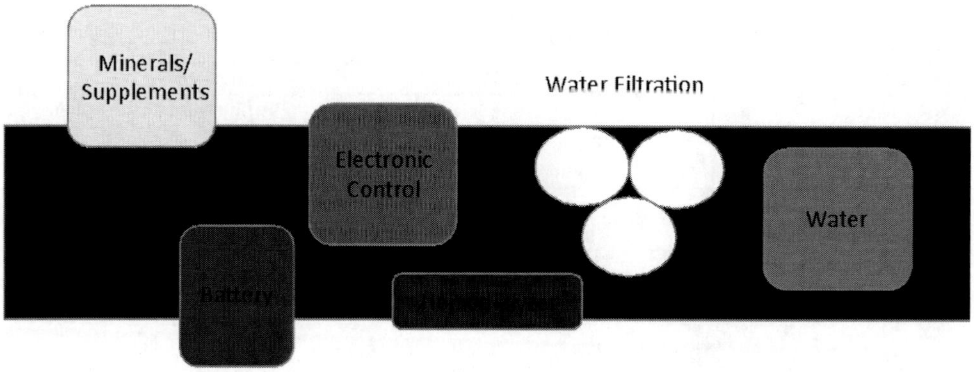

Figure 1. Schematic of the WAK.

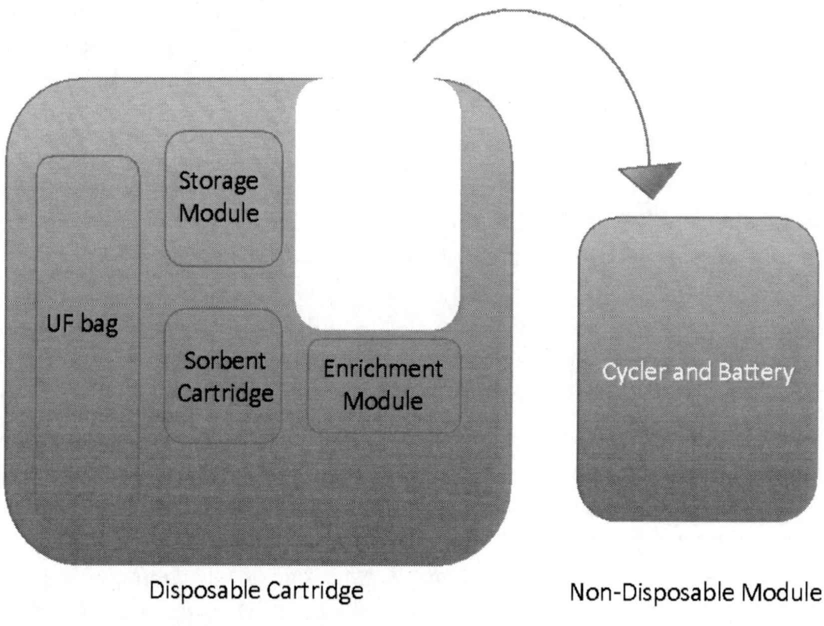

Figure 2. Schematic of the AWAK.

Automated Wearable Artificial Kidney

AWAK Technologies Pte. Ltd. utilizes sorbent technology to develop portable hemodialysis and peritoneal dialysis (PD) systems. The AWAK PD is a tidal PD-based artificial kidney designed to be worn like a purse (Figure 2). Initially, 1 to 1.5L of dialysate is placed in the peritoneal cavity. The AWAK system drains 500 mL of equilibrated dialysate into the storage module. The dialysate goes through the sorbents for toxin removal as described above. The sorbent system can release hydrogen that can bind carbonate and form carbon dioxide bubbles. The fluid is degassed before being supplemented with electrolytes and returning to the peritoneal cavity. Each of these exchanges takes 7.5 minutes with 8 exchanges per hour. The reserve volume is returned to the peritoneal cavity and the remaining fluid drains into an ultrafiltration bag from which the ultrafiltrate can eventually be discarded. The sorbent cartridge can be used for 6-8 hours before being discarded. In a study of 20 patients, the AWAK was worn for 4-24 hours at a time and provided an average urea clearance of 31.5 mL/min [2]. There were no safety issues during this short window; the consequences of continuous fluid exchange and regenerated dialysate and how this affects the risk for peritonitis, hyperglycemia, membrane failure, and encapsulating peritoneal sclerosis are not yet known. The use of tidal PD and small dwell volumes may help reduce drain-related pain and risk for hernias. The use of a single cartridge per day with or without a long dwell could allow for adequate clearance without being tethered to a machine or the need for multiple manual exchanges.

Implantable Artificial Kidney

The IAK (Vanderbilt University Medical Center and University of California, San Francisco) is designed to be surgically implanted to mimic a native kidney. The IAK combines a high-efficiency filter (the HemoCartridge) with a bioreactor of cultured renal tubule epithelial cells (the BioCartridge) as shown in Figure 3. The device would be connected to the arterial vasculature and would use the patient's own blood pressure to pump blood through the filter. The HemoCartridge is made of silicon membranes that form filters; each microchip has slit-shaped pores similar to glomerular slit diaphragms [8-10]. The ultrafiltrate generated in the HemoCartridge is processed by the BioCartridge, which contains tubular cells from human cadaver kidneys grown in cell culture on a scaffolding of silicon membranes. The BioCartridge returns salt, water, and glucose to the blood and progressively concentrates toxins into a small volume of fluid similar to urine. The scaffold allows the device to be implanted without the need for immunosuppression and the blood conduits are designed to protect blood from stagnation and shear so that it can be used without anticoagulation [11-13]. The device has been implanted in experimental animals for up to a month but has not yet been studied in humans [14]. It is possible that the IAK could be implanted with the toxin-laden ultrafiltrate directed to the bladder. The patients may excrete 2-4 liters of ultrafiltrate daily and would need to weigh themselves often to determine fluid intake goals. Close monitoring of electrolytes and urea clearance could guide the need for dietary restrictions or supplement needs. If this is successfully implemented in humans, one drawback to its use is the possible need for surgical intervention for thrombosis or device failure since it is implanted.

Conclusion

The research and development of renal replacement therapy devices provide promise for a better life for dialysis patients in the near future. Some of the models in preclinical and clinical trials have been addressed, yet even these may continue to evolve before being ready for widespread use. It is also yet to be seen how other new technologies will be used in artificial kidneys, such as the activated wafer deionization (AWEDI) technology, which uses an electrical field to drive ion transport through ion exchange wafers, simulating the ion transport function of the nephron [15].

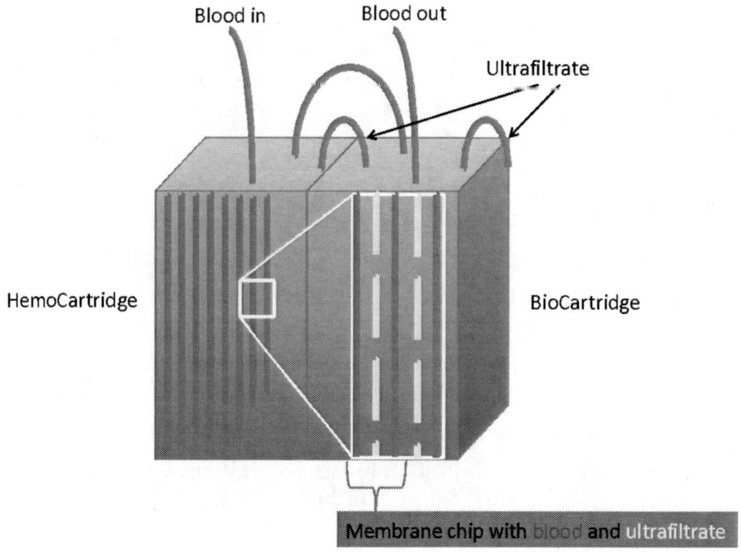

Figure 3. Schematic of the IAK.

Innovative devices may allow home dialysis to be more accessible and/or enticing and address several of the factors that patients receiving dialysis rate as most important, i.e., fatigue and energy, ability to travel, resilience and coping, and stress on family. Increased treatment time and higher clearance may improve middle molecule clearance compared with current therapies and may help mitigate dialysis-related hypotension and myocardial stunning. To be acceptable for patients, the wearable devices will need to be lightweight and easy to use. The implantable device will need to have a long service life to minimize the need for recurrent procedures. The risks of such technologies are not completely defined at this time pending additional safety and efficacy trials.

Given the reduction of water use, the devices discussed in this chapter could be used in arid areas where water is scarce. Even where water is not a barrier to dialysis, such devices can help to reduce water consumption, which is substantial with current dialysis practices. In-center dialysis also has significant carbon emissions so the reduction in electricity use with these technologies may have important environmental implications if they become available for widespread use. Successful implementation may also lead to reduced healthcare costs for both the patient and the healthcare system.

REFERENCES

[1] Gura V, Beizai M, Ezon C, Polaschegg HD. Continuous renal replacement therapy for end-stage renal disease. The wearable artificial kidney (WAK). *Contrib Nephrol* 2005;149:325-333.

[2] Lee DB, Roberts M, Lee DBN, Roberts M. A peritoneal-based automated wearable artificial kidney. *Clin Exp Nephrol*. 2008;12(3):171-180.

[3] Lewin AJ, Greenbaum MA, Gordon A, Maxwell MH. Current status of the clinical application of the Redy R dialysate delivery system. *Proc Clin Dial Transplant Forum.* 1972;2:52-56.

[4] Gura V, Macy AS, Beizai M, Ezon C, Golper TA. Technical breakthroughs in the wearable artificial kidney (WAK). *Clin J Am Soc Nephrol.* 2009;4(9):1441-1448.

[5] Davenport A, Gura V, Ronco C, et al. A wearable haemodialysis device for patients with end-stage renal failure: a pilot study. *Lancet.* 2007;370(9604):2005-2010.

[6] Gura V, Davenport A, Beizai M, Ezon C, Ronco C. Beta2-microglobulin and phosphate clearances using a wearable artificial kidney: a pilot study. *Am J Kidney Dis.* 2009;54(1): 104-111.

[7] Gura V, Rivara MB, Bieber S, et al. A wearable artificial kidney for patients with end-stage renal disease. *JCI Insight.* 2016;1(8):e86397. Q2.

[8] Li L, Marchant RE, Dubnisheva A, Roy S, Fissell WH. Antibiofouling sulfobetaine polymer thin films on silicon and silicon nanopore membranes. *J Biomat Sci Polym. Ed.* 2011;22(1-3): 91-106.

[9] Kanani DM, Fissell WH, Roy S, Dubnisheva A, Fleischman A, Zydney AL. Permeability-selectivity analysis for ultrafiltration: effect of pore geometry. *J Membr Sci.* 2010;349(1-2): 405-410.

[10] Fissell WH, Dubnisheva A, Eldridge AN, Fleischman AJ, Zydney AL, Roy S. High-performance silicon nanopore hemo-filtration membranes. *J Membr Sci.* 2009;326(1):58-63.

[11] Melvin ME, Fissell WH, Roy S, Brown DL. Silicon induces minimal thromboinflammatory response during 28-day intravascular implant testing. *ASAIO J.* 2010;56(4):344-348.

[12] Iqbal Z, Moses W, Kim S, Kim EJ, Fissell WH, Roy S. Sterilization effects on ultrathin film polymer coatings for silicon-based implantable medical devices. *J Biomed Materials Res B Appl Biomater.* 2018; 106(6): 2327-2336.

[13] Muthusubramaniam L, Lowe R, Fissell W, et al. Hemocompatibility of silicon-based substrates for biomedical implant applications. *Ann Biomed Eng.* 2011;39(4):1296-1305.

[14] Kensinger C, Karp S, Kant R, et al. First implantation of silicon nanopore membrane hemofilters. *ASAIO J.* 2016;62(4): 491-495.

[15] Hestekin CN, Hestekin JA, Paracha S. et al. Simulating nephron ion transport function using activated wafer electrodeionization. *Commun Mater.* 1, 20 (2020).

In: Issues in Kidney Disease – Dialysis
Editors: Stephen Z. Fadem and José A. Moura-Neto
ISBN: 978-1-68507-000-7

Chapter 19

Green Dialysis: A Necessary Trend

José A. Moura-Neto[1,*], MD, Ana Flavia Moura[1], MD, Cassiano Augusto Braga Silva[2], MD and John W. M. Agar[3], MBBS

[1]Department of Internal Medicine, Bahiana School of Medicine and Public Health, Salvador, Bahia, Brazil

[2]Hospital Dom Pedro de Alcântara, Santa Casa de Misericordia de Feira de Santana, Feira de Santana, Bahia, Brazil

[3]Renal Services, University Hospital Geelong, Geelong, Australia

Abstract

Climate change is frequently discussed at global meetings and can increase the prevalence of several diseases. Ironically, healthcare can play an important role in aggravating climate change, and dialysis is one of the activities that most contributes to that environmental impact. Several measures have been proposed in the past years to reduce these adverse effects with 'Green Dialysis' emerging as a key environmental concept. This chapter aims to discuss the environmental impact of global dialysis, in addition to proposing measures that may reduce the carbon footprint, as well as waste generation, by individual dialysis centers.

Keywords: dialysis, hemodialysis, sustainability, nephrology, eco-dialysis, green nephrology, green dialysis, ecology, waste, water, energy

Introduction

Dialysis is one of the healthcare activities with the greatest environmental impact. This results from both the high resource consumption and significant waste generation of the process. Current estimates suggest that more than three million people are under dialysis in the world [1]. Further, not only has the global dialysis patient population rapidly increased in the

* Corresponding Author's E-mail: moura@nephrologyworldwide.com.

last decade, but data trends suggest an acceleration in coming years due to the combined effects of ageing in the global population and an increasing prevalence of chronic diseases, such as hypertension and diabetes mellitus, which are major risk factors for kidney disease [2]

The concept of "Green Dialysis" or "Eco-dialysis" has emerged and gained ground in nephrology around the world in the last decade. In some countries, such as Australia and the United Kingdom (UK), studies have been carried out to map the environmental impact of dialysis, as well as to implement measures aimed at reducing this impact. This chapter will discuss this concept and suggest opportunities for sustainable practices in Renal Replacement Therapy (RRT) centers.

Environmental Impact of Dialysis

Dialysis treatment results in an excessive generation of disposable waste (mainly plastics) and a high consumption of resource utilities, such as water and energy. Of these, water is perhaps the most important resource expended by the dialysis process, especially in hemodialysis (HD), the predominant RRT modality in the world.

Conventional maintenance HD with an average dialysate flow rate of 500 ml / min, 4 hours per session, results in an estimated total expenditure of 400 to 500 liters of water per session when all water used for dialysate production is considered. In the traditional regime of three weekly sessions, 63 to 78 thousand liters of water are spent annually per patient treated. This value may vary depending not only on the frequency and duration of the sessions, but also on the model of the dialysis machine used and the efficiency of the reverse osmosis (RO) system. The estimate is based on: a) the volume of pure water generated by the RO for the production of dialysate (about 120 liters = 500ml / min x 240min); b) the volume of water 'rejected' (about 240 liters) by RO, which typically rejects up to 60-70% of the water used in the production of pure water; c) other water expenditures, such as re-use, sterilization, pre-HD priming and post-HD rinse, inter-treatment 'idle,' and any addition potential losses resulting from the leakage [3, 4].

The consumption of 63 to 78 thousand liters per patient per year on HD may represent an estimated expenditure of 29.5 to 36.5 billion liters of water per year in the United States of America (USA) alone, based on an estimated 468,000 patients on hemodialysis in 2017 [5]. To understand the magnitude of these numbers, annual water consumption per capita in all domestic activities is about 210,000 liters in the USA, 54,500 in Australia, and 55,000 in France [6, 7]. Worldwide, estimated HD water consumption is likely to exceed 200 billion liters per year. What makes the scenario even more concerning is that most of this water is discarded, despite that it is safe to drink; i.e., potable water [8, 9].

Peritoneal dialysis (PD) requires less water than HD. Although treatment is daily, patients typically use only 6 to 12 liters of sterile PD solution, well below 400-500 liters per HD session. However, there are still no estimates of the volume of mains water needed to produce this sterile solution, it is likely far greater than 12 liters per day [3, 8, 10].

Energy consumption is also impressive. An Australian study calculated the energy expenditure per patient per hour to be 1.3 kWh in 2012 [9]. In a rough estimate, based on some three million HD patients in 2020, and assuming a three 4-hour sessions per week regime, energy expenditure likely exceeds 2 billion kWh (2.43 billion) worldwide. This figure is much higher than the annual energy consumption of some populous countries in Africa such as Mali (~18 million inhabitants: 1.4 billion kWh), Madagascar (~25 million inhabitants: 1.3 billion kWh), and Niger (~20 million inhabitants: 1.2 billion kWh).

Another factor that contributes to the environmental impact of dialysis is the vast quantitiers of disposable 'waste' that is produced. A 2011 British case study estimated the generation of solid clinical waste at 2.5 kg per HD session, 38% of which is plastic waste. This equates to an annual generation of 390 kg of plastic waste per patient under treatment [11]. PD produced almost twice as much waste, about 617 kg per patient per year. None of these estimates included packaging [12]. Again, the numbers are alarming when multiplied by the total number of global RRT patients with 1.35 million tons of waste produced annually by the sector.

Table 1 summarizes the estimates presented in this section regarding global water expenditure, energy consumption, and waste generation. The calculations were based on an estimated total of 4 million dialysis patients in the world in 2021 [1]. In 2008, only 11% of the population on dialysis was on PD [13]. For this reason, we have considered 3,560,000 HD patients and 440,000 PD patients, worldwide.

Of note, differences in local practices may constitute bias in the calculations. Examples of such differences include whether they reuse dialyzers and lines, use of convective techniques (hemodiafiltration and hemofiltration), model of dialysis machines used, use of generator, RO system, dialysate flow prescribed, time and frequency of sessions.

Table 1. Estimated environmental impact of dialysis per year in 2021

	World	
	HD (3,560,000)	PD (440,000)
Water (liters)	224 – 270.5 billions	NC
Power (kWh)	2.88 billions	NC
Waste (ton)	1.39 millions	271,480

NC = Not Calculated; HD = Hemodialysis; PD = Peritoneal Dialysis.

CARBON FOOTPRINT

The carbon footprint (CF) is a recent environmental indicator that is particularly useful for evaluating environmental and sustainability performance, and for formulating policy [14, 15]. It originates from the concept of the ecological footprint - a measure of the environment impact expressed as the area of land required to maintain the natural resources it utilizes [16]. Many countries have an estimated ecological footprint above both the ideal (1.8 gha - global hectares) and the world average (2.7 gha) [17]. The Brazilian ecological footprint, for example, was estimated at 2.9 (gha) per individual, well below countries like the USA (11.6 gha) and Denmark (8.22 gha) [17]. In practice, this means that if all the inhabitants of the world lived and consumed like Brazilians, 1.6 planets would be needed in order to keep the supply of natural resources stable. Applying the same logic, if all global citizens expended the same carbon footprint as the US average, 10.3 planets would be needed for stabilization of natural resources.

The carbon footprint, unlike the ecological footprint, refers only to the carbon dioxide (CO_2) emissions produced by an activity, be it a product, a process, or the provision of a service

[18]. Although there is no universal concept, it can be defined as the total amount of CO2 emissions generated, directly and indirectly, by an activity over the entire cycle of a service or product, including its recovery and disposal at the end of life – a holistic process sometimes referred to as a cradle-to-grave analysis. The unit of measure is the ton of carbon dioxide equivalent (ton CO2 Eq).

Some studies have assessed the CF of dialysis in recent years. A UK study published in 2011 showed a CF of 3.8 ton CO2 Eq (t-CO2-eq) per patient per year on a conventional maintenance HD regimen of three times a week at the center. Most emissions came from medical equipment (37%), energy use (21%), and displacement of patients (20%) [11].

That same study also evaluated the CF in patients on home HD. The results varied substantially according to the dialysis prescription and the machine used. In patients on dialysis on conventional machines and at four times a week, four and a half hours per session, the CF was 4.3 t-CO2-eq. At five times a week, four hours per session, the measured value was 5.1 t-CO2-eq. In HD patients six times a week, with shorter sessions (two hours), the CF was 5.2 t-CO2-eq. The authors also assessed the annual CF of patients in nocturnal HD in three times (3 days x 7 hours: 3.9 t-CO2-eq) or six times a week (6 days x 7 hours: 7.2 t-CO2-eq). As expected, the frequency of treatment had a greater influence on the CF than the duration of treatment [11].

Another aspect addressed in the British study was the assessment of patients in home HD with machines from the NxStage system (NxStage Medical Inc., Lawrence, Massachusetts, USA). In addition to reduced water consumption, the machine had a relatively smaller CF than conventional machines on similar dialysis schemes, both in the short daily regime (5.5 days x 6 hours: 1.8 t-CO2-eq) and in nocturnal HD (6 days x 7 hours: 2.1 t-CO2-eq) [16]. It is suggested, therefore, that if new machines and emerging technologies could officially map and disclose the carbon footprint, this might become an important element for decision-making [19].

A later Australian study, which evaluated an HD satellite unit, showed a different result. It found a larger CF of 10.2 t-CO2-eq per patient per year from the dialysis process, a figure that compares with CF of an average Australian of 18 t-CO2-eq. A significant difference between the UK and the Australian study was seen in water procurement, in which the distance and topographical characteristics of water transport were key factors in the higher Australian figure. In this study, the major contributors were pharmaceutical products (35.7%), medical equipment (23.4%), energy use (18.6%), and displacement of patients and employees (8.8%) [19].

Green Dialysis and Green Nephrology Around the World

Some publications have already addressed sustainability in dialysis and nephrology in the previous decade [20-24]. However, the term "Green Dialysis" was first introduced in 2009 when the article "Conserving water in and applying solar power to haemodialysis: 'Green Dialysis' through wiser resource utilization" was published online in the prestigious journal Nephrology [4]. Since then, other articles have also incorporated the newly created term in their titles [8, 25, 26].

In the same year, the "Green Nephrology Network" of doctors, nurses, patients, suppliers, and other stakeholders was created in the UK. This initiative was responsible for profound cultural changes in a short period of 3 to 4 years related to the environmental impact of dialysis.

Based on 20 sustainable practices, a potential annual savings of 7 million pounds sterling (about USD 9.52 million), 11,000 t-CO2-eq and 470 million liters of water were estimated if these initiatives, already tested and validated, could be widely replicated in nephrology services throughout the UK [27].

In April 2017, the Lancet started to publish the journal, The Lancet Planetary Health [28], an initiative that suggests the theme is now broadly valued in the academic field. In the same vein, the Australia and New Zealand Society of Nephrology (ANZSN), in partnership with Kidney Health Australia, began to offer incentives and awards for research in nephrology with the theme of sustainability and environmental development [29].

In 2018, an international group was formed with representatives from several countries to debate and promote sustainability in nephrology ('Green Nephrology'). This initiative, led by Australians Katherine Barraclough and John Agar, was supported by the International Society of Nephrology (ISN). This group first met at Kidney Week 2018, the annual congress of the American Society of Nephrology (ASN), bringing together nephrologists of several different nationalities to discuss global initiatives in sustainable nephrology and to plan the dissemination of this mission [30]. A position statement on sustainability in nephrology was subsequently formulated for presentation to the ISN. The document was a collaborative effort and was intended to include sustainable practices in ISN's activities, for later extension to other regional societies.

At the 2019 World Nephrology Congress (WCN) in Melbourne, Australia, environmental activist Tim Flannery was invited to present the opening plenary lecture of the event, entitled "Keeping the Climate Safe," confirming the importance that the theme has now achieved in nephrology worldwide [31].

In 2020, an interesting, published review discussed the environmental impact of dialysis on climate change, and outlined some of the global data related to waste generation, water and power usage; in particular its impact on the global carbon footprint [32]. In the same year, Yau et al. listed some of the early responses from dialysis centers worldwide, particularly focusing on the capture and reuse of RO reject water, the installation of solar power systems in new unit builds, and the progressive replacement of dialysis machines with more energy-efficient alternatives [33].

From the beginning of 2020, the pandemic has forced every country in the world to rethink and adopt measures which minimize human environmental impacts. Virtual meetings, more carefully controlled admission of temporary patients in hemodialysis centers (especially if coming from another city or as a tourist from another country) and, when possible, virtual medical visits via telemedicine have all rapidly transformed practice in dialysis centers. As a by-product, these new behaviors will likely help reduce the carbon footprint and may become part of routine future practice in these centers.

Sustainable Measures

Several sustainable practices can be adopted in dialysis. In addition to the environmental benefit, these initiatives must be a strategic competitive differential. On one hand, they may promote cost savings and yield economic benefits. On the other, they can add value to the brand image and contribute to a more efficient and up-to-date marketing positioning, differentially attracting and retaining customers. Both strategies promise to enhance environmental and social responsibility.

Reuse of Reject Water from Reverse Osmosis

Two water components are generated by the HD process: 1) the water rejected by the RO; and 2) the effluent from the used dialysate. While there remain several potential risks with re-use and/or re-purposing the dialysate effluent, RO reject water is created by the pre-dialysis filtration process and is formed from pure, filtered mains water that has not been exposed to blood or blood products. Despite the common application of the term 'reject' to the water discarded by the RO, using the word 'reject' to describe water of such high quality is both inappropriate and counterproductive [21]. The water discarded at the RO, according to all standards, is drinking quality (potable) water, as shown in Table 2 [34].

Unfortunately, most dialysis centers dispose their RO reject water directly to the sewer. Some re-use systems have been described [3, 25, 26] with multiple re-purposing options available: redirecting water to flush toilets, sinks, watering gardens, washing floors or outside areas, using in autoclave systems, as drinking water in animal water-troughs, or even in human drinking fountains, although some controversy remains regarding this latter use, due to the slight metallic flavor and greater conductivity of the discard product [22]. A few years ago, a blinding "taste test" was conducted in an Australian hospital: a pitcher containing commercially sold mineral water was compared to another containing a random sample of water from RO waste. Interestingly, the test participants were unable to taste-distinguish between the two water samples [34].

The reuse of reject water for agriculture has also been practiced for some years in Morocco and Australia [20, 36, 37]. During the 2018 construction of a dialysis center in Salvador, Brazil, a system for reusing the reject water from the first step of the RO was designed. It works as follows:

1. The double-step RO is located on the fourth floor of the building. A water reservoir (Reservoir 1) was installed on the first floor. Water from the tailing [discarded RO reject water] descends under gravity from the first step of the RO into this reservoir.
2. In the Penthouse (sixth floor), another reservoir (Reservoir 2) with a capacity of 5,000 liters was installed to receive the water from 'Reservoir 1' and distribute it via plumbing installed in the building.
3. The reject water stored in 'Reservoir 2' is directed to general purpose taps, garden, sinks, and flushes.
4. Water is directed from 'Reservoir 1' to 'Reservoir 2' via a set of pumps.
5. From 'Reservoir 2' the water feeds by gravity to supply the branches.
6. 'Reservoir 2' is electronically controlled by the main reservoir such that if the system detects that the reject water from the first step of the RO is insufficient to supply the building demand, Reservoir 2 can then be supplied with treated water from the water utility company.

Table 2. Water analysis for multiple analyte concentrations

Analyte	Units	Reporting units	Mains HD Unit #1	RO RW Unit #1	Mains HD Unit #2	RO RW Unit #2	US EPA Standard	Pass/Fail US EPA Standard
Aluminium	mg/L	0.005	0.01	0.01	0.01	0.01	0.2	Pass
Arsenic	mg/L	0.001	0.001	0.001	0.001	0.001	0.01	Pass
Cadmium	mg/L	0.0002	0.0002	0.002	0.0002	0.0002	0.005	Pass
Copper	mg/L	0.001	0.021	0.009	1.3	0.01	1.3	Pass
Iron	mg/L	0.06	0.05	0.02	0.02	0.002	0.3	Pass
Lead	mg/L	0.001	0.002	0.001	0.003	0.002	0.015	Pass
Manganese	mg/L	0.001	0.001	0.01	0.001	0.002	0.05	Pass
Mercury	mg/L	0.0001	0.0001	0.0001	0.0001	0.0001	0.002	Pass
Zinc	mg/L	0.002	0.014	0.002	0.055	0.008	5	Pass
Calcium	mg/L	0.1	8.4	0.1	8.3	0.1	No standard	Pass
Magnesium	mg/L	0.1	5.3	0.1	5.3	0.1	No standard	Pass
Sodium	mg/L	0.1	34	140	33	68	200	Pass
Total Hardness	mg/L	0.1	43	0.1	43	0.1	No standard	Pass
Chloride	mg/L	1	60	150	61	74	250	Pass
Nitrate	mg/L	0.01	0.01	0.01	0.01	0.01	10	Pass
Nitrite	mg/L	0.01	0.01	0.01	0.01	0.023	1	Pass
Sulphate	mg/L	1	9.4	23	9.5	11	250	Pass
Dichloramine	mg/L	0.1	0.01	0.1	0.1	0.1	08	Pass
Conductivity	μS/cm	0.1	280	680	280	340	2500	Pass
Fluoride	mg/L	0.05	0.06	0.15	0.07	0.06	2	Pass
Free Chlorine	mg/L	0.1	0.1	0.1	0.1	0.1	4	Pass
Monochloramine	mg/L	0.1	0.1	0.1	0.1	0.1	4	Pass
pH	pH units		7.3	7.5	7.2	7.5	7.5±1.0	Pass
Dissolved Solids	mg/L	5	110	320	150	200	500	Pass
Trichloramine	mg/L	0.1	0.1	0.1	0.1	0.1	Uncertain	Pass
Turbidity	NTU	0.1	0.2	0.1	0.1	0.1	2	Pass

Table 2. Water analysis for multiple analyte concentrations, sampled from the mains water inflow of two separate suburban satellite dialysis units (Mains HD Unit #1 and Mains HD Unit #2) when compared with the same concentrations of the same analytes in the reverse osmosis reject water (RO RW) of their respective reverse osmosis plants (RO Unit #1 and RO Unit #2). The USA Environmental Protection Authority (EPA) Standards for potable water are given *. A 'Pass' is recorded where both RO RW Unit #1 and RO RW Unit #2 satisfy US EPA standards for potable water. A 'Fail' is recorded if one or other of RO RW Unit #1 and/or RO RW Unit #2 fail potable standards. Water analysis was provided by the Barwon Regional Water Authority ^: 2004.
*https://www.epa.gov/ground-water-and-drinking-water/national-primary-drinking-water-regulations.
(Table adapted from the chapter by Agar JWM. *Diálise e meio ambiente: em busca de um futuro mais sustentável.* In "Terapia Renal Susbtitutiva 2" José A. Moura-Neto (ed)/São Paulo: Livraria Balieiro, 2019) [34, 35].

In this example, the reject water re-use system was installed during the construction of the center as part of the original project design. However, this may not always be possible. When the installation of a re-use system requires structural modifications, it is important to first evaluate the installation costs to assess the cost/benefit ratio. However, it almost always proves to be a good medium term investment. One case described in a hospital in Australia consisted of installing tanks on the terrace and a simple piping system to direct the reject water to the autoclaves in the central sterilization department, and to ward toilets. Payback was achieved in less than three years (30 months) [34].

A city (population: 80,000) located 375 km from Salvador, Brazil, with a hot climate and suffering from drought and water scarcity, has reported another positive experience. The city's RRT center, responsible for the dialysis treatment of 250 patients, has been redirecting RO reject water from pipes to irrigate a small garden in front of the clinic since 2016. The 600 liters of reject water generated per day is divided into two daily waterings (morning and late afternoon) through a hose coupled to an automatic irrigator. The garden has since been transformed into a pleasant place for family members of patients to wait for the end of the dialysis session on days when the weather is mild. It has also become a meeting point for the traditional ride on World Kidney Day (WKD) [38] and is used for an annual patient bazaar, as well as for birthday celebrations.

"Recycling" of Tailings Water

In addition to the re-use of reject water, it is possible to reduce the total volume of water rejected by the RO. A dialysis center in Bahia, Brazil, has installed a system to "recycle" their RO reject water back through the RO.

With 400 HD patients, water consumption is particularly high at this facility. Before this system was installed, their double-step RO system processed 66% of the total water draw into pure water for HD. While 30% of the water was rejected by the first step, a further 20% was subsequently rejected in the second step (Figure 1A) [39].

The amendment provides for two separate changes. The first consisted of attaching an accessory RO to "recycle" the waste from the first step. This RO is smaller (in quantity and in the size of the membranes), has a single step and acts exclusively in the rejection of the first step of the main RO, being therefore called "RO of the Reject" or "Accessory RO." The second change consisted of diverting the waste from the second step to the feed tank, diluting the drinking water that arrives from the water utility company. With these changes, at the end of the water treatment process, there is a rejection of only 9% of the water used to produce pure water for HD, since the final waste corresponds to 30% of the accessory RO from 30% of the rejected water discarded in the first step of the main RO. The changes were outlined in Figure 1B. The production data, in liters per hour (L / h), of the RO system are represented in Figure 2 [39].

These changes require some financial investment. However, environmental and economic benefits tend to outweigh this initial investment. In the case reported, the waste from the RO system went from 44% to just 9% of the water used [39].

The decrease in the useful life of the main RO membrane is an existing concern. As the recycled RO reject water from the second step is mixed with water from the water utility company, the water being re-treated will thus have a higher conductivity. This, in turn, may result in a more frequent turnover of the RO membranes. Even so, the financial savings and the environmental benefits of lower water expenditure may outweigh any costs incurred from membrane replacement.

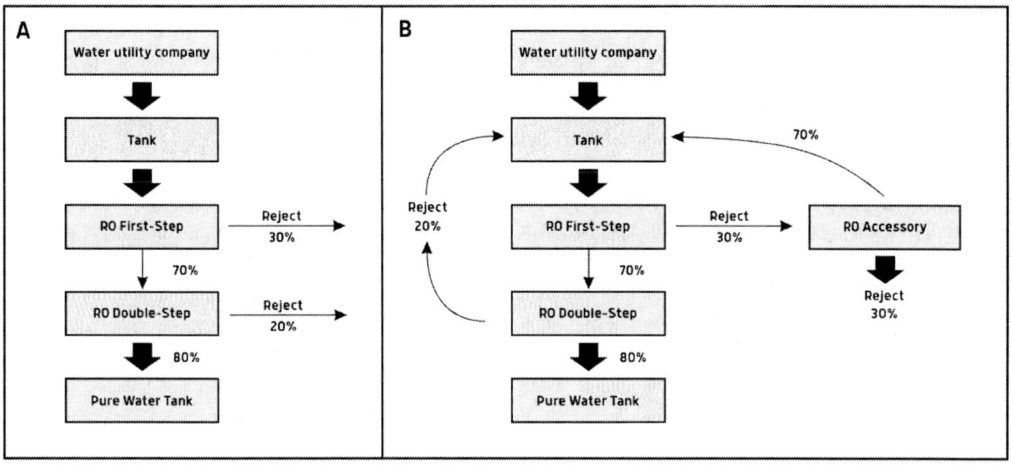

Figure 1. "Recycling" of reject water.

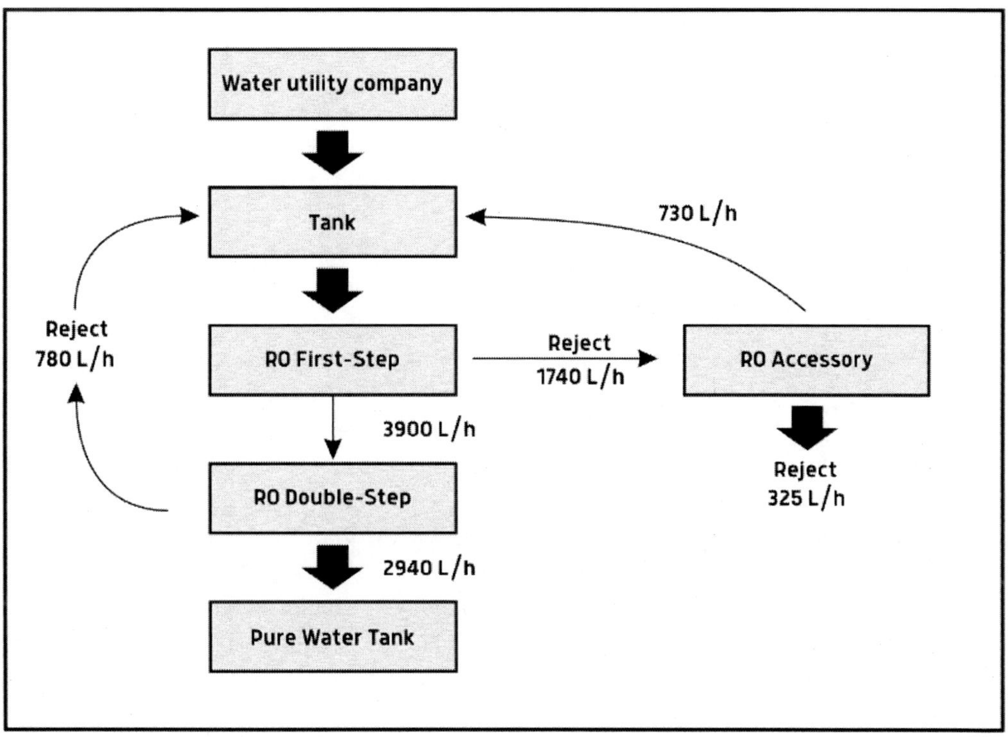

Figure 2. "Recycling" of reject water.

It should be noted that the "recycling" of reject water does not prevent the re-use of the final discard volume. As discussed above, these are complementary and not competing initiatives. Nevertheless, the objective of a sustainable dialysis center in relation to water must be to waste as little as possible and reuse as much of the "reject" as possible.

The double-step RO would reject 44% of the water used to produce pure water for HD (A). The modification consisted of: 1) coupling an accessory RO for the treatment of tailings from the first step of the main RO; 2) Divert the waste from the second step, in its entirety, to the feed tank, which receives drinking water from the water utility company. After the modifications, the RO system started to reject only 9% of the water used to produce pure water for HD (B). (Figure adapted from the chapter by Moura-Neto JA & Silva CAB. *Diálise sustentável – entre a teoria e a prática*. In "Atualidades em Nefrologia 16." Jenner Cruz / São Paulo: Savier, 2020) [39].

These are the production data, in L/h, of the RO system after modifications have been made. In the end, even so, 325 liters per hour is rejected, which is also reused in sinks, flushes and for cleaning the external area.

Renewable Energy Sources

Despite a growing interest in renewable energy, there is still little data available on the use of solar and wind energy in dialysis centers. Solar energy has the advantage of being a clean and inexhaustible source, in addition to being silent. The average life expectancy of current solar arrays is 25 to 30 years [40].

A feasibility study prior to installation is important. The calculations must be based on the solar exposure of each location, which can be easily measured by directly recording solar radiation or by calculating solar insolation (energy from solar radiation received in an area at a given time). Estimates of these exposure levels can be found on the internet. After providing the local latitude and longitude coordinates, tables and graphs can be obtained for the average daily, weekly, monthly, or annual sun exposure [9, 40].

An Australian experiment for using solar energy in a home HD unit resulted in a 78% reduction in energy costs only in the first year of operation, projecting the return on the invested amount (payback) in just under 8 years (7.7) [40]. The charges associated with the purchase of materials, installation cost, as well as the possibility of sharing surplus energy via a buy-back scheme with area energy providers [22, 40] were included in the calculation. The final amount also depends on government policy, regulation, and the attitudes of local energy utilities.

One possibility for larger groups is to tap into remote energy generation from area photovoltaic arrays - also known as 'solar plants' or 'solar farm.' However, in some countries, more incentives are still needed for initiatives like these to become viable and attractive for small and medium-sized business ventures.

The application of wind energy in dialysis centers is still incipient, and reports in literature are scarce. Despite wind energy being a clean and renewable source, there are some negative aspects that might impact the popularization of wind technology; in particular, noise and visual pollution, greater susceptibility to environmental influences, and unpredictability in relation to the amount of energy generated [40].

In the USA, in a note released to the press in 2019, a transnational dialysis provider shared an ambitious plan to use 100% renewable energy by 2022. There are two projects in Texas - a wind farm and a solar plant – that are expected to generate approximately 625,000 MWh per year [41]. In Brazil, there are still no published plans to augmented renewable energy in dialysis services, and all investments from transnational companies currently seem focused on the acquisition of dialysis units and the consolidation of the sector.

Waste Management

The amount of waste generated in a HD session depends on the appropriate choice of materials and local practices. Currently, a percentage of discarded materials is unnecessarily disposed of as hospital waste, ignoring recycling opportunities.

The recycling process must start at the units themselves, with the material segregated by trained employees through careful inspection, aiming at the disposal of contaminated and sharps waste. An Italian study pointed out that it only takes 1 minute for an adequate differentiation of the discarded waste [42]. In addition to inspection training, for greater team engagement, it is essential to make employees aware of the environmental importance of this initiative which, in turn, will mean some additional work in their daily routines.

In Australia, an innovative process is under investigation in Geelong, Victoria, by a tri-partite group comprising a dialysis service, a university department of engineering, and a major dialysis provider, whereby all used post-dialysis plastic [average plastic weight per patient per treatment = 2.5 kg: or 7.5 kg per patient per week] is autoclave-sterilized, shredded into a confetti-sized shreddate, then incorporated via a cold-chain process into concrete. The early results have been promising, with significant interest from the construction industry, given that the product appears to lose none of its tensile strength but is significantly less water-permeable. This has implications for the preservation of concrete rebar – the metal strengthening used in concrete construction – and may yet prove to be a useful product for use in seawalls and other marine situations [43].

Meantime, other exciting possibilities remain to be explored.

Other Measures

There are many simple and easy-to-implement generic measures in dialysis centers that, when taken together, can have a significant positive environmental impact. Video-conferencing meetings, in addition to reducing costs and optimizing employees' time, reduce the frequency of travel and commuting and, consequently, the emission of greenhouse gases. Telemedicine also promises to reduce health costs and reduce the environmental impact of travel.

Encouraging clean means of transport, such as bicycles, is another opportunity to be explored. The installation of a bicycle rack at the dialysis units, and the provision of a suitable changing room for bathing and changing clothes, may be the best way to encourage the use of bicycles among employees. An educational campaign about the benefits to the environment and health also contributes to awareness. In countries where physical safety or climate extremes are barriers, an encouragement of car-pooling between employees, or the use of public transportation (subway and bus) in place of private vehicles, are alternatives.

Other measures can also have a positive impact on the unit. Selective garbage collection, flushing of double-acting or single-command toilets with reduced flush-volumes (4.8 liters), and the responsible use of printers (reducing the use of paper, double-sided printing, wax printers), are some examples of sustainable practices that are easy to implement.

Dialysis unit design aimed at minimizing energy expenditure offers another an under-utilized potential. The thermal insulation of buildings can be optimized to minimize heat loss during winter and indoor temperatures during summer, thus reducing heating and cooling needs. A greater use of natural light is desirable despite creating an architectural challenge: the desire for greater natural lighting must be balanced against the privacy and security requirements of the health center. The use of light colors to reflect sunlight, i.e., instead of dark colors that absorb, is both simple and useful. Other options to reduce energy consumption include the use of timers, motion sensors, or automation for lighting, including the choice of LED lamps in place of incandescent globes. Finally, the roof of the building can be used for photovoltaic panels installation, or even for planting and providing vegetables for patient and staff consumption.

Providers

The dialysis equipment companies can – and must – play a key role. The nephrology community must apply pressure to industry providers to present transparent data on the cradle-to-grave environmental impact of their products: the materials used, the manufacturing process, and the disposal policies at the end of the useful life of their product. In turn, this will reflect well on the environmental performance and standing of their organization.

An objective way of searching the market for companies that are more engaged in sustainable practices is to evaluate the holders of the ISO 14001 seal, version 2015. This standard incorporates, in addition to strategic issues, an environmental management system that prioritizes environmental policies, and demonstrates compliance with sustainable practices, customers, and outside organizations.

Climate Change and Nephrology

Climate change can also influence kidney disease. Despite the constant debate, climate change is already considered a global public health emergency due to the impact on human health, whether by spreading climate-related vectors and diseases, decreasing the production of food and agricultural inputs, lowering the availability of drinking water and extreme weather events [44].

The pattern of distribution of kidney disease also tends to change with ongoing climate change. Some studies associate an increase in hospital admissions due to acute kidney injury in regions prone to periodic heat waves [45-49]. Higher temperatures are known to be related to a higher incidence of nephrolithiasis [50]. The increased prevalence of chronic kidney disease in some regions of the world has been linked to a lack of access to drinking water, in combination with prolonged exposure to higher temperatures [51]. Climate change increases the propensity to flooding [52], which, in turn, correlates with diarrheal disease and the spread of vector-borne diseases, both major causes of acute kidney injury in low-income tropical regions [53-55].

In addition, climate change also impacts the treatment of patients with kidney disease. Extreme weather events can hinder the satisfactory supply of drinking water, the adequate supply of energy for HD sessions, the transport of supplies, and even make it difficult or – in major catastrophic storm, flood, or fire – impossible for patients to access RRT [56, 57].

CONCLUSION

Dialysis, while maintaining the lives of more than three million individuals, paradoxically causes a significant environmental impact. High energy consumption, high water consumption, and excessive waste generation make dialysis treatment one of the most aggressive threats to the environment within the health sector. In addition, climate change also alters the epidemiological profile of some kidney diseases. The good news is that there are opportunities to minimize the damage done. Most of these options are easy to implement and economically viable. Sustainable practices must be part of the nephrology strategy in its various spheres; in the individual sphere (nephrologists), organizational (renal replacement therapy centers), and as a society (government, professional bodies, and professional entities).

REFERENCES

[1] Moura-Neto JA, Divino-Filho JC, Ronco C. Nephrology Worldwide: the Vision, the Project, and the Mission. In: Moura-Neto JA, Divino-Filho JC, Ronco C, editors. *Nephrology Worldwide*. Basel: Springer Nature Switzerland AG; 2021. p. 1-9.

[2] Lv JC, Zhang LX. Prevalence and Disease Burden of Chronic Kidney Disease. *Adv Exp Med Biol.* 2019; 1165:3-15.

[3] Agar JWM. Reusing and Recycling Dialysis Reverse Osmosis Reject Water. *Kidney Int.* 2015;88:653-657.

[4] Agar JWM. Conserving water in and applying solar power to haemodialysis: "Green Dialysis" through wiser resource utilisation. *Nephrology* (Carlton). 2010; 15:448–453.

[5] Anumudu SJ, Fadem SZ. Nephrology in the United States of America. In: Moura-Neto JA, Divino-Filho JC, Ronco C, editors. *Nephrology Worldwide.* Basel: Springer Nature Switzerland AG; 2021. p. 173-184.

[6] FAO. AQUASTAT website. *Food and Agriculture Organization of the United Nations* (FAO) 2016. Accessed 10 Nov 2020.

[7] Service de l'observation et des statistiques – Service des statistiques et de la prospective (SOeS-SSP). *Enquête Eau 2008.* http://www.developpementdurable.gouv.fr/IMG/pdf/LPS67b.pdf. [Service de l'observation et des statistiques – Service des statistiques et de la prospective (SOeS-SSP). *Enquête Eau 2008.*]

[8] Agar JW. Green dialysis: the environmental challenges ahead. *Semin Dial.* 2015;28:186-92.

[9] Agar JW. Personal Viewpoint: hemodialysis-water, power, and waste disposal: rethinking our environmental responsibilities. *Hemodial Int.* 2012;16:6-10.

[10] Moura-Neto JA, Barraclough K, Agar JWM. A call to action for sustainability in dialysis in Brazil. *Braz J Nephrol*. 2019; 41(4): 560-563.

[11] Connor A, Lillywhite R, Cooke MW. The carbon footprints of home and in-center maintenance hemodialysis in the United Kingdom. *Hemodial Int.* 2011; 15:39–51.

[12] Mortimer F. Reduce, reuse, recycle in the dialysis unit: a case study and how-to guide. *The Centre for Sustainable Healthcare—Green Nephrology.* http://www.sustainable healthcare.org.uk/nephrology-resources/reduce-reuse-recycle. Accessed 7 Dec 2020.

[13] Jain AK, Blake P, Cordy P, Garg AX. Global Trends in Rates of Peritoneal Dialysis. *J Am Soc Nephrol.* 2012 Mar; 23(3): 533–544.

[14] Wiedmann T, Minx J. A definition of 'carbon footprint.' *Ecol Econ Res Trends.* 2018; 1: 1–11.

[15] Abeydeera LHU, Mesthrige JW, Samarasinghalage TI. Global Research on Carbon Emissions: A Scientometric Review. *Sustainability.* 2019; 11: 3972.

[16] Peters, G. P. Carbon footprints and embodied carbon at multiple scales. *Curr Opin Environ Sustain.* 2010; 2: 245–250.

[17] World Wildlife Fund. *Pegada Brasileira.* https://www.wwf.org.br/natureza_brasileira/especiais/pegada_ecologica/pegada_brasileira/. [*Brazilian Footprint.*]

[18] Geng Y, Dong H, Xi F et al. A review of carbon footprint research on climate change. *China Population, Resources and Environment* 2010; 20(10):6–12.

[19] Lim AE, Perkins A, Agar JWM. The carbon footprint of an Australian satellite haemodialysis unit. *Aust Health Rev.* 2013; 37(3):369–74.

[20] Tarrass F, Benjelloun M, Benjelloun O. Recycling wastewater after hemodialysis: an environmental analysis for alternative water sources in arid regions. *Am J Kid Dis.* 2008;52(1):54-8.

[21] Agar JWM. Reusing dialysis wastewater: The elephant in the room. *Am J Kidney Dis.* 2008; 52 (1): 10–2.

[22] Agar JWM, Simmonds RE, Knight R. Using water wisely: New, essential and affordable water conservation practices for both facility and home hemodialysis. *Hemodial Int.* 2009; 13 (1):32–7.

[23] Agar JWM, Wilson S, Magoffin J, Knight R, Somerville CA. Recycling reject water: A new essential for all facility-based dialysis services. *Nephrology* (Carlton) 2007; 12 (2) Abstract. A4:1012.

[24] Agar JWM, Wilson S, Simmonds RE, Boddington JM, Magoffin J, Somerville CA. Water-wise home dialysis: New essentials for home-based dialysis installations. *Nephrology* (Carlton). 2007; 12 (2) Abstract. A4: 1013.

[25] Ponson L, Arkouche W, Laville M. Toward green dialysis: focus on water savings. *Hemodial Int* 2014;18(1):7-14.

[26] Agar JWM. It is time for "Green Dialysis." *Hemodialysis Int.* 2013; 17(4):474 – 478.

[27] Limb M. NHS could save 1bn by adopting green strategies used in kidney units. *BMJ* 2013; 346: f588–f588.

[28] The Lancet Planetary Health. *Welcome to the Lancet Planetary Health Inaugural Edition of Lancet Planetary Health: Editorial.* https://www.thelancet.com/journals/ lanplh/article/PIIS2542-5196(17)30013-X/fulltext.

[29] *Australian and New Zealand Society of Nephrology–ANZSN Awards* (2019). https://www.nephrology.edu.au/awardsfellowshipsandgrants/anzsnawards.asp. Accessed 8 Dec 2020.

[30] Moura Neto, JA. Diálise Sustentável – Uma proposta para o Brasil. *SBN Informa 2019*; 117 (26): 22-23. https://arquivos.sbn.org.br/uploads/SBN-Informa-Ed-117.pdf. Accessed 10 Dec 2020. [Sustainable Dialysis - A proposal for Brazil]

[31] Flannery T. *Keeping the climate safe.* Available from: https://cm.theisn.org/cmPortal/searchable/WCN2019/config/normal#!sessiondetails/0000009350_0.

[32] Barraclough KA, Agar JWM. Green nephrology. *Nat Rev Nephrol.* 2020;16: 257–268.

[33] Yau A, Agar JWM, Barraclough KA. Addressing the Environmental Impact of Kidney Care. *Am J Kidney Dis*. 2021 Mar;77(3):406-409.

[34] Agar JWM. Diálise e meio ambiente: em busca de um futuro mais sustentável. In Moura-Neto JA (ed). *Terapia Renal Substitutiva 2 – Controvérsias e Tendências*. Livraria Balieiro: São Paulo, 2019, pp 105-116. [Dialysis and the environment: in search of a more sustainable future. In Moura-Neto JA (ed). *Renal Replacement Therapy 2 – Controversies and Trends*.]

[35] Moura-Neto JA (ed). *Terapia Renal Substitutiva 2 – Controvérsias e Tendências*. Livraria Balieiro: São Paulo, 2019, pp 1-444. [*Renal Replacement Therapy 2 – Controversies and Trends*].

[36] Tarrass F. Research Needs: Treatment of Hemodialysis Wastewater for Agricultural Reuse. *Water Environment Research* 2010;82(4):291-293.

[37] Agar JWM. *A holiday gift to the planet from the Outback*. Available from: http://www.homedialysis.org/news-and-research/blog/80-a-holiday-gift-to-the-planet-from-the-outback.

[38] Brazilian Society of Nephrology *Eventos do Dia Mundial do Rim – Clinefro – Senhor do Bonfim – Bahia* https://sbn.org.br/eventos-do-dia-mundial-do-rim-clinefro-senhor-do-bonfim-bahia/ Accessed 10 Dec 2020. [*World Kidney Day Events – Clinefro – Senhor do Bonfim – Bahia*]

[39] Moura-Neto JA, Silva CAB. Diálise sustentável – entre a teoria e a prática. In Cruz J, Cruz HMM, Kirsztajn GM, Oliveira RB, Barros RT (eds). *Atualidades em Nefrologia* 16. Editora Savier: São Paulo, 2020, pp 304-16. [Sustainable dialysis – between theory and practice. In Cruz J, Cruz HMM, Kirsztajn GM, Oliveira RB, Barros RT (eds). *News in Nephrology*]

[40] Agar JWM, Perkins A, Tjipto A. Solar-Assisted Hemodialysis. *Clin J Am Soc Nephrol*. 2012; 7: 310–314.

[41] DaVita Kidney Care. *DaVita to use 100 percent renewable energy*. https://pressreleases.davita.com/2019-04-25-DaVita-to-Use-100-Percent-Renewable-Energy. Accessed 4 Dec 2020.

[42] Piccoli GB, Nazha M, Ferraresi M, Vigotti FN, Pereno A, Barbero S. Eco-dialysis: the financial and ecological costs of dialysis waste products: is a 'cradle-to-cradle' model feasible for planet-friendly haemodialysis waste management? *Nephrol Dial Transplant*. 2015; 30: 1018–1027.

[43] Agar JWM, Barraclough KA and Al-Ameri R. *Dialysis plastic waste recycled as a concrete incorporative. Abstract presented at the ANZSN ASM*, 2019. Available from: http://www.anzsnasm.com/4609.

[44] Watts N, Adger WN, Agnolucci P, et al. Health and climate change: policy responses to protect public health. *Lancet*. 2015;386(10006):1861-1914.

[45] Knowlton K, Rotkin-Ellman M, King G, et al. The 2006 California heat wave: impacts on hospitalizations and emergency department visits. *Environ Health Perspect*. 2009;117(1):61-67.

[46] Semenza JC, McCullough JE, Flanders WD, McGeehin MA, Lumpkin JR. Excess hospital admissions during the July 1995 heat wave in Chicago. *Am J Prev Med*. 1999;16(4):269-277.

[47] Kovats RS, Hajat S, Wilkinson P. Contrasting patterns of mortality and hospital admissions during hot weather and heat waves in Greater London, UK. *Occup Environ Med*. 2004;61(11):893-898.

[48] Mastrangelo G, Fedeli U, Visentin C, Milan G, Fadda E, Spolaore P. Pattern and determinants of hospitalization during heat waves: an ecologic study. *BMC Public Health*. 2007;7:200.

[49] Hansen AL, Bi P, Ryan P, Nitschke M, Pisaniello D, Tucker G. The effect of heat waves on hospital admissions for renal disease in a temperate city of Australia. *Int J Epidemiol.* 2008;37(6):1359-1365.

[50] Brikowski TH, Lotan Y, Pearle MS. Climate-related increase in the prevalence of urolithiasis in the United States. *Proc Natl Acad Sci USA*. 2008;105(28):9841-9846.

[51] Glaser J, Lemery J, Rajagopalan B, et al. Climate Change and the Emergent Epidemic of CKD from Heat Stress in Rural Communities: The Case for Heat Stress Nephropathy. *Clin J Am Soc Nephrol*. 2016; 11(8):1472-83.

[52] Intergovernmental Panel on Climate Change. *Fifth Assessment Report. Summary for Policy Makers + Longer Report*. https://www.ipcc.ch/pdf/assessment-report/ar5/syr/SYR_AR5_FINAL_full_wcover.pdf. Accessed 10 Oct 2020.

[53] Jha V, Parameswaran S. Community-acquired acute kidney injury in tropical countries. *Nat Rev Nephrol*. 2013;9(5):278-290.

[54] Lameire NH, Bagga A, Cruz D, et al. Acute kidney injury: an increasing global concern. *Lancet*. 2013;382(9887):170-179.

[55] Campbell-Lendrum D, Manga L, Bagayoko M, J S. Climate change and vector-borne diseases: what are the implications for public health research and policy? *Phil Trans R Soc B*. 2015;370(20130552).

[56] Kopp JB, Ball LK, Cohen A, et al. Kidney patient care in disasters: lessons from the hurricanes and earthquake of 2005. *Clin J Am Soc Nephrol*. 2007;2(4):814-824.

[57] Anderson AH, Cohen AJ, Kutner NG, Kopp JB, Kimmel PL, Muntner P. Missed dialysis sessions and hospitalization in hemodialysis patients after Hurricane Katrina. *Kidney Int*. 2009;75(11):1202-1208.

INDEX

A

B

D

E

F

G

H

I

K

L

M

N

O

P

Q

R

S

T

U

V

W